Safety and Biological Effects in MRI

eMagRes Books

eMagRes (formerly the *Encyclopedia of Magnetic Resonance*) publishes a wide range of online articles on all aspects of magnetic resonance in physics, chemistry, biology and medicine. The existence of this large number of articles, written by experts in various fields, is enabling the publication of a series of *eMagRes* Books – handbooks on specific areas of NMR and MRI. The chapters of each of these handbooks will comprise a carefully chosen selection of *eMagRes* articles.

Published *eMagRes* Books

NMR Crystallography
Edited by Robin K. Harris, Roderick E. Wasylishen, Melinda J. Duer
ISBN 978-0-470-69961-4

Multidimensional NMR Methods for the Solution State
Edited by Gareth A. Morris, James W. Emsley
ISBN 978-0-470-77075-7

Solid-State NMR Studies of Biopolymers
Edited by Ann E. McDermott, Tatyana Polenova
ISBN 978-0-470-72122-3

NMR of Quadrupolar Nuclei in Solid Materials
Edited by Roderick E. Wasylishen, Sharon E. Ashbrook, Stephen Wimperis
ISBN 978-0-470-97398-1

RF Coils for MRI
Edited by John T. Vaughan, John R. Griffiths
ISBN 978-0-470-77076-4

*MRI of Tissues with Short T_2s or T_2*s*
Edited by Graeme M. Bydder, Gary D. Fullerton, Ian R. Young
ISBN 978-0-470-68835-9

NMR Spectroscopy: A Versatile Tool for Environmental Research
Edited by Myrna J. Simpson, André J. Simpson
ISBN 978-1-118-61647-5

NMR in Pharmaceutical Sciences
Edited by Jeremy R. Everett, Robin K. Harris, John C. Lindon, Ian D. Wilson
ISBN 978-1-118-66025-6

Handbook of Magnetic Resonance Spectroscopy In Vivo: MRS Theory, Practice and Applications
Edited by Paul A. Bottomley, John R. Griffiths
ISBN 978-1-118-99766-6

EPR Spectroscopy: Fundamentals and Methods
Edited by Daniella Goldfarb, Stefan Stoll
ISBN 978-1-119-16299-5

Handbook of High Field Dynamic Nuclear Polarization
Edited by Vladimir K. Michaelis, Robert G. Griffin, Björn Corzilius, Shimon Vega
ISBN 978-1-119-44164-9

Safety and Biological Effects in MRI
Edited by Devashish Shrivastava, J. Thomas
ISBN 978-1-118-82130-5

eMagRes

Edited by Sharon Ashbrook, Bela Bode, George A. Gray, John R. Griffiths, Tatyana Polenova, Roberta Pieratelli, Thomas Prisner, André J. Simpson, Myrna J. Simpson.

eMagRes (formerly the *Encyclopedia of Magnetic Resonance*) is based on the original publication of the *Encyclopedia of Nuclear Magnetic Resonance*, first published in 1996 with an updated volume added in 2000. The *Encyclopedia of Magnetic Resonance* was launched in 2007 online with all the existing published material, and was later relaunched as *eMagRes* in 2013. *eMagRes* captures every aspect of the interdisciplinary nature of magnetic resonance, providing all the essential information on the science, methodologies, engineering, technologies, applications, and the history of magnetic resonance, whilst encompassing a whole range of techniques, including MRI, MRS, NMR, and EPR/ESR.

For more information see: http://www.wileyonlinelibrary.com/ref/eMagRes.

Safety and Biological Effects in MRI

Editors

Devashish Shrivastava

US Food and Drug Administration, Silver Spring, MD, USA &
In Vivo Temperatures, LLC, Burnsville, MN, USA

J. Thomas Vaughan

Director of Magnetic Resonance Research, School of Engineering and Applied Sciences, Columbia University, New York, NY, USA

WILEY

This edition first published 2021

Registered Office
John Wiley & Sons Ltd, The Atrium, Southern Gate, Chichester, West Sussex, PO19 8SQ, UK

Library of Congress Cataloging-in-Publication Data

Names: Shrivastava, Devashish, 1976- editor. | Vaughan, J. Thomas (John Thomas), 1957- editor.
Title: Safety and biological effects in MRI / editors, Devashish Shrivastava, J. Thomas Vaughan.
Other titles: Safety and biological aspects in MRI | eMagRes books.
Description: First edition. | Chichester, West Sussex ; Hoboken : John Wiley & Sons Ltd, 2021. | Series: eMagRes books | Includes bibliographical references and index.
Identifiers: LCCN 2020042302 (print) | LCCN 2020042303 (ebook) | ISBN 9781118821305 (cloth) | ISBN 9781118821299 (adobe pdf) | ISBN 9781118821282 (epub)
Subjects: MESH: Magnetic Resonance Imaging | Patient Safety | Magnetic Fields–adverse effects | Radio Waves–adverse effects
Classification: LCC RC386.6.M34 (print) | LCC RC386.6.M34 (ebook) | NLM WN 185 | DDC 616.07/548–dc23
LC record available at https://lccn.loc.gov/2020042302
LC ebook record available at https://lccn.loc.gov/2020042303

Cover Design: Wiley
Cover Images: Courtesy of Malgorzata Kloc; Courtesy of Lawrence L. Wald; Courtesy of Devashish Shrivastava; Background © kWaiGon / Getty Images

Set in 9.5/11.5pt TimesLTStd by SPi Global, Chennai, India

10 9 8 7 6 5 4 3 2 1

To our children Athena Rachana Devashish, Minerva Rachana Devashish,
John Thomas Vaughan, Dylan Amelia Vaughan, and Charles Robert Vaughan;

&

To all those engineers, physicists, biologists, clinicians, MR techs, and numerous others
who toil everyday to make MRI safer for everyone.

eMagRes

International Advisory Board

Contents

Contributors

Volkan Açıkel
ASELSAN, Ankara, Turkey
Chapter 23: RF Safety of Active Implantable Medical Devices

Oktay Algın
Atatürk Training and Research Hospital, Ankara, Turkey
Chapter 15: RF Heating Due to a 3T Birdcage Whole-body Transmit Coil in Anesthetized Sheep

Philipp Amrein
University of Freiburg, Freiburg, Germany
Chapter 34: Gradient Coils

Leonardo M. Angelone
Division of Biomedical Physics, Office of Science and Engineering Laboratories, CDRH/FDA, Silver Spring, MD, USA
Chapter 21: RF-Induced Heating in Bare and Covered Stainless Steel Rods: Effect of Length, Covering, and Diameter

Ergin Atalar
Bilkent University, Ankara, Turkey
Chapter 23: RF Safety of Active Implantable Medical Devices

John C. Bischof
University of Minnesota, Minneapolis, MN, USA
Chapter 27: The Use and Safety of Iron-Oxide Nanoparticles in MRI and MFH

Bruce Breneman
Breneman Consulting, Rancho Santa Fe, CA, USA
Chapter 31: History, Physics, and Design of Superconducting Magnets for MRI
Chapter 32: Fabrication of Superconducting Magnets for MRI
Chapter 33: Magnet Field Shimming and External Ferromagnetic Influences on the Homogeneity and Site Shielding of Superconducting MRI Magnets

Marjean H. Cefaratti
Children's National Medical Center, Washington, DC, USA
Chapter 17: Temperature Management and Radiofrequency Heating During Pediatric MRI Scans

Ji Chen
University of Houston, Houston, TX, USA; IEEE, Houston, TX, USA
Chapter 16: In Vivo Radiofrequency Heating due to 1.5, 3, and 7 T Whole-body Volume Coils
Chapter 22: On the Development of a Novel Leg Phantom for RF Safety Assessment for Circular Ring External Fixation Devices in 1.5 T
Chapter 24: An Analysis of Factors Influencing MRI RF Safety for Patients with AIMDs

Mathias Davids
Heidelberg University, Heidelberg, Germany; Massachusetts General Hospital, Charlestown, MA, USA
Chapter 5: Peripheral Nerve Stimulation Modeling for MRI

Kathleen Durkin
Columbia University, New York, NY, USA
Chapter 30: Safety Practices and Protocols in the MR Research Center of the Columbia University in the City of New York

Dania Elder
Columbia University, New York, NY, USA
Chapter 30: Safety Practices and Protocols in the MR Research Center of the Columbia University in the City of New York

Hamza Ergüder
Yildiz Technical University, Istanbul, Turkey
Chapter 15: RF Heating Due to a 3T Birdcage Whole-body Transmit Coil in Anesthetized Sheep

Stuart Feltham
MR Science & Technology, GE Healthcare, Florence, SC, USA
Chapter 1: Static and Low Frequency Electromagnetic Fields and Their Effects in MRIs

Stanley Thomas Fricke
Georgetown University Medical Center, Washington, DC, USA; Children's National Medical Center, Washington, DC, USA
Chapter 17: Temperature Management and Radiofrequency Heating During Pediatric MRI Scans

Kyoko Fujimoto
Division of Biomedical Physics, Office of Science and Engineering Laboratories, CDRH/FDA, Silver Spring, MD, USA
Chapter 21: RF-Induced Heating in Bare and Covered Stainless Steel Rods: Effect of Length, Covering, and Diameter

Michael Garwood
University of Minnesota, Minneapolis, MN, USA
Chapter 27: The Use and Safety of Iron-Oxide Nanoparticles in MRI and MFH

Sairam Geethanath
Columbia Magnetic Resonance Research Center, Columbia University in the City of New York, New York, NY, USA
Chapter 14: Radio Frequency Safety Assessment for Open Source Pulse Sequence Programming

Rafik M. Ghobrial
The Houston Methodist Research Institute, Houston, TX, USA; Department of Surgery, The Houston Methodist Hospital, Houston, TX, USA
Chapter 3: Effects of Magnetic Fields and Field Gradients on Living Cells

Paul Glover
University of Nottingham, Nottingham, UK
Chapter 2: Magnetic-field-induced Vertigo in the MR Environment

Anand Gopinath
University of Minnesota, Minneapolis, MN, USA
Chapter 28: Numerical Simulation for MRI RF Coils and Safety
Chapter 29: Integral Equation Approach to Modeling RF Fields in Human Body in MRI Systems for Safety

Christopher J. Gordon
Retired, U.S. Environmental Protection Agency, Research Triangle Park, NC, USA
Chapter 18: Failure to Monitor and Maintain Thermal Comfort During an MRI Scan: A Perspective from a Thermal Physiologist Turned Patient

David Gross
MED Institute Inc., West Lafayette, IN, USA
Chapter 4: Effect of Strong Time-varying Magnetic Field Gradients on Humans

Joshua Guag
Division of Biomedical Physics, Office of Science and Engineering Laboratories, CDRH/FDA, Silver Spring, MD, USA
Chapter 21: RF-induced Heating in Bare and Covered Stainless Steel Rods: Effect of Length, Covering, and Diameter

Bastien Guérin
Massachusetts General Hospital, Charlestown, MA, USA; Harvard Medical School, Boston, MA, USA
Chapter 5: Peripheral Nerve Stimulation Modeling for MRI

David H. Gultekin
Columbia University, New York, NY, USA
Chapter 30: Safety Practices and Protocols in the MR Research Center of the Columbia University in the City of New York

Qiang He
Shanghai United Imaging Healthcare Co., Ltd, Shanghai, China
Chapter 16: In Vivo Radiofrequency Heating due to 1.5, 3, and 7 T Whole-body Volume Coils

Xing Huang
Abbott Laboratories, Chicago, IL, USA
Chapter 22: On the Development of a Novel Leg Phantom for RF Safety Assessment for Circular Ring External Fixation Devices in 1.5 T

Maria Ida Iacono
Division of Biomedical Physics, Office of Science and Engineering Laboratories, CDRH/FDA, Silver Spring, MD, USA
Chapter 21: RF-Induced Heating in Bare and Covered Stainless Steel Rods: Effect of Length, Covering, and Diameter

Feng Jia
University of Freiburg, Freiburg, Germany
Chapter 34: Gradient Coils

Julie Kabil
Columbia Magnetic Resonance Research Center, Columbia University in the City of New York, New York, NY, USA
Chapter 14: Radio Frequency Safety Assessment for Open Source Pulse Sequence Programming

Julie M. Kabil
Columbia University, New York, NY, USA
Chapter 28: Numerical Simulation for MRI RF Coils and Safety

Malgorzata Kloc
The Houston Methodist Research Institute, Houston, TX, USA; Department of Surgery, The Houston Methodist Hospital, Houston, TX, USA; M.D. Anderson Cancer Center, Department of Genetics, The University of Texas, Houston, TX, USA
Chapter 3: Effects of Magnetic Fields and Field Gradients on Living Cells

Russell Lagore *University of Minnesota, Minneapolis, MN, USA*
Chapter 35: RF Coil Construction for MRI

Charles A. Lemaire *In Vivo Temperatures, LLC, Burnsville, MN, USA*
Chapter 25: On Using Fluoroptic Thermometry to Measure Time-varying Temperatures in MRI

Sebastian Littin *University of Freiburg, Freiburg, Germany*
Chapter 34: Gradient Coils

Jingshen Liu *IEEE, Calabasas, CA, USA*
Chapter 24: An Analysis of Factors Influencing MRI RF Safety for Patients with AIMDs

Sreeparna Majee *Jadavpur University, Kolkata, India*
Chapter 9: Effect of Magnetic Field on Blood Flow

Tahir Malas *Lorentz Solution, Santa Clara, CA, USA*
Chapter 15: RF Heating Due to a 3T Birdcage Whole-body Transmit Coil in Anesthetized Sheep

Andrew Matisoff *Children's National Medical Center, Washington, DC, USA*
Chapter 17: Temperature Management and Radiofrequency Heating During Pediatric MRI Scans

John H. Miller Jr *Texas Center for Superconductivity, University of Houston, Houston, TX, USA; Department of Physics, University of Houston, Houston, TX, USA*
Chapter 3: Effects of Magnetic Fields and Field Gradients on Living Cells

Joseph Murphy-Boesch *National Institutes of Health, NINDS, Bethesda, MD, USA*
Chapter 20: Heating of RF Coil

Mykhaylo Nosovskyy *In Vivo Temperatures, LLC, Burnsville, MN, USA*
Chapter 25: On Using Fluoroptic Thermometry to Measure Time-varying Temperatures in MRI

John Nyenhuis *Purdue University, West Lafayette, IN, USA*
Chapter 4: Effect of Strong Time-varying Magnetic Field Gradients on Humans

Henrik Odéen *University of Utah, Salt Lake City, UT, USA*
Chapter 19: MR Thermometry to Assess Heating Induced by RF Coils Used in MRI

Çağdaş Oto *Ankara University, Ankara, Turkey*
Chapter 15: RF Heating Due to a 3T Birdcage Whole-body Transmit Coil in Anesthetized Sheep

Dylan Palomino *University of Utah, Salt Lake City, UT, USA*
Chapter 19: MR Thermometry to Assess Heating Induced by RF Coils Used in MRI

Dennis L. Parker
University of Utah, Salt Lake City, UT, USA
Chapter 19: MR Thermometry to Assess Heating Induced by RF Coils Used in MRI

Alexander J.E. Raaijmakers
University Medical Center Utrecht, Utrecht, The Netherlands; Eindhoven University of Technology, Eindhoven, The Netherlands
Chapter 13: Local SAR Assessment for Multitransmit Systems: A Study on the Peak Local SAR Value as a Function of Magnetic Field Strength

Sunder Rajan
Division of Biomedical Physics, Office of Science and Engineering Laboratories, CDRH/FDA, Silver Spring, MD, USA
Chapter 21: RF-Induced Heating in Bare and Covered Stainless Steel Rods: Effect of Length, Covering, and Diameter

Hattie L. Ring
University of Minnesota, Minneapolis, MN, USA
Chapter 27: The Use and Safety of Iron-Oxide Nanoparticles in MRI and MFH

John Rock Hadley
University of Utah, Salt Lake City, UT, USA
Chapter 19: MR Thermometry to Assess Heating Induced by RF Coils Used in MRI

Lothar R. Schad
Heidelberg University, Heidelberg, Germany
Chapter 5: Peripheral Nerve Stimulation Modeling for MRI

Peter Serano
Division of Biomedical Physics, Office of Science and Engineering Laboratories, CDRH/FDA, Silver Spring, MD, USA
Chapter 21: RF-Induced Heating in Bare and Covered Stainless Steel Rods: Effect of Length, Covering, and Diameter

Michael Keith Sharp
University of Louisville, Louisville, KY, USA
Chapter 8: Modeling Blood Flow

G.C. Shit
Jadavpur University, Kolkata, India
Chapter 9: Effect of Magnetic Field on Blood Flow

Devashish Shrivastava
In Vivo Temperatures, LLC, Burnsville, MN, USA
Chapter 11: On the Choice of RF Safety Metric in MRI: Temperature, SAR, or Thermal Dose
Chapter 16: In Vivo Radiofrequency Heating due to 1.5, 3, and 7 T Whole-body Volume Coils
Chapter 25: On Using Fluoroptic Thermometry to Measure Time-varying Temperatures in MRI
Chapter 26: On Using Magnetic Resonance Thermometry to Measure 'Strong' Spatio-temporal Tissue Temperature Variations and Compute Thermal Dose

Berk Silemek
Bilkent University, Ankara, Turkey
Chapter 23: RF Safety of Active Implantable Medical Devices

Shuo Song
University of Houston, Houston, TX, USA
Chapter 16: In Vivo Radiofrequency Heating due to 1.5, 3, and 7 T Whole-body Volume Coils

Michael C. Steckner
Canon Medical Research USA, Inc., Mayfield Village, OH, USA
Chapter 7: A Review of MRI Acoustic Noise and its Potential Impact on Patient and Worker Health
Chapter 10: Safety Standards for MRI

Bart R. Steensma
University Medical Center Utrecht, Utrecht, The Netherlands
Chapter 13: Local SAR Assessment for Multitransmit Systems: A Study on the Peak Local SAR Value as a Function of Magnetic Field Strength

Katelynn Stroth
University of Utah, Salt Lake City, UT, USA
Chapter 19: MR Thermometry to Assess Heating Induced by RF Coils Used in MRI

Samat Turdumamatov
University of Central Asia, Bishkek, Kyrgyzstan
Chapter 15: RF Heating Due to a 3T Birdcage Whole-body Transmit Coil in Anesthetized Sheep

Ahmed Uosef
Ain Shams University School of Medicine, Cairo, Egypt; The Houston Methodist Research Institute, Houston, TX, USA
Chapter 3: Effects of Magnetic Fields and Field Gradients on Living Cells

J. Thomas Vaughan
Columbia University in the City of New York, New York, NY, USA
Chapter 12: RF Coil and MR Safety
Chapter 14: Radio Frequency Safety Assessment for Open Source Pulse Sequence Programming
Chapter 16: In Vivo Radiofrequency Heating due to 1.5, 3, and 7 T Whole-body Volume Coils
Chapter 35: RF Coil Construction for MRI

Martha Villagran
Texas Center for Superconductivity, University of Houston, Houston, TX, USA; Department of Physics, University of Houston, Houston, TX, USA
Chapter 3: Effects of Magnetic Fields and Field Gradients on Living Cells

Lawrence L. Wald
Massachusetts General Hospital, Charlestown, MA, USA; Harvard Medical School, Boston, MA, USA; Harvard-MIT Health Sciences and Technology, Cambridge, MA, USA
Chapter 5: Peripheral Nerve Stimulation Modeling for MRI

Qingyan Wang
IEEE, Houston, TX, USA
Chapter 24: An Analysis of Factors Influencing MRI RF Safety for Patients with AIMDs

Terry O. Woods
Office of Science and Engineering Laboratories, Center for Devices and Radiological Health, Silver Spring, MD, USA
Chapter 6: Magnetically Induced Force and Torque on Medical Devices

Jarek Wosik
Department of Electrical and Computer Engineering, University of Houston, Houston, TX, USA; Texas Center for Superconductivity, University of Houston, Houston, TX, USA
Chapter 3: Effects of Magnetic Fields and Field Gradients on Living Cells

Tayeb Zaidi
Division of Biomedical Physics, Office of Science and Engineering Laboratories, CDRH/FDA, Silver Spring, MD, USA
Chapter 21: RF-Induced Heating in Bare and Covered Stainless Steel Rods: Effect of Length, Covering, and Diameter

Maxim Zaitsev
University of Freiburg, Freiburg, Germany
Chapter 34: Gradient Coils

Rongxing Zhang
Shanghai United Imaging Healthcare Co., Ltd, Shanghai, China
Chapter 16: In Vivo Radiofrequency Heating due to 1.5, 3, and 7 T Whole-body Volume Coils

Zhenyu Zhang
MR Science & Technology, GE Healthcare, Florence, SC, USA
Chapter 1: Static and Low Frequency Electromagnetic Fields and Their Effects in MRIs

Jianfeng Zheng
IEEE, Houston, TX, USA
Chapter 24: An Analysis of Factors Influencing MRI RF Safety for Patients with AIMDs

Series Preface

The *Encyclopedia of Nuclear Magnetic Resonance* was originally published in eight volumes in 1996, in part to celebrate the fiftieth anniversary of the first publications describing the discovery of NMR (nuclear magnetic resonance) in January 1946. Volume 1 contained a historical overview and 200 articles by prominent NMR practitioners, while the remaining seven volumes consisted of 500 articles on a wide variety of topics in NMR, including MRI (magnetic resonance imaging). A ninth volume was brought out in 2000 and two 'spin-off' volumes incorporating the articles on MRI and MRS (together with some new ones) were published in 2002. In 2006, the decision was taken to publish all the articles electronically with the resulting Encyclopedia becoming available online in 2007. Since then, new articles have been published online every 3 months and many of the original articles have been updated. To recognize the fact that the *Encyclopedia of Magnetic Resonance* is a true online resource, the website was redesigned and new functionalities added, with a relaunch in January 2013 in a new Volume and Issue format, under the new name *eMagRes*. In December 2012, a new print edition of the *Encyclopedia of Nuclear Magnetic Resonance* edited by Robin K. Harris and Roderick E. Wasylishen was published in 10 volumes (6200 pages). This much needed update of the 1996 edition of the Encyclopedia encompassed the entire field of NMR.

As part of the development of *eMagRes*, a series of printed handbooks on specific areas of magnetic resonance have been introduced. The handbooks are planned in advance by specially selected editors, and new articles written to give appropriate complete coverage of the subject area. The handbooks are intended to be of value and interest to research students, postdoctoral fellows, and other researchers learning about the topic in question and undertaking relevant experiments, whether in academia or industry.

This new handbook *Safety and Biological Effects in MRI* edited by Devashish Shrivastava and J. Thomas Vaughan is the third handbook of special interest to researchers working in the field of magnetic resonance imaging. The previous two MRI handbooks, *MRI of Tissues with Short* T_2 *and* T_2* edited by G. Bydder, G. Fullerton and I.R. Young and *RF Coils for MRI* edited by J.T. Vaughan and J.R. Griffiths will also be of interest to the MRI community. Obviously, safety and biological effects are critically important in MRI and in fact to the entire magnetic resonance community; particularly relevant to the broader magnetic resonance community is the third section of this handbook titled, *Engineering*. We thank the editors, D. Shrivastava and J.T. Vaughan, for their efforts in assembling this authoritative handbook which will be an important resource for the MRI community. Finally, I wish to thank Jenny Cossham at Wiley for her assistance and patience in helping editors of this and previous Handbooks associated with *eMagRes*.

Roderick E. Wasylishen

May 2020

Preface

The goal of this book is to present the effect of the magnetic resonance imaging (MRI) environment on the human body, and tools and methods to quantify such effects. By presenting such information all in one place, the expectation is that this book will help everyone interested in the Safety and Biological Effects in MRI find relevant information relatively quickly and know where we stand as a community. The information is expected to bring engineers, physicists, biologist, clinicians, MR technologists, and other healthcare professionals closer together and foster collaborations to develop new ways to improve patient safety in MR scanners of today, and develop faster, yet more powerful, but safer MR scanners of tomorrow.

The book is arranged in three sections. The first section, named 'Static and Gradient Fields' (Chapters 1–9), presents the effects of static magnetic field and the gradients of magnetic field, in time and space, on the human body. The second section, named 'Radiofrequency Fields' (Chapters 10–30), presents ways to quantify radiofrequency (RF) field induced heating in patients undergoing MRI. The effect of the three fields (i.e., Static Magnetic Field, Time-varying Gradient Magnetic Field, and RF Field) on medical devices, that may be brought into the MRI environment with patients, is also included. Finally, the third section, named 'Engineering' (Chapters 31–35), presents the basic background engineering information regarding the equipment (i.e., superconducting magnets, gradient coils, and RF coils) that produce the Static Magnetic Field, Time-varying Gradient Magnetic Field, and RF Field.

The book is intended for engineers, physicists, biologists, clinicians, MR technologists, other healthcare professionals, and everyone else who might be interested in looking into the role of MRI environment on patient safety.

Writing this book has been a rewarding experience. Tommy and I are deeply indebted to all our expert friends and colleagues who took time out from their busy schedules to contribute to this book and who responded gently to all my sobbing, prodding, and threats. We also appreciate the support of those who promised to contribute but for some reason failed to follow through. Next, we would like to acknowledge the enthusiastic support of Dr. Michael Steckner throughout this project. His help was instrumental in finding experts in a timely fashion on many occasions. We are also immensely thankful to the kind staff members of John Wiley and Sons (Jenny Cossham and Joshua Charles) who were quick, efficient, and always ready to help. Finally, I would like to thank my friend, colleague, and the most ardent supporter of 21 years (and wife for 19 or so years) Dr. Rachana Visaria, for making sure that Tommy and I kept making progress and finished in time.

Devashish Shrivastava, PhD
Clarksville, MD

Acknowledgments

The editors would like to acknowledge the many authors who have contributed their time and energy assisting in bringing a unique handbook to the DNP community. The editors thank Professor Roderick E. Wasylishen who commissioned the content for this book as Editor-in-Chief of *eMagRes* and who is now co-chairman of the advisory board through Wiley. The editors dedicate this book to the memory of Professor Charles P. Slichter in acknowledgment of his pioneering efforts in NMR spectroscopy. Finally, the many past, present, and future colleagues and students who will continue to advance the DNP research field are thanked for their efforts.

PART A
Static and Gradient Fields

Chapter 1

Static and Low Frequency Electromagnetic Fields and Their Effects in MRIs

Zhenyu Zhang and Stuart Feltham

MR Science & Technology, GE Healthcare, Florence, SC, USA

Magnetic resonance (MR) scanners employ three distinct magnetic field types to make the noninvasive imaging possible. First, a static magnetic field (B_0) is used to align hydrogen atoms (which are actually just protons) in the patient's body. This magnetic field is very strong (most clinical imaging is carried out in the 1.5–3 T range) and is highly uniform in the imaging field of view (FOV), typically ~10 ppm variation over a 50 cm diameter sphere. Second, a low-frequency switching magnetic field, normally in kHz range, that produces a three-dimensional spatial gradient inside the FOV, this operation distinguishes each point in the FOV enabling spatial encoding. Lastly, radio frequency magnetic fields (B_1) are used to perturb the polarized hydrogen atoms from their equilibrium positions. At a specific resonant frequency, the energy of the RF pulse can be absorbed by an atom and then released shortly after the RF is turned off. The resonant frequency is the so-called Larmor frequency (42.5 MHz T^{-1} for hydrogen) which is determined by the B_0 field strength and the nuclei of observation.

The three magnetic fields work together to produce an RF output that can be reconstructed into MR images. Each of these three magnetic fields can be a source of safety concerns during MR scans and operations. For instance, some physiological or sensory effects and projectile motion of ferromagnetic objects are related to the static B_0 field; peripheral nerve stimulation (PNS), helium boil-off, and excessive noise are related to the switching gradient fields, conductor heating, and electromagnetic interference with other high-frequency equipment are related to the RF field. Moreover, the image quality (IQ) can be affected by external electromagnetic interferences, especially at low frequencies. Some safety and IQ aspects of static and low-frequency magnetic fields are discussed here.

1.1 STATIC MAGNETIC FIELD AND ITS EFFECTS

Higher B_0 field strength brings higher signal-to-noise ratio (SNR), along with the potential for better image resolution (IQ) and faster image processing; therefore, MR scanners with stronger B_0 field are strongly desired. In today's clinical applications, the mainstream of MRI systems has 1.5 or 3.0 T static fields. MR scanners with even higher field strengths of 7.0, 9.4, and 10.5 T have been producing human images mostly in

Safety and Biological Effects in MRI.
Edited by Devashish Shrivastava and J. Thomas Vaughan
 ISBN: 978-1-118-82130-5
Also published in eMagRes (online edition)
DOI: 10.1002/9780470034590.emrstm1611

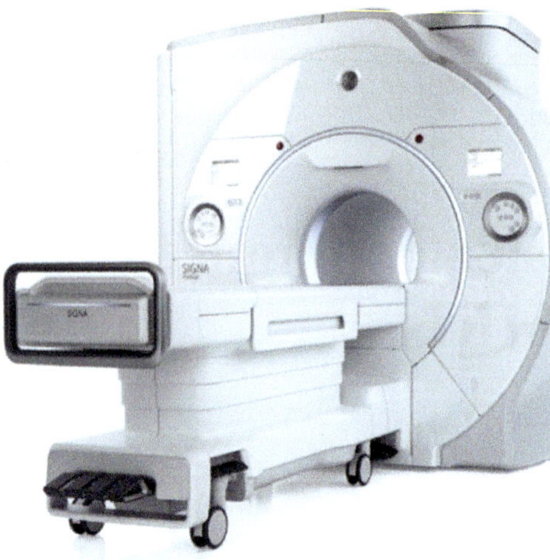

Figure 1.1. A 3.0 T MRI scanner

research environment and an 11.7 T MR scanner will be in operation in the next few years.[1] These are very strong magnetic fields compared with our daily experiences and exposure. For example, the center magnet field produced by a 3.0 T MRI scanner is 60 000 times stronger than the Earth's magnetic field which is *strong enough to navigate by compass and shield our planet from harmful cosmic radiation.* While resistive, permanent and hybrid magnets all exist in MRI scanners, field strength of 1.5 T and above can only be practically generated by superconducting magnets. These magnets made by industry vendors, with few exceptions, are cylindrical in shape and horizontally placed (Figure 1.1).

1.1.1 Physiological Effects of B_0 Field

With such a strong B_0 field produced by MR scanners, the first concern is what potential physiological effects could result from exposure. Fortunately, there is no proof of permanent deleterious effects from MRI scans or their operations.[2–4] This was summarized in 2000 by Schenck,[5] who wrote '*… it should not be concluded that it has been proved that there are no significant biological effects of static magnetic fields. However, it does appear correct to say that the work performed to date has yet to provide a single example of a scientifically sound and rigorously verified pathological effect of such fields. The steadily increasing capability of producing ever stronger magnets gives reason to believe that such effects will eventually be established, but probably at field strengths well above those currently used in MRI.*' In fact, the risk assessment around strong magnetic fields continues to be questioned and evaluated as MR scanners with higher fields become available for research and clinical purposes. FDA established safety guideline for MR scanner up to 2.0 T to be nonsignificant risk device in 1987, the limit increased to 4.0 T in 1996 and 8.0 T in 2003. This positive conclusion is largely due to the static nature of B_0 field. Although it is very strong, the electromagnetic interaction between the magnet and human body is minimized because the field is not a function of time, i.e., $\mathbf{d}\boldsymbol{B}_0/\mathbf{d}\boldsymbol{t} = \mathbf{0}$.

Nevertheless, there are several widely reported sensory effects associated with the strong B_0 fields produced by MR magnets. This could be traced back to two mechanisms: (i) motion of human body such as head shaking, eyeball rotating, and heart beating; because B_0 field is a function of space, i.e., $\nabla\boldsymbol{B}_0 \neq \mathbf{0}$, the motion results in a time changing B_0 field, which induces currents in human tissues and creates stimulations; (ii) there are natural electrical currents existing in human body, these micro-currents can experience Lorentz forces in an external magnetic field, if the field is strong enough, the resultant force could exceed thresholds and cause stimulations.

For example, magnetophosphene, it is a phenomenon of flashes of light that are seen when one is subjected to a time-varying magnetic field. This changing field induces electric fields and therefore currents within the retina or visual cortex resulting in the illusion of light.[6] A clinical study reported 8 out of 1023 people having experienced flashing lights during 1.5 and 3.0 T MR scans.[7] Strong B_0 field can also affect vestibular function, which could incur the feeling of vertigo.[8,9] Ward *et al.*[10] provided an explanation using Lorentz force. Ward argues the interaction between a static magnetic field and the ionic current existing naturally in inner ear endolymph results in Lorentz force. Observations have been made in human's and mice demonstrating this force is strong enough to agitate the lateral semicircular canal cupula to induce vertigo. Since the Lorentz force of such a stimulation is proportional to the magnetic field strength, MRI scanners with higher field strength have a higher probability of causing such an effect. Currently, the FDA safety guideline[11] suggests MRI scanners up to 8.0 T can operate with nonsignificant risk. With few 9.4 and 10.5 T systems in operation and (soon the) 11.7 T system, it is yet to see if these guidelines will be increased.

A widely known sensory effect is taste perversion or metallic taste, which is a sensation that can occur when one moves around in a high magnetic field.[12] The mechanism of this effect is related to a direct nerve stimulation or electrolysis of saliva or both.[13,14] The first can explain why this occurs with a magnetic field present, the second mechanism may describe how the metallic taste remains for a short time after the magnet field is removed. An experimental study was carried out by Cavin *et al.*[15] to assess this effect using a 7 T MRI scanner. This investigation revealed several interesting results: (i) the metallic taste is caused by motion in B_0 field; (ii) it is a common phenomenon, 12 of 21 test participants experienced a metallic taste; (iii) the effect has a $\mathbf{d}\boldsymbol{B_0}/\mathbf{d}\boldsymbol{t}$ dependence, the authors found normal motions in the field of 7 T magnet could result in field change $\mathbf{d}\boldsymbol{B_0}/\mathbf{d}\boldsymbol{t}$ at about 2 T s^{-1}, for example, if one shakes head with 1.5 s period, the resulting field change rate can be as high as 2.3 T s^{-1} and about 50% of the test subjects could feel a metallic taste under this condition.

Another issue caused by exposure to a strong B_0 field has the potential to alter electrocardiogram (ECG) waveforms. ECG monitoring during MRI scan is often needed for clinical purpose. When a patient is placed in the magnetic field of an MR scanner, an elevation of the T-wave of the EKG is often observed.[16–18] These effects may result in faulty cardiac triggering, especially in stronger magnetic fields. In fact, this magnetic field generated effect on the EKG does not originate in the heart itself, instead by a voltage that develops in blood as it flows down the thoracic aorta, which has been induced by its flow in the magnetic field. An induced electrical field developing in a conductive fluid flowing through a magnetic field is a well-known phenomenon in fluid mechanics called the magnetohydrodynamic (MHD) effect.[19]

In summary, the strong B_0 field has some temporary physiology effects, but there is no evidence that these effects are dangerous or have long-lasting impact to health. Nevertheless, one should avoid quick body motion in high field magnets (3 T and above) to minimize the probability of having magnetophosphene, a metallic taste, or the more unpleasant effects of vertigo or nausea. Patients with implants (i.e., cardiac pacemaker, insulin pumps, clips) need to be strictly screened before MR scan. Ferromagnetic components in various implants could experience high magnetic forces and torques[5] in strong magnetic field and cause unexpected implant motion inside human body. This could be a life-threatening risk and must be controlled. In addition, there is an annoying effect associated with MR's strong magnetic field called 'Gaussian Carditis,'[20] which refers to a phenomenon of the magnetic strip on one's credit card being erased when it is accidentally brought too close to MRI's powerful magnetic field. This is not exactly a human safety concern but could be very disruptive to one's life.

1.1.2 Magnetic Forces of B_0 Field

While much attention has been paid to physiological effects of B_0 field, these effects do not appear to be true safety risks for mainstream 1.5 and 3 T clinical MR scanners. The projectile motion of ferromagnetic objects, however, has proven to be a real threat which has resulted in serious injuries and sometimes death in MR scan rooms.[21,22] This is mainly due to the fact that one cannot see or feel the magnetic field directly until it is too late (Figure 1.2).

From both design and operation point of view, the safety of superconducting MR magnets is a central concern and needs to be addressed at several different levels. First, the magnetic dipole moments of these magnets are huge; therefore, the stray field can extend far away from the magnet. This is not only a threat to

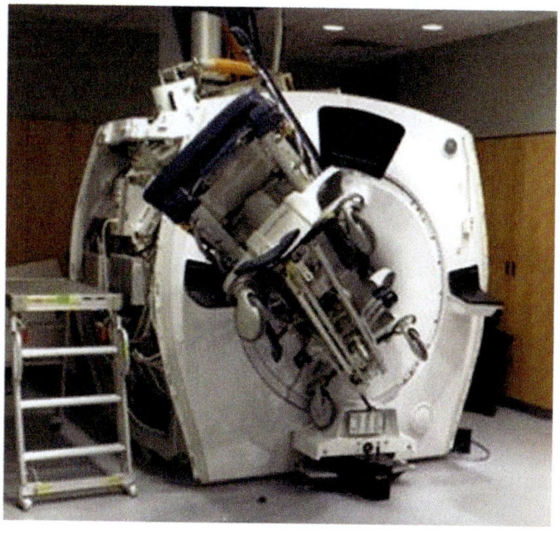

Figure 1.2. A cart with ferromagnetic material attracted to a 3 T MR scanner

personnel and electronic equipment in the vicinity but also can be a safety risk in the adjacent facilities. Modern superconducting magnet designs utilize shielding coils to control the footprint of stray field.[23,24] For a 1.5 T magnet, the 0.5 mT (5 G) line can be maintained within an area of 2.5 m (R) × 4.0 m (Z), which is fairly close to the size of most MR scan rooms. If the 0.5 mT line extends beyond the MRI suite, passive magnetic shielding material can be employed for confinement. Carbon-steel or silicon-steel based metal sheets are typically built into walls of magnet room for shielding purpose. If shielding is not possible, warning signs and physical barriers can be arranged to prevent people from entering an area of >0.5 mT background field.

Second, in case of emergency, if the B_0 magnetic field of an MR scanner needs to be removed, all superconducting magnets are equipped with a magnet run-down unit (MRU), which once activated, can eliminate the field within half a minute or so by quenching the supercomputing magnet in a controlled manner. The MRU is a critical safety component for MRI magnets and modern MRI scanners periodically monitor its status to make sure it is functioning.[25]

Third, when a ferromagnetic object is placed near an MR scanner, it experiences magnetic forces and can be attracted to the magnet if this force exceeds its weight. The high-speed motion of ferromagnetic objects is highly dangerous, they must be controlled. These objects are typically prohibited in the MR scan room. Nevertheless, in many cases, traditional tools for clinical or maintenance operations are ferrous, and therefore at risk of being carried into an MR scan room accidentally. Less frequently, there can be a need to use ferrous tools at which time it is important to be able to calculate or estimate the magnetic force exerted on such objects and how close they can approach the magnets.

1.1.3 Evaluation of Magnetic Forces

In electromagnetic analysis, ferromagnetic objects can be equated to a localized current distribution of the same magnetic moment. For a localized current distribution in an external magnetic field, the following relationship[26] can be obtained from the Lorenz formula $\mathbf{J} \times \mathbf{B}$:

$$\boldsymbol{F} = \nabla(\mathbf{m} \cdot \boldsymbol{B}) \tag{1.1}$$

where $\boldsymbol{J}$ is the current density, $\boldsymbol{F}$ is the magnetic force, $\mathbf{m}$ is the total magnetic moment, $\boldsymbol{B}$ is external magnetic field flux density. Note, all these physical quantities are vectors and functions of space. In general, the external field $\boldsymbol{B}$ is not uniform and has a three-dimensional structure, magnetic moment $\boldsymbol{m}$ is the same and determined by knowing the external field, material properties, and geometry of the object. The total magnetic force is the integration of $\boldsymbol{F}$ over the volume of the object. To accurately calculate the magnetic force on a ferromagnetic object can be quite involved.

Equation (1.1) can be simplified into a more explicit format in some special cases. First, since superconducting magnets are mostly cylindrical, the magnet field produced by these magnets possess rotational symmetry and can be described in 2D. In this case, equation (1.1) is expanded as follows:

$$\boldsymbol{F} = \nabla[m_z(r,z)B_z(r,z) + m_r(r,z)B_r(r,z)] \tag{1.2}$$

If one assumes magnetization is not a function of space, i.e., $m_z(r,z) = \text{constant}$ and $m_r(r,z) = \text{constant}$,

$$\boldsymbol{F} = m_z\nabla[B_z(r,z)] + m_r\nabla[B_r(r,z)] \tag{1.3}$$

Expand equation (1.3), we arrive at:

$$\boldsymbol{F} = \hat{\boldsymbol{r}}\left(m_z\frac{\partial B_z}{\partial r} + m_r\frac{\partial B_r}{\partial r}\right) + \hat{z}\left(m_z\frac{\partial B_z}{\partial z} + m_r\frac{\partial B_r}{\partial z}\right) \tag{1.4}$$

Equation (1.4) reveals the gradient terms of the B_0 field, such as $\frac{\partial B_z}{\partial z}$ and $\frac{\partial B_z}{\partial r}$ that are important to magnetic force calculations.

On the other hand, since both magnetic moment and magnetic field are vectors,

$$\mathbf{m} \cdot \boldsymbol{B} = |\mathbf{m}||\boldsymbol{B}|\cos\theta \tag{1.5}$$

If one assumes $\mathbf{m}$ and $\boldsymbol{B}$ are parallel, then $\cos\theta = 1$, equation (1.1) can be written as:

$$\boldsymbol{F} = |\mathbf{m}|\nabla(|\boldsymbol{B}|) + |\mathbf{B}|\nabla(|\mathbf{m}|) \tag{1.6}$$

Now if $\mathbf{m}$ is not spatial dependent, $\nabla(|\mathbf{m}|) = 0$, we arrive at:

$$\boldsymbol{F} = |\mathbf{m}|\nabla(|\boldsymbol{B}|) \tag{1.7}$$

If $\mathbf{m}$ is spatial dependent but linearly related to $\boldsymbol{B}$, so $\mathbf{m} = k\boldsymbol{B}$, where k is a scaler constant, then:

$$\boldsymbol{F} = k|\boldsymbol{B}|\nabla(|\boldsymbol{B}|) + |\mathbf{B}|\nabla(|\mathrm{k}\boldsymbol{B}|) \tag{1.8}$$

We arrive at:

$$|\boldsymbol{F}| = 2k|\boldsymbol{B}||\nabla(|\boldsymbol{B}|)| \tag{1.9}$$

Equation (1.9) is important, as it indicates the magnetic force can be determined by the product of the magnitude and gradient of B_0 field.

Now let us pursue some analytical expressions of magnetic force for special cases. First, if one assumes the ferromagnetic object is fully saturated, the total magnetic moment can be approximated by using the saturation magnetization, such as illustrated in equation (1.10).

$$\iiint \mathbf{m} dV \cong \frac{M_s}{\mu_0} \iiint \hat{\mathbf{m}} dV \tag{1.10}$$

where M_s is the saturation magnetization, μ_0 is the permeability of free space, $\hat{\mathbf{m}}$ is the unit vector representing the direction of the magnetization at any point within the object. Here, the object is highly magnetized due to the external field, in addition, the magnetization can be assumed to be uniform within the object. In this situation, the magnetization is determined by the magnetic property of the object only, which allows the external field structure and geometry of the object to be neglected.

$$m = \frac{M_s \times V}{\mu_0} \tag{1.11}$$

Furthermore, as a reasonable approximation for the worse scenario, one can assume the magnetization is along the maximum field gradient direction, so equation (1.1) becomes

$$F = \frac{M_s \times V}{\mu_0} \times \max(\nabla|B|) \tag{1.12}$$

Now we can normalize equation (1.12) with regard to the force of gravity (weight) of the object:

$$\frac{F_m}{F_g} = \frac{M_s \times V \times \max(\nabla|B|)}{\mu_0 \times \rho \times g \times V} = \frac{M_s}{\mu_0} \frac{\max(\nabla|B|)}{\rho \times g} \tag{1.13}$$

where ρ is the density of ferromagnetic material (i.e., 7870 kg m^{-3} for iron), g is local gravitational acceleration (9.8 m s^{-2}). In equation (1.13), M_s is part of the ferromagnetic material property (usually about 2.0 T for iron-based material), max($\nabla|B|$) is determined by the electromagnetic design of the magnet and the information typically provided by MRI system vendors, all other parameters are known constants. Equation (1.13) can be used to provide a fast yet conservative estimation on magnetic forces.

On the other hand, if the ferrous objects possess simple geometry (i.e., ellipsoid), the analytical solution of magnetization is known as[27]:

$$M_z = \frac{\aleph B_0}{\mu_0} \left[\frac{\cos^2\theta}{1 + \aleph D_a} + \frac{\sin^2\theta}{1 + \aleph D_r} \right] \tag{1.14}$$

where B_0 is the external field, $\aleph$ is the magnetic susceptibility, D_a and D_r are geometry-related factors, θ is the angle between the symmetry axis of the object and the magnetic field. This expression is further simplified by considering a sphere ($D_a = D_r = 1/3$):

$$M_z = \frac{\aleph B_0}{\mu_0} \frac{3}{3 + \aleph} \tag{1.15}$$

Then following a similar logic as in equations (1.12) and (1.13), one can get:

$$\frac{F_m}{F_g} = \frac{M_z * V * \max(\nabla|B|)}{\rho * g * V} = \frac{3\aleph}{3 + \aleph} \frac{B_0}{\mu_0} \frac{\max(\nabla|B|)}{\rho * g} \tag{1.16}$$

For soft magnetic material, equation (1.13) can be written as follows due to $\aleph \gg 1$:

$$\frac{F_m}{F_g} = \frac{3B_0}{\mu_0} \frac{\max(\nabla|B|)}{\rho \times g} \tag{1.17}$$

In this case, the magnetization is a linear function of external field only, not depending on the material properties. Equation (1.17) can be used for analytically calculating magnetic forces, but it tends to underestimate the magnetic force due to its assumptions and can only be applied to some special cases when the objects are spherical.

To accurately compute magnetic forces for general cases, one needs to solve Maxwell's equations numerically using a finite element method. This is mainly due to (i) nonlinear magnetic properties of ferromagnetic material; (ii) geometrical dependence of the object' magnetization; (iii) both external field and magnetization have spatial dependencies. To illustrate this, several objects with the same ferromagnetic material property (B–H curve) but different geometries have been positioned at the same location (object center) around a MR magnet, the magnetic flux density distribution inside these objects as the result of magnetization are calculated using the commercial FEM OPERA 3D package developed by Vector Field.[28] The results are shown in Figure 1.3.

The plot of the magnetic field in the area where the ferromagnetic objects are placed is shown in Figure 1.3(a). It can be seen the field is not uniform, the field strength is between 270 and 280 G with an average value around 275 G. Figure 1.3(b) shows the magnetic field across a steel plate placed at the same location, due to magnetization, the field strength increases to ~600–5300 G, with an averaged value at ~4000 G. It is not uniform due to the external field as well as the geometry of a plate, but the magnetization approximately follows the pattern of the external

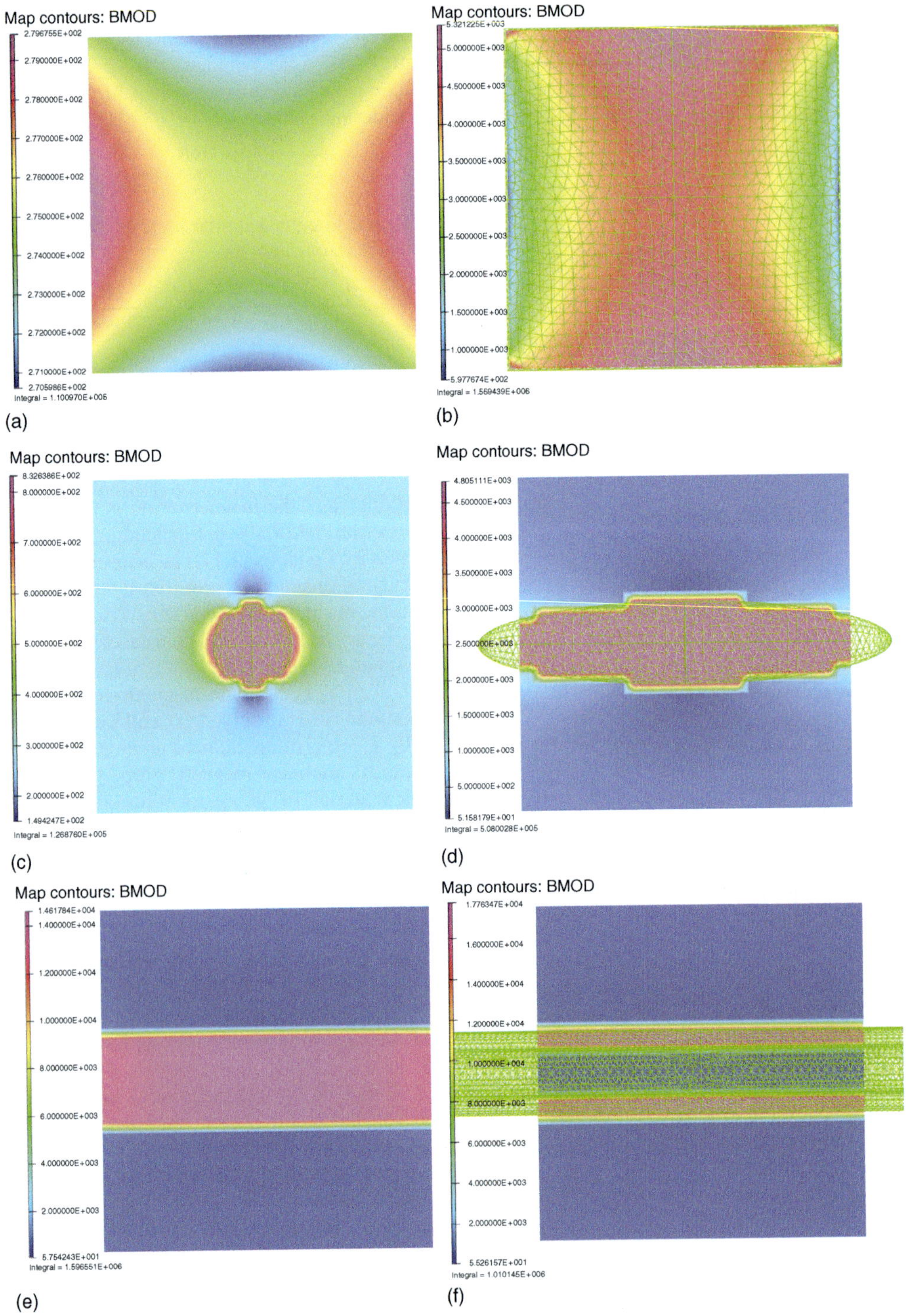

Figure 1.3. FEM simulated magnetic flux density distribution inside ferromagnetic objects with different geometry next to a magnet

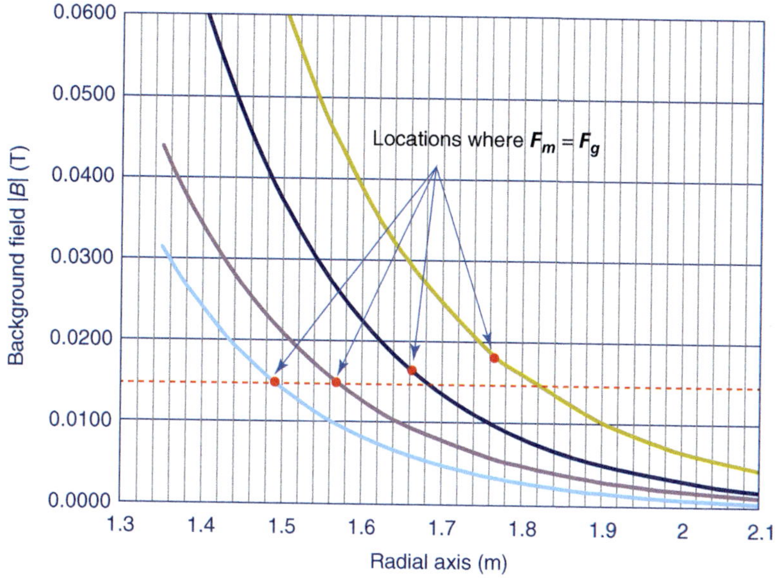

Figure 1.4. Measured radial locations where $F_m = F_g$ for a cylindrical ferromagnetic object next to different magnets

field. Figure 1.4(c) presents the field strength inside a metallic sphere when placed at the center of the external field, where the field has better uniformity. In this case, the magnetization of the sphere agrees with analytical solution well: (i) the magnetization inside the sphere is uniform; (ii) the effective permittivity μ_{eff} is 3. The field strength is around 830 G, which is very close to the theoretical numbers $275 \times 3 = 825$ G. Similarly, an ellipsoid is placed in the same location as illustrated in Figure 1.4(d), the magnetization across the ellipsoid is mostly uniform and at about 4700 G, the effective permeability μ_{eff} is calculated at 17. In Figure 1.3(e) and (f), a rod and a cylindrical tube are placed in the external field, it can be seen the magnetizations inside the objects are very uniform and reach to a much higher magnitude at 1.45 and 1.75 T, respectively. The magnetization density inside these objects is summarized in Table 1.1. For a sphere, it is true that $\mu_{\text{eff}} = 3$, but for a rod μ_{eff} is around 50. Since they have the same material property (B–H curve), this means they operate at different points on the B–H curve. It is mainly driven by their different geometries, as the required solution of Maxwell's equation is determined by the external field distribution, object's material property, and object's geometry. It is worth noting that the magnetization of a tube (iron pipe for example) is approximately *20 times higher* than the magnetization of a sphere. Thus, the force on a tube could be 20 times higher than a sphere, this makes gas cylinders particularly dangerous.

Table 1.1. Magnetization in object with different geometry

Simulation cases	Magnetization (Gauss)
Baseline	275
Sphere	820
Ellipsoid	4800
Plate	4000
Rod	14 300
Tube	17 000

1.1.4 Estimation and Guidelines

As discussed earlier, accurate calculation of the magnetic force on ferrous objects is difficult for general cases. Most of the time, what can be provided are estimations. In a weak field (100 ~ 200 G), the B–H relation is close to linear. The μ_{eff} strongly depends on the object's shape, size, and orientation, and does not strictly follow the material's B–H curve but is governed by the Laplace's equation and boundary conditions. Magnetization can be very high even in a relatively weak field, therefore, conservative estimation is necessary.

For a ferromagnetic object to be dangerous, the magnetic force exerted on it must be equal or larger than its gravitational force. The locations where $F_m = F_g$ for a cylindrical object measured for several different magnets are shown in Figure 1.4. In the plot, the magnetic fields naturally decay when moving away from the magnet radially. Although the field strength and decay rate are different for each magnet, the field strength where the magnetic force exerted on the object is equal to objects' weight is between 150 and 200 G. It is, therefore, necessary to keep ferromagnetic objects outside 100 G line of MR magnets.

From equations (1.7) and (1.9), it can be interpreted the magnetic force is dependent on the magnitude of field $|\boldsymbol{B}|$ and the magnitude of field gradient $|\nabla(|\boldsymbol{B}|)|$. These two values are often provided by MRI system vendors and recommended by industrial standards such as IEC 60601-2-33. In practice, the first value is very straightforward, but the second value often causes some confusion on how it is calculated. In the following, the expression to calculate $|\nabla(|\boldsymbol{B}|)|$ in 2D is derived. In 2D with rotational symmetry, the magnetic field is

$$\boldsymbol{B} = \hat{\boldsymbol{z}}B_z + \hat{\boldsymbol{r}}B_r \tag{1.18}$$

So we have $\nabla(|\boldsymbol{B}|) = \nabla|\hat{\boldsymbol{z}}B_z + \hat{\boldsymbol{r}}B_r| = \nabla(\sqrt{B_Z^2 + B_r^2})$, then the partial differentiation is

$$\frac{\partial\left(\sqrt{B_Z^2 + B_r^2}\right)}{\partial r} = \frac{1}{2\sqrt{B_Z^2 + B_r^2}}\left(2B_z\frac{\partial B_z}{\partial r} + 2B_r\frac{\partial B_r}{\partial r}\right) \tag{1.19}$$

$$\frac{\partial\left(\sqrt{B_Z^2 + B_r^2}\right)}{\partial r} = \frac{1}{2|\boldsymbol{B}|}\left(2B_z\frac{\partial B_z}{\partial r} + 2B_r\frac{\partial B_r}{\partial r}\right) \tag{1.20}$$

Similarly:

$$\frac{\partial\left(\sqrt{B_Z^2 + B_r^2}\right)}{\partial z} = \frac{1}{2|\boldsymbol{B}|}\left(2B_z\frac{\partial B_z}{\partial z} + 2B_r\frac{\partial B_r}{\partial z}\right) \tag{1.21}$$

Now $\nabla(|\boldsymbol{B}|)$ can be written as:

$$\nabla(|\boldsymbol{B}|) = \hat{\boldsymbol{z}}\frac{B_z\frac{\partial B_z}{\partial z} + B_r\frac{\partial B_r}{\partial z}}{|\boldsymbol{B}|} + \hat{\boldsymbol{r}}\frac{B_z\frac{\partial B_z}{\partial r} + B_r\frac{\partial B_r}{\partial r}}{|\boldsymbol{B}|} \tag{1.22}$$

Take the magnitude of equation (1.22):

$$|\nabla(|\boldsymbol{B}|)| = \sqrt{\frac{\left(B_z\frac{\partial B_z}{\partial z} + B_r\frac{\partial B_r}{\partial z}\right)^2}{|\boldsymbol{B}|^2} + \frac{\left(B_z\frac{\partial B_z}{\partial r} + B_r\frac{\partial B_r}{\partial r}\right)^2}{|\boldsymbol{B}|^2}} \tag{1.23}$$

Using a linear relation between $\boldsymbol{B}$ and $\boldsymbol{H}$ in free space, finally, we get

$$|\nabla(|\boldsymbol{B}|)| = \frac{\mu_0}{|\boldsymbol{B}|}\sqrt{\left(B_z\frac{\partial H_z}{\partial z} + B_r\frac{\partial H_r}{\partial z}\right)^2 + \left(B_z\frac{\partial H_z}{\partial r} + B_r\frac{\partial H_r}{\partial r}\right)^2} \tag{1.24}$$

Equation (1.24) is the definition of $|\nabla(|\boldsymbol{B}|)|$, which can be calculated numerically or directly by using an electromagnetic FEA package. In Figure 1.5, as an example, the calculation using equation (1.24) is performed for a 3.0 T magnet and shows both the strength and gradient of the B_0 field. Figure 1.5(a) is the plot along the main axis of the magnet where $R = 0$ and Figure 1.5(a) is for $R = 0.3$ m. It can be observed that the gradient profile along the main axis has a peak located approximately 0.9 m from the magnet center, this occurs near the largest coil block (the majority of amp turns on a magnet are at the ends) and the physical end of the magnet itself. As one moves from the center line toward the coils themselves the rate of change of the field increases substantially.

1.1.5 B_0 Homogeneity Impact to IQ

To obtain high-quality MR images, the B_0 field (as well as being very strong) must be very homogenous. There are several methods to homogenize a magnetic field but all act to smooth out the imperfections (primarily from the manufacturing process) within the static field magnet. Passive shimming is an industry standard technique used across a large range of field strengths for MR imaging. Characterizing the inhomogeneity and the shimming process used for correcting it can be carried out in many different formats. For example, the homogeneity can be characterized by peak-to-peak value (see equation (1.25), which is defined by the difference between maximum and minimum field points on the surface of FOV.

$$H|_{pk-pk} = \frac{\max B_z(r,\theta,\varphi) - \min B_z(r,\theta,\varphi)}{B_0}, \quad (r,\theta,\varphi) \in S \tag{1.25}$$

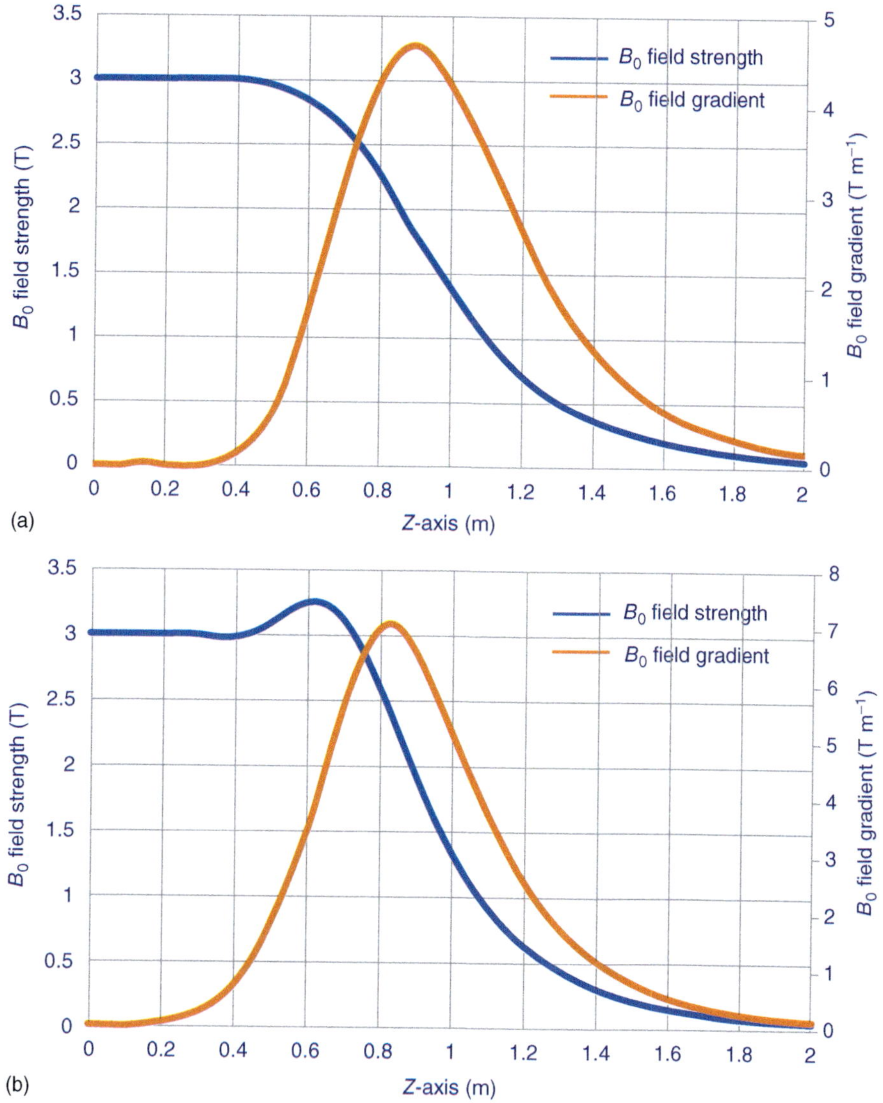

Figure 1.5. (a) B_0 field strength $|\boldsymbol{B}|$ and field gradient $|\nabla(|B|)|$ of a 3T MRI magnet along z-axis ($R = 0$). (b) B_0 field strength $|\mathbf{B}|$ and field gradient $|\nabla(|B|)|$ of a 3 T MRI magnet along z-axis ($R = 0.3$ m)

Alternatively, the homogeneity can be defined by using VRMS (volume root-mean-square) value as shown in equation (1.26).

$$H|_{\mathrm{VRMS}} = \sqrt{\frac{\int_V [B_z(r,\theta,\varphi) - B_0]^2 \mathrm{d}V}{V}}, \quad (r,\theta,\varphi) \in V \tag{1.26}$$

The VRMS value can also be express by using spherical harmonics as demonstrated in[29]:

$$H|_{\mathrm{VRMS}} = \sqrt{\frac{3}{2}\sum_{n=1}^{\infty}\sum_{m=0}^{n}\frac{(n+m)!}{(n-m)!}\frac{1}{(2n+1)(2n+3)}\left(\frac{r}{R}\right)^{2n}[\varepsilon_m C_{n,m}^2 + S_{n,m}^2]} \tag{1.27}$$

and

$$B_z(r,\theta,\varphi) = \sum_{n=0}^{\infty}\sum_{m=0}^{n}\left(\frac{r}{R}\right)^2 P_{n,m}(\cos\theta)$$
$$[C_{n,m}\cos(m\varphi) + S_{n,m}\sin(m\varphi] \quad (1.28)$$

where $P_{n,m}$ are the associated Legendre polynomials and R is the reference radius of the volume on which the expansion coefficients $C_{n,m}$ and $S_{n,m}$ are computed. Similarly, several shimming techniques have been developed to obtain the desired homogeneity for MR magnets. Two of the more popular methods are compared here to show their relative benefits: (i) peak-to-peak magnetic field-based method (p-method) which aims to minimize the maximum amplitude of magnetic field difference over the surface of a FOV and (ii) spherical harmonics based method (h-method) which optimizes a shim distribution to minimize difference between targeted and measured field harmonics. Both methods have their merits and drawbacks. In general, p-method can effectively control pk-pk values but could leave unexpected harmonic components since for any given pk–pk homogeneity, there are infinite number of harmonic combinations. The h-method controls harmonics directly, but often require more passive shims and sometimes have trouble to find a solution if the virgin inhomogeneity is high. In this chapter, a constructed 3T initial map is theoretically shimmed by the abovementioned methods and then imaging simulations are conducted to study the performances of these two shimming schemes in terms of IQ of a single shot Echo planar imaging (EPI) image, which is the most sensitive sequence to B_0 field inhomogeneity.[30]

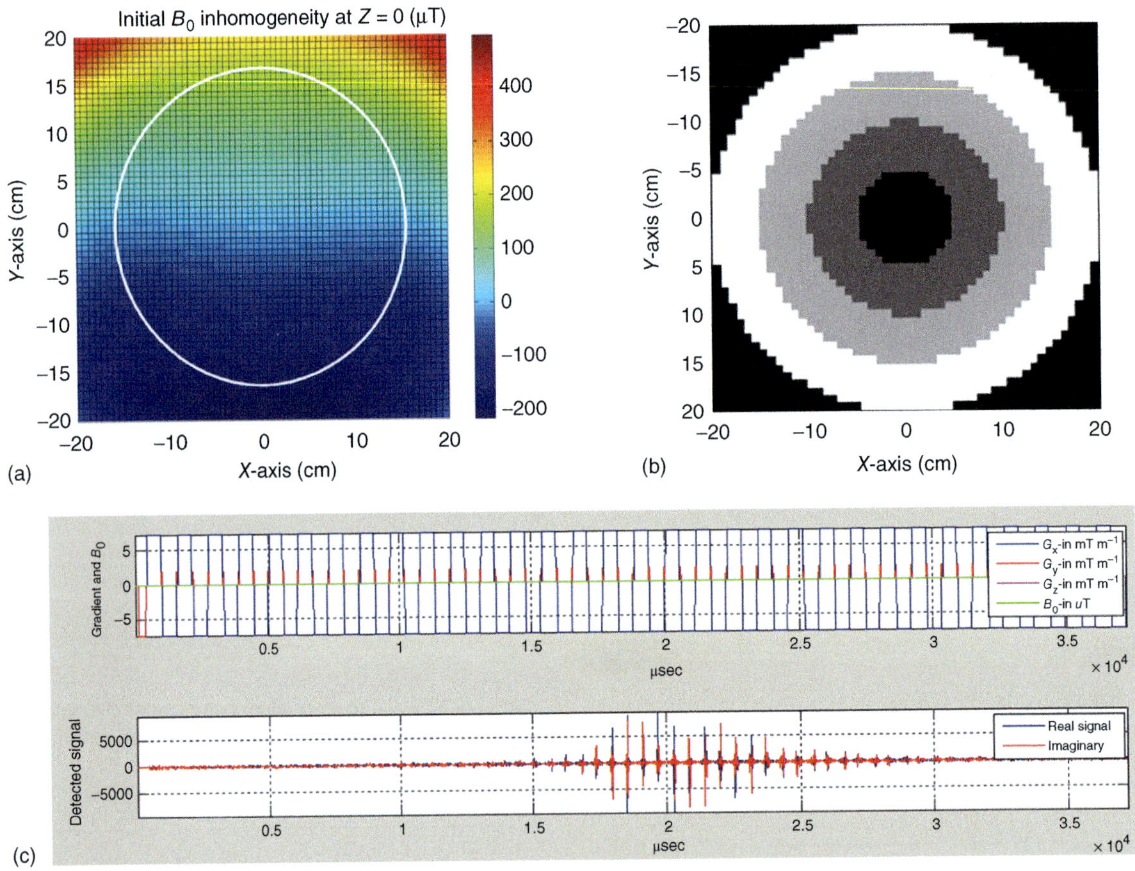

Figure 1.6. Simulation set up: (a) virgin field homogeneity, (b) subject under simulation, and (c) single Shot EPI pulse sequence

The shimming optimization can be constructed as a linear programming (LP) problem which includes a linear cost function and a set of linear constraints, a detailed mathematical description can be found in reference.[31] The simulation is realized in MATLAB.[32] The case study assumes 1000 shim pockets (25 pockets in phi-direction and 40 pockets in Z-direction) and 576 field sampling points (24 points in phi-direction and 24 points in theta-direction). Each shim pocket allows maximum 12 mm thickness with 5 cm by 3 cm cross sectional area. The initial map has pk–pk inhomogeneity of 520 ppm on the 45 cm DSV, the reconstructed inhomogeneity on a 40 cm by 40 cm FOV at $Z = 0$ is shown Figure 1.6(a). The shimming target is set at 5 ppm pk–pk on 40 DSV and harmonics are allowed to have 0.5 ppm deviation from their desired values.

In image simulations, a 64×64 subject is created in a 40 DSV volume as shown in Figure 1.6(b). The proton density (PD) distribution of the subject is shown in Figure 1.6(b). A single shot EPI sequence used in this simulation is shown in Figure 1.6(c) with maximum gradient strength of 33 mT m^{-1} and 64 kHz receiver bandwidth. To this end, the phenomenological Bloch equation is solved against the as-shimmed B_0 inhomogeneity.[33] No phase correction is applied during image reconstruction.

Simulation results are illustrated in Figure 1.7. As far as shimming is concerned, at 40 DSV, the p-method results in a pk–pk inhomogeneity 4.32 ppm while the h-method produces 4.05 ppm. However, h-method employs about 1.5 times of the shim mass that needed for p-method. Theoretical shimmed B_0 inhomogeneity is reconstructed on the 40 cm by 40 cm FOV at $Z = 0$ plane for both h-method and p-methods which are shown in Figure 1.7(b) and (d) respectively. Inside the FOV, the inhomogeneity of p-method and h-method are -3.41 μT ± 8.34 μT and -0.20 μT ± 2.25 μT, respectively which indicates h-method produced better homogeneity. Mean and standard deviations in the region of interest (ROI) of Figure 1.7(b) are 0.07 and 0.44 Hz respectively; and −0.19 and 0.30 Hz respectively in Figure 1.7(c). ROI's are drawn at maximum ghosting regions in Figure 1.7(c) and (e) and the calculated maximum ghosting levels are 18.4% and 7.4%.

The results indicate that h-method generates better mean field homogeneity compared to the p-method in the imaging region. However, the p-method offers better symmetry and smaller standard deviation in the imaging volume (32 DSV). As a result, maximum ghosting in the h-method is higher than the p-method. This phenomenon can be explained as follows. The p-method allows some higher order harmonics to stay with relatively large magnitudes but strictly limits low order harmonics. The h-method, on the other hand, has good control on overall harmonics, especially high order harmonics but can leave some room for low order harmonics. So, for a smaller FOV, the higher order harmonics decay very fast, where the p-method show advantages over the h-method.

1.2 ENVIRONMENTAL LOW-FREQUENCY FIELD AND ITS EFFECTS

MR scanners are a strong source of electromagnetic signals; at the same time, they are sensitive to electromagnetic interferences (EMI) from the environment in which they operate. Without proper mitigations, these EMI's can cause significant IQ degradation. For instance, external RF signals (10^6 Hz and above) could directly interact with the RF field of the transmission/receiving chain during image acquisition and corrupt images. The well-established mitigation is to install a Faraday cage to act as an RF shield around the MR room, in this way, the two-way interference is eliminated. There are other environmental sources of EMI's at much lower frequency, could cause artifacts and IQ issues. For example, disturbances can be caused by large objects with significant ferrous or conductive materials or electrical motors; elevators close to scan room, nearby traffic, trams, and subways.[34] These scenarios can be considered as magnetic moments moving in the vicinity of MR scanners, which create temporary and random disturbances to magnetic fields inside FOV. Two distinct features separate these EMI signals from others: (i) these signals have small magnetic field magnitudes (mGauss or less); (ii) their frequency range is extremely low (10^0–10^2 Hz) and somewhat random in nature. Because of the later fact, these low-frequency EMI's could induce phase errors and result in artifacts in the reconstructed images such as ringing, ghosting, signal losses, etc.[35–40] In addition, advanced imaging schemes such as fast pulse sequences,[41,42] phase array coils,[43] and parallel imaging techniques[44–47] have more stringent requirements on stability and homogeneity of the B_0 field to produce high-quality images. Therefore, they are more sensitive to low-frequency EMI signals. This presents

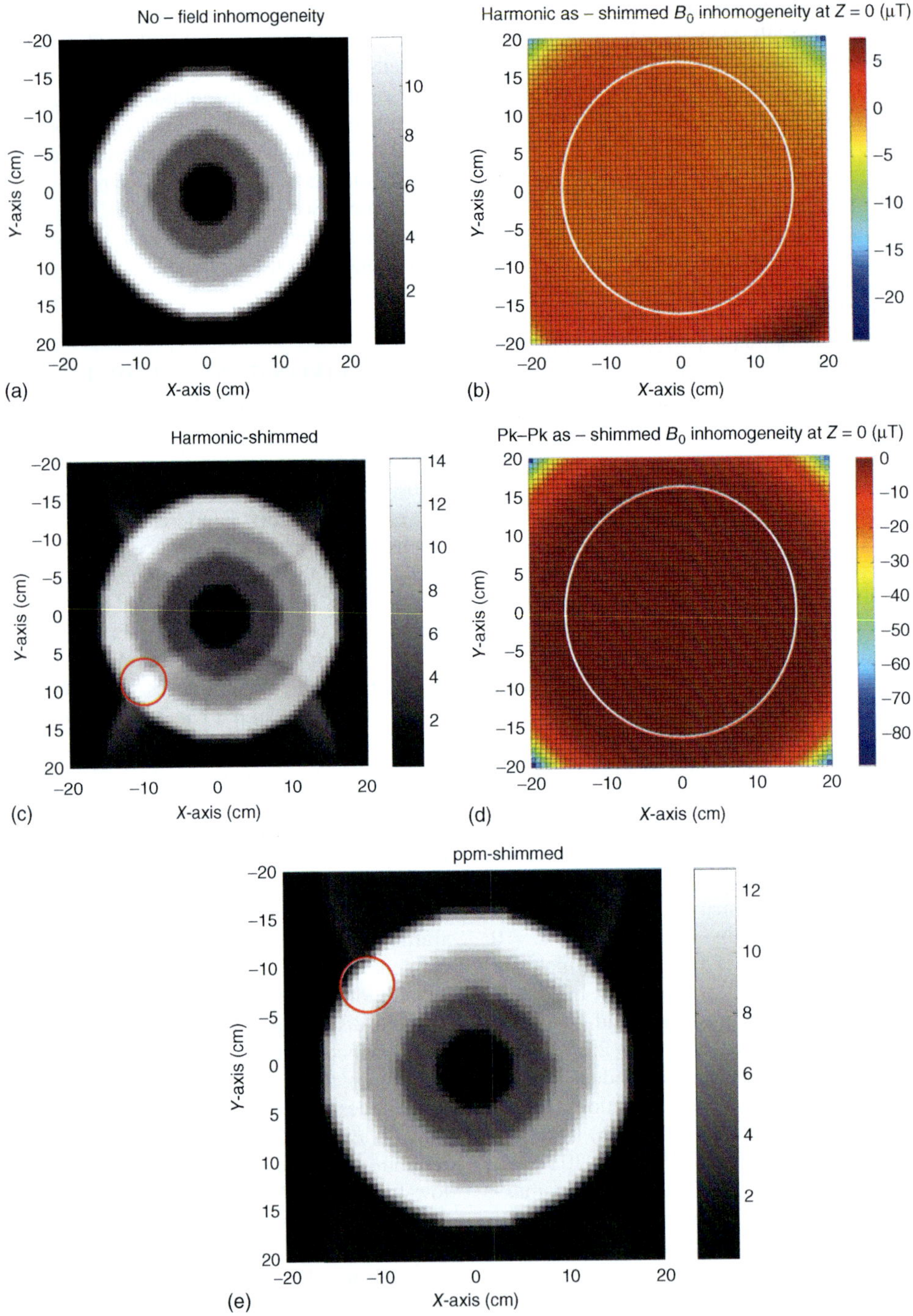

Figure 1.7. Simulation results: (a) EPI image with zero inhomogeneity; (b) harmonic shimmed B_0 inhomogeneity; (c) EPI image with harmonic shimmed B_0 inhomogeneity; (d) pk-pk shimmed B_0 inhomogeneity; (e) EPI image with pk-pk shimmed B_0 inhomogeneity. ROIs are drawn at maximum ghost levels in (b) and (e).

considerable challenges to hardware component design, and hardware solutions to minimize the impact of these low-frequency EMI signals are expensive and have low ROI (return on investment). Nevertheless, the artifacts may be reduced or eliminated by carefully optimized pulse sequences and novel post-processing correction algorithms. This would need prior knowledge and characterization of the low-frequency signals and determination of critical parameters to remove the artifacts. Therefore, it is critical to be able to quantify how the low-frequency EMI signals affect IQ.

In this study, the fast spin echo (FSE) sequence is used to quantitatively investigate the impact to quality of received echo signals caused by different interference *or similar*.... The phase errors are computed by numerically solving the phenomenological Bloch equation for different receiver bandwidths, with low-frequency field signals having different frequencies. To this end, the Bloch equation can be written as follows for a time-dependent magnetic field in a rotating framework[48]:

$$\frac{d\mathbf{M}}{dt} = \gamma \cdot (\mathbf{M} \times \mathbf{B}) - \begin{pmatrix} \frac{M_x}{T_2} \\ \frac{M_y}{T_2} \\ \frac{(M_z - M_0)}{T_1} \end{pmatrix} \quad (1.29)$$

the magnetic flux density $\overline{B}$ represents the total magnetic field in Z direction in FOV and has the following components:

$$\mathbf{B}(\mathbf{r}, t) = \mathbf{B}_0 + \Delta\mathbf{B}(\mathbf{r}) + (\mathbf{G}(t) \cdot \mathbf{r})\vec{e}_z + \mathbf{B}_1(t) \quad (1.30)$$

where $\overline{B}_0$ is the constant term of the static B_0 field, $\Delta\overline{B}$ represents the spatial-dependent inhomogeneity of B_0 field, $\overline{G}(t)$ is the applied gradients, $\overline{r} = (x, y, z)^T$ is the position vector, and $\overline{B}_1(t)$ is the magnetic flux density of the RF field. In the time domain, equation (1.29) can be solved with an incremental time-step Δt, for which magnetization vector $\overline{M}(\overline{r}, t)$ and next step $\overline{M}(\overline{r}, t + \Delta t)$ are linked by:

$$\mathbf{M}(\mathbf{r}, t + \Delta t) = R_{\text{grad}} \cdot R_{\text{inh}} \cdot R_{\text{relax}} \cdot R_{\text{RF}} \cdot \mathbf{M}(\mathbf{r}, t) + M_0(\mathbf{r})\left(1 - e^{-\frac{t}{T_1(\mathbf{r})}}\right)\vec{e}_z \quad (1.31)$$

In Formula (1.31), matrices R_{grad}, R_{inh}, R_{relax}, and R_{RF} represent the effect of the applied gradients, main-field inhomogeneity, relaxation, and rotating properties of the RF pulse, respectively. The approach to solve equations (1.29)–(1.31) is thoroughly covered in the paper by Brenner *et al.*[48]

To investigate the impact of low-frequency field signals, the main-field inhomogeneity $\Delta\overline{B}(\overline{r})$ is made to be time-dependent $\Delta\overline{B}(\overline{r}, t)$. In our simulation, $\Delta\overline{B}(\overline{r}, t)$ is modeled as a sinusoidal signal with a 1 Hz amplitude and the frequency is in the range (10^0–10^2 Hz):

$$\Delta\overline{B}(\overline{r}, t) = B_{\text{EMI}} \sin(\omega_{\text{EMI}} t) \quad (1.32)$$

and its rotation matrix R_{inh} can be expressed as:

$$R_{\text{inh}} = \begin{pmatrix} \cos\varphi_{\text{inh}} & \sin\varphi_{\text{inh}} & 0 \\ -\sin\varphi_{\text{inh}} & \cos\varphi_{\text{inh}} & 0 \\ 0 & 0 & 1 \end{pmatrix} \quad (1.33)$$

where φ_{inh} is given by:

$$\varphi_{\text{inh}} = \gamma \cdot \Delta B(\mathbf{r}, t) \cdot \Delta t. \quad (1.34)$$

In the simulation, the subject is modeled as a single spin with steady state magnetization $M_0 = 10$ (arbitrary unit along Z-axis) located at (10 cm, 0 cm, 0 cm). To ignore relaxation effects, T_1 and T_2 are set at 500-second and 1000-second, respectively. Under this condition, the steady-state magnetization M_0 is proportional to proton density, so the reconstructed signals are noted as PD signals. The spin is set to go through two different FSE pulse sequences with echo train length (ETL) equal to 8 as shown in Figure 1.8. In Sequence-1, time step $\Delta t = 32$ μs which is corresponding to ~16 kHz bandwidth; in Sequence-2, $\Delta t = 8$ μs which is corresponding to ~62 kHz bandwidth.

In Sequence-1, the 90-degree flip angle pulse is applied with 15.3 μT amplitude and 180-degree flip angle pulse (with 90-degree phase) is applied with 30.6 μT amplitude for 384 μs duration. In sequence-2, the 90-degree flip angle pulse is applied with *61.2* μT amplitude and 180-degrees flip angle pulse (with 90-degree phase) is applied with 122.4 μT amplitude for 96 μs duration. For Sequences 1 and 2, the half of the echo times (*TE*) are set to 4096 μs and 1024 μs respectively. As far as gradient pulses are concerned, the x-gradient amplitudes are set to 1.84 mT m^{-1} with 16384 μs readout duration and 7.34 mT m^{-1} with 4096 μs readout duration for Sequences 1 and 2, respectively.

Solving equations (1.30)–(1.34) with modeling set up discussed above, the magnetization $\overline{M}$ can be obtained for every time step. The transverse magnetization M_{xy} signals are shown in Figure 1.8 (real and imaginary parts). The phase errors (PEs) in the received signal is defined as:

$$\text{PEs} = \text{rms}[\text{Phase}(M_{xy}) - \text{Phase}(M_{xy0})] \quad (1.35)$$

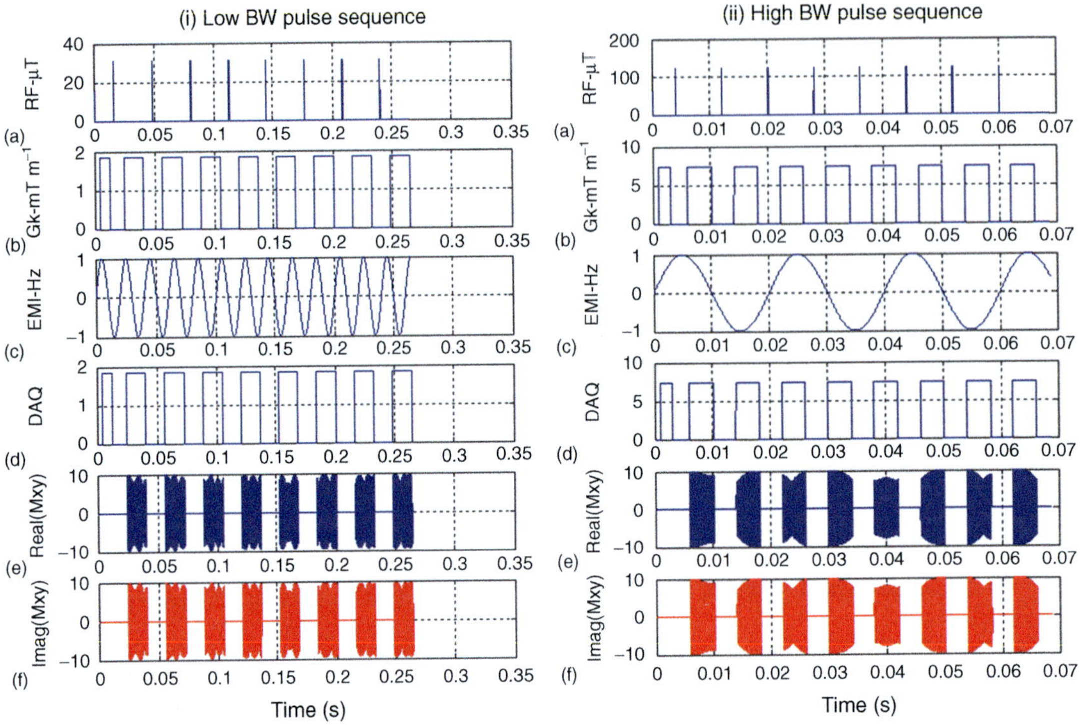

Figure 1.8. Pulse sequences definition: Low (16 kHz) and high (62 kHz) bandwidth pulse sequences are shown in (i) and (ii), respectively. Both sequences are designed to acquire signals from a spin @ $x = 10$ cm in a 20-cm FOV. RF transmit pulse amplitude is shown in (a); x-Gradient amplitude in (b); AC EMI signals in (c); data acquisition windows in (d); real and imaginary simulated signals in (e) and (f), respectively

where M_{xy0} is the reconstructed signal without low-frequency EMI signals.

PEs as a function of frequency and bandwidths for different echo signals are shown in Figure 1.9. It is clear for all eight echoes: (i) PEs are more pronounced at lower frequencies (<100 Hz) rather than higher frequencies (>200 Hz), this manifests the fact that with similar field strength, the low-frequency EMI's can be more detrimental to IQ than higher frequency EMI's; (ii) PEs are heavily dependent on the receiving bandwidth, higher BW produces fewer errors than lower BW, especially for the EMI signals under 100 Hz.

To illustrate the relationship between PEs and time, Figure 1.10 shows PEs vs echo time (proportional to echo number) at various EMI signal frequencies. At very low frequency (1 Hz, see Figure 1.10a), the PEs monotonically increase with echo numbers and Sequence-2 exhibits much lesser PEs than Sequence-1. However, this characteristic gradually changes when the frequency increases. At high frequency (1000 Hz, see Figure 1.10d), the PEs keep almost constant over different echo numbers and Sequence-1 shows lesser phase error than Sequence-2, although both are very small in magnitudes. In the intermediate frequencies (100–200 Hz, see Figure 1.10b and c), the relationship between phase errors and echo numbers are nonlinear and bandwidth of the sequence does not play a significant role in terms of the magnitude of phase errors. In addition, it is evident from Figure 1.10(a) to (d), as EMI frequency increases, the magnitude of phase errors decays significantly.

To understand why phase errors introduced by an EMI signal are more pronounced at lower frequencies, let us have a closer look at how PEs evolve with time. Phase errors of Sequence-1 (bandwidth ~16 kHz) vs time for different f_{EMI} are shown in Figure 1.11. When the frequency is very low (1 Hz), phase error is by-and-large linearly correlated with time, so it can increase to high magnitude during signal acquisition.

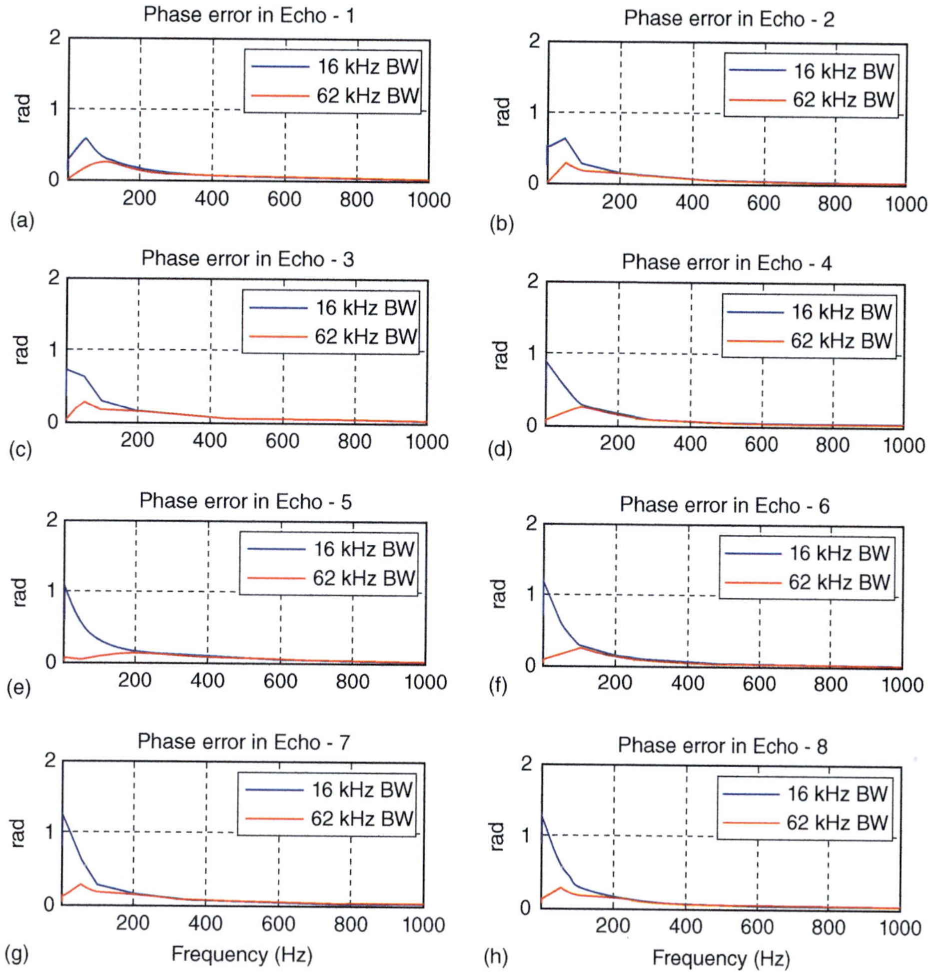

Figure 1.9. Frequency vs Phase error in echo signals: Phase errors in eight different echo signals are shown in (a)–(h) for two different bandwidths

This characteristic becomes oscillatory at higher frequency (>200 Hz), the self-cancelation effect limits the magnitudes of the resultant phase errors, which are irrelevant with respect to time. Indeed, at 1 Hz, the period (1 s) of the EMI signal is significantly longer than the read-out duration (*16.384* ms) of the data acquisition window, while at 1200 Hz, the period (0.83 ms) is very short in comparison to the read-out duration.

Once phase errors are introduced in received echoes, several artifacts can be produced such as ringing, ghosting, signal loss, etc. To demonstrate these artifacts, echo signals are first generated with influence from low-frequency EMI signal at the location (10 cm, 0 cm, 0 cm) with amplitude $B_{\mathrm{EMI}} = 1$ Hz and frequency $f_{\mathrm{EMI}} = 10$ Hz, inverse Fourier transform is then applied to these echo signals to reconstruct the 1D signal and the resultant signals for Sequence-1 (low BW) and Sequence-2 (high BW) are shown in Figure 1.12.

In the ideal situation when there is no EMI signal, all eight reconstructed 1D signals should have the same amplitude of 10 at location $x = 10$ cm. However, when the low-frequency EMI signals are present, with low bandwidth the received echoes have inconsistent amplitudes and the peaks move away from $x = 10$ cm as

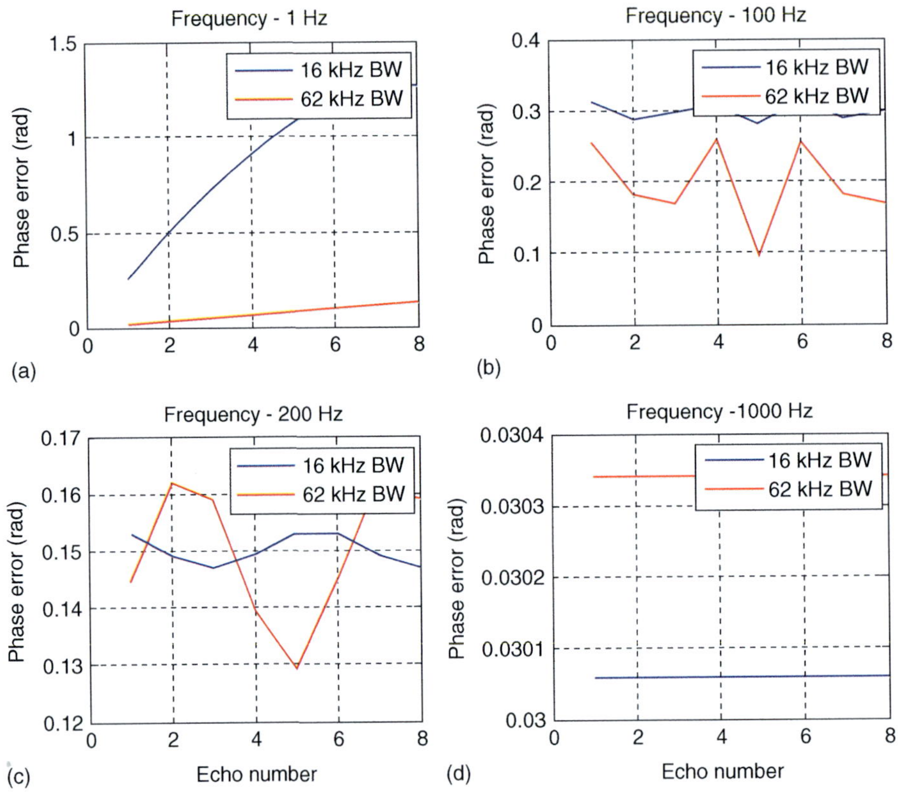

Figure 1.10. Phase error vs echo number: Phase errors for 1, 100, 200 and 1000 Hz EMI frequencies are shown in (a)–(d)

seen in Figure 1.12(a), resulting in positional inaccuracies. With higher bandwidth, the reconstructed 1D signal amplitudes and locations are more consistent (see Figure 1.12b). Comparing Figure 1.12(a) and (b), higher bandwidth demonstrates an advantage to reduce the IQ impact of EMI signals. The slight positional shift in Figure 1.12(b) can be interpreted as linear phase offset in the received k-space signals due to low-frequency EMI signals. Higher bandwidth clearly shows an advantage to reduce the IQ impact of EMI signals.

Low-frequency EMI signals induced artifacts depends on pulse sequence designs. Some PSDs (gradient echo, conventional spin echo, etc.) contain only one echo signal in one repetition time (TR) and some other PSDs (FSE, EPI, etc.) contain multiple echo signals. Multiple echo signals are often used to reduce scan time by filling multiple lines in k-space along the phase encoding direction.[42–47] When only one echo is acquired in one TR, the reconstructed image could have shifted pixels (ringing) in the frequency readout direction. If multiple echoes are acquired to fill in multiple k-space lines, phase errors in the received signals could result in both ringing (in frequency encoding direction) and ghosting (in the phase encoding direction) effects.

Some methods to minimize phase distortions due to B_0 fluctuations and corresponding artifacts have been previously proposed.[41,49–51] In one study, an interleaved navigator echo from an offset location was sampled immediately after the image echo is acquired, and the phase of the navigator signal was used as a reference to correct the imaging data.[49] In another study, view-to-view phase shifts due to B_0 instability are corrected by applying a phase correction to the low-spatial-frequency views.[50] Both these techniques estimate B_0 fluctuation from the acquired NMR data to correct the phase distortions. In contrast to software-based correction methods, a magnetic active compensation system has been proposed.[51] In this

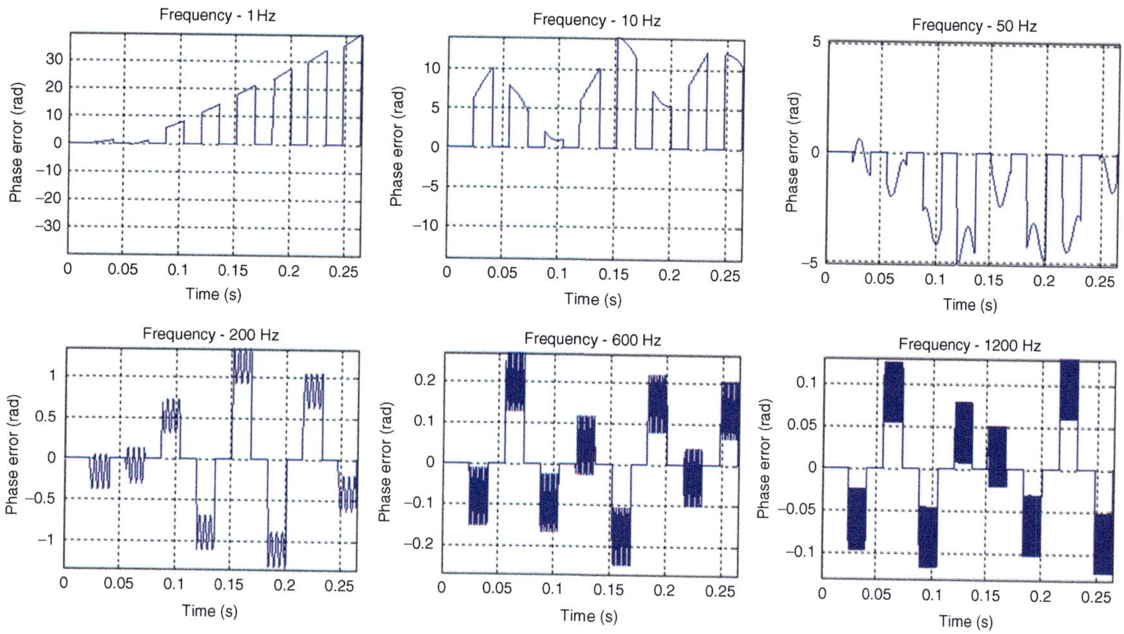

Figure 1.11. Phase error for different EMI frequencies: When the frequency is increased, the phase error has changed from linear (1 Hz) to oscillatory (1200 Hz)

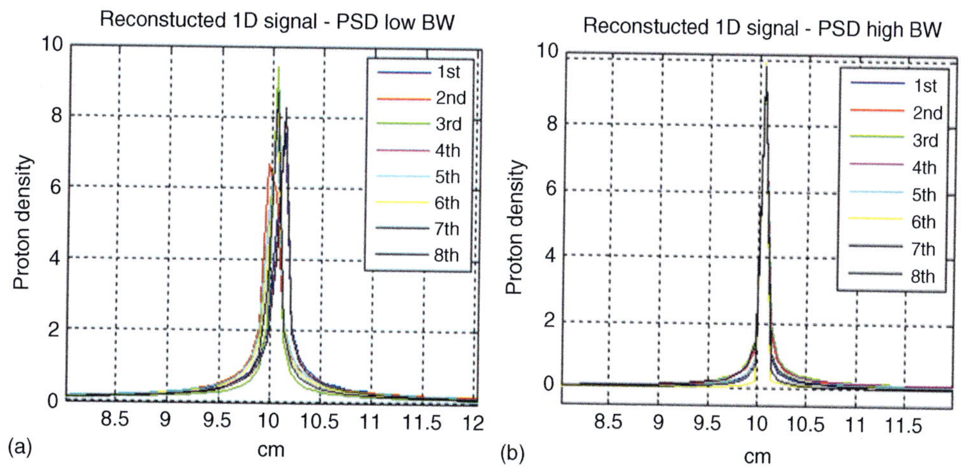

Figure 1.12. Reconstructed 1D signal: Low and high BW inverse Fourier transformed signals are shown in (a) and (b) respectively

active method, B_0 compensation coils can be strategically placed inside the system to offset the field disturbances from external sources. All these techniques are important to improve IQ for all systems regardless of field strength or if active shielding coils are utilized.

Either to correct the phase distortions by innovative post processing techniques or by designing compensation hardware, knowledge about the sensitivity of the phase errors to low- and high-frequency EMI is useful. The detailed simulation results presented here could be useful to other researchers in developing new methods to improve IQ.

RELATED ARTICLES IN EMAGRES

Shimming of Superconducting Magnets

Shimming for High-Resolution NMR Spectroscopy

Safety Considerations in MRI

Metals in the Environment

REFERENCES

1. A. Nowogrodzki, *Nature*, 2018, **563**, 24.
2. E. Kanal, F. G. Shellock, and L. Talagala, *Radiology*, 1990, **176**, 593.
3. F. G. Shellock and J. V. Crues, *Radiology*, 2004, **232**, 635.
4. J. Zhuo and R. P. Gullapalli, *Radiographics*, 2006, **26**, 275.
5. J. F. Schenck, *J. Magn. Reson. Imaging*, 2000, **12**, 2.
6. P. Lövsund, P. Å. Öberg, S. E. G. Nilsson, and T. Reuter, *Med. Biol. Eng. Comput.*, 1980, **18**, 326.
7. M. I. Weintraub, A. Khoury, and S. P. Cole, *J. Neuroimaging.*, 2007, **17**, 241.
8. A. Kangarlu *et al.*, *Magn. Reson. Imaging.*, 1999, **17**, 1407.
9. D. W. Chakeres, R. Bornstein, and A. Kangarlu, *J. Magn. Reson. Imaging.*, 2003, **18**, 342.
10. B. K. Ward, D. C. Roberts, C. C. Della Santina, J. P. Carey, and D. S. Zee, *Ann. N. Y. Acad. Sci.*, 2015, **1343**, 69.
11. U.S. Department of Health and Human Services, Food and Drug Administration, Center for Devices and Radiological Health, Guidance for Industry and FDA Staff. Criteria for Significant Risk Investigations of Magnetic Resonance Diagnostic Devices, Jun 20, 2014
12. P. Erhard, W. Chen, J.-H. Lee, and K. Ugurbil, in 'Proceedings of the 3rd Annual Meeting of ISMRM': Nice, France, 1995.
13. M. Frank, T. Hettinger, M. Herness, and C. Pfaffman, in 'Clinical Measurement of Taste and Smell', eds H. Meiselman and R. Rivlin, Macmillan: New York, 1986, p 187.
14. Z. Bujas, in 'Handbook of Sensory Physiology', ed L. M. Beidler, Springer: Berlin, 1971, Vol. **4**, p 180.
15. I. D. Cavin, P. M. Glover, R. W. Bowtell, and P. A. Gowland, *J. Magn. Reson. Imaging*, 2007 Nov, **26**, 1357.
16. D. W. Chakeres, A. Kanarlu, H. Boudoulas, and D. C. Young, *J. Magn. Reson. Imaging*, 2003, **18**, 346.
17. M. Jekic, Y. Ding, R. Dzwonczyk, *et al.*, *Magn. Reson. Med.*, 2010, **64**, 1586.
18. J. W. Krug and G. Rose, *Comput. Cardiol. IEEE.*, 2011, 769.
19. Niendorf, Thoralf and Lukas Winter, in 'Electrocardiogram in an MRI Environment: Clinical Needs, Practical Considerations, Safety Implications, Technical Solutions and Future Directions.' (2014).
20. G. Carditis, *N. Engl. J. Med.*, 1982, **307**, 448.
21. C. Landrigan, *N. Engl. J. Med.*, 2001, **345**, 1000.
22. Family gets $2.9M in 6-year-old boy's MRI death, February 5, 2010. https://nypost.com/2010/02/05/family-gets-2-9m-in-6-year-old-boys-mri-death/
23. Y. Lvovsky and P. Jarvis, *IEEE Trans. Appil. Supercond.*, 2005, **15**, 1317.
24. Y. Lvovsky, E. W. Stautner, and T. Zhang, *Supercond. Sci. Technol.*, 2013, **26**, 093001.
25. Gebhardt M.L. and McGregor R.J., Emergency run-down unit for superconducting magnets, U.S. Pat. Specification US 20080169889 A1.
26. J. D. Jackson, Classical Electrodynamics, 3rd edn, John Wiley Sons: New York, 1999.
27. L. D. Landau and E. M. Lifshitz, Electrodynamics of Continuous Media, Addison-Wesley: Massachusetts, Reading, 1960.
28. Vector Fields, Cobham Technical Services, Network House, Langford Locks Kidlington, Oxfordshire, OX5 1LH, UK.
29. T. J. Havens, T. Duby, and J. Huang, *Proc. Intl. Soc. Mag. Reson. Med.*, 2002, **10**, 29501.
30. H. Zeng *et al.*, *MRM*, 2002, **48**, 137.
31. B. Dorri *et al.*, *IEEE Trans. Appl. Supercond.*, 1993, **3**, 254.
32. MATLAB Release 2016, The MathWorks, Inc., Natick, MA.
33. A. R. Brenner *et al.*, *MAGMA*, 1997, **5**, 129.

34. D. Le Bihan, C. Poupon, A. Amadon, *et al.*, *J. Magn. Reson.*, 2006, **24**, 478.

35. S. Ardekani and U. Sinha, *Magn. Reson. Med.*, 2005, **54**, 1163.

36. X. Wan, D. L. Parker, J. N. Lee, H. R. Buswell, and G. T. Gullberg, *Magn. Reson. Med.*, 1995, **34**, 632.

37. P. Jezzard, A. S. Barnett, and C. Pierpaoli, *Magn. Reson. Med.*, 1998, **39**, 801.

38. N. G. Papadakis, K. M. Martin, J. D. Pickard, L. D. Hall, T. A. Carpenter, and C. L.-H. Huang, *Magn. Reson. Med.*, 2000, **44**, 616.

39. F. Calamante, D. A. Porter, D. G. Gadian, and A. Connelly, *Magn. Reson. Med.*, 1999, **41**, 95.

40. L. Jiang and T. J. Havens, *IEEE Trans. Appl. Supercond.*, 2012, **22**, 4400704.

41. E. Durand, P.-F. van de Moortele, M. Pachot-Clouard, and D. Le Bihan, *Magn. Reson. Med.*, 2001, **46**, 198.

42. P. Mansfield, *J. Phys. C: Solid State Phys.*, 1977, **10**, L55. DOI: 10.1088/0022-3719/10/3/004.

43. J. Hennig, A. Nauerth, and H. Friedburg, *Magn. Reson. Med.*, 1986, **3**, 823.

44. P. B. Roemer, W. A. Edelstein, C. E. Hayes, S. P. Souza, and O. M. Mueller, *Magn. Reson. Med.*, 1990, **16**, 192.

45. D. K. Sodickson and W. J. Manning, *Magn. Reson. Med.*, 1997, **38**, 591.

46. K. P. Pruessmann, M. Weiger, M. B. Scheidegger, *et al.*, *Magn Reson Med*, 1999, **42**, 952.

47. M. A. Griswold, P. M. Jakob, R. M. Heidemann, *et al.*, *Magn Reson Med*, 2002, **47**, 1202.

48. A. R. Brenner, J. Kürsch, and T. G. Noll, *Magnetic Reson. Mater. Phys., Biol. Med.*, 1997, **5**, 129.

49. J. Li, Y. Wang, Y. Jiang, H. Xie, and G. Li, *Magn Reson Imaging*, 2009, **27**, 988.

50. T. K. Foo and C. E. Hayes, *J Magn Reson Imaging*, 1993, **3**, 676.

51. K. Kazimierczuk and W. Kozminski, *J Magn Reson*, 2005, **174**, 287.

Chapter 2

Magnetic-field-induced Vertigo in the MR Environment

Paul Glover

University of Nottingham, Nottingham, UK

2.1 INTRODUCTION

Since the start of the twenty-first century, there has been a growing number of magnetic resonance imaging (MRI) facilities having scanners operating above 3 T. There are around 50 seven tesla systems worldwide, together with an increasing number of scanners operating at 9.4 T or above, mainly within research focused environments. Elsewhere in the related articles, the effects of time-varying magnetic fields used for MRI have been discussed; being a function of induced currents in the case of magneto-phosphenes, peripheral nerve stimulation (PNS), and radio frequency (RF) heating (depending on the specific absorption rate (SAR)). The physics and biology of these interactions are well known, if not always easy to predict due to the varying geometry of the human body in the population, position in the scanner, etc.

Static fields (including natural movements in their presence) present a much larger unknown in terms of interactions with the human body. Much of the literature historically discussing magnetic field safety has concentrated on power-line or micro-tesla levels of magnetic field. It is no surprise that there are very few biological effects due to magnetic fields have been reliably observed in vitro, and none in vivo (as yet). There is evidence for some avian sensitivity to earth's field levels due to polarization effects in the retina cryptochromes.[1] Magnetite particles embedded in cellular organs have all been cited as potential 'sensors' of magnetic fields in birds, insects, or fish. There do not appear to be any (or even remnants of any) such mechanism in higher mammals.

However, users of high-field systems do report feeling slightly dizzy or disorientated. Patients do have to steady themselves after getting out of such a scanner. While not a true clinical definition of 'vertigo,' it is useful to describe these nonveridical sensations with such a term. In its mild form, and probably the most common, it is just a sensation that something is 'not quite right.' Scanner technicians working in and around the bore of high-field scanners do have to take rest-breaks if they feel giddy. It is noted that experienced operators may adjust or learn so the effects are minimized. Whether that is by avoiding particular

Safety and Biological Effects in MRI.
Edited by Devashish Shrivastava and J. Thomas Vaughan

ISBN: 978-1-118-82130-5
Also published in eMagRes (online edition)
DOI: 10.1002/9780470034590.emrstm1607

movements or activities, or if some neural level of processing is involved is not known. This would be akin to aircrew or sailors adjusting to the motions of their craft.

It was initially thought that movements in the magnetic field, and therefore the small electrical currents induced in the head or the fluids of the semi-circular canals, were the cause of magnetic-field-induced vertigo (MFIV). The term for magnetic field fluid interactions is magnetohydrodynamics (MHD). The obvious conclusion to make is that a conductor moving in a magnetic field experiences a force opposing that motion (Lenz's law). A similar effect is that of a Lorentz force acting on the ionic currents flowing in the endolymph of the vestibular system. Another potential mechanism is susceptibility related forces in the vestibular maculae. In this chapter, the physical basis for the biological effects is described together with a brief description of the inner ear. The evidence for each possible interaction mechanism is discussed in the light of experimental evidence. As the user base of 7-T installations has increased, it is now possible to find literature reporting subjective experiences. These data are usually collected from the subjects undergoing the study itself.

2.2 HUMAN INNER EAR PHYSIOLOGY

It is useful to review the basics of the vestibular system biology for those readers unfamiliar with the physiology and function. The reader is encouraged to consult a suitable physiology textbook for further details.[2] The inner ear comprises the cochlea (responsible for hearing), three semi-circular canals each incorporating an ampulla which houses the cupula and hair cells (responsible for the three orthogonal rotational velocity components), and saccules containing the maculae (which are responsible for gravitational orientation and linear accelerations). The maculae are L-shaped plates having embedded otoliths (calcium carbonate crystals) to give a relatively high mass. The shapes, mass, and spring constants of the two maculae allow all three linear acceleration directions to be determined from the plate deflections giving a person orientation information. Hair cells have their stereocilia (hair cell extensions) embedded in the gel of the maculae. Deflection of the stereocilia causes the potassium channels to either open or close, thus increasing or decreasing the firing rate of the hair cell afferent axons.

Likewise, the positional displacement of the cupulae are sensed by hair cells. In both sensory mechanisms, the hair cells are biased into a linear region of operation and are able to adjust their firing rate according to both positive (higher rate) and negative (lower) displacement. A high potassium ion-flux maintains this bias (called the dark current) and is supplied by stria cells on the walls of the ampullae and saccule. These specialized cells can be thought of as a potential source and current sink.

The inertia of the fluid in the canals under angular acceleration creates a pressure on the cupula causing it to deflect slightly which is then sensed by the hair cells. The normal cupula forms a sealed flap across the ampulla. The geometry of the canal, the viscosity of the endolymph, and the spring constant of the cupula result in a system which responds as an integrator of the inertial acceleration, therefore, acting as a sensor of angular velocity (for frequency ranges encompassing normal movements of the head).[3,4] Linear and angular movement sensors have a direct coupling to ocular response in mammals.

2.3 THE PHYSICS OF MAGNETIC FIELD INTERACTIONS

Likewise, with the biology, it is useful to collect together here the basic physical principles which govern magnetic field interactions with biological matter. Again for expansion of any of these topics a suitable textbook on electromagnetism can be consulted.[5]

2.3.1 Magnetic Susceptibility

Biological materials have a magnetic susceptibility χ, which is small and can be either positive (paramagnetic) or, more usually for organic compounds, negative (diamagnetic). Iron in the form of hemoglobin or ferritin is present in the body, but there is no indication that these have any transduction effects. For most materials, magnetic susceptibility is measured in parts-per-million and is sometimes either a nuisance or of interest to the MRI community (quantitative susceptibility mapping might be an example of the latter). Placed in a strong inhomogeneous magnetic field, a diamagnetic material will be subject to a force directed

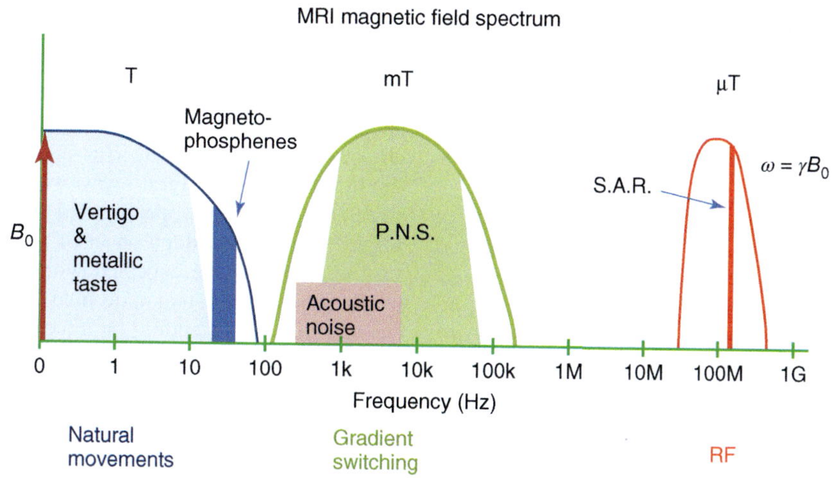

Figure 2.1. Figurative graphic depicting the range of frequencies and magnetic field amplitudes present in an MRI scanner. In this chapter, it is the frequency range of the natural movements which are of interest

toward a lower field region. The force, **F**, on an object having a difference in susceptibility from the surrounding medium $\Delta\chi$ is $\mathbf{F} = \Delta\chi\tau\,\nabla\,(B^2)/2\mu_0$, where τ is the object volume, $\mu_0 = 4\pi\,10^{-7}\,\mathrm{N\,A^{-2}}$ is the permeability of free space and B is the magnitude of the magnetic field. Note that the term $\nabla(B^2)/2$ is equal in magnitude to the product of the magnitudes of the magnetic field (B) and the spatial magnetic field gradient (G) at that point. For example, a field-gradient ($B{\cdot}G$) product of $1470\,\mathrm{T^2\,m^{-1}}$ would produce a force sufficient to balance the force due to gravity and potentially 'levitate' water or biological tissue in air.[6]

2.3.2 Electric Fields Induced by Movement in a Magnetic Field

In an isotropic conductive medium, the induced current density, **J**, is given by the electric field, **E**, multiplied by the conductivity, σ. The general expression for the induced electric field may be given by, $E = -\nabla V - \partial\mathbf{A}/\partial t - \mathbf{v}\times\mathbf{B}$, where V is a scalar potential and **A** is a vector potential such that the magnetic field, **B**, is defined as $\mathbf{B} = \nabla\times\mathbf{A}$. For an isolated, rigid body moving at velocity, **v**, in a static magnetic field, the final term is nonzero. Translational movements in an in-homogeneous, or rotations in a uniform, magnetic field can equally give rise to an induced electric field.[7] In low conductivity biological tissues, where σ is of order unity, the main magnetic field is not perturbed by the additional magnetic field caused by the current density itself. Note that it is the middle term (i.e., time-varying magnetic fields) that gives rise to the driving term which results in PNS and SAR. Figure 2.1 shows the spectrum of magnetic field effects in MRI. In this chapter, it is the low-frequency effects in the 0–20 Hz range which are significant – either due to the static field itself or due to natural movements. So here, the time varying vector potential term $\partial\mathbf{A}/\partial t$ is zero and $\mathbf{v}\times\mathbf{B}$ is finite.

2.3.3 Magnetohydrodynamics

MHD usually relates to a conductive fluid flow and the modification of that flow by the presence of a magnetic field. If the current induced by movement of a conductive medium in a magnetic field is large enough, then that current itself generates a magnetic field which will oppose the main magnetic field. The net force is given by the volume integral of the Lorentz force $\mathbf{F} = \int(\mathbf{J}\times\mathbf{B})\mathrm{d}\tau$. For fluids, this force can be added into the Navier–Stokes' flow equation. Hence a net increase in pressure can be calculated for a given flow velocity and magnetic field. In addition, if there is an external applied net potential, V, driving a current density (either electrons and/or ions), **J**, through the medium, then there will be a force generated which is perpendicular to both **J** and **B**.

2.4 MAGNETIC-FIELD-INDUCED VERTIGO

In a series of informative animal experiments, rodents show circular swimming behavior and taste aversion after exposure to high magnetic fields.[8,9] After destruction in vivo of the labyrinth organs, the animals appear to be are oblivious to the field exposure. The vertigo effect has thus been confirmed as an action of the magnetic field on the primary transducer – rather than directly on the central nervous system (CNS)[10] or mediated through another sense organ such as the eyes or olfactory system as in birds.

In the light of the physics of magnetic field interactions, it is now possible to discuss four likely candidates for the sensation of MFIV which have their origins in the vestibular system: forces due to the susceptibility of vestibular structures[11]; current flow due to a net rate of change of magnetic flux[11]; MHD due to head movement[11,12]; and fluid pressure due to Lorentz forces.[13]

2.4.1 Susceptibility-induced Forces

The force due to differences in magnetic susceptibility (and density) between the vestibular endolymph and the cupulae or maculae structures could effectively generate a mechanical displacement which would be sensed by the brain as an effective motion. The otoliths which make up the utricle and saccule maculae have a susceptibility and density close to that of the aragonite form of calcium carbonate. For these structures, a magnetic field × gradient product of $46\,T^2\ m^{-1}$ would effectively produce a perceived acceleration of $0.1\,m\,s^{-2}$.[11] This mechanism would imply that a subject could sense (but not necessarily perceive) an effective acceleration in areas where such a field-gradient product exists – even if the subject is not moving at all. In the case of a 7 T magnet, this field-gradient product is similar to the maximum value on-axis just inside the bore, having maximal values up against the bore edge near to the magnet coil windings. The polarity of the effect would, in general, indicate that the perception of acceleration would be toward regions of higher field. In addition, the polarity of the field is not relevant to the polarity of the effect – as the forces are dependent on the spatial derivative of the square of the magnetic field magnitude. For the cupulae, the perceived rotational acceleration in a similar magnetic field gradient may be assumed to be negligible because the gel-like structure of the cupula has a similar susceptibility and density to that of the surrounding fluid. The susceptibility mechanism is a strong candidate as there are a small number of subjects who claim to perceive 'falling' when standing adjacent to a 7 T magnet. This can be measured by monitoring their postural sway while they fix their gaze on a spot while opening and closing their eyes. Subjects report a sudden onset of the effect near the magnet as would be expected with an effect related to the square of the magnetic field.[11] The effects can be 'amplified' by standing on a foam or spongy base as this reduces the effectiveness of the balance proprioception mechanisms (in feet, ankles, and knees). Usually, such a task of balancing on such a base is easy for subjects with normal vestibular function, but in the magnetic field, it is very much harder. As such this effect on the vestibular system is at such a low frequency, it precludes any temporal derivative term as is required with induced currents as mediator.

2.4.2 Magneto-hydrodynamic Effect (MHD)

The net pressure due to velocity-generated magneto-hydrodynamic effects can be calculated for given angular accelerations. For a fluid-filled toroid, representing the semi-circular canal, the pressure generated is mostly radial which does not couple to the cupula in that canal. Induced pressure will also largely cancel in orthogonal canals. Calculations of the effective pressure indicate that even for high magnetic fields (>4 T) the effect would only be at the limits of perception for very high angular accelerations such as vigorous shaking of the head.[12] For a fuller discussion and derivation of the radial and tangential pressures experienced during angular accelerations in a closed loop of conductive fluid see Ref. 11. The radial pressures are greater than the tangential pressures by a factor equal to the ratio of the radii of the structure to the tube inner diameter. However, it is the tangential pressure which would cause the cupula to deflect. This mechanism does not have any experimental support as real effects are perceived at very low frequency of movement, or even when the subject is stationary or only moving very slowly.

2.4.3 Directly Applied or Induced Currents

Galvanic vestibular stimulation (GVS) and inner vestibule stimulation experiments demonstrate the linearity of hair cell nerve firing and subject response directly modulates the firing rate of the cell. Hence it is possible to hypothesize that quite small rotations and movements in the magnetic field can generate electric fields of the order of magnitude to generate the GVS effects. Experiments in a 7-T magnetic field show that a magnetic field change of the order of 4 T during a period of 2 s are required for subjects to perceive an effect.[11] This measured response of subjects is sensitive to the polarity of the field as well as the direction of travel. The sense of the direction of perception of movement reverses if the sense of the current flow around the head reverses. However, it has been noted that large peak rates of change of magnetic field are not in themselves enough to induce vertigo,[11] leading to the anomaly that vertigo can be perceived by a subject at head rotation velocities and accelerations which are a lot lower than are expected from calculation.

2.4.4 Lorentz Force Mechanism

Roberts *et al.*[13] demonstrated that horizontal slow-phase eye nystagmus velocity (H-SPV) produced by exposure to a strong magnetic field is directly proportional to the magnetic field strength, with a response which has an adaption component and a linear response to field. This linear response measurement provided a new and vital piece of objective evidence. The experiment does not depend on a scored subjective response as the subject has no control over the reflex if there is no visual reference. They measured the SPV of the eye nystagmus in the dark as a function of time and related it to the applied magnetic field. A typical set of response data which reproduces this experiment is shown in Figure 2.2. These data show the initial response to the magnetic field change and the slow adaption process which does not return to zero until the subject is removed from the field. The adaption (habituation) process takes place in the hair cell nerve afferents is shown occurring both after the start of the exposure period and after the field reduces to zero (where it is temporarily reversed in polarity). Subjects report a reversal of apparent rotation during this latter period when compared to the initial exposure period response. There is, therefore, an element of incomplete DC cancellation in the ocular response where the response does not return to zero whilst the exposure is maintained. In addition, Roberts *et al.* proposed a mechanism based on a Lorentz force, where the current does not come from induction but that the dark current has a high enough current density to elicit a pressure change in the semi-circular canals.

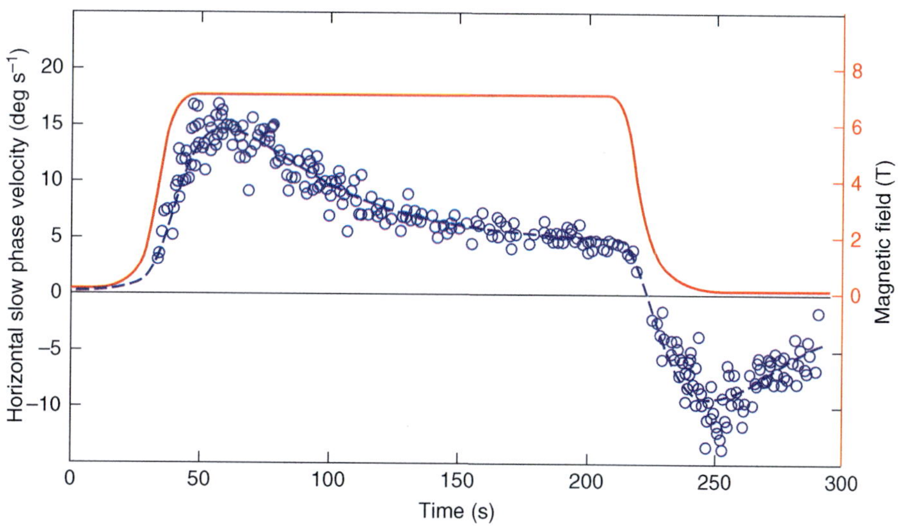

Figure 2.2. The experimentally measured horizontal slow phase velocity (crosses) of eye nystagmus as a response to an exposure period of 7 T magnetic field change. This response demonstrates the adaption phase of the response, the response to a static field (from about 150 to 225 s), and the nystagmus reversal on removal from the field. The dashed line shows the model fit response as described by Glover *et al.* (Modified from Glover *et al.*[14])

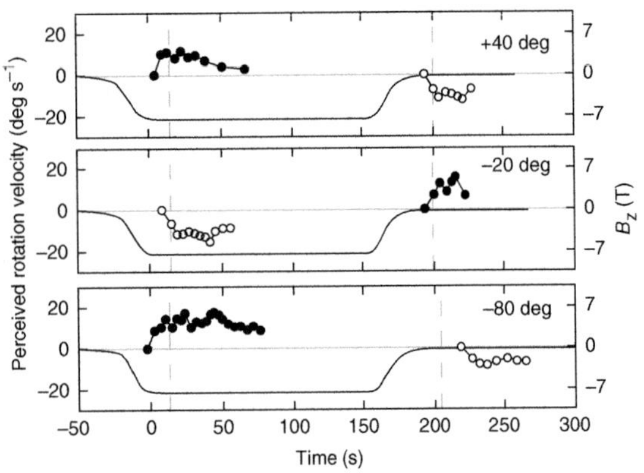

Figure 2.3. A graph showing perception of rotational velocity due to a period of exposure to 7 T. The solid lines indicate the subjects exposure to magnetic field. The dots indicate a velocity to the left (open) or right (solid) and the 3 graphs show results for different angles of head pitch relative to the direction of magnetic field. Note the 'phase' of response, both for different orientations, and the alternation of phase at the end of the exposure as also shown in Figure 2.2. (Mian *et al.*, 2013. https://journals.plos.org/plosone/article?id=10.1371/journal.pone.0078748. Licensed under CC0)

Antunes *et al.*[14] refined the calculation by Roberts *et al.* by modeling the canals, currents, and forces and confirmed that this mechanism is plausible and gives a realistic prediction of both the magnitude and direction of perception. As the Lorentz force is dependent on magnitude and directions of both magnetic field and orientation of the cupula then the SPV response is highly directional with both peaks and nulls in the response dependent upon head orientation.[13,15] The dynamics of the response may be modeled in terms of a low pass and high pass (partial) adaption model. The time constants of the model used to fit to experimental data give characteristics similar to those measured experimentally for rotational motion[16] and shown as a dashed line in Figure 2.3. These data fit a mechanical transduction model for the canal–cupula system which includes a partial habituation stage based on a hair cell response.

In addition to the eye nystagmus measurements (purely involuntary), it is possible for the subjects to report the magnitude and direction of their perceived rotation. For example, on introduction to the magnet bore of a 7 T Philips magnet installation, the perception of rotation is that the lower half of the body is moving to the right in the horizontal plane. The rate of movement can be recorded by button presses as shown in Figure 2.3.[15,17,18] It is interesting to note that the perception of movement ceases after an adaption period yet the nystagmus does not. Either the perception threshold and/or the adaption mechanism is different between the ocular and perception response. It might be that this question is answered by experiments (or subject responses) at higher fields than 7 T in future.

As expected, when a vector product term determines the magnitude and polarity of the effect, then it is possible to demonstrate that head position relative to the magnetic field direction does follow a 'sinusoidal' type of response. Clearly, this type of experiment is limited by the angles at which the head can be oriented in the magnetic field of a horizontal bore of a typical magnet. However, data show that the standard supine position that patients assume during scans is actually quite benign relative to other possible orientations. For example, a more head-up prone position (i.e., looking along the field direction) has potential for severe effects. Keeping the eyes open during field exposure is certainly a factor in perception effects. The ability for the eyes to fixate usually 'destroys' any perception effects. All the measurements of nystagmus and perception are carried out in complete darkness.

Using the Lorentz mechanism as a model, it is possible to explain the pattern of responses measured in previous studies. For example, it explains why a slowly changing field can elicit a strong response, determines how the 'polarity' of response varies, and why there is a response to a field. The habituation mechanism of the primary afferent explains the reversal in polarity after the exposure returns to zero.

2.5 SUBJECT RESPONSE

2.5.1 Physiological Response

Ward *et al.*[19] produce further compelling evidence for a Lorentz force mechanism. Firstly, they demonstrate that subjects without any vestibular function show no response, and subjects having a unilateral functional deficit have a modified response consistent with the orientation of the head in the magnetic field as expected from the model. These authors also raise the possibility of using magnetic fields as either a diagnostic tool to assess vestibular function, either in the clinic or for vestibular function research. Effectively the magnetic field provides a rotational velocity profile that it is not possible to generate mechanically. Theysohn *et al.*[20] demonstrate that there is a significant postural sway effect (employing Unterberger's stepping test) 1 min post exposure to a 7-T magnetic field which is absent 15 min later and not observed at all for exposure to 1.5 T. They also note that very short exposures do not elicit a sway response. Such an observation is entirely consistent with an adaption mechanism. In a paper by van Nierop *et al.*[21] postural body sway is measured outside a 7-T magnet at magnetic field strengths of the order of 0.5 T and recorded rates of change of $0.7\,\mathrm{T\,s^{-1}}$. Their conclusion was that body sway area had a significant correlation with exposure and that this was on a par with a blood alcohol concentration of 0.09% which would be well above the maximum legal limit for driving in the UK. The authors aim was to assess the effect of magnetic fields (static and time-varying) on human performance (e.g., surgeons performing interventional MRI) rather than determine a mechanism of interaction.

2.5.2 Acceptance by Subjects

Since the introduction of the first high-field (7 T or above) scanners, there are now a number of studies which report on the acceptance of 7 T (or 9.4 T) amongst both clinical and healthy volunteer subjects. These studies attempt to understand the influence of the higher field on aspects of the scan experience such as claustrophobia, PNS, RF SAR. Some of the questions posed to subjects, depending on study, ask about the prevalence of vertigo or movement-like sensations. It is important to note that, amongst most of the studies cited below, there is no mention of, or recording of, the lighting used, or the state of the subject's eyes (open, closed). To elicit SPV nystagmus there is a requirement for the subject to be in total darkness. Sensations of nonveridical movement (leaning, bending, curving) are largely suppressed if there are visual cues.[15] Hence, in the dark, nearly 100% of subjects report sensations,[15] but only around 15–25% of subjects notice these effects in the ordinary light conditions in the reports cited. This discrepancy highlights the difference between findings of experiments which test mechanisms and those which are looking for responses during standard protocols. In addition, the standard protocols are carried out with the subject supine in the normal scanning position, whereas the maximum vertigo response might be with the head pitched upward with the body prone.[15] There is, undoubtedly, an effect linked with head attitude and even body position. These latter effects are more likely to be relevant to operators (and hence of interest to regulators) than the responses of subjects being scanned.

One of the first papers to appear on the levels of acceptance of 7 T MRI was by Theysohn *et al.*[22] which reported vertigo sensations in 26% of subjects ($N = 142$) with 5% rating it as very unpleasant. These figures appear to be consistent across a range of subsequent studies. However, in these various studies, the questions used and subjective grade scales range from simple yes-no[23] to more complex grades.[24] In the Uwano *et al.* study,[24] reports of vertigo or nonveridical movements (such as 'curving' or 'leaning' which are perceived during magnet entry) are reported in around 10% of subjects. This is lower than in previous studies but could occur for a number of reasons, such as the lighting conditions as well as head positioning. Another more subtle reason, demonstrated in a single-center study by Cosottini *et al.*[25] is an apparent decline in scores to a lower reporting of vertigo by subjects across the study. They attribute this to a better understanding of the effects by operators. This is possibly the first measured evidence of something which is largely anecdotal amongst the high-field community – that operators adapt their behavior to, and expectations of, working in and around high-field magnets. However, this 'expectation' seems to have transmitted itself to the subjects. It may be that the way subjects are treated or that information given, either unconsciously or deliberately, reduces anxiety about the perceived movements and increases acceptability. Studies such as those by Rauschenberg *et al.*[26] and Uwano *et al.*[24] discriminate between the periods where subjects are being moved into the magnet and periods where they remain stationary in the static field (during the scanning process). Clearly, the vertigo effect is lower while at iso-center (during the scan) but can clearly be explained by the adaption process and the static field Lorentz mechanism so there is no inconsistency. Uwano *et al.*[24] attribute the high degree of acceptability and tolerance to vertigo amongst subjects to a low table speed. If the introduction time is of similar order to the adaption time (of order 40–100 s) then the perception will be minimized. Rauschenberg *et al.*[26] (surveying responses from over 3000 subjects) also compare data from subjects undergoing scans at the higher field strength of 9.4 T. A higher level of discomfort related to vertigo at the higher field was recorded but did not lead to a higher rejection rate by subjects.

It is not known, as yet, what the subjective effect of high magnetic fields might be on children. The only paper to broach this subject by Chou *et al.*[27] 'interpolate' a level of acceptance from responses of experienced adults. There is certainly no reason to worry regarding likelihood of damage to the vestibular system as any of the mechanisms discussed above point to the vestibular system working well within its dynamic range. However, the variation observed in the magnitude of the SPV responses across the measured populations are large – it is not known at present if these vary with age of subject.

What is still lacking is any reliable evidence for vertigo effects on operators and the issue of exposure on cognition, although some effects might be mediated through a balance mechanism.[28,29]

2.6 SUMMARY

It appears from the experimental evidence that the major sensory effects observed at field strengths up to 7 T are largely mediated through a Lorentz force acting on the dark ionic currents in the vestibular system. These effects are larger and more sustained than electric fields which are induced by rotation or translation of the subject in magnetic fields. Magnetic susceptibility of sensory tissues in the vestibular system may also be responsible for some of the perceived magnetic field effect on humans, but this is likely to be translational rather than the experimentally perceived rotations. This effect requires there to be high levels of both magnetic field and associated gradient and hence at its highest magnitudes in and around the bore entrance rather than at iso-center. MHD due to movement is unlikely to have a role in such small vestibular structures and there is no need to invoke a direct magnetic effect on the CNS. There is agreement across a number of surveys involving a total of over 4000 subjects that the incidence of vertigo or nonveridical perception at high fields (>3 T) is about 10–25% but this will depend on local conditions (eyes open and closed or lighting), protocols, and positioning of subjects. A better understanding of high-field effects by operators and other personnel may lead to a reduction in the anxiety about vertigo effects. There is no evidence of long-term (beyond 20 min after exposure) of a vertigo effect on balance or sway. A high field is a pre-requisite for subject reported vertigo-like effects and although the rate of change of field is important for the perception of that field, a similar rate of change around zero mean or at low field does not elicit the same effect.

RELATED ARTICLES IN EMAGRES

Bioeffects and Safety of Radiofrequency Electromagnetic Fields

High-Field Whole Body Systems

Radiofrequency Fields: Interactions, Biological Effects, and Safety Issues

REFERENCES

1. C. T. Rodgers and P. J. Hore, *Proc. Natl. Acad. Sci. U. S. A.*, 2009, **106**, 353.
2. J. F. Lamb, in 'Essentials of Physiology', eds J. F. Lamb, C. G. Ingram, I. A. Johnston, and R. M. Pitman, Blackwell Scientific: Oxford, 1991.
3. C. M. Oman, E. N. Marcus, and I. S. Curthoys, *Acta Otolaryngol.*, 1987, **103**, 1.
4. A. A. J. van Egmond, J. J. Groen, and L. B. W. Jongkees, *J. Physiol. Lond.*, 1949, **110**, 1.
5. J. D. Jackson, Classical Electrodynamics, Wiley: New York, 1998.
6. R. Herranz, O. J. Larkin, C. E. Dijkstra, R. J. Hill, P. Anthony, M. R. Davey, L. Eaves, J. J. W. A. van Loon, F. J. Medina, and R. Marco, *BMC Genomics*, 2012, **13**, Article no 52. DOI: 10.1186/1471-2164-13-52.
7. C. Cobos Sanchez, P. Glover, H. Power, and R. Bowtell, *Phys. Med. Biol.*, 2012, **57**, 4739.
8. T. A. Houpt, B. Kwon, C. E. Houpt, B. Neth, and J. C. Smith, *Am. J. Phys. Regul. Integr. Comp. Phys.*, 2013, **305**, R793.
9. T. A. Houpt, D. W. Pittman, C. Riccardi, J. A. Cassell, D. R. Lockwood, J. M. Barranco, B. Kwon, and J. C. Smith, *Physiol. Behav.*, 2005, **86**, 379.
10. A. M. Cason, B. Kwon, J. C. Smith, and T. A. Houpt, *Physiol. Behav.*, 2009, **97**, 36.
11. P. M. Glover, I. Cavin, W. Qian, R. Bowtell, and P. A. Gowland, *Bioelectromagnetics*, 2007, **28**, 349.
12. J. F. Schenck, *Prog. Biophys. Mol. Biol.*, 2005, **87**, 185.

13. D. C. Roberts, V. Marcelli, J. S. Gillen, J. P. Carey, C. C. Della Santina, and D. S. Zee, *Curr. Biol.*, 2011, **21**, 1635.
14. A. Antunes, P. M. Glover, Y. Li, O. S. Mian, and B. L. Day, *Phys. Med. Biol.*, 2012, **57**, 4477.
15. O. S. Mian, Y. Li, A. Antunes, P. M. Glover, and B. L. Day, *PLoS One*, 2013, **8**, e78748.
16. P. M. Glover, Y. Li, A. Antunes, O. S. Mian, and B. L. Day, *Phys. Med. Biol.*, 2014, **59**, 631.
17. O. S. Mian, P. M. Glover, and B. L. Day, *Front. Neurol.*, 2015, **6**, 201.
18. O. S. Mian, Y. Li, A. Antunes, P. M. Glover, and B. L. Day, *J. Physiol.*, 2015, **594**, 1051.
19. B. K. Ward, D. C. Roberts, C. C. Della Santina, J. P. Carey, and D. S. Zee, *Front. Neurol.*, 2014, **5**, 28.
20. J. M. Theysohn, O. Kraff, K. Eilers, D. Andrade, M. Gerwig, D. Timmann, F. Schmitt, M. E. Ladd, S. C. Ladd, and A. K. Bitz, *PLoS One*, 2014, **9**, e92104.
21. L. E. van Nierop, P. Slottje, H. Kingma, and H. Kromhout, *Magn. Reson. Med.*, 2013, **70**, 232.
22. J. M. Theysohn, S. Maderwald, O. Kraff, C. Moenninghoff, M. E. Ladd, and S. C. Ladd, *Magn. Reson. Mater. Phys. Biol. Med.*, 2008, **21**, 63.
23. S. Klix, A. Els, K. Paul, A. Graessl, C. Oezerdem, O. Weinberger, L. Winter, C. Thalhammer, T. Huelnhagen, J. Rieger, H. Mehling, J. Schulz-Menger, and T. Niendorf, *PLoS One*, 2015, **10**, e0117095. DOI: 10.1371/journal.pone.0117095.
24. I. Uwano, T. Metki, F. Sendai, R. Yoshida, K. Kudo, F. Yamashita, S. Higuchi, K. Ito, T. Harada, J. Goodwin, A. Ogawa, and M. Sasaki, *Magn. Reson. Med. Sci.*, 2015, **14**, 35.
25. M. Cosottini, D. Frosini, L. Biagi, I. Pesaresi, M. Costagli, G. Tiberi, M. Symms, and M. Tosetti, *Eur. Radiol.*, 2014, **24**, 1923.
26. J. Rauschenberg, A. M. Nagel, S. C. Ladd, J. M. Theysohn, M. E. Ladd, H. E. Moller, R. Trampel, R. Turner, R. Pohmann, K. Scheffler, A. Brechmann, J. Stadler, J. Felder, N. J. Shah, and W. Semmler, *Investig. Radiol.*, 2014, **49**, 249.
27. I. J. Chou, C. R. Tench, P. Gowland, T. Jaspan, R. A. Dineen, N. Evangelou, R. Abdel-Fahim, W. P. Whitehouse, and C. S. Constantinescu, *BMJ Open*, 2014, **4** (10), e006094. DOI: 10.1136/bmjopen-2014-006094.
28. A. Heinrich, A. Szostek, F. Nees, P. Meyer, W. Semmler, and H. Flor, *J. Magn. Reson. Imaging*, 2011, **34**, 758.
29. M. Schlamann, M. A. Voigt, S. Maderwald, A. K. Bitz, O. Kraff, S. C. Ladd, M. E. Ladd, M. Forsting, and H. Wilhelm, *J. Magn. Reson. Imaging*, 2010, **31**, 1061.

Chapter 3

Effects of Magnetic Fields and Field Gradients on Living Cells

Jarek Wosik[1,2], Martha Villagran[2,3], Ahmed Uosef[4,5], Rafik M. Ghobrial[5,6], John H. Miller Jr[2,3], and Malgorzata Kloc[5,6,7]

[1]*Department of Electrical and Computer Engineering, University of Houston, Houston, TX, USA*
[2]*Texas Center for Superconductivity, University of Houston, Houston, TX, USA*
[3]*Department of Physics, University of Houston, Houston, TX, USA*
[4]*Ain Shams University School of Medicine, Cairo, Egypt*
[5]*The Houston Methodist Research Institute, Houston, TX, USA*
[6]*Department of Surgery, The Houston Methodist Hospital, Houston, TX, USA*
[7]*M.D. Anderson Cancer Center, Department of Genetics, The University of Texas, Houston, TX, USA*

3.1 INTRODUCTION

Magnetic resonance imaging (MRI) has proven to be a great success as a nondestructive, nonionizing, and noninvasive imaging modality widely used as a diagnostic medical technique in hospitals and in animal research. The possibility that the exposure of the human body to the strong magnetic and electromagnetic fields required for MRI may be harmful has been voiced since this powerful imaging modality was introduced in the 1970s. MRI relies not only on the use of a static magnetic field B_0 to polarize nuclei spins but also on switching magnetic field gradients to provide spatial and temporal information and radiofrequency (RF) electromagnetic signals to manipulate the spins' orientations and precessions. The RF and switching gradient fields are applied only during the image acquisition process, whereas the high static magnetic field, usually generated by a superconducting magnet, is always present. All these fields interact with biological matter, so MRI safety considerations should take these three types of exposure into account. Physical effects induced by RF and switching gradient fields are easier to observe than the effects introduced by the static fields. It is already well known that the exposure of the human body to excessive RF field amplitudes and excessively rapid switching gradient fields must be limited because of heating effects and stimulation of nerves, respectively. Table 3.1 describes the known

Safety and Biological Effects in MRI.
Edited by Devashish Shrivastava and J. Thomas Vaughan
 ISBN: 978-1-118-82130-5
Also published in eMagRes (online edition)
DOI: 10.1002/9780470034590.emrstm1609

Table 3.1. Comparison of the biological effects of the low-frequency switching gradients, RF electromagnetic and static magnetic fields during MRI scans

Type of field	Physical effects
Low-frequency gradient fields (1 Hz-kHz)	Peripheral nerve stimulation
Radiofrequency B_{rf} fields (up to hundreds MHz)	Tissue RF electric field heating
Static B_0 fields	Not fully explored and known

physical effects resulting from static, low frequency, and RF fields.[1]

All living organisms, including humans, have adapted to the relatively weak Earth's magnetic field (30–70 μT) and occasionally to slightly stronger magnetic fields from naturally occurring magnetic minerals. The invention of the electromagnet in the nineteenth century[2] and its subsequent development[3,4] when resistive wires were replaced with superconducting wires, introduced much stronger sources of the magnetic field. In the last couple of decades, this has enabled the development of whole-body clinical and research MRI scanners. Magnetic fields currently used for research are higher than for clinical applications and can now exceed even 11.5 T (230 000 times higher than the Earth's magnetic field) in commercially available imaging scanners. In Europe and in the United States, there are individual units for spectroscopy and imaging of small animals with the magnetic fields above 30 T.[5] Such ultra-high fields can be generated due to the discovery, in 1986, of high-critical temperature superconductors (HTS), which have extremely high critical fields. Recent developments, in the deposition of HTS (rare earth barium cuprate) thin films on flexible tapes,[6] have enabled production of magnets with critical magnetic fields above 23 T. HTS tapes are used to build inserts whenever the required field value exceeds the critical magnetic fields of low-temperature superconductors, such as Nb_3Sn and Nb-Ti.

Such progress in magnet technology has opened a new chapter in the exposure of living organisms to magnetic fields, which far exceed any naturally occurring field found on Earth. In MRI, the RF signal is intrinsically weak because of its proportionality to the difference between the number of protons aligned with and against the applied dc magnetic field, and this number is very small at human body temperatures. For example, at 3 T only 18 protons out of two million participate in signal generation, which makes MRI a signal-to-noise ratio (SNR) 'hungry' modality.[7] The SNR is proportional to the magnetic field strength. This dependence indicates that the use of stronger magnets should allow for higher SNR, which consequently would result either in higher resolution or shorter scanning time. Spectral dispersion and susceptibility contrast, in addition to SNR, also improve with increasing static magnetic field strength. Such a trend of increasing static magnetic fields in MRI magnets is clearly seen from the early 1980s, when a standard clinical whole-body scanners magnetic field strength was 1.5 T, to the present day, when the 3-T whole-body clinical scanners have become an industry standard. In 2017, the first clinical whole-body 7-T scanner, the Magnetom Terra by Siemens Medical Solutions, Inc., was cleared to be used in both the United States and Europe. Further advances, in high field magnet, gradient, and RF hardware technologies, have led on the extreme end to the development of 10.5-T whole-body MRI scanner currently installed at the Center for Magnetic Resonance Research (CMRR) at University of Minnesota, which is the strongest whole-body MRI machine available to date for human applications. Furthermore, two 11.7 T wide-bore scanners for people were built and are readying for imaging human brains.[8,9] The first one is located at the NeuroSpin Centre at CEA Saclay outside Paris, and the second one at the US National Institutes of Health (NIH) in Bethesda in Maryland.

While such ultra-high field scanners are currently used in human and animal research, their effects on the human body are still not fully explored nor understood. The field strengths of MRI magnets are much higher than those any other magnetic field sources that would normally be encountered by humans. Other objects in our environment, such as permanent magnet-based devices, electric motors, and power transmission lines, can locally generate static magnetic fields, but such fields rarely exceed 100 mT.

Modern MRI magnets are shielded by a set of coils placed next to the primary superconducting coil. Such secondary coils produce a magnetic field opposite to that generated by the primary coil. This creates a much faster rate of decay of the magnetic field outside of the main magnet. The U.S. Food and Drug Administration (FDA) guidelines[10] refer to 5G as the upper limit when the field strength is considered as benign for the general public, including persons with implanted electronic devices.[11,12] In such a shielded configuration, MRI scanner operators, patients, and medical personnel are exposed to the static magnetic fields only in the very proximity and inside of the magnet.

Several early investigations, which focused on the bio effects of magnetic fields and their interactions with living organisms, showed lack of any harmful effects for a broad range of magnetic fields.[1,13,14] Clinical epidemiological MRI studies showed that the static fields of 1.5–7 T do not have any significant effects on the human body with the exception of short-lasting vertigo in a small percentage of participants exposed to 7 T field.[15]

The data on the magnetic field interaction with the cell nucleus, chromosomes, and deoxyribonucleic acid (DNA) are often inconsistent and contradictory. Many studies indicate that the magnetic field of 1–10 T does not cause nuclear changes or DNA damage, does not affect chromosomal crossover and does not increase the rate of mutations in healthy cells with properly functioning anti-oxidative stress and DNA damage control,[16] but some studies show exactly the opposite.[16–18] The main reason behind these conflicting findings is a very small diamagnetic susceptibility of living organisms. Most likely some effects are below the threshold of significance, especially in cases when the magnetic field-generated forces are smaller than the gravitationally generated forces. Most of these studies do not describe the quantitative characteristics of the effect, that is, the dependence on field parameters and the duration of the exposure, making comparisons of the results very difficult.

However, the MRI industry trend of using ever-stronger superconducting magnets increases the chances that such effects may become noticeable. The best example of the effects, which started to be noticeable when the ultra-high field was applied, is the interaction of the static magnetic field with the purified microtubules. It has been shown that in vitro, the microtubules align along the static magnetic field due to their diamagnetic anisotropy.[19] It was also reported that the mitotic spindles (which are composed of microtubules) in dividing mammalian cells align along the magnetic field and that the degree of the alignment depends on the magnetic field magnitude and exposure time. The effect of MRI field below 9 T was weak and only partial alignment was reported. However, the exposure of CNE-2Z and RPE1 human cells to 9 T field and the ultra-high field of 27 T aligned spindles and chromosomes along the direction of the magnetic field.[20] In addition, such ultra-high field also perturbed the morphology of the spindle.

It is known that the strong magnetic field gradients when interacting with the diamagnetic structures, cause an effect analogous to negative microgravity.[21–23] This effect is recognized as a diamagnetic levitation[24] and results in a significant force applied to the cells, affecting their morphology and differentiation.[25,26] Such levitation can take place even at low-strength but highly nonuniform fields because the force acting on biological material depends also on the degree of the field nonuniformity. Static fields in the range of 15 T affect cell differentiation and viability.[27] Studies of the interaction of the magnetic nanoparticles (NP) with cells showed the magnetic field effects were caused either by local NP magnetic fields or by the mechanical forces enhanced by the presence of NP.[28–32]

3.2 EFFECTS OF STATIC MAGNETIC FIELDS ON CELLS AND TISSUES

There are a number of mechanisms that could lead to effects of the magnetic field on cells and tissues, which we outline in the following sections.

3.2.1 Magnetic Susceptibilities of Materials and Their Classification

The interaction of the electromagnetic fields with cells or tissues depends on the electric- and magnetic-field-induced polarizations. The degree of polarization depends on the electric and magnetic susceptibilities of the biological object. For a typical cell/tissue, the electric susceptibility is 10^5-10^6 times greater than the magnetic susceptibility. For this reason, an applied electric field can cause significant damage to cells or tissue, whereas magnetic field effects are usually weak.

If an object is placed in a magnetic field $\boldsymbol{H}$, its magnetic response will lead to a magnetic induction $\boldsymbol{B}$, which is composed of two parts, $\vec{B} = \mu_0(\vec{H} + \vec{M})$. Here μ_0 is the permeability of free space, equal to $4\pi\ 10^{-7}\,\boldsymbol{H}\,\mathrm{m}^{-1}$, and $\boldsymbol{M}$ is the magnetization. In general, all materials, on the basis of their response to the magnetic field are classified into three groups: diamagnetic, paramagnetic, and ferromagnetic. In the diamagnetic and paramagnetic materials, the magnetization is linearly proportional to $\boldsymbol{H}$, as $\boldsymbol{M} = \chi\ \boldsymbol{H}$. Here χ is expressed as a dimensionless, substance-specific quantity and is called the volume susceptibility. The molar magnetic susceptibility χ_m is more commonly used and is defined as the product of the volume susceptibility χ and the molar volume V_m of a substance, $\chi_m = \chi V_m = (\chi \text{ mol})/\rho$, where mol indicates molar mass, and ρ is the density of the substance. The diamagnetic materials have negative values of χ_m, so the magnetic induction $\boldsymbol{B}$ inside the object will be reduced as compared to the field outside the object. The para- and ferromagnetic materials have positive values of χ_m, so the magnetic induction in such objects is higher. The ferromagnetic materials have χ values much greater than one. This is why the static magnetic fields can strongly affect implanted devices, especially those containing ferromagnetic components.

Living cells and tissues are mostly diamagnetic, usually having small, negative magnetic susceptibilities.[14] Such cells/tissues when experiencing nonuniform field will be repelled by regions of high magnetic field toward the regions with lower fields. By contrast, paramagnetic materials, which have a positive magnetic susceptibility, will be attracted to the regions with higher magnetic fields.

3.2.2 Translational and Rotational Forces Acting on Cells and Tissues

In a uniform field, diamagnetic or paramagnetic cells, which do not have a permanent magnetic moment, will not experience a translational force but will only disturb field homogeneity. A nonuniform magnetic field is needed to produce a translational force (F_{mag}), which pushes diamagnetic or paramagnetic cells from the strong toward the weak fields, or vice versa. In order to calculate the force F_{mag} we begin with the expression for the magnetic energy of a cell placed in a magnetic field:

$$U = -\frac{\vec{m}\vec{B}}{2} \tag{3.1}$$

where magnetic dipole moment $\vec{m} = -(\chi V\vec{B}/\mu_0)$, and χ, $\boldsymbol{B}$, and V are representing the susceptibility, magnetic induction, and volume of the cell, respectively. We assume that the magnetic field and susceptibility are constant over the cell volume because it is relatively small. The magnetic energy equation can be rewritten as $U = -(\chi VB^2/2\mu_0)$, and the use of the magnetic force function defined as $\vec{F}(x,y,z) = \nabla U$, results in the following expression:

$$\vec{F}(x,y,z) = -\frac{V\chi_c}{\mu_0}\vec{B}\cdot(\nabla\vec{B}) \tag{3.2}$$

The response of cells to a magnetic field gradient often depends on the difference between the susceptibilities of the cells and the surrounding buffer medium.[33,34] This can be expressed as:

$$\vec{F}(x,y,z) = \frac{V(\chi_M - \chi_c)}{\mu_0}\vec{B}\cdot(\nabla\vec{B}) \tag{3.3}$$

where ∇ is the del operator and V is the cell volume. $\Delta\chi = (\chi_c - \chi_M)$ describes the difference in magnetic susceptibilities between the cell and the surrounding buffer medium. Equation (3.3) shows that the magnetic force depends on the product of the magnetic induction $\vec{B}$ (in T units) and the magnetic field gradient $\nabla\vec{B}$ (in T m^{-1}). Such magnetic force is therefore often denoted as the magnetic force product, given in units of T^2 m^{-1}.[13] Expanding the force product in rectangular coordinates, and after normalization to $V(\chi_M - \chi_c)/\mu_0$, a second-order tensor is obtained. Its magnitude can be expressed as:

$$\begin{aligned} |F(\vec{B})| &= |\vec{B}\cdot\nabla(\vec{B})| \\ &= \sqrt{[F_x(B_x)]^2 + [F_y(B_y)]^2 + [F_z(B_z)]^2} \end{aligned} \tag{3.4}$$

where B_x, B_y, B_z and F_x, F_y, F_z are x, y, z components of magnetic induction and magnetic force, respectively.

The susceptibility of human cells (both in vitro and in vivo) is in a range between -7.0 and -11.0×10^{-6}. Application of the nonuniform magnetic field can introduce the mechanical force applied to the cell and as a result, can create some internal forces that propagate into the cell via its cytoskeleton. For the actin filament network, the magnitude of such forces is believed to be in a range from 10 pN to several nN.[35,36] Another force is the adhesion force exerted by the cell on a substrate to which it is attached through focal adhesions. This force typically ranges from 1 to 100 nN.[37,38] For comparison purposes, a single protein unfolding and stretching process is known to require 2–10 pN,[39] while stretching of a complete actin filament, which consists of many protein monomers, requires a much larger force of about 10 nN.[40,41] By comparison, the forces produced by a set of rare earth permanent magnets with 1 T fields and acting on a cell will be about 10 pN.[42] In addition to the magnetic force F_{mag}, the cells in a buffer medium also experience a buoyancy force (F_b), which can be written[43] as:

$$\vec{F_b} = V\Delta\rho\vec{g} \tag{3.5}$$

Here $\boldsymbol{g}$ is the gravitational acceleration in z direction and ρ is the difference between the volumetric densities of the cell and the buffer medium. After the cell achieves a velocity $\vec{v}$, it will also experience a drag force F_d as it moves through the medium. Such a force, when a spherical shape of the object is assumed, can be calculated[17,44,45] using the following equation:

$$\vec{F_d} = 6\pi f_D r\eta\vec{v} \tag{3.6}$$

Here r is the radius of the cell, η indicates the dynamic viscosity of the buffer medium, and f_D is the drag coefficient, which is equal to one when the cell is not in proximity to the container wall. All the above-defined forces are shown schematically in Figure 3.1 where the cells are placed in a medium above two permanent south-north (SN) and north-south (NS) magnetized magnets placed side by side. The direction and magnitude of the magnetic force on a cell, in addition to depending strongly on the magnetic field and field gradient, also depends on the difference in susceptibilities of the cell and its surrounding (a medium or a tissue).

The animal cells are usually weakly diamagnetic. The surrounding tissue can be slightly less diamagnetic than the cell itself or, in some cases, nonmagnetic or even paramagnetic. The force direction will, in this case, depend on the sign of the magnetic susceptibility difference $\Delta\chi$. For positive $\Delta\chi$, cells will be attracted to the regions of highest fields and field gradients as it is marked in Figure 3.1; whereas negative $\Delta\chi$ will lead to a repulsive force away from those regions. The same mechanism will be working with the static magnetic field gradients present in MRI magnets.

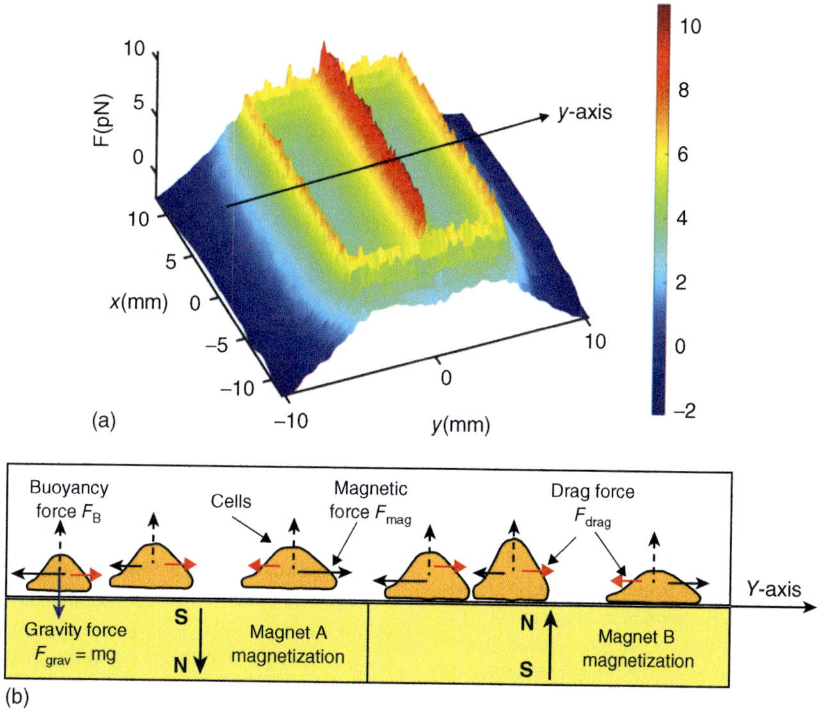

Figure 3.1. A sketch of forces acting on cells in the nonuniform magnetic field. For simplicity purposes, NS-SN anti-parallel magnetization arrangement of two magnets is assumed, and magnetic force F_{mag} along the y-axis is plotted to show where the strongest force above the two magnets is created. Forces exerted to cells due to the presence of the magnetic field gradient, gravity, and surrounding cells media are shown with different color arrows (magnetic (F_{mag}, black), gravity (F_{grav}, blue), buoyancy (F_B, dashed), and drag (F_{drag}, red).

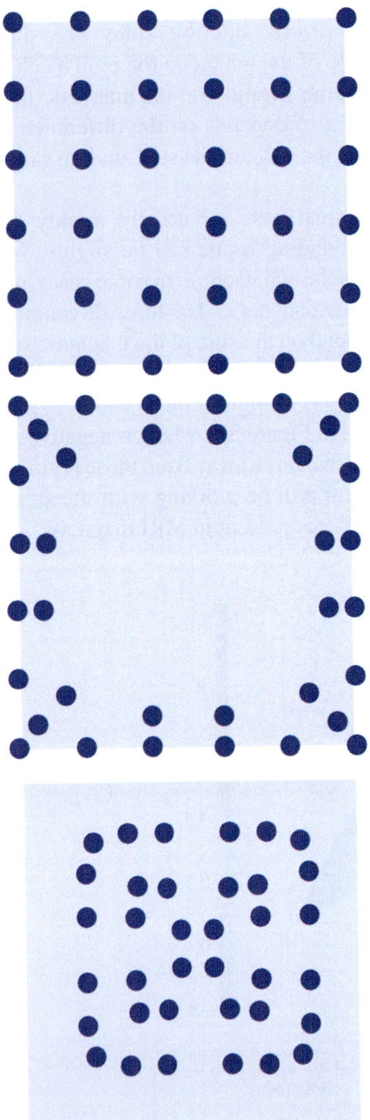

(a) (b) (c)

Figure 3.2. Cells are either repelled or attracted to the highest magnetic field gradient lines. Simulated distribution of the cells located above a permanent magnet with 1.2 T field at the surface and vertical N-S magnetization. Three cases are shown: (a) cells are uniformly distributed indicating no translation force observed in either uniform or no magnetic field applied; (b) and (c) in nonuniform magnetic field, the cells are either repelled from (b) or attracted (c) to the highest-gradient present above the edges of a permanent magnet. Sign of the force depends on the sign of $\Delta\chi$, which was selected as negative for (b) and positive fore (c).

We have simulated the movement of the cells for two directions of the F_{mag} [equation (3.3)] force, as determined by either positive or negative $\Delta\chi$ susceptibility differences. Cells were represented as spherical particles. The mass of each particle was selected to be equal to that of a cell, about $(70-80) \times 10^{-12}$ g. We compared the results of this simulation with the behavior of mouse macrophages exposed to magnetic field gradients.[42] We found a very good correlation between the calculated directions of magnetic field-induced forces and experimentally observed alignment of the macrophages exposed to the gradients created by multiple permanent magnets. The example of such an alignment is shown in Figure 3.2 where the 3.2b and 3.2c cases represent repulsive and attractive forces, respectively, from or toward the high gradient regions. In these configurations, we observed the highest density of macrophages right above the edges of permanent magnets (Figure 3.2a) what indicates that, in this case, $\Delta\chi$ is positive, i.e. the macrophages have higher susceptibilities than the medium. For negative $\Delta\chi$, the macrophages should congregate near the center of each magnet, since they would be pushed away from the region of the highest magnetic field gradient. This is shown in the simulated cell alignments in Figure 3.2b, in which no cells are present above the highest gradient areas of the magnet. In general, the total force combines magnetic buoyancy with diamagnetic repulsive forces; however, the buoyancy force is much smaller and can be neglected.

3.2.3 MRI Scanner Gradients

MRI scanners are equipped with three sets of electromagnetic coils, which produce linear known gradients in the magnetic field along three orthogonal directions (G_x, G_y, and G_z). These are added to the main magnetic field B_0, thus enabling MRI signals to be spatially encoded. The gradient power supplies enable rapid, fully controlled magnetic field generation with precise control of their field strengths and directions.

The quality of MR imaging can be improved through a better resolution, which is proportional to gradient strength and, in addition, by increasing the gradients' switching frequency the image acquisition time can be reduced. However, there is an upper limit for the switching frequency because of neural and cardiac bio-effects induced by nerve stimulation at higher frequencies or when a certain combination of gradient strength, duration time and frequency occurs. Requirements regarding technical limitations, which have to be applied to gradients in the medical MRI scanners are provided by IEC released standard IEC 60601-2-33.[46] This standard is a generally accepted document regulating medical electrical equipment parameters. There are also reports indicating that, for much higher switching frequency, nerves stimulation can be suppressed.[47] Typical gradient systems in 1.5 T and 3 T clinical scanners can generate gradient fields up to 100 mT m^{-1} and slew rates (ramp time normalized to the maximum achievable gradient field strength) in 150–200 mT m^{-1} s^{-1} range. Strength of magnetic field generated by switching gradients is usually below 100 mT.[48] Static magnetic field force generated by such gradients is relatively small and below the threshold of significance.

Much larger magnetic static field gradients values are generated outside or close to edge of the magnet because of the fringe field, which can reach, depending on magnetic field strength and the magnet construction, tens of the T m^{-1}. The magnetic field in high (1.5 T, 3 T) and ultra-high field (above 3 T) MRI systems is produced by superconducting electromagnets. Horizontal bore magnets produce magnetic field lines, with the highest density and uniformity in the magnet center, which go out of the one end of the magnet's bore to the other creating the fringe fields around the magnet. The largest magnetic field forces acting on the diamagnetic, paramagnetic, or ferromagnetic objects will, therefore, occur on edge of the magnet where the largest special magnetic field gradients exist.

To get some perspective on the gradient strength it needs to be mentioned that for example gradients of 10 T m^{-1} could be obtained in laboratory electromagnets with tapered inserts generating fields exceeding 3–4 T and force product BdB dz^{-1} can be of an order of 30–40 T^2 m^{-1}.[49] There is a big difference between such static field gradients magnitude in clinical and small bore magnet scanners. The clinical superconducting magnets have force products of 50 T^2 m^{-1} at 7 T; however, the small-bore 11.7 T magnets have force product as high as 3500 T^2 m^{-1}. Levitation in such strong, but nonuniform field requires the force product to be at least equal to 2500 T^2 m^{-1}. In Figures 3.3 and 3.4, static spatial gradients created in 11.7 T and 3.0 T shielded superconducting magnets are plotted along the magnet axis. In Figure 3.5 functions of $|B_x|$, $|\nabla \vec{B}_x|$ $|B \cdot \nabla \vec{B}_x|$ versus distance from the magnet center are plotted for different strength of the magnetic field. This comparison shows that magnitude of gradients due to fringe fields shown in Figure 3.5 for high-field research scanners are comparable with the gradients used in in vitro experiments in which strong effects of the applied magnetic field were reported.

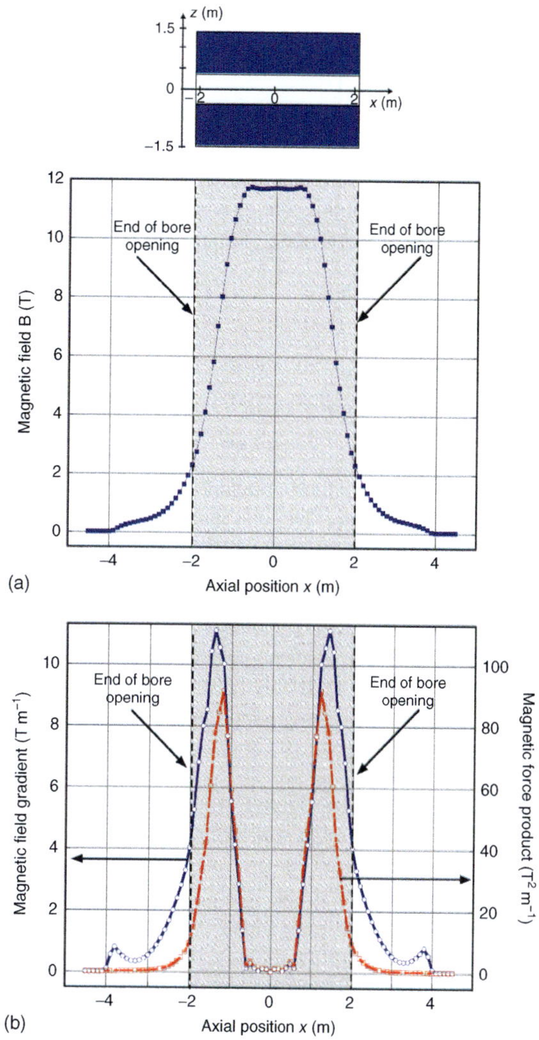

Figure 3.3. Static magnetic field gradient inside of 11.7 T whole-body scanner. A sketch of a vertical cross-section of the 11.7 T whole-body magnet with 60 cm bore opening. (a) Plots of the dependence of the magnetic inductance B_x component; (b) field gradient and force product on axial position x are shown. They were calculated along the horizontal magnet axis x, for $z = 0$. Magnet overall length is around 4 m.

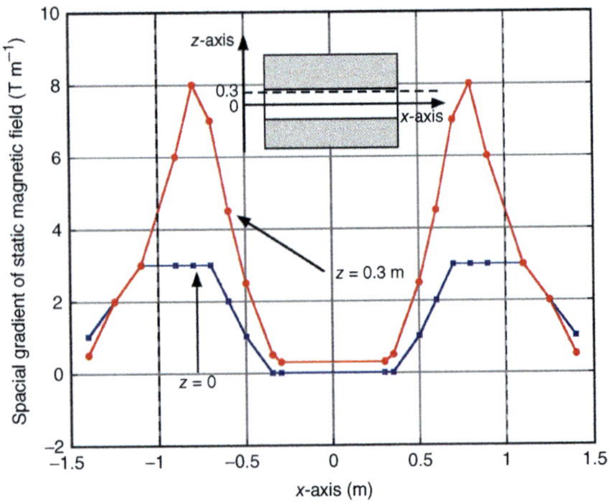

Figure 3.4. The gradient magnetic field of 3.0 T whole-body scanners. Plots of spatial magnetic field gradient along the x-axis of 3.0 T Phillips clinical magnets are shown. Two z-axis values were selected: $z = 0$, which is 0.15 m above the lower opening surface of the magnet and $z = 0.3$ m, which is close to the upper surface of the magnet opening. The highest gradient, which can be observed locally on the cover's surface is listed for this magnet as 17 T m^{-1}.

Much stronger gradients, above 10^5 T m^{-1}, can be produced in very small, micron-scale, regions at the cellular level. Such gradients can produce very large forces, in the range 10^5–10^6 T^2 m^{-1}.[50,51] The gradients can be created, for example, by applying a strong external magnetic field to meshes of very thin (10 μm) ferromagnetic wires, or by using rare earth NdFeB magnetic thin films with 20–50 μm gaps.[50,51] A few in vitro studies carried out recently for spatially modulated magnetic fields, where very thin, micro-scale magnetic field sources were involved, showed a clear strong field–cell interaction.[34,52–55] Such locally created, both uniform and nonuniform, fields were proven to generate sufficiently large magnetically induced mechanical forces to profoundly affect cell morphology, differentiation, and functionality.[25,26]

It was also shown that the magnetic-field gradients interacting with diamagnetic structures cause an effect analogous to microgravity.[21–23] Making the surrounding medium/tissue more paramagnetic can increase magnetic force acting on cells. MRI contrast agents such as paramagnetic gadolinium will increase the magnetic force on cells due to its positive magnetic susceptibility.[55]

3.2.4 Rotational Force

The translational force acting on a biological object will reach maximum near the opening of the magnet and will vanish inside the magnet, where the field is uniform (Figure 3.1). A rotational force (torque) will be generated when the object has either susceptibility- or shape-related anisotropy and will be strongest inside the magnet. Upon careful analysis, one finds that, for the case of shape anisotropy, the torque is proportional to χ^2.[56] This makes shape-dependent alignment negligible. When the torque is due to anisotropic susceptibility, however, it will be larger. In this case, the diamagnetic object will tend to align itself such that the field points along an axial region where the susceptibility has the least negative value.

3.2.5 Lorentz Force Acting on Moving Charges

The Lorentz force is produced whenever a magnetic field interacts with moving charged particles, such as for example ionic currents flowing through a membrane. There are reports about the influence of static magnetic fields on cells, in which magnetic fields have been found to modify cell shape, structurally alter the plasma membrane, and increase the levels of intracellular Ca^{2+} current. Examples of such changes were found by Chionna *et al.*,[57] which reported that a static magnetic field strongly affects lymphocytes and U937 cells when exposed to drug-induced apoptosis.

3.3 EFFECTS OF DC MAGNETIC FIELD ON CELLS

There are contradictory data on the effects of the strong static magnetic field on cells.[16] Although some studies show that the magnetic field of strength between 1.5 and 7 T does not affect the timing of cell cycle phases, growth rate or cell proliferation other studies indicate otherwise. It seems, that the effects of the magnetic field depend very much on the type of cells used in the studies. For example, application of 0.2–1.5 T had no effect on the cell cycle and proliferation of human fetal[58] or gingival fibroblasts,[59] but decreased proliferation and increased necrosis of cultured rat astrocytes and kidney epithelial cells (Vero cell line) derived from an African green monkey.[17] A stronger

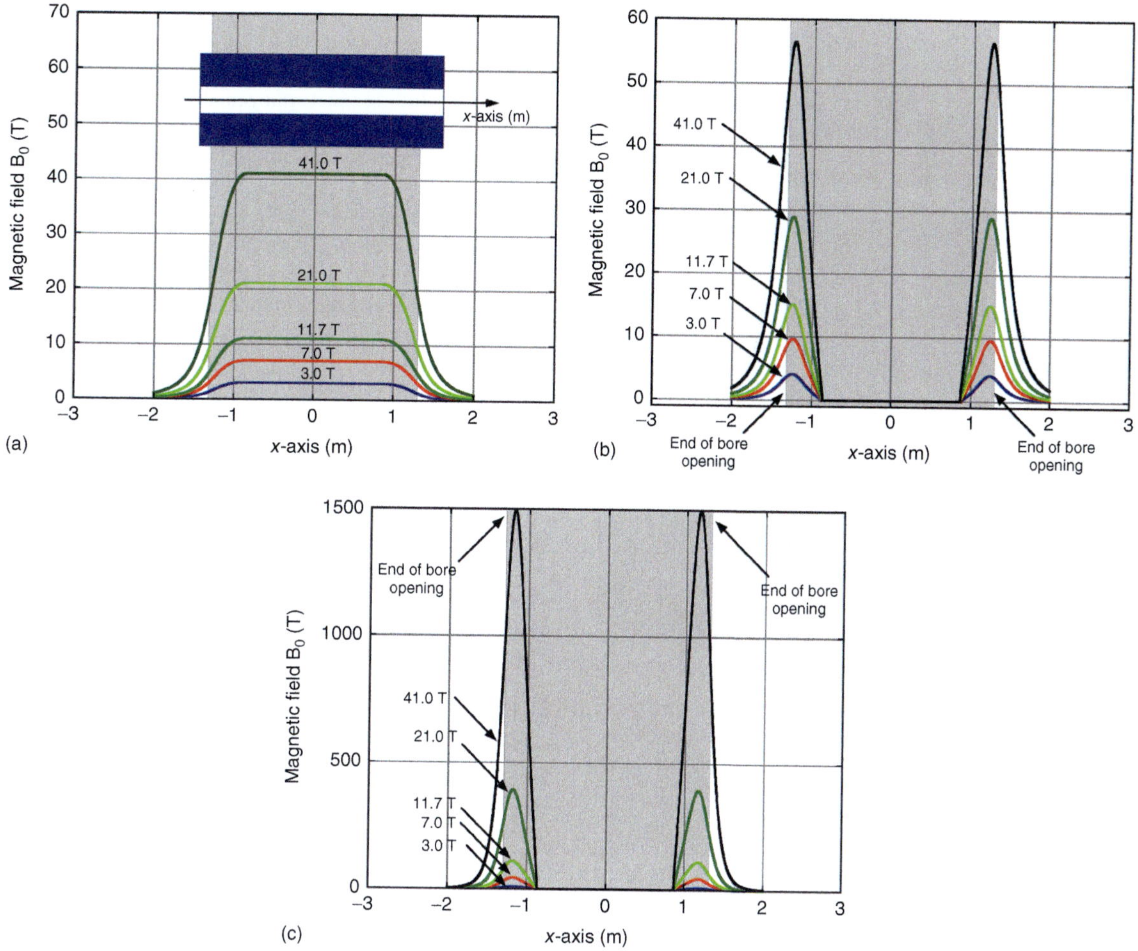

Figure 3.5. Magnetic field gradients and magnetic force products in high field magnets. A sketch of the field flux lines inside and outside (fringe field) of a solenoid is shown. Plots of the magnetic field inductance $|B_x|$ component (a); magnetic field gradient $|\nabla \vec{B}_x|$ (b); and magnetic force product $|B \cdot \nabla \vec{B}_x|$ (c) along horizontal magnet axis are shown. They were calculated for different magnetic field strength magnets. Magnets length and opening diameter were assumed to be around 3 m and 0.3 m, respectively.

field of 7–7.5 T affected proliferation and growth of human B lymphocytes from Burkitt's lymphoma (CCL86), human ovarian carcinoma (HTB77IP3), and human melanoma (HTB63) cells[18] but not of human promyeloblasts (HL60) from peripheral blood.[60] No influence of magnetic fields on cell cycle progression was noticed using conditions relevant for patients during MRI preparation and scans.[61] Exposure to a magnetic field of 10 T increased apoptosis and death of dividing (activated) but not the nondividing immune cells.[62]

There are also contradictory data on if/how the magnetic field affects cell nucleus, chromosomes, and DNA. Many studies indicate that the magnetic field of 1–10 T does not cause nuclear changes or DNA damage, does not affect chromosomal crossover and does not increase the rate of mutations in healthy cells with properly functioning anti-oxidative stress and DNA damage response.[16,63–67]

There are also reports of the effects of the strong magnetic field on the cell shape and morphology. Exposure of human skin fibroblasts (Ditroit 550

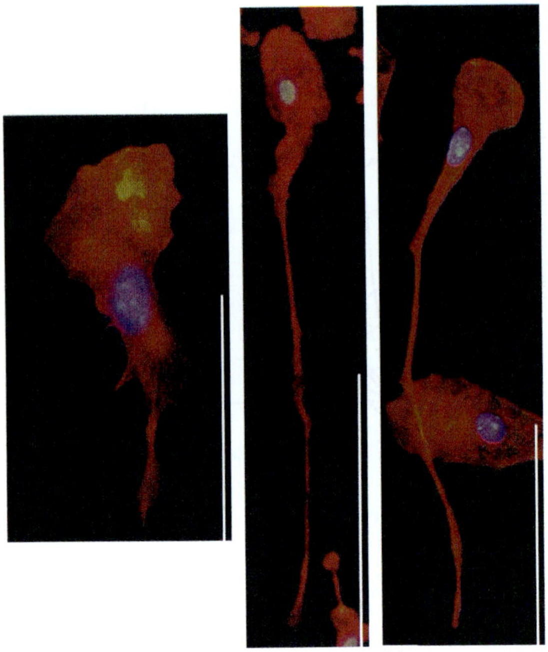

Figure 3.6. Hummingbird phenotype of magnetic field-exposed and RhoA-inhibited macrophages. Macrophages were stained with rhodamine-phalloidin (red) to visualize actin. (a) Control macrophage grown without magnetic field exposure is slightly elongated, whereas magnetic field-grown (b) and RhoA inhibited; incubated with RhoA GEF inhibitor Y16 (c) macrophages are extremely elongated, acquiring a hummingbird phenotype. Nuclei are stained with DAPI (blue). Panel a–c are merged images of actin and DAPI staining. The bar represents 50 μm in panel a and 100 μm in panel b and c. Panel b is the image from Figure 3.6 in.[42]

cell line) to 0.2 T resulted in the change of shape from a polygonal to a spindle-like, and the formation of many thin, sharp, and elongated cytoplasmic extensions.[68] The same intensity of magnetic field had also effect on the morphology of human neuronal cells (FNC-B4) causing an extensive branching.[69] Exposure of the chick embryo dorsal root ganglia (DRG) neurons to the magnetic field caused extreme elongation of their neurites,[70] and induced directional growth of neurites in the neuron-like cell culture[71] and cultured human neuronal cells.[72] In contrast, the exposure of HeLa cells and the exposure of mouse macrophages to the magnetic field of 1.2 T caused their extreme elongation (Figure 3.6).[12,42] Very often the elongation was so extensive that it led to the breakage of the cell (Figure 3.7). The shape and morphology of all eukaryotic cells, including macrophages, depend on the cellular cytoskeleton, especially on the actin cytoskeleton, which is regulated by calcium (Ca^{2+}) ion current and small GTPase RhoA pathway.[12] We showed that the magnetic field exposure changed (probably though the mechanotransduction, i.e. the force acting on the cell membrane) the distribution of calcium channel receptors (TRPM2) in the macrophages.[12]

In addition to the effects on morphology and shape of the individual cells, the magnetic field can also change the distribution of cells by aligning individual cells or the groups of cells along the direction of the magnetic field. We showed that mouse macrophages exposed to the magnetic field align in the rows or waves where the cells follow each other in the orderly fashion (Figure 3.8).[12]

The studies from other laboratories showed that erythrocytes and Schwann cells align parallel to the direction of 1–4 T and 8 T magnetic fields, respectively.[33,73,74] In contrast, human glioblastoma[75] and bull sperms[76] became oriented perpendicularly to the 10 T and 1.7 T magnetic field, respectively. Iwasaka *et al.*,[77] showed that the magnetic field of 10–14 T changed the morphology of whole colonies of muscle cells, which aligned along the direction of the magnetic field.

The question arises how the magnetic field can change the shape and/or the alignment of cells or/and groups of cells, and how is it possible that in response to the magnetic field the individual cells form rows or waves in which they follow each other? The observation from our laboratories that the exposure of mouse macrophages to the magnetic field resulted in macrophage elongation and clustering of cation channel receptors (TRPM2), which are indispensable for the proper functioning of ion homeostasis and the RhoA- and calcium-dependent polymerization of actin filaments[12,78,79] led us to propose the preliminary hypothesis that the magnetic-field forces through the mechanical distortion of cellular[60,80–82] membrane, cause clustering of calcium receptors, which in turn disrupts Ca^{2+} homeostasis and affects current-dependent actin polymerization resulting in macrophage elongation (Figure 3.6).[12,42] Studies on the effect of the magnetic field on the Ca^{2+}, ion current, and ion homeostasis indicated that even very low strength of magnetic field may have a profound effect on these processes in certain types

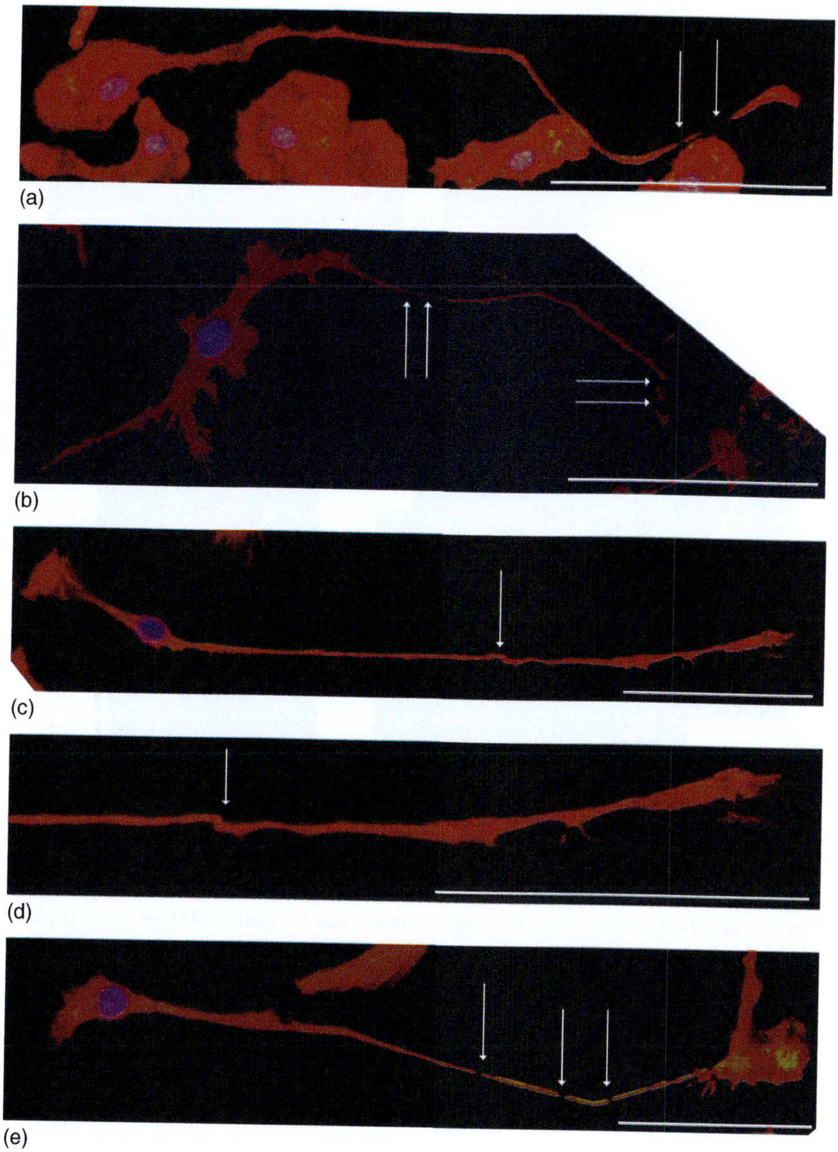

Figure 3.7. Magnetic force induced the cells breaking. (a–e) Cells stained with rhodamine-phalloidin (red) for actin. The nucleus is stained with DAPI (blue). Exposure to the magnetic field (a, b) or RhoA deletion (c–e) causes extreme elongation to the point of cell breakage (arrows). (a) Mouse peritoneal macrophage grown on the magnet for 48 h. Bar is equal to 100 μm; (b) RAW 264 cell (Abelson murine leukemia virus-transformed mouse macrophage) grown on the magnet for 72 h. Bar is equal to 50 μm; (c) RhoA-deleted mouse peritoneal macrophage. Bar is equal to 50 μm; (d) Higher magnification of the breakage point in macrophage shown in panel c. Bar is equal to 50 μm; (e) RhoA-deleted mouse peritoneal macrophage. Bar is equal to 50 μm.

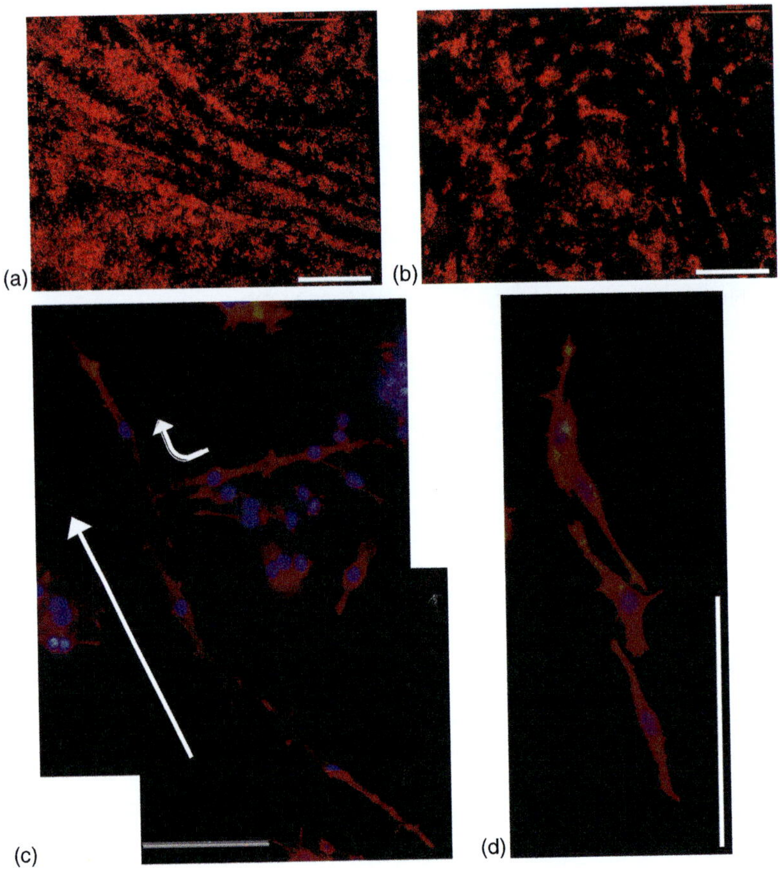

Figure 3.8. The long-range alignment of cells. (a–d) RAW 264 cells (Abelson murine leukemia virus-transformed mouse macrophages) grown on the magnet for 72 h. stained with rhodamine-phalloidin (red) for actin. The nucleus is stained with DAPI (blue); (a,b) Cells aligned in the rows (waves), which follow the magnetic force distribution pattern. (a) The area at the magnet corner, and (b) the area further away from the magnet corner. Bar is equal to 500 µm; (c,d) Higher magnification of cells following the 'leader' cell. Arrows indicate the direction of cells' movement. Bar is equal to 100 µm.

of cultured cells[16,83] but no visible effect on other cell types.[84] The mechanical (magnetic) force applied to the cell membrane acts on the mechanosensitive (stretch-gated) ion channels, which are present in the membrane of all prokaryotic and eukaryotic cells, and sense and respond to mechanical stimuli and membrane deformation.[60,80–82,85–90] The examples of the mechanosensitive channels involved in the mechanotransduction are the TRP channels, which include, mentioned earlier, TRPM2 channels.[12,42,91] Upon mechanical stimulation, the mechanosensitive-gated channels open and initiate the influx of Ca^{2+} into the cell. The effect of Ca^{2+} on actin cytoskeleton can be either direct or indirect. In the direct effect, the increase in intracellular Ca^{2+} induces actin polymerization (Figure 3.9)[92] and/or actin filament bundling.[93–95] In the indirect effect, the Ca^{2+} regulate, through the calcium activated-phosphorylating enzymes (Figure 3.9)[96–99] the activity of RhoA/Rac pathway, which is the master regulator of actin polymerization.

The explanation for the alignment of cells or groups of cells along the magnetic field forces can be deduced from the analysis of the behavior of cells during the wound healing. Studies of Gov[100] and Omelchenko *et al.*,[101] showed that the wound-healing fibroblasts form the columns of cells. Within each column,

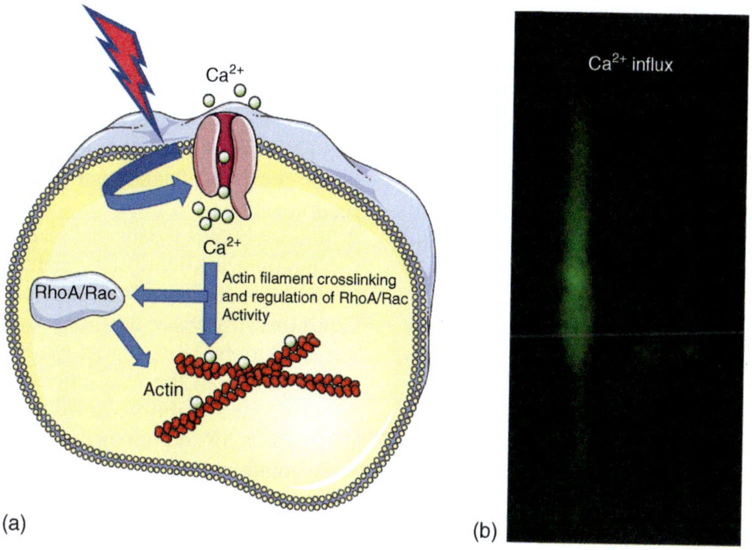

Figure 3.9. The diagram of the mechanotransduction pathway in the cell exposed to the magnetic force. (a). The magnetic (mechanical force) acting (red arrow) on the cell membrane causes the opening of stress-sensitive mechano-gated ion (including Ca^{+2}) channels. The influx of the Ca^{+2} into the cell influences, directly and indirectly, the actin filament cytoskeleton, which controls cell elongation and movement. In the direct effect, the Ca^{+2} induces actin filament crosslinking and the formation of thick actin cables. In the indirect effect, the Ca^{+2} regulates the activity of RhoA/Rac1 pathway, which in turn regulates actin polymerization/depolymerization status. (b) Image of live RAW 264.7 cells exposed to the magnet and stained with Fluo-8 AM green fluorescent calcium-binding dye (Abcam ab142773). Green color indicates Ca^{2+} influx. The cell on the left is highly elongated and brightly stained; the cell on the right is roundish and unstained. Bar is equal to 85 μm.

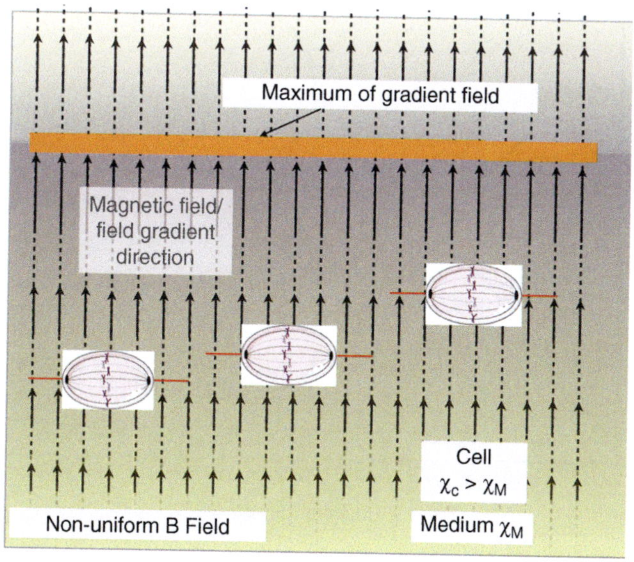

Figure 3.10. Mitotic spindles rotation by a magnetic force. The nonhomogeneous magnetic field will create the magnetic force acting on the dividing cells and moving them towards the maximum of the gradient field. In addition, due to the anisotropy of the dividing cells, a rotational force will be acting on mitotic spindles of dividing cells aligning them toward perpendicular direction relative to magnetic field lines direction.

there is a leader fibroblast, which is the first cell that reorganized its cytoskeleton, followed by the following cells, which reorganized their cytoskeletons accordingly.[12,42]

The mechanical/magnetic forces not only affect the actin cytoskeleton but also the microtubular cytoskeleton, which plays a role in cell motility, intracellular transport, and cell division. The cancer formation and metastasis depend on the uncontrolled divisions of cells and the orientation of their mitotic spindles.[102–104] Thus, the interference with the divisions of cancer cells may inhibit cancer development and/or metastasis.

Cell division occurs through the formation of the mitotic spindle, which is built of microtubules and separates chromosomes to the opposite poles of the dividing cell. The microtubules, which are the polymers of tubulin, are diamagnetically anisotropic,[19] which makes them sensitive to the magnetic field forces, and purified microtubules align along the magnetic field.[105–107] Valles *et al.*,[108] showed that the magnetic field affects spindle orientation in dividing early Xenopus embryos. Thus, in contrast to the other effects, the effect of the magnetic field on the dividing cells and spindles is undisputable and one of very few magnetic field effect consensuses.

As discussed earlier, when a diamagnetic material such as cells is placed in an inhomogeneous magnetic field then it is subjected to a translational and/or rotational force. Its magnitude is strongly dependent on the magnetic field and magnetic field gradient. The direction of this force depends on the susceptibility χ difference between cells and medium. If the surrounding medium is slightly less diamagnetic than the cell itself, it results in a positive sign of the magnetic susceptibility difference $\Delta\chi$. For positive $\Delta\chi$, cells will be attracted to the highest gradient lines.

In addition to the translational force, if cells have intrinsic susceptibility anisotropy, then either homogeneous or inhomogeneous magnetic field will exert rotational force. Such experimentally confirmed behavior is sketched in Figure 3.10 where the mitotic spindles of dividing cells exhibit tendency to be aligned perpendicular to the magnetic field/magnetic field gradient direction.

The magnetic field gradient erases division randomness and all dividing cells have longitudinal axes of the spindles oriented perpendicular to the magnetic

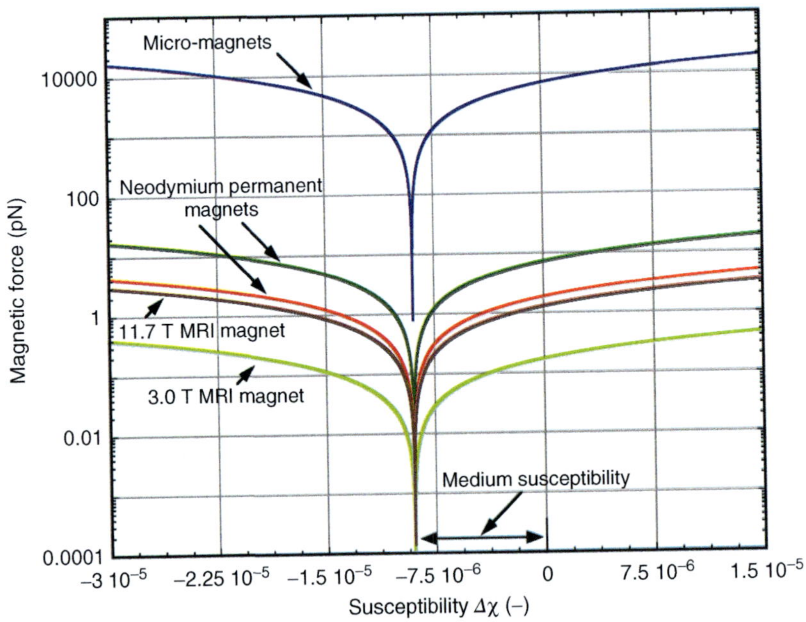

Figure 3.11. Magnetic force versus magnetic susceptibility plots. The magnetic force acting on a single cell is plotted as a function of magnetic susceptibility difference $\Delta\chi$ between a cell and medium. A typical range of susceptibility ranging from -3.5×10^{-5} till $+1.5\times10^{-5}$ was selected. Medium susceptibility was assumed to be -9.0×10^{-6} as marked on the graph. The cases of the static magnetic field gradients introducing magnetic force in 3.0 T and 11.7 T superconducting magnets are compared with such forces existing above the surface of rare-earth and micro-magnets used in in vitro experiments.

field lines. As a result of this magnetic interference, all cells will divide in the same direction. Recently Zhang *et al.*,[79] showed that the static magnetic field of 27 T aligns spindles and affects chromosomes in dividing CNE-2Z and R PE1 human cells. They also showed that the magnetic field of 27 T changes the spindle morphology. In addition, prolonged exposure to the magnetic field of 1 T causes multipolar spindles.[103] These data indicate that the magnetic field exposure may have negative consequences on any highly dividing healthy cells (such as cells in the embryos or naturally replenishing tissues) and has a potential to be used to interfere with the divisions of the cancer cells.

3.4 SUMMARY

The studies reviewed above indicate very clearly that the magnetic field gradient and a strong uniform magnetic field have a profound effect on the cellular cytoskeleton (actin filaments and tubulin microtubules) in resting and dividing cells. Figure 3.11 shows the plots of the magnetic force magnitude as a function of magnetic susceptibility. All these data indicate that with the current trend to introduce stronger and stronger MRI magnets the further studies are necessary to assess the danger of the high uniform and nonuniform magnetic fields to patients and MRI personnel. On the brighter side, there is potential to use magnetic forces for the disruption of division and metastasis of cancer cells, which would lead to new anti-cancer therapies.

ACKNOWLEDGMENT

The authors gratefully acknowledge support from the William Stamps Farish Fund, the William and Ella Owens Medical Research Foundation and the Center for Bioenergetics at Houston Methodist Research Institute.

RELATED ARTICLES IN EMAGRES

Magnetic Resonance Imaging: A Historical Overview

Safety Considerations in MRI

Garroway, Allen N.: Origins of MRI—A Personal View

Applications of Preclinical MRI/MRS in the Evaluation of Drug Efficacy and Safety

Breast Magnetic Resonance Imaging (MRI)

Hinshaw, Waldo: Notes on the History of MR Imaging from my Perspective

Koretsky, A.P.: Contributions to Functional, Cellular, and Molecular Imaging with MRI

Lauterbur, Paul C.: One Path out of Many—How MRI Actually Began

Macovski, Albert: My MRI Journey

REFERENCES

1. J. F. Schenck, *J Magn. Reson. Imag.*, 2000, **12**, 2.
2. W. Sturgeon, Oxford Dictionary of National Biography, online edn, Oxford University Press, 2004.
3. G. B. Yntema, *Phys. Rev.*, 1955:1197. DOI: 1955PhRv ... 98.1144.
4. J. E. Kunzler, E. Buehler, F. S. L. Hsu, and J. H. Wernick, *Phys. Rev. Lett.*, 1961, **7**, 215. DOI: 10.1103/PhysRevLett.7.215.
5. D. C. Larbalestier, J. Jiang, U. P. Trociewitz, F. Kametani, C. Scheuerlein, M. DalbanCanassy, M. Matras, P. Chen, N. C. Craig, P. J. Lee, and E. E. Hellstrom, *Nat. Mater.*, 2014, **13**, 375.
6. G. Majkic, E. Galstyan, and V. Selvamanickam, *IEEE T. Appl. Supercon.*, 2015, **25**, 1. DOI: 10.1109/tasc.2014.2372902.
7. M. S. NessAiver and M. N. Aiver, All You Really Need to Know About MRI Physics, 1st edn, Simply Physics, 1997. ISBN: 10:096609820X.
8. F. Schmitt, A. Potthast, B. Stoeckel, C. Triantafyllou, C. J. Wiggins, G. Wiggins, and G. Wiggins, *Bio. Magn. Reson.*, 2006, **26**, 59.
9. P. Vedrine, G. Aubert, J. Belorgey, C. Berriaud, A. Bourquard, P. Bredy, A. Donati, O. Dubois, F. Elefant, G. Gilgrass, F. P. Juster, H. Lannou, F. Molinié, M. Nusbaum, F. Nunio, A. Payn, L. Quettier, T. Schild, L. Scola, and A. Sinanna, *IEEE T. Appl. Supercon.*, 2014, **24**, 1. DOI: 10.1109/tasc.2013.2286256.
10. Administration. USFaD. A primer on medical device interactions with magnetic resonance imaging systems. [FDA Guidance Document]. U.S. Food and Drug Administration Web site. 1997. http://www.fda.gov/MedicalDevices/DeviceRegulationandGuidance/GuidanceDocuments/ucm107721.htm.

11. L. L. Tsai, A. K. Grant, K. J. Mortele, J. W. Kung, and M. P. Smith, *Radiographics*, 2015, **35**, 1722. DOI: 10.1148/rg.2015150108.
12. J. Wosik, W. Chen, K. Qin, R. M. Ghobrial, J. Z. Kubiak, and M. Kloc, *Biophys. J.*, 2018, **114**, 2001. DOI: 10.1016/j.bpj.2018.03.002.
13. J. F. Schenck, C. Dumoulin, R. Redington, H. Kressel, R. Elliott, and I. McDougall, *Med. Phys.*, 1992, **19**, 1089.
14. J. F. Schenck, *Med. Phys.*, 1996, **23**, 815. DOI: 10.1118/1.597854.
15. J. M. Theysohn, S. Maderwald, O. Kraff, C. Moenninghoff, M. E. Ladd, and S. C. Ladd, *MAGMA*, 2008, **21**, 63. DOI: 10.1007/s10334-007-0095-x.
16. J. Miyakoshi, *Prog. Biophys. Mol. Biol.*, 2005, **87**, 213. DOI: 10.1016/j.pbiomolbio.2004.08.008.
17. M. Buemi, D. Marino, G. Di Pasquale, F. Floccari, M. Senatore, C. Aloisi, F. Grasso, G. Mondio, P. Perillo, N. Frisina, and F. Corica, *Nephron*, 2001, **87**, 269. DOI: 10.1159/000045925.
18. R. R. Raylman, A. C. Clavo, and R. L. Wahl, *Bioelectromagnetics*, 1996, **17**, 358. DOI: 10.1002/(SICI)1521-186X(1996)17:5<358::AID-BEM2>3.0.CO;2-2.
19. W. Bras, J. Torbet, G. P. Diakun, G. L. Rikken, and J. F. Diaz, *J. Biophys.*, 2014, **2014**, 985082. DOI: 10.1155/2014/985082.
20. L. Zhang, Y. Hou, Z. Li, X. Ji, Z. Wang, H. Wang, X. Tian, F. Yu, Z. Yang, L. Pi, T. J. Mitchison, Q. Lu, and X. Zhang, *Elife*, 2017, **6**. DOI: 10.7554/eLife.22911.
21. E. Beaugnon and R. Tournier, *Nature*, 1991, **349**, 1. DOI: 10.7554/eLife.22911.
22. O. A. Kuznetsov and K. H. Hasenstein, *Planta*, 1996, **198**, 87.
23. M. Yamaguchi and Y. Tanimoto, in 'Magneto-Science: Magnetic Field Effects on Materials: Fundamentals and Applications, Springer Series in Materials Science', Kodansha Ltd and Springer-Verlag: Berlin Heidelberg, 2006, Vol. 89. ISBN: 978-3-540-37061-1.
24. A. K. Geim, M. D. Simon, M. I. Boamfa, and L. O. Heflinge, *Nature*, 1999, **400**, 323.
25. A.-R. Qian, X. Gao, W. Zhang, J.-B. Li, Y. Wang, S.-M. Di, L. F. Hu, and P. Shang, *PloS one*, 2013, **8**, e51036.
26. D. Shi, R. Meng, W. Deng, W. Ding, Q. Zheng, W. Yuan, L. Liu, C. Zong, P. Shang, and J. Wang, *Stem Cell Rev. Rep.*, 2010, **6**, 567.
27. O. Valiron, L. Peris, G. Rikken, A. Schweitzer, Y. Saoudi, C. Rémy, and J. Didier, *J. Magn. Reson. Imaging*, 2005, **22**, 334.
28. J. Dobson, *Nat. Nano.*, 2008, **3**, 139.
29. J. Dobson, S. H. Cartmell, A. Keramane, and A. J. E. Haj, *IEEE Trans. NanoBiosci.*, 2006, **5**, 173. DOI: 10.1109/tnb.2006.880823.
30. S. Hughes, A. J. El Haj, and J. Dobson, *Med. Eng. Phys.*, 2005, **27**, 754. DOI: 10.1016/j.medengphy.2005.04.006.
31. R. J. Mannix, S. Kumar, F. Cassiola, M. Montoya-Zavala, E. Feinstein, M. Prentiss, and D. E. Ingber, *Nat. Nano.*, 2008, **3**, 36. DOI: http://www.nature.com/nnano/journal/v3/n1/suppinfo/nnano.2007.418_S1.html.
32. N. J. Sniadecki, *Endocrinology*, 2010, **151**, 451. DOI: 10.1210/en.2009-0932.
33. Y. Eguchi, S. Ueno, C. Kaito, K. Sekimizu, and K. Shiokawa, *Bioelectromagnetics.*, 2006, **27**, 307. DOI: 10.1002/bem.20215.
34. J. M. Denegre, J. M. Valles Jr., K. Lin, W. B. Jordan, and K. L. Mowry, *Proc. Natl. Acad. Sci. U S A.*, 1998, **95**, 14729.
35. P. A. Giardini, D. A. Fletcher, and J. A. Theriot, *Proc. Natl. Acad. Sci. U S A.*, 2003, **100**, 6493. DOI: 10.1073/pnas.1031670100.
36. V. Noireaux, R. M. Golsteyn, E. Friederich, J. Prost, C. Antony, D. Louvard, and C. Sykes, *Biophys. J.*, **78**, 1643. DOI: 10.1016/S0006-3495(00)76716-6.
37. N. Q. Balaban, U. S. Schwarz, D. Riveline, P. Goichberg, G. Tzur, I. Sabanay, D. Mahalu, S. Safran, A. Bershadsky, L. Addadi, and B. Geiger, *Nat. Cell Biol.*, 2001, **3**, 466.
38. J. Stricker, Y. Aratyn-Schaus, W. Oakes Patrick, and L. Gardel Margaret, *Biophys. J.*, 2011, **100**, 2883. DOI: 10.1016/j.bpj.2011.05.023.
39. C. Grashoff, B. D. Hoffman, M. D. Brenner, R. Zhou, M. Parsons, M. T. Yang, M. L. MA, S. G. Sligar, C. S. Chen, T. Ha, and M. A. Schwartz, *Nature*, 2010, **466**, 263.
40. S. Deguchi, T. Ohashi, and M. Sato, *J. Biomech.*, 2005, **39**, 2603. DOI: 10.1016/j.jbiomech.2005.08.026.
41. V. Zablotskii, O. Lunov, S. Kubinova, T. Polyakova, E. Sykova, and A. Dejneka, *J. Phys. D: Appl. Phys.*, 2016, **49**, 493003. DOI: 10.1088/0022-3727/49/49/493003.
42. J. Wosik, M. Suarez-Villagran, J. H. Miller Jr., R. M. Ghobrial, and M. Kloc, *Immunol. Res.*, 2019. DOI: 10.1007/s12026-019-9066-3.

43. M. A. Gijs, F. Lacharme, and U. Lehmann, *Chem. Rev.*, 2010, **110**, 1518. DOI: 10.1021/cr9001929.
44. M. Kloc, X. Li, and R. Ghobrial, *J. Immuno. Biol.*, 2016, **1**, 103. DOI: 10.4172/jib.1000103.
45. H. C. Tekin, M. Cornaglia, and M. A. Gijs, *Lab. Chip.*, 2013, **13**, 1053. DOI: 10.1039/c3lc41285g.
46. Commission IE. IEC 60601-2-33, Edition 3.2 2015-06. Medical electrical equipment – Part 2-33: Particular requirements for the basic safety and essential performance of magnetic resonance equipment for medical diagnosis, 2015.
47. I. N. Weinberg, P. Y. Stepanov, S. T. Fricke, R. Probst, M. Urdaneta, D. Warnow, H. Sanders, S. C. Glidden, A. McMillan, P. M. Starewicz, and J. P. Reilly, *Med. Phys.*, 2012, **39**, 2578. DOI: 10.1118/1.3702775.
48. D. W. McRobbie, *Br. J. Radiol.*, 2012, **85**, 293. DOI: 10.1259/bjr/30146162.
49. H. Nakamura, T. Takayama, H. Uetake, N. Hirota, and A. K. Kitazawa, *Phys. Rev. Lett.*, 2005, **94**, 144501. DOI: 10.1103/PhysRevLett.94.144501.
50. D. Kelland, H. Kolm, C. de Latour, E. Maxwell, and J. Oberteuffer, in 'Superconducting Machines and Devices', Springer: Boston, MA, 1974, Vol. 1, p 581.
51. V. Zablotskii, A. Dejneka, S. Kubinova, D. Le-Roy, F. Dumas-Bouchiat, D. Givord, N. M. Dempsey, and E. Sykovál, *PLoS One*, 2013, **8**, e70416. DOI: 10.1371/journal.pone.0070416.
52. P. Kauffmann, A. Ith, D. O'Brien, V. Gaude, F. Boue, S. Combe, F. Bruckert, B. Schaack, N. M. Dempsey, V. Haguet, and G. Reyne, *Lab Chip*, 2011, **11**, 3153. DOI: 10.1039/c1lc20232d.
53. A. L. Gassner, M. Abonnenc, H. X. Chen, J. Morandini, J. Josserand, J. S. Rossier, J. M. Busnel, and H. H. Girault, *Lab Chip*, 2009, **9**, 2356. DOI: 10.1039/b901865d.
54. V Zablotskii, JMn Pastor, S Larumbe, JI Pérez-Landazábal, V Recarte, C Gómez-Polo High-Field Gradient Permanent Micromagnets for Targeted Drug Delivery with Magnetic Nanoparticles, In *AIP Conference Proceedings,* 2010, 152–7. DOI: 10.1063/1.3530005.
55. A. Winkleman, K. L. Gudiksen, D. Ryan, G. M. Whitesides, D. Greenfield, and M. Prentiss, *Appl. Phys. Lett.*, 2004, **85**, 2411. DOI: 10.1063/1.1794372.
56. F. G. Shellock, Magnetic Resonance Procedures: Health Effects and Safety, CRC Press: Boca Raton, 2001.
57. A. Chionna, M. Dwikat, E. Panzarini, B. Tenuzzo, E. C. Carla, T. Verri, H. P. Rodemann, C. D. Claussen, and S. H. Duda, *Eur. J. Histochem.*, 2003, **47**, 299.
58. J. Wiskirchen, E. F. Gronewaller, F. Heinzelmann, R. Kehlbach, E. Rodegerdts, M. Wittau, H. P. Rodemann, C. D. Claussen, and S. H. Duda, *Radiology*, 2000, **215**, 858. DOI: 10.1148/radiology.215.3.r00jn11858.
59. H. Yamaguchi, K. Hosokawa, A. Soda, H. Miyamoto, and Y. Kinouchi, *BBA – Gen. Subjects*, 1993, **1156**, 302. DOI: 10.1016/0304-4165(93)90047-C.
60. C. D. Pivetti, M. R. Yen, S. Miller, W. Busch, Y. H. Tseng, I. R. Booth, and M. H. Saier, *Microbiol. Mol. Biol. R.*, 2003, **67**, 66. DOI: 10.1128/MMBR.67.1.66-85.2003.
61. I. B. Schiffer, W. G. Schreiber, R. Graf, E. M. Schreiber, D. Jung, D. M. Rose, M. Hehn, S. Gebhard, J. Sagemüller, H. W. Spiess, F. Oesch, M. Thelen, and J. G. Hengstler, *Bioelectromagnetics*, 2003, **24**, 241. DOI: 10.1002/bem.10097.
62. H. Onodera, Z. Jin, S. Chida, Y. Suzuki, H. Tago, and Y. Itoyama, *Radiat. Res.*, 2003, **159**, 775. DOI: 10.1667/0033-7587(2003)159[0775:EOTSMF]2.0.CO;2.
63. P. Cooke and P. G. Morris, *Br. J. Radiol.*, 1981, **54**, 622. DOI: 10.1259/0007-1285-54-643-622.
64. M. Ikehata, T. Koana, Y. Suzuki, H. Shimizu, and M. Nakagawa, *Mutat. Res./Fund. Mol. M.*, 1999, **427**, 147. DOI: 10.1016/S0027-5107(99)00087-1.
65. M. Zmyślony, J. Palus, J. Jajte, E. Dziubaltowska, and E. Rajkowska, *Mutat. Res./Fund. Mol. M.*, 2000, **453**, 89. DOI: 10.1016/S0027-5107(00)00094-4.
66. Q. M. Zhang, M. Tokiwa, T. Doi, T. Nakahara, P. W. Chang, N. Nakamura, M. Hori, J. Miyakoshi, and S. Yonei, *Int. J. Radiat. Biol.*, 2003, **79**, 281. DOI: 10.1080/0955300031000096289.
67. T. Nakahara, H. Yaguchi, M. Yoshida, and J. Miyakoshi, *Radiology*, 2002, **224**, 817. DOI: 10.1148/radiol.2243011300.
68. S. Pacini, M. Gulisano, B. Peruzzi, E. Sgambati, G. Gheri, S. Gheri Bryk, S. Vannucchi, G. Polli, and M. Ruggiero, *Cancer Detect. Prev.*, 2003, **27**, 327. DOI: 10.1016/S0361-090X(03)00124-7.
69. S. Pacini, G. B. Vannelli, T. Barni, M. Ruggiero, I. Sardi, P. Pacini, and M. Gulisano, *Neurosci. Lett.*, 1999, **267**, 185. DOI: 10.1016/S0304-3940(99)00362-6.
70. N. Dubey, P. C. Letourneau, and R. T. Tranquillo, *Exp. Neurol.*, 1999, **158**, 338. DOI: 10.1006/exnr.1999.7095.
71. C. Riggio, M. P. Calatayud, M. Giannaccini, B. Sanz, T. E. Torres, R. Fernandez-Pacheco, A. Ripoli, M. R. Ibarra, L. Dente, A. Cuschieri, G. F. Goya,

and V. Raffa, *Nanomedicine*, 2014, **10**, 1549. DOI: 10.1016/j.nano.2013.12.008.

72. S. Kim, W. S. Im, L. Kang, S. T. Lee, K. Chu, and B. I. Kim, *J. Neurosci. Meth.*, 2008, **174**, 91. DOI: 10.1016/j.jneumeth.2008.07.005.

73. T. Higashi, N. Ashida, and T. Takeuchi, *Physica B*, 1997, **237-238**, 616. DOI: 10.1016/S0921-4526(97)00276-7.

74. T. Higashi, S. Sagawa, N. Ashida, and T. Takeuchi, *Bioelectromagnetics*, 1996, **17**, 335. DOI: 10.1002/(SICI)1521-186X(1996)17:4<335::AID-BEM10>3.0.CO;2-N.

75. H. Hirose, T. Nakahara, and J. Miyakoshi, *Neurosci. Lett.*, 2003, **338**, 88. DOI: 10.1016/S0304-3940(02)01363-0.

76. R. Emura, T. Takeuchi, Y. Nakaoka, and T. Higashi, *Bioelectromagnetics*, 2003, **24**, 347. DOI: 10.1002/bem.10109.

77. M. Iwasaka, J. Miyakoshi, and S. Ueno, *In Vitro Cell. Dev. Biol. Anim.*, 2003, **39**, 120. DOI: 10.1007/s11626-003-0005-0.

78. C. S. Bascom Jr., L. J. Winship, and M. Bezanilla, *Proc. Natl. Acad. Sci. U S A.*, 2018, **115**, E2869. DOI: 10.1073/pnas.1711037115.

79. L. Zhang, T. Ji, Q. Wang, K. Meng, R. Zhang, H. Yang, C. Liao, L. Ma, and J. Jiao, *Cell Physiol. Biochem.*, 2017, **43**, 1777. DOI: 10.1159/000484064.

80. V. S. Markin and F. Sachs, in 'Mechanosensitive Ion Channels, Part A. Current Topics in Membranes', Academic Press, 2007, Vol. 58, p 87.

81. C. Kung, *Nature*, 2005, **436**, 647. DOI: 10.1038/nature03896.

82. C. M. Hackney and D. N. Furness, *Am. J. Physiol.*, 1995, **268**, C1. DOI: 10.1152/ajpcell.1995.268.1.C1.

83. A. R. Liboff, S. Cherng, K. A. Jenrow, and A. Bull, *Bioelectromagnetics*, 2003, **24**, 32. DOI: 10.1002/bem.10063.

84. M. Rubio Ayala, T. Syrovets, S. Hafner, V. Zablotskii, A. Dejneka, and T. Simmet, *Biomaterials*, 2018, **163**, 174. DOI: 10.1016/j.biomaterials.2018.02.031.

85. S. Sukharev and F. Sachs, *J. Cell Sci.*, 2012, **125**, 3075. DOI: 10.1242/jcs.092353.

86. P. A. Gottlieb and F. Sachs, *Channels (Austin)*, 2012, **6**, 214. DOI: 10.4161/chan.21050.

87. F. Sachs, *Physiology (Bethesda)*, 2010, **25**, 50. DOI: 10.1152/physiol.00042.2009.

88. C. L. Bowman, P. A. Gottlieb, T. M. Suchyna, Y. K. Murphy, and F. Sachs, *Toxicon*, 2007, **49**, 249. DOI: 10.1016/j.toxicon.2006.09.030.

89. T. M. Suchyna and F. Sachs, *J. Physiol.*, 2007, **581**, 369. DOI: 10.1113/jphysiol.2006.125021.

90. V. S. Markin and F. Sachs, *Phys. Biol.*, 2004, **1**, 110. DOI: 10.1088/1478-3967/1/2/007.

91. J. Yin and W. M. Kuebler, *Cell Biochem. Biophys.*, 2010, **56**, 1. DOI: 10.1007/s12013-009-9067-2.

92. O. Dushek, S. Mueller, S. Soubies, D. Depoil, I. Caramalho, D. Coombs, and S. Valitutti, *PLoS One*, 2008, **3**, e3913. DOI: 10.1371/journal.pone.0003913.

93. N. W. Ikebuchi and D. M. Waisman, *J. Biol. Chem.*, 1990, **265**, 3392.

94. C. L. Schwebach, R. Agrawal, S. Lindert, E. Kudryashova, and D. S. Kudryashov, *J. Mol. Biol.*, 2017, **429**, 2490. DOI: 10.1016/j.jmb.2017.06.021.

95. H. Ishida, K. V. Jensen, A. G. Woodman, M. E. Hyndman, and H. J. Vogel, *Sci. Rep.*, 2017, **7**, 40662. DOI: 10.1038/srep40662.

96. C. Gonzalez-Billault, P. Munoz-Llancao, D. R. Henriquez, J. Wojnacki, C. Conde, and A. Caceres, *Cytoskeleton (Hoboken)*, 2012, **69**, 464. DOI: 10.1002/cm.21034.

97. Y. R. Jin, M. R. Cho, C. K. Ryu, J. H. Chung, D. Y. Yuk, J. T. Hong, K. S. Lee, J. J. Lee, M. Y. Lee, Y. Lim, and Y. YPI, *J. Pharmacol. Exp. Ther.*, 2005, **312**, 214. DOI: 10.1124/jpet.104.073718.

98. R. J. Gasperini, M. Pavez, A. C. Thompson, C. B. Mitchell, H. Hardy, K. M. Young, J. K. Chilton, and L. Foa, *Mol. Cell Neurosci.*, 2017, **84**, 29. DOI: 10.1016/j.mcn.2017.07.006.

99. L. Masiero, K. A. Lapidos, I. Ambudkar, and E. C. Kohn, *J. Cell Sci.*, 1999, **112**, 3205.

100. N. S. Gov, *Proc. Natl. Acad. Sci. U S A.*, 2007, **104**, 15970. DOI: 10.1073/pnas.0708037104.

101. T. Omelchenko, J. M. Vasiliev, I. M. Gelfand, H. H. Feder, and E. M. Bonder, *Proc. Natl. Acad. Sci. U S A.*, 2003, **100**, 10788. DOI: 10.1073/pnas.1834401100.

102. J. A. Knoblich, *Nat. Rev. Mol. Cell Biol.*, 2010, **11**, 849. DOI: 10.1038/nrm3010.

103. J. C. Pease and J. S. Tirnauer, *J. Cell Sci.*, 2011, **124**, 1007. DOI: 10.1242/jcs.081406.

104. V. Yong-Gonzalez, B. D. Wang, P. Butylin, I. Ouspenski, and A. Strunnikov, *Genes Cells*, 2007, **12**, 1075. DOI: 10.1111/j.1365-2443.2007.01109.x.

105. P. M. Vassilev, R. T. Dronzine, M. P. Vassileva, and G. A. Georgiev, *Bioscience Rep.*, 1982, **2**, 1025. DOI: 10.1007/BF01122171.

106. W. Bras, G. P. Diakun, J. F. Díaz, G. Maret, H. Kramer, J. Bordas, and F. J. Medrano, *Biophys. J.*, 1998, **74**, 1509. DOI: 10.1016/S0006-3495(98)77863-4.

107. N. Glade and J. Tabony, *Biophys. Chem.*, 2005, **115**, 29. DOI: 10.1016/j.bpc.2004.12.048.

108. J. M. Valles Jr., S. R. Wasserman, C. Schweidenback, J. Edwardson, J. M. Denegre, and K. L. Mowry, *Exp. Cell Res.*, 2002, **274**, 112. DOI: 10.1006/excr.2001.5456.

Chapter 4

Effect of Strong Time-varying Magnetic Field Gradients on Humans

John Nyenhuis[1] and David Gross[2]

[1]*Purdue University, West Lafayette, IN, USA*
[2]*MED Institute Inc., West Lafayette, IN, USA*

Safety and Biological Effects in MRI.
Edited by Devashish Shrivastava and J. Thomas Vaughan

ISBN: 978-1-118-82130-5
Also published in eMagRes (online edition)
DOI: 10.1002/9780470034590.emrstm1575

4.1 INTRODUCTION

The time-varying magnetic field gradients in a magnetic resonance imaging (MRI) system expose patients to time-varying magnetic (d*B*/d*t*) fields of audio frequency. The corresponding induced electric fields may be of sufficient intensity to induce peripheral nerve stimulation (PNS) in patients. Regulatory standards limit the gradient intensity to avoid painful stimulation.

The time-varying magnetic field gradients can also interact with implanted medical devices. The interactions may be due to direct exposure of the device to time-varying magnetic field d*B*/d*t*. Interactions of this type include heating due to induction of eddy currents and mechanical vibration due to torque from eddy currents and the static magnetic field. The interactions may also be due to the exposure of the devices to induced eddy currents in the body. These interactions may be most significant for electrically active implants with lead wires (e.g., cardiac pacemakers).

In this chapter, we undertake the following:

1. Describe MRI gradient coils and the associated magnetic field patterns.
2. Calculate the electric fields that are induced in an ASTM F2182 phantom and the patient.
3. Summarize measurements of physiologic interactions of the time-varying gradients with the patient.

4. Discuss potential for cardiac stimulation by the time-varying gradients.
5. Discuss regulatory limits on the time-varying gradients.
6. Briefly discuss interactions of the time-varying gradients with implanted medical devices.

4.2 DESCRIPTIONS OF MRI GRADIENT COILS

Time-varying current in MRI gradient coils produces variation in the intensity of the static field B_0 in the three principal directions. The spatial variation in B_0 results in a change in frequency of precessing spins, and these changes are used for purposes of slice selection, frequency encode, and phase encode. We assume B_0 to be in the z-direction.

$$G_x = \frac{\partial B_z}{\partial x}, \quad G_y = \frac{\partial B_z}{\partial y}, \quad G_z = \frac{\partial B_z}{\partial z} \tag{4.1}$$

The gradients G_x, G_y, and G_z will be approximately uniform over the imaging volume. The slew rate is defined as the time derivative of the gradient intensity, with $S_x = \mathrm{d}G_x/\mathrm{d}t$ and similarly for S_y and S_z. The technical specification for the MR system provides the maximal slew rate in the three gradient axes. This quantity has units of $\mathrm{T\,m^{-1}\,s^{-1}}$ and is defined at the isocenter. Another relevant parameter for gradient interactions is the minimal ramp time from the maximal negative gradient amplitude to maximal positive gradient amplitude. The time-varying magnetic field $\mathrm{d}B/\mathrm{d}t$ at some point in the scanner will be proportional to the slew rate. The time-varying magnetic fields may be expressed as:

$$\begin{pmatrix} \dfrac{\mathrm{d}B_x}{\mathrm{d}t} \\ \dfrac{\mathrm{d}B_y}{\mathrm{d}t} \\ \dfrac{\mathrm{d}B_z}{\mathrm{d}t} \end{pmatrix} = \begin{pmatrix} f_{xx} & f_{xy} & f_{xz} \\ f_{yx} & f_{yy} & f_{yz} \\ f_{zx} & f_{zy} & f_{zz} \end{pmatrix} \begin{pmatrix} S_x \\ S_y \\ S_z \end{pmatrix} \tag{4.2}$$

where the elements of the f matrix are functions of position inside the bore. In the imaging region of uniform gradients,

$$f_{xx}(0,0,z) = f_{yy}(0,0,z) = f_{zz}(0,0,z) = z \quad \text{(in imaging regions)}$$

Other terms in the f matrix in the imaging region are negligible.

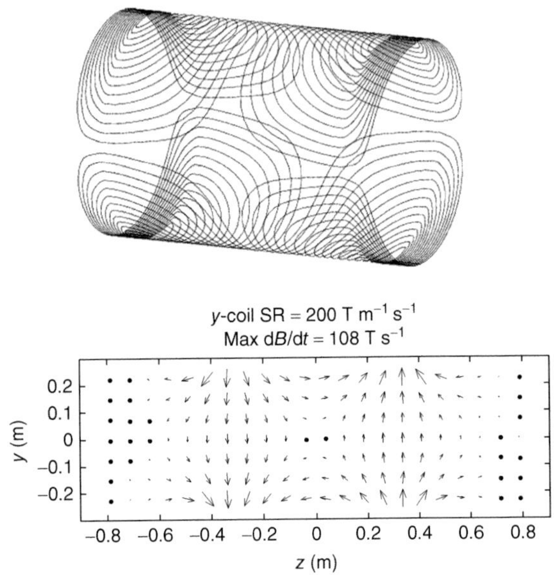

Figure 4.1. Model for a y-gradient coil and $\mathrm{d}B/\mathrm{d}t$ map at a slew rate of $200\,\mathrm{T\,m^{-1}\,s^{-1}}$. Maximum $\mathrm{d}B/\mathrm{d}t$ at a radial distance of 25 cm from the centerline is $108\,\mathrm{T\,s^{-1}}$. At a radial distance of 20 cm, $\mathrm{d}B/\mathrm{d}t = 75.1\,\mathrm{T\,s^{-1}}$

Figure 4.1 depicts a y-gradient coil and the associated magnetic field pattern. (The y-gradient coil pattern was developed by Jonathon Edmonson of Medtronic.) Near the isocenter, the magnetic field is along z. With increasing distance from the isocenter, the y-component in B increases in magnitude, and the maximum intensity of B_y occurs at z approximately ± 35 cm. The x-gradient coil is the same as the y-coil, but rotated by 90°.

Figure 4.2 depicts a z-gradient coil and the associated magnetic field pattern.[1] For this coil, B_z is a maximum at a distance of approximately 38 cm from the centerline.

The winding patterns in Figures 4.1 and 4.2 represent unshielded gradient coils. Shielded coils have an additional metal pattern on a second cylinder of greater radius. A shielded coil has a reduced magnetic field outside of the bore and will induce fewer eddy currents in the inner wall of the magnet and other components of the MR system.

Note that the terms of the f matrix in equation (4.2) for a practical whole-body MR system will be similar inside the imaging volume. Thus, gradient coils with similar diameter and field of view are expected to generate similar $\mathrm{d}B/\mathrm{d}t$ distributions in the bore and induced electric fields in the patient. Outside the imaging

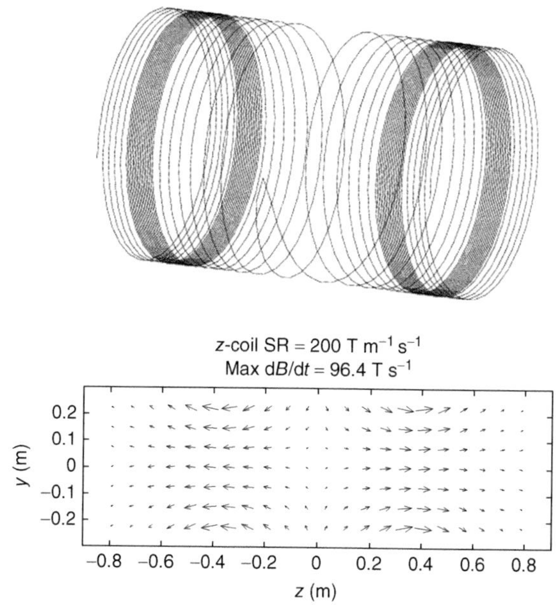

Figure 4.2. Model for a *z*-gradient coil and d*B*/d*t* map at a slew rate of $200\,\mathrm{T\,m^{-1}\,s^{-1}}$. Maximum d*B*/d*t* at a radial distance of 25 cm from the centerline is $96.4\,\mathrm{T\,s^{-1}}$. At a radial distance of 20 cm, d*B*/d*t* = $77.7\,\mathrm{T\,s^{-1}}$

volume, and especially near the wall of the bore, the terms of the *f* matrix may depend on the details of the gradient coil design (e.g., shielded vs unshielded).

Figure 4.3 depicts the representative current, *I*, and d*I*/d*t* through windings of a gradient coil. The gradient strength is proportional to the current in the windings, and d*B*/d*t* is proportional to the time derivative of the coil current. The purpose of the gradient amplifier is to produce currents in the windings of the coil. The load posed by a gradient coil is both resistive and inductive. Peak power delivered by the gradient amplifier is of the order of kilowatts.

A switched amplifier may be used to produce the gradient waveforms. Figure 4.4 shows the d*B*/d*t* that was measured with a search coil during a linear ramp in a GE 3 T MR system. d*B*/d*t* ranges from approximately 0 to $40\,\mathrm{T\,s^{-1}}$ with a waveform period of 16.2 μs.

Since the currents in the gradient coils change with time, the patient is exposed to a time-varying magnetic field, with representative effective frequency of a few kilohertz. The maximum d*B*/d*t* at a radial distance of 20 cm from the axial centerline for the *x*-, *y*-, and *z*-gradient coils will be about 0.4 m times the slew rate. In a cylindrical bore MR system, typical maximum slew rate S_{max} per axis ranges from 100 to $200\,\mathrm{T\,m^{-1}\,s^{-1}}$. For $S_{max} = 200\,\mathrm{T\,m^{-1}\,s^{-1}}$, maximum d*B*/d*t* at radial distance of 20 cm will be about $80\,\mathrm{T\,s^{-1}}$ for *x*-, *y*-, and *z*-gradient coils. At a radial distance of 25 cm, maximum d*B*/d*t* will be about $100\,\mathrm{T\,s^{-1}}$ for the *z* coil and about $110\,\mathrm{T\,s^{-1}}$ for the *x*- and *y*-gradient coils. The actual maximum d*B*/d*t* will depend on the details of the coil-winding pattern. Table A2 in ISO/TS 10974, 2nd Edition,[2] presents maximum d*B*/d*t* in gradient coils at a slew rate of $200\,\mathrm{T\,m^{-1}\,s^{-1}}$ for different radial distances.

Hardware limits on gradient output are described in the MR compatibility data sheet that is provided by the manufacturer of the MR system. Annex D of ISO/TS 10974 presents a survey of gradient outputs for several clinical MR systems. For the systems that are considered, the maximum available slew rate is $200\,\mathrm{T\,m^{-1}\,s^{-1}}$, and the maximum gradient amplitude is $45\,\mathrm{mT\,m^{-1}}$. Thus, for these systems, assuming that the gradient on an axis is switched from −45 to $+45\,\mathrm{mT\,m^{-1}}$, the maximum slew rate may be applied for a pulse duration of 450 μs. The maximum slew rate is determined by the voltage limit of the gradient amplifier, and the maximum gradient amplitude is determined by the current limit.

4.3 CALCULATION OF ELECTRIC FIELD AND d*B*/d*t* IN THE ASTM PHANTOM

The so-called ASTM phantom is used for testing of implants in an MR system and is described in ASTM F2182-11a.[3] It has a rectangular container with dimensions for the phantom materials of 65 cm long, 42 cm wide, and 9 cm deep. This phantom couples with the time-varying magnetic field, at both RF and gradient frequencies, to produce a background electric field that serves for in vitro testing of medical implants.

Calculations of induced electric fields in the phantom and the patient that are presented here were performed with a relaxation algorithm, similar to that described by Liu *et al.*[4] The body or phantom in the coil was modeled by 5 mm cubic voxels. Each of the voxels is a circuit element in which the sum of currents entering from neighboring voxels is zero. A time-varying current of 1 A at 1 kHz was assumed in the winding of the coil. The driving electric field *e* force in each cube is:

$$e = -j\omega \frac{\mathrm{d}\mathbf{A}}{\mathrm{d}t} d \tag{4.3}$$

where *ω* is the angular frequency, **A** is the magnetic vector potential, and *d* is the voxel dimension.

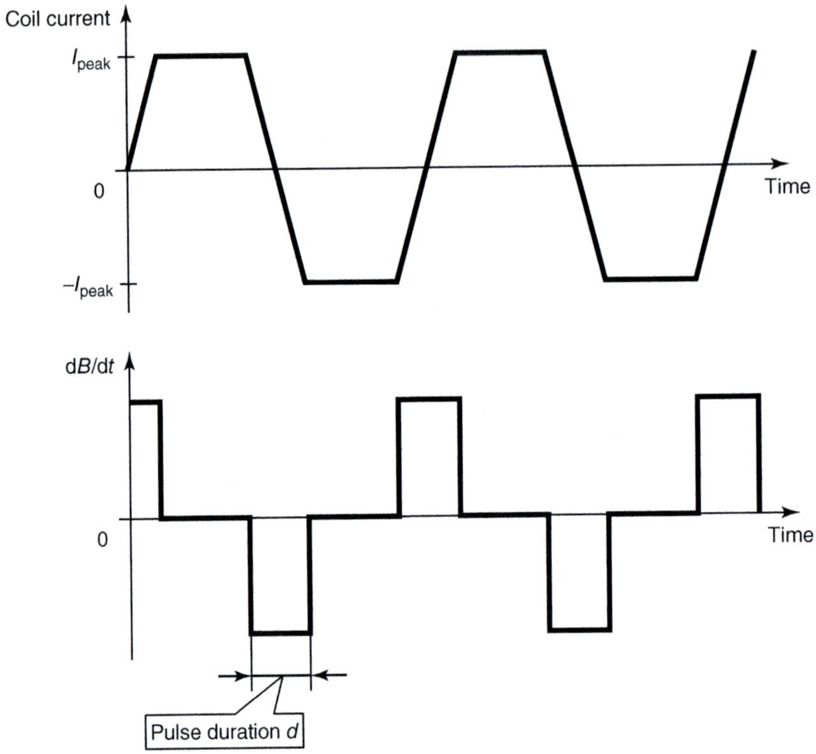

Figure 4.3. Waveforms for current and dB/dt for a gradient coil. The gradient strength is proportional to the current in the windings, and dB/dt is proportional to the time derivative of the coil current

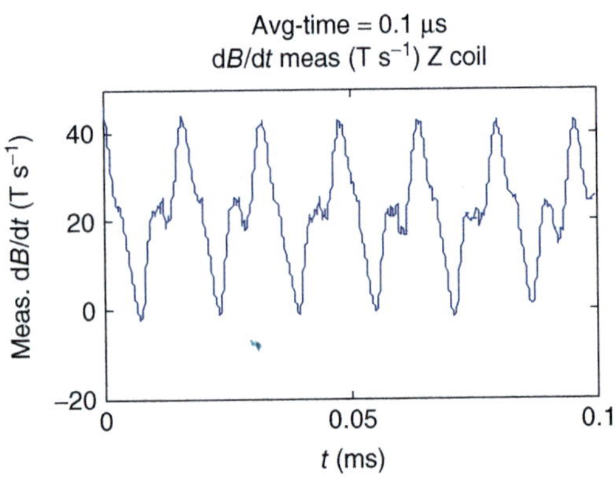

Figure 4.4. dB/dt during a linear ramp for a switched amplifier. Measurement made with a search coil in a GE 3 T system. Sample window for the measurement is 0.1 ms. Period of waveform is 16.2 µs

For the calculation of the vector potential, the coil is divided into line segments, and the magnetic vector potential is obtained as described by Nyenhuis *et al.*[5] Consider a straight line carrying a current I along vector $\mathbf{L}$ from (x_1, y_1, z_1) to (x_2, y_2, z_2). The evaluation point $\mathbf{P}$ is (x, y, z), and vector $\mathbf{r}$ connects (x_1, y_1, z_1) to (x, y, z). The vector potential is then:

$$\mathbf{A}(x, y, z) = \frac{\mu_0 I \mathbf{L}}{4\pi L} \ln \left[\frac{|\mathbf{L} - \mathbf{r}| + L - \frac{\mathbf{L}\cdot\mathbf{r}}{L}}{r - \frac{\mathbf{L}\cdot\mathbf{r}}{L}} \right] \quad (4.4)$$

Figure 4.5 shows the calculated induced electric field in the ASTM phantom with the top of the phantom at the center of the y-coil in Figure 4.1 (i.e., landmark LM = 0). The electric field pattern is primarily due to the y-component of dB/dt. The most intense electric field occurs near the side of the walls. For the assumed slew $S_y = 200\,\mathrm{T\,m^{-1}\,s^{-1}}$, maximum electric field intensity in the phantom is $7.1\,\mathrm{V\,m^{-1}}$. In contrast, in an ASTM F2182-11a heating test, a representative maximum specific absorption rate (SAR) in the phantom is $10\,\mathrm{W\,kg^{-1}}$, which corresponds to an rms electric field of $146\,\mathrm{V\,m^{-1}}$.

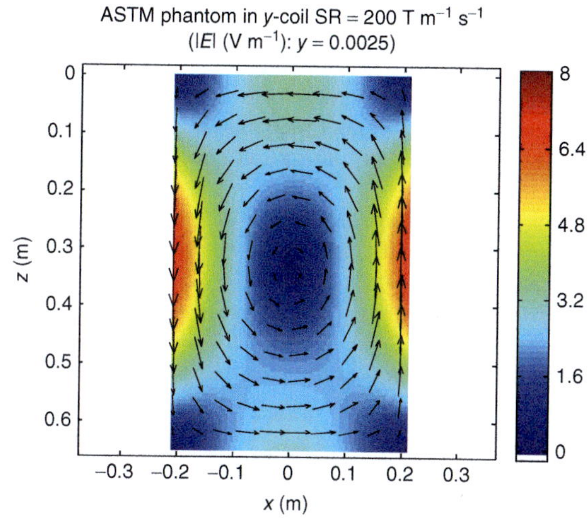

Figure 4.5. Electric field intensity in the ASTM phantom inside the y-coil. The top of the phantom is longitudinally centered in the coil. The conductivity of phantom material is $0.47\,\mathrm{S\,m^{-1}}$

Figure 4.6 shows $\mathrm{d}B_y/\mathrm{d}t$ in the midplane of the phantom. The maximum intensity is $51.3\,\mathrm{T\,s^{-1}}$, and this occurs at a distance of approximately 30 cm from the isocenter.

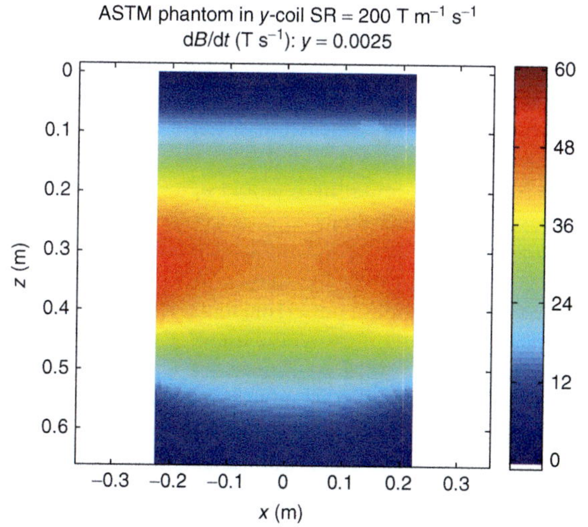

Figure 4.6. $\mathrm{d}B_y/\mathrm{d}t$ in vertical centerline of ASTM phantom inside y-gradient coil. The top of the phantom is longitudinally centered in the coil. Slew rate = $200\,\mathrm{T\,m^{-1}\,s^{-1}}$. Maximum $\mathrm{d}B_y/\mathrm{d}t$ is $51.3\,\mathrm{T\,s^{-1}}$

The electric field pattern in Figure 4.5 can be used to design tests for gradient exposure of implants. The implant is exposed to the most intense electric field when it is near the wall of the phantom. For example, greatest coupling will occur with the implant near the wall of the phantom with its long axis parallel to the wall. If the implant is active with a lead wire, maximum induced voltage occurs for the lead wire parallel to the wall of the phantom.

4.4 GRADIENT-INDUCED ELECTRIC FIELD IN THE PATIENT

In this section, we calculate the electric fields that are induced in the patient by the gradient-induced $\mathrm{d}B/\mathrm{d}t$. The virtual human model Hugo was used and is derived from the US National Library of Medicine Visible Human project.

Figure 4.7 shows sections of the Hugo model. Table 4.1 lists the conductivities for principal tissues

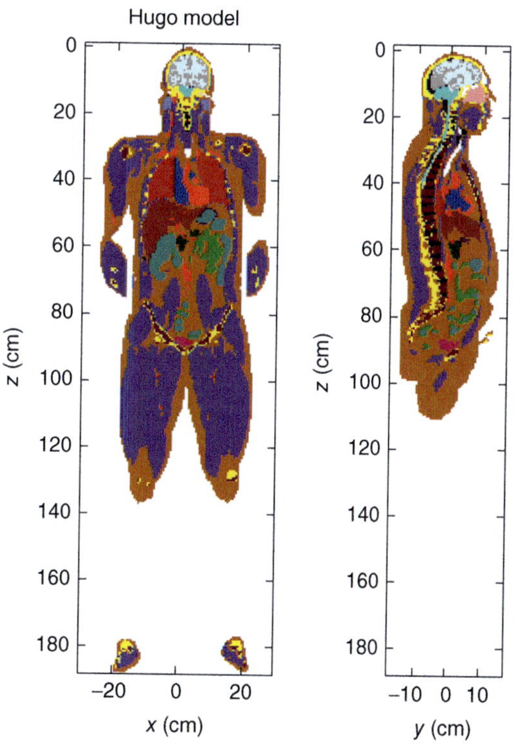

Figure 4.7. Hugo model for calculation of gradient-induced voltage

Table 4.1. Conductivity values in the Hugo model for the calculations in this chapter

Tissue	Conductivity ($S\,m^{-1}$)
Fat	0.022
Cortical bone	0.0202
Muscle	0.321
Blood	0.7
Right ventricle	0.11
Left ventricle	0.11
Right atrium	0.11
Right ventricle	0.11
Brain – white	0.063
Brain – gray	0.099
Cerebellum	0.03

for the calculations. Figure 4.8 shows the electric field intensity at the centerline for Hugo placement in the *x*-, *y*-, and *z*-gradient coils. The greatest electric field intensity tends to occur at the periphery of the body.

Figure 4.9 plots the 99.5 percentile electric field vs the landmark for fat in Hugo. The greatest electric fields occur for the *y*-coil at landmarks of 60 and 70 cm, which correspond to the approximate level of the umbilicus being at the center of the coil. At the slew rate of $200\,T\,m^{-1}\,s^{-1}$, maximum electric fields for the *x*-, *y*-, and *z*-gradient coils are 10.9, 20.0, and $13.7\,V\,m^{-1}$, respectively.

Figure 4.10 plots the 99.5 percentile electric field vs the landmark for muscle in Hugo. As for fat, the greatest electric fields occur for the *y*-coil. However, the maximum electric field of $5.9\,V\,m^{-1}$ is less than the one-third of the maximum electric field of $20\,V\,m^{-1}$ for fat.

Similarly, Figure 4.11 plots the 99.5 percentile electric field vs the landmark for the heart. The maximum electric field of $7.6\,V\,m^{-1}$ occurs for the *y*-gradient coil.

Figure 4.12 plots the 99.5 percentile electric field vs the landmark for the brain. The electric field intensities vs landmark range from approximately 2 to $4\,V\,m^{-1}$, with a maximum of $4.5\,V\,m^{-1}$ for the *y*-coil at a landmark in the head.

Table 4.2 lists maximum calculated 99.5 percentile electric fields for different tissues in the Hugo model.

Discussion on the plots of 99.5 percentile electric field vs landmark is as follows. Electric fields in fat are greater than in muscle owing to the lower electrical conductivity of fat. At planar interfaces between two materials, the normal component of the current density and the tangential component of electric field are continuous. The geometry of the fat and electric field distribution is of course complex. However, the greater conductivity of muscle, which in these calculations is 14.6 times greater than that of fat, results in fat having a considerably larger maximum electric field than muscle.

The intensity of electric field in the heart is important for understanding the potential for cardiac stimulation. The maximum electric field in the heart is $7.6\,V\,m^{-1}$ versus a maximum of $5.9\,V\,m^{-1}$ in muscle. It is possible that the calculated electric field for the heart is an overestimate given that the conductivity in the calculation is $0.11\,S\,m^{-1}$, which is likely less than the true value.

Electric field in the brain is less than in other tissues. This is likely a consequence of the diameter of the head being less than the effective diameter of the torso.

4.5 PERIPHERAL NERVE STIMULATION IN THE PATIENT BY INTENSE PULSED GRADIENTS

It was observed experimentally and predicted theoretically somewhat early in the history of clinical MRI that modern gradient coil hardware may produce dB/dt intensity sufficient to induce a physiological response. The lowest level of response will be PNS, the lowest level sensation which can be felt by the patient. The first report of physiological response was perhaps by Cohen *et al.*[6] who reported sensation in the noses of subjects exposed to transverse gradients in a prototype fast scan system. Another early report was by Budinger *et al.*[7] who reported neuromuscular stimulation by rapidly oscillating gradient fields created by an experimental echo planar gradient coil. A stimulus of about twice the sensation induced pain. Ueno *et al.*[8] made a coil to fit over the human head and applied a train of 64 trapezoidal pulsed currents, which produced rectangular dB/dt pulses with a duration d of 200 μs. A threshold of $80–100\,T\,s^{-1}$ was observed for sensation in the middle of the forehead.

Ham *et al.*[9] measured stimulation thresholds vs risetime for volunteers for a bipolar gradient waveform with gradient coils energized either singly or simultaneously. At a 200 μs risetime, stimulation threshold for a single *y*-coil was $dB/dt = 43\,T\,s^{-1}$. With three axes simultaneously energerized, the threshold dB/dt was $57\,T\,s^{-1}$. Abart *et al.*[10] studied PNS with the *y*-gradient in 113 human subjects with a sinusoidally

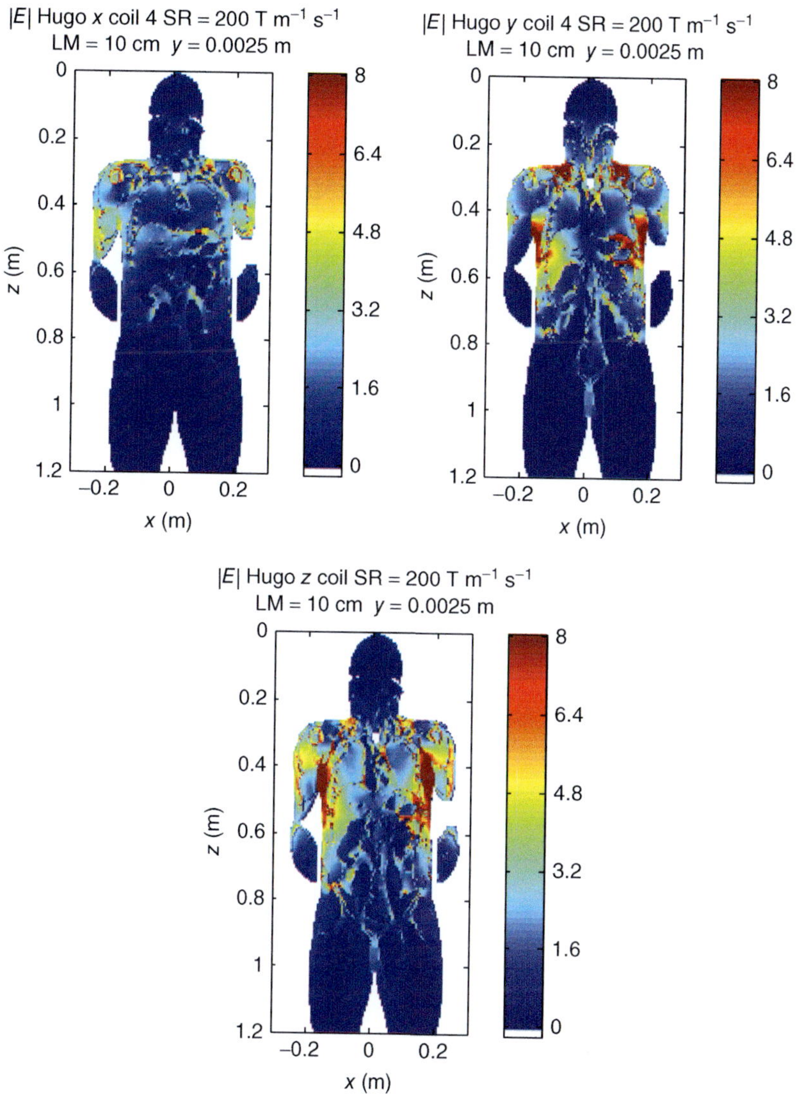

Figure 4.8. Electric field distribution in center plane for Hugo for x, y, and z-gradient coils. Landmark is 10 cm, i.e. section of Hugo 10 cm below the top of the head at the coil center

ramped gradient with a period of 1200 μs and effective ramp time of 300 μs. The sensation thresholds were expressed in millitesla per meter units, but the mean threshold can be inferred to be about 45 T s^{-1}. Studies of stimulation thresholds were also undertaken by Ehrhardt *et al.*[11] and Frese *et al.*[12]

Hebrank *et al.*[13] measured PNS thresholds for a y-coil in 65 volunteers at eight pulse durations from 200 to 1000 μs. The thresholds ranged from 24.3 T s^{-1} at a duration of 1000 μs to 57.6 T s^{-1} at a duration of 1000 μs.

Schaefer *et al.*[14] measured PNS thresholds for trapezoidal pulse trains in a whole-body cylindrical coil. z-Axis sensation thresholds at a pulse duration of 200 μs ranged from 50 to 100 T s^{-1}. Stimulation sites included the scapula and other sites on the back, bridge of the nose, upper arms, legs, hands, buttocks, head, and xyphoid. For the AP (y) gradient, clasping

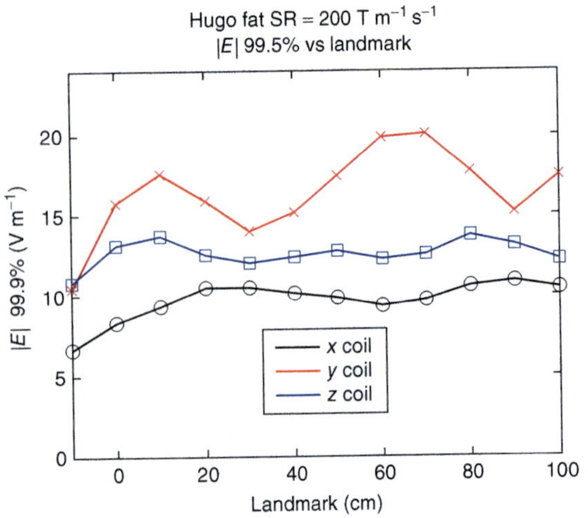

Figure 4.9. 99.5th percentile magnitude of gradient-induced electric field in the fat of Hugo. The slew rate is $200\,\mathrm{T\,m^{-1}\,s^{-1}}$

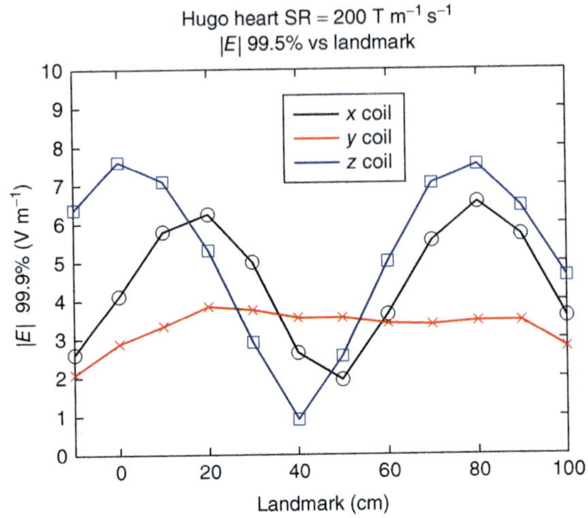

Figure 4.11. 99.5th percentile magnitude of gradient-induced electric field in the heart of Hugo. The slew rate is $200\,\mathrm{T\,m^{-1}\,s^{-1}}$

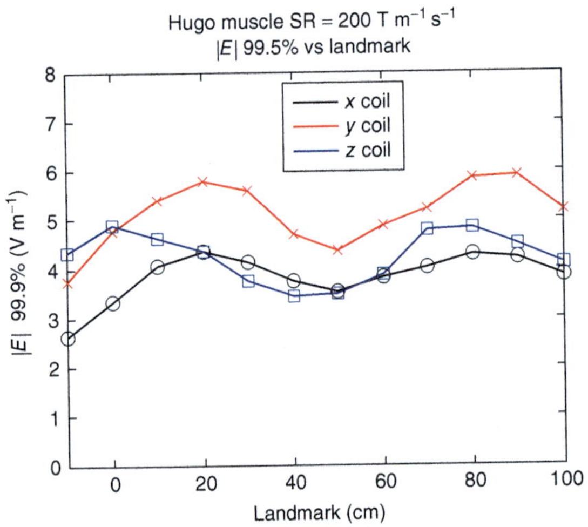

Figure 4.10. 99.5th percentile magnitude of gradient-induced electric field in the muscle of Hugo. The slew rate is $200\,\mathrm{T\,m^{-1}\,s^{-1}}$

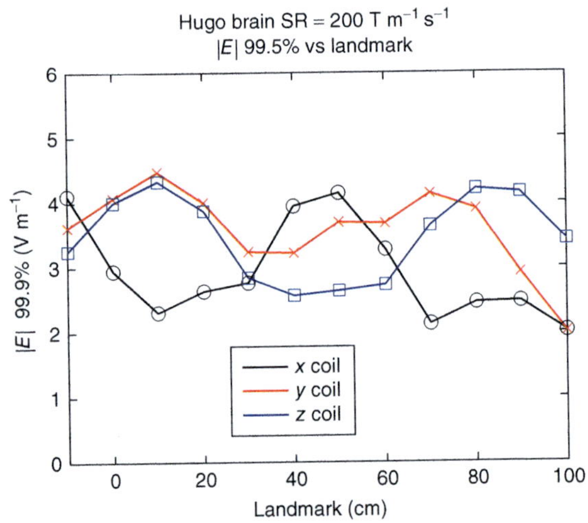

Figure 4.12. 99.5th percentile magnitude of gradient-induced electric field in the brain of Hugo. The slew rate is $200\,\mathrm{T\,m^{-1}\,s^{-1}}$

of the hands caused an approximately 30% reduction in the threshold.

Zhang *et al*. measured PNS properties of head and body gradient coils of various sizes.[15] It was found that the average stimulation threshold increases while gradient-region-of-uniformity size decreases. Also minimum slew rate and gradient step for stimulation were found to vary inversely with the diameter of the homogeneous gradient spherical volume.

Chronik and collaborators reported on stimulation by pulsed gradients in a series of papers.[16–18] Schaefer *et al.*[19] provided a detailed review of the present understanding of patient safety in time-varying gradient fields in MRI.

Table 4.2. Maximum calculated 99.5 percentile electric fields in units of $V\,m^{-1}$ in the Hugo model for the gradient coils

Tissue	Maximum 99.5%. $\|E\|$ for x-coil	Maximum 99.5%. $\|E\|$ for y-coil	Maximum 99.5%. $\|E\|$ for z-coil
Fat	10.9	20.0	13.7
Muscle	4.3	5.9	4.9
Heart	6.5	3.8	7.6
Brain	4.1	4.5	4.3

Slew rate is $200\,T\,m^{-1}\,s^{-1}$, and coils are those shown in Figures 4.1 and 4.2.

Den Boer *et al.*[20] made a comparison of the threshold for PNS during gradient switching in whole-body MR systems. The conclusion was, when expressed in the appropriate format, the thresholds for PNS in volunteers for whole-body MR equipment can be described with a hyperbolic threshold curve with rheobase 18.8 ± 0.6 T s and chronaxie 0.36 ± 0.02 ms.

Bourland *et al.* from Purdue University performed a study of stimulation by MRI pulsed gradient fields in 84 human subjects.[21,22] Trains of 128 rectangular d*B*/d*t* pulses similar to those used in echo planar imaging were applied with coils simulating the magnetic field patterns produced by MRI z- and y-gradient coils. Pulse durations ranged from 50 to 1000 μs. The amplitude of d*B*/d*t* vs pulse width was measured for the physiological endpoints of sensation (score = 1), discomfort (score = 5), and intolerance (score = 10). The experimental data were fitted to the Lapique[23,24] (hyperbolic) form of the strength duration relationship to determine the population average and standard deviation for physiologic response:

$$\frac{dB}{dt} = b\left(1 + \frac{c}{d}\right) \tag{4.5}$$

where b represents the rheobase for long duration pulses, c is chronaxie, and d is the duration of a rectangular pulse. Figure 4.13 shows responses for a subject in the Purdue study on physiologic effects of pulsed gradients. The points are d*B*/d*t* values vs duration of a single pulse in the 128 pulse train. The curves are fit according to equation (4.5) and the indicated rheobase b and chronaxie c values. Figure 4.14 shows rank-ordered intensities required from the Purdue study to achieve response scores of 1, 5, and 10 for y-thresholds at a pulse duration of 300 μs for the y-coil. Approximately, uncomfortable stimulation (score = 5) required d*B*/d*t* that is about 50% above the threshold level (score = 1), and painful stimulation (score = 10) required d*B*/d*t* that is twice the threshold level. Table 2.2 in Ref. 22 lists population median rheobases calculated from the d*B*/d*t* intensity for the Purdue study. A chronaxie of 380 μs described well the response vs pulse duration thresholds. The rheobase for PNS was $18.8\,T\,s^{-1}$ for the y-gradient coil and $28.8\,T\,s^{-1}$ for the z-coil. These d*B*/d*t* values were evaluated at a radial distance of 20 cm from the axes of the coils.

So *et al.* undertook the calculation of the electric fields in the patient for the coils used in the Purdue gradient study.[25] Table 4.3 lists the calculated electric fields in fat at the rheobase levels for PNS in the Purdue study. For the So calculations, the 99.5 percentile electric fields in fat for the y and z coils were 4.4 and $4.6\,V\,m^{-1}$. The rheobase electric fields based on calculations in Hugo as described above agree to within 14%. Given the differences in coil geometry, human model, and electrical properties for tissues, the agreement in electric fields in fat for the two calculations is considered to be good.

4.6 POTENTIAL FOR CARDIAC STIMULATION IN THE PATIENT BY INTENSE PULSED GRADIENTS

Early in the development of fast-scan MRI, there was concern that the heart could be at risk with respect to stimulation by the pulsed gradients. Accordingly, Bourland and collaborators[22,26,27] measured thresholds for cardiac stimulation (induction of ectopic beats) by pulsed magnetic fields in anesthetized dogs. The coils they used induced eddy currents similar to what would be induced by MRI transverse and z-gradient coils. Because of the very high intensities of d*B*/d*t* that are required for cardiac stimulation, only single pulses of d*B*/d*t* were applied. The projected median threshold for a pulse duration of 530 μs was $2700\,T\,s^{-1}$. Assuming a representative cardiac chronaxie of 3 ms and scaling the numbers to typical human geometry result in an estimate of 0.43 T for the minimal ramp in magnetic field for a typical human subject. The lowest 1-percentile is projected to require a minimal ramp of 0.215 T. This ramp is more than a factor of 5 greater than the ramp that would cause significant discomfort to the patient. At a duration of 450 μs, a ramp of 0.215 T corresponds to d*B*/d*t* in a rectangular pulse of $478\,T\,s^{-1}$.

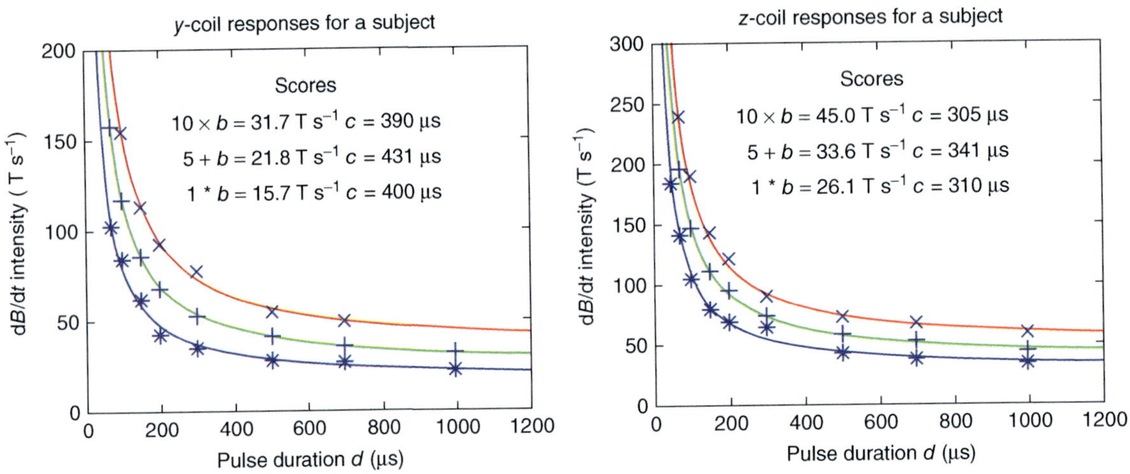

Figure 4.13. Responses for a subject in the Purdue study on physiologic effects of pulsed gradients

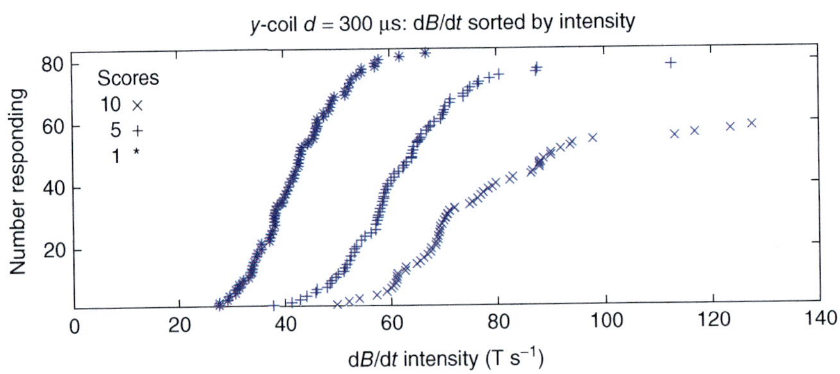

Figure 4.14. Rank-ordered intensities required from the Purdue study to achieve response scores of 1, 5, and 10 at a pulse duration of 300 μs for the *y*-coil

Reilly used the results from his SENN model and the results from a number of studies to predict electric thresholds for nerve and cardiac stimulation.[28] He predicted that rheobase electric field thresholds for PNS and the 1-percentile cardiac thresholds will both be about $6.2\,\mathrm{V\,m^{-1}}$.

Several investigators have undertaken calculation of the induced eddy currents in the heart due to pulsed magnetic fields. Ragan *et al.*[29] determined the fields and currents induced by a time-varying magnetic field produced by a pair of coplanar coils that had been shown to cause irregular heart beats in canines. An electric field of about $100\,\mathrm{V\,m^{-1}}$ resulted in cardiac simulation for the waveform considered. Mouchawar *et al.*[30] used a finite element model to calculate the electric field that was applied to the heart in specially made coils that simulated the stimulating characteristics of an MRI *z*-gradient coil. For a 540 μs pulse, the required electric field in the heart was $86\,\mathrm{V\,m^{-1}}$. This is an average electric field. If we use the Reilly estimate that the 1-percentile is 1/2 of the average, this would be a field of $43\,\mathrm{V\,m^{-1}}$. Assuming a chronaxie c of 3 ms for cardiac muscle and using equation (4.5) result in a rheobase of $6.6\,\mathrm{V\,m^{-1}}$, in good agreement with Reilly's predicted value of $6.2\,\mathrm{V\,m^{-1}}$.

Assuming $b = 6.6\,\mathrm{V\,m^{-1}}$, $c = 3\,\mathrm{ms}$, and gradient pulse width of 450 μs results in an electric field following equation (4.5) of $50.6\,\mathrm{V\,m^{-1}}$. This is a factor of 6.7 greater than the maximum electric field in the heart (Table 4.2) of $7.6\,\mathrm{V\,m^{-1}}$ at slew rate of $200\,\mathrm{T\,m^{-1}\,s^{-1}}$. The slew rate in the

Table 4.3. Calculated electric fields in fat in human models in gradient coils

Coil type	Rheobase dB/dt ($T s^{-1}$)	99.5%. $\|E\|$ in fat Tab. V in So *et al.* (Ref. 26) ($V m^{-1}$)	99.5% $\|E\|$ in fat Hugo ($V m^{-1}$)
z-coil	28.8	4.6	5.1
y-coil	18.8	4.4	5.0

For the So *et al.* results, the electric field is maximum for one human model for the z-coil and average for three human models for the y-coil. The Hugo results are maximum for the coils in Figures 4.1 and 4.2 and maximum electric fields in fat from Figure 4.9.

z-coil to produce cardiac stimulation is then (6.7) ($200\,T\,m^{-1}\,s^{-1}$) = $1340\,T\,m^{-1}\,s^{-1}$. From the above, dB/dt for the z-coil at a radial distance of 20 cm from the coil center at S_z at $200\,T\,m^{-1}\,s^{-1}$ is $77.7\,T\,s^{-1}$. The time-varying magnetic field for achieving cardiac stimulation at a pulse duration of 450 μs is then (6.7) ($77.7\,T\,s^{-1}$) = $521\,T\,s^{-1}$.

4.7 REGULATORY LIMITS ON PULSED GRADIENTS IN MRI

Early regulatory standards[31] limited pulsed gradient intensities dB/dt to $20\,T\,s^{-1}$ in order to avoid nerve stimulation.[32,33] The present-day limits on gradient intensity are described in the MRI standard IEC 60601-2-33, 3rd edition.[34]

The gradient intensity in normal operating mode is to be limited to 80% of the average PNS threshold level. In the first-level controlled mode, the gradient intensity is limited to 100% of the average PNS threshold.

Thresholds for PNS may be determined by a study on human volunteers or by application of the formula of equation (4.5) using chronaxie of 360 μs and specified default values of rheobase. The default rheobase in terms of dB/dt is $20\,T\,s^{-1}$, close to the value of $18.8\,T\,s^{-1}$ for the y-coil from the Purdue study. The default rheobase expressed in terms of electric field is $2.2\,V\,m^{-1}$. This electric field is determined for a uniform patient model. If we model the body as a cylindrical conductor, dB/dt of $20\,T\,s^{-1}$ along the axis will produce a maximum electric field of $2.2\,V\,m^{-1}$ at a circumference of 1.38 m, which is the girth of a large person.

To avoid cardiac stimulation, it is specified in 60601-2-33, 3rd edition, that

$$\frac{dB}{dt} < \frac{20\ T\ s^{-1}}{1-\exp\left(-\frac{t_{s,\text{eff}}}{3}\right)} \tag{4.6}$$

where $t_{s,\text{eff}}$ is the effective duration in milliseconds of the gradient pulse. The electric field rheobase for avoiding cardiac stimulation is specified to be $2\,V\,m^{-1}$. With $t_{s,\text{eff}} = 0.45$ ms, the limit in 60601-2-33 on dB/dt to avoid cardiac stimulation is $144\,T\,s^{-1}$. This compares to the predicted threshold of $521\,T\,s^{-1}$ based on the discussion in the prior section. Thus, the limit on gradient output in IEC 60601-2-33 for avoidance of cardiac stimulation appears to have a safety margin of approximately 3.7. It should be noted that the applied dB/dt by the gradients is biphasic with separation between pulses less than the cardiac chronaxie. This will tend to increase the cardiac threshold,[35] providing additional safety margin.

4.8 DETERMINATION OF PNS THRESHOLDS FOR NONRECTANGULAR WAVEFORMS

The convolution method described in IEC 60601-2-33, 3rd edition, is a means to determine the relative amplitude of the gradients relative to threshold. Following Eq. AA.22 in the standard, the stimulation integral R_x is defined:

$$R_x(t) = \frac{1}{b}\int_0^t \frac{dB_x/dt(\theta)c}{(c+t-\theta)^2}d\theta \tag{4.7}$$

where b is the chronaxie, t is the duration of the waveform, and θ is the time during the waveform. Similar expressions apply for R_y and R_z. The total stimulation integral is then

$$R_{\text{total}} = \sqrt{R_x^2 + R_y^2 + R_z^2} \tag{4.8}$$

Excitation will occur when $R_{\text{total}} > 1$.

4.9 IMPLANT INTERACTIONS

ISO 10974/TS, 2nd edition,[2] describes the potential interactions with an implant of the dB/dt and electric fields from the pulsed gradients. A brief summary of the interactions of gradients with implants is presented in this section.

4.9.1 Concentration of Electric Field and Induced Current with Conducting Implants

A conducting implant will interact with the electric field induced in the body by the pulsed gradients. For an elongated implant, there will be a concentration of electric current in the tissue surrounding the ends. To illustrate quantitatively the current concentration, Figure 4.15 shows the electric field intensity surrounding the ends of bare and insulated wires 20 cm in length. The wires are based on the standard implant that was presented by FDA. The length is 20 cm, and the metal diameter is 1.5 mm. The insulated wire has an insulation outer diameter of 2.5 mm, and 1 cm of insulation is removed from each end. In the calculation, a uniform tangential electric field of frequency 10 kHz was applied. For the insulated wire, the electric field intensity was in excess of 10 times the background within 2 mm from the tip. The bare wire yields less electric field.

It seems possible that concentration of background electric field by a conducting implant could result in nerve stimulation. The greatest likelihood for stimulation is expected for an elongated implant near the surface of the body. However, reports in the literature of gradients interacting with implants to induce stimulation appear to be rare.

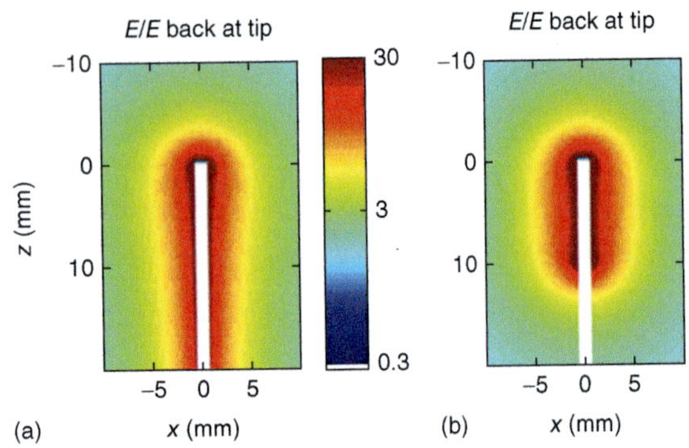

Figure 4.15. Electric field around the end of wires relative to background for 20 cm long wires: (a) bare and (b) insulated with 1 cm insulation removed from each end

4.9.2 Induction of Voltage Along a Lead Wire

For an active implant with a lead wire, the gradient electric field will induce a voltage between the proximal and distal ends. This voltage will produce in the lead a current that depends on the electrode impedance on the distal end and the generator impedance at the proximal end. The driving voltage ΔV for the current is the integrated tangential electric field along the length of the lead. The voltage is calculated as:

$$\Delta V = \int_0^L E_{\tan}(\tau)\mathrm{d}\tau \tag{4.9}$$

where $E_{\tan}$ is the tangential electric field, and τ is the distance along the lead, with $\tau = 0$ at the distal end of the lead and $\tau = L$ at the generator.

Gradient voltage will depend on the coil, the slew rate, and the landmark of the patient. The current induced through an electrode by gradient voltage should be below the stimulation threshold, especially for electrodes that are implanted in the heart. ISO/TS 10974 provides methods for testing the response of a pulse generator to gradient-induced ΔV.

The gradient voltage could also be calculated with the loop area method that is described in ISO/TS 10974.

$$\Delta V = \frac{L^2}{4\pi}\frac{\mathrm{d}B}{\mathrm{d}t} \tag{4.10}$$

where L is the circumference. The loop area calculation of equation (10) is expected to provide a greater value for ΔV than that provided by the direct integration of equation (9).

4.9.3 Gradient Heating of a Metallic Implant

The time-varying gradient field will induce eddy currents when normally incident on a planar surface of an implant. These eddy currents will produce a power dissipation that may produce a measurable temperature rise. Heating will tend to be greatest for large implants, a geometry that provides easy pathways for flow of eddy currents, a larger electrical conductivity, and a thickness that is approximately the same or greater than the electrical skin depth. The calculation of gradient heating of model implants was described in a thesis by Stem.[36] ISO/TS 10974 provides an equation that shows that power dissipation is proportional to the fourth power of the radius of a disk-shaped implant. Thus, gradient heating is expected to be small for a small implant.

4.9.4 Gradient-induced Vibration of a Metallic Implant

There will be torque induced on a metallic implant due to the Lorentz forces that are exerted by the eddy currents that are induced by d*B*/d*t*. The torque is greatest when d*B*/d*t* is normally incident on an implant, and the static field is parallel to the plane. The torque will be greatest for the same device parameters that maximize the heating. ISO/TS 10974 provides an equation that shows that the gradient torque on a circular disk is proportional to the fourth power of its radius. The standard describes tests to confirm reliability of an active implant in response to the gradient vibrations.

4.10 SOME POINTS OF DISCUSSION

In this chapter, we describe the magnitude of d*B*/d*t* produced by the gradient coils in a pulsed MR system. For a patient without implants, the main physiologic effect will be PNS. There have been a number of studies on stimulation with the pulsed gradients, and the intensity level of d*B*/d*t* vs duration for PNS, as quantified in equation (4.5), appears to be well enough understood. Less well understood is how the background electric field in the patient couples with neurons to elicit stimulation. Reilly has provided a good review that describes mechanisms for nerve stimulation by time-varying magnetic fields.[35]

As per IEC 60601-2-33, the normal mode operation of the MR system limits d*B*/d*t* to 80% of the PNS threshold level and the first-level controlled mode limits d*B*/d*t* to 100% of the PNS threshold level. At the currently maximum available slew rate of $200\,\mathrm{T\,m\,s^{-1}}$ at pulse duration of 450 μs, PNS thresholds using rheobase and chronaxie from the Purdue study and equation (4.5) are $34.7\,\mathrm{T\,s^{-1}}$ for the *y*-coil and $53.1\,\mathrm{T\,s^{-1}}$ for the *z*-coil, at a radial distance $r = 20$ cm. These values are compared to the calculated d*B*/d*t* for the coils of Figures 4.1 and 4.2 at $200\,\mathrm{T\,m^{-1}\,s^{-1}}$ and $r = 20$ cm of $75.1\,\mathrm{T\,s^{-1}}$ for the *y*-coil and $77.7\,\mathrm{T\,s^{-1}}$ for the *z*-coil. Thus, the peak output of presently available gradient systems seems sufficient to elicit PNS for some patients and positions in the coil.

As illustrated in Figure 4.4, gradient amplifiers are expected to be the switched mode, and the impact of the switching on the d*B*/d*t* waveform varies across MR systems. The switching will add peaks to the d*B*/d*t* waveform, but average d*B*/d*t* is preserved. Presumably, peak d*B*/d*t* is still limited by the peak slew rate of the gradient system. Given that the effective frequency of the switching is of the order 100 kHz, we expect that PNS threshold will be influenced by average d*B*/d*t* and not the peak d*B*/d*t*. Given that the electrical skin depth decreases with increasing frequency, we expect that higher frequency content in the switched d*B*/d*t* will not result in significant additional heating or vibration of the case. The input impedance at the header connection of a generator will likely be less at the switching frequency than at the fundamental gradient frequency, and this factor should be considered when evaluating the interaction of the generator circuitry with the pulsed gradients.

Cardiac stimulation of the patient during MRI by the d*B*/d*t* from the pulsed gradients appears to be avoided with a safety factor of at least 7.6. Implants will locally concentrate in their vicinity the electric field that is produced by the pulsed gradients. The authors are not aware of the cardiac simulation induced by a passive implant. Nonetheless, the potential for a metallic implant in the heart to concentrate the electric field to the point that cardiac stimulation occurs should be considered.

ACKNOWLEDGMENTS

JN is grateful to have been a member of the Purdue team that determined the strength–duration relationship for patients in response to the MRI pulsed gradients and expresses thanks to J.D. Bourland, D.J. Schaefer, and other team members.

The program for the gradient calculations presented here was developed by R. Kamondetdacha.

DISCLAIMER

The subject matter, content, and views presented do not represent the views of the Department of Health and Human Services (HHS), US Food and Drug Administration (FDA), and/or the United States.

REFERENCES

1. J. A. Nyenhuis, J. D. Bourland, and D. J. Schaefer, *J. Appl. Phys.*, 1997, **81**, 4314.
2. ISO/IEC, Assessment of the Safety of Magnetic Resonance Imaging for Patients with an Active Implantable Medical Device, Technical Specification

ISO/TS 10974, 2nd edn, ISO: Geneva, 2018, Reference No. ISO/TS 10974:2018(E).

3. ASTM International, Standard Test Method for Measurement of Radio Frequency Induced Heating Near Passive Implants During Magnetic Resonance Imaging, Standard F2182-11a, West Conshohocken, PA, 2011.
4. F. Liu, H. Zhao, and S. Crozier, *IEEE Trans. Biomed. Eng.*, 2003, **50**, 804.
5. J. A. Nyenhuis, G. A. Mouchawar, J. D. Bourland, and L. A. Geddes, *IEEE Trans. Magn.*, 1991, **27**, 680.
6. M. S. Cohen, M. R. Weisskopf, and R. R. Rzedian, *Magn. Reson. Med.*, 1990, **14**, 409.
7. T. F. Budinger, H. Fischer, D. Hentshel, *et al.*, *J. Comput. Assist. Tomogr.*, 1991, **15**, 609.
8. S. Ueno, O. Hiwaki, T. Matsuda, *et al.*, *Ann. N. Y. Acad. Sci.*, 1992, **369**, 96.
9. C. L. G. Ham, J. M. L. Engels, G. T. van de Weil, and A. Machielsen, *J. Magn. Res. Imaging*, 1997, **7**, 933.
10. J. Abart, K. Eberhardt, H. Fischer, *et al.*, *J. Comput. Assist. Tomogr.*, 1997, **21**, 532.
11. J. C. Ehrhardt, C. S. Lin, V. A. Magnotta, D. J. Fisher, and W. T. C. Yuh, *J. Magn. Reson. Imaging*, 1997, **7**, 405.
12. G. Frese, F. X. Hebrank, W. Renz, and T. Storch, *Radiologe*, 1998, **38**, 750.
13. X. Hebrank Franz and M. Gebhardt, *Proc. Int. Soc. Magn. Reson. Med.*, 2000, **8**, 2007.
14. D. J. Schaefer, J. D. Bourland, J. A. Nyenhuis, *et al.*, *Proc. Int. Soc. Magn. Reson. Med.*, 1994, **2**, 104.
15. B. Zhang, Y. Yen, B. A. Chronik, G. C. McKinnon, D. J. Schaefer, and B. K. Rutt, *Magn. Reson. Med.*, 2003, **50**, 50.
16. B. A. Chonik and B. K. Rutt, *Magn. Reson. Med.*, 2001, **45**, 916.
17. B. A. Chronik and M. Ramachandran, *J. Magn. Reson. Imaging*, 2003, **17**, 716.
18. B. A. Chonik and B. K. Rutt, *Magn. Reson. Med.*, 2001, **46**, 386.
19. D. J. Schaefer, J. D. Bouland, and J. A. Nyenhuis, *J. Magn. Reson. Imaging*, 2000, **12**, 20.
20. J. A. Den Boer, J. D. Bourland, J. A. Nyenhuis, C. L. G. Ham, J. M. L. Engels, F. X. Hebrank, G. Frese, and D. J. Schaefer, *J. Magn. Reson. Imaging*, 2002, **15**, 520.
21. J. D. Bourland, J. A. Nyenhuis, and D. J. Schaefer, *Neuroimaging Clin. N. Am.*, 1999, **9**, 363.
22. J. Nyenhuis, J. D. Bourland, A. V. Kildishev, and D. J. Schaefer, in 'Magnetic Resonance Procedures: Health Effects and Safety', ed. F. G. Shellock, CRC Press: Boca Raton, FL, 2001, Chapter 2.
23. L. Lapicque, *Comp. R. Acad. Sci.*, 1909, **67**, 280.
24. W. Irnich and F. Schmitt, *Magn. Reson. Med.*, 1995, **33**, 619.
25. P. So, M. A. Stuchly, and J. A. Nyenhuis, *IEEE Trans. Biol. Med. Eng.*, 2004, **51**, 1907.
26. J. D. Bourland, J. A. Nyenhuis, G. A. Mouchawar, *et al.*, In *Proceedings of 10th Annual Meeting of the Society of Magnetic Resonance in Medicine*, San Francisco, 1991, 969.
27. J. A. Nyenhuis, J. D. Bourland, D. J. Schaefer, *et al.*, In *Proceedings of 11th Annual Meeting of the Society of Magnetic Resonance in Medicine*, 1991, 586.
28. J. P. Reilly, *Ann. N. Y. Acad. Sci.*, 1992, **649**, 96.
29. P. M. Ragan, W. Wang, and S. R. Eisenberg, *IEEE Trans. Biomed. Eng.*, 1995, **42**, 1110.
30. G. A. Mouchawar, J. A. Nyenhuis, J. D. Bourland, L. A. Geddes, D. J. Schaefer, and M. E. Riehl, *IEEE Trans. Magn.*, 1993, **29**, 3355.
31. T. W. Athey, *Ann. N. Y. Acad. Sci.*, 1992, **649**, 96.
32. A. T. Barker, *J. Clin. Neurophysiol.*, 1991, **8**, 26.
33. S. Ueno and M. Iwasaka, in 'Biological Effects of Magnetic and Electromagnetic Fields', ed. S. Ueno, Plenum Press: New York, 1996, Vol. **1**.
34. International Electrotechnical Commission, 'IEC 60601-2-33, Medical Electrical Equipment – Part 2-33: Particular Requirements for the Basic Safety and Essential Performance of Magnetic Resonance Equipment for Medical Diagnosis', 3rd edn, International Electrotechnical Commission, 2010.
35. J. P. Reilly, *Med. Biol. Eng. Comput.*, 1989, **27**, 101.
36. B. Stem, Computer Modeling and Simulation of Implantable Medical Device Heating Due to MRI Gradient Coil Fields, MS Thesis, Purdue University, 2014.

Chapter 5

Peripheral Nerve Stimulation Modeling for MRI

Mathias Davids[1,2], Bastien Guérin[2,3], Lothar R. Schad[1], and Lawrence L. Wald[2,3,4]

[1]*Heidelberg University, Heidelberg, Germany*
[2]*Massachusetts General Hospital, Charlestown, MA, USA*
[3]*Harvard Medical School, Boston, MA, USA*
[4]*Harvard-MIT Health Sciences and Technology, Cambridge, MA, USA*

Safety and Biological Effects in MRI.
Edited by Devashish Shrivastava and J. Thomas Vaughan

ISBN: 978-1-118-82130-5
Also published in eMagRes (online edition)
DOI: 10.1002/9780470034590.emrstm1586

5.1 INTRODUCTION

Understanding and predicting peripheral nerve stimulation (PNS)[1] created by MR gradient coils requires a detailed understanding of the induction of electromagnetic fields in the body and their interaction with the nerve fibers. The goal of modeling PNS is an improved understanding of its origins and mechanisms, and ultimately improved characterization and control of this important biological limitation to magnetic resonance imaging (MRI) gradient coil strength and switching rates. Other goals for better understanding magneto-stimulation include improved targeted magneto-stimulation of nerve fibers to assess nerve viability or suppress or evoke function. Fortunately, the needed understanding can be built on comprehensive research over the last century on how nerves interact with electromagnetic fields and our ever-improving ability to model induced electric fields within the body.

The earliest experiments of electrical stimulation of peripheral nerves focused on the properties of nerve impulse propagation. Currently, stimulation and nerve conduction velocity experiments are widely used to interrogate diseases of the peripheral nerves.[2,3] In magneto-stimulation, the electric field

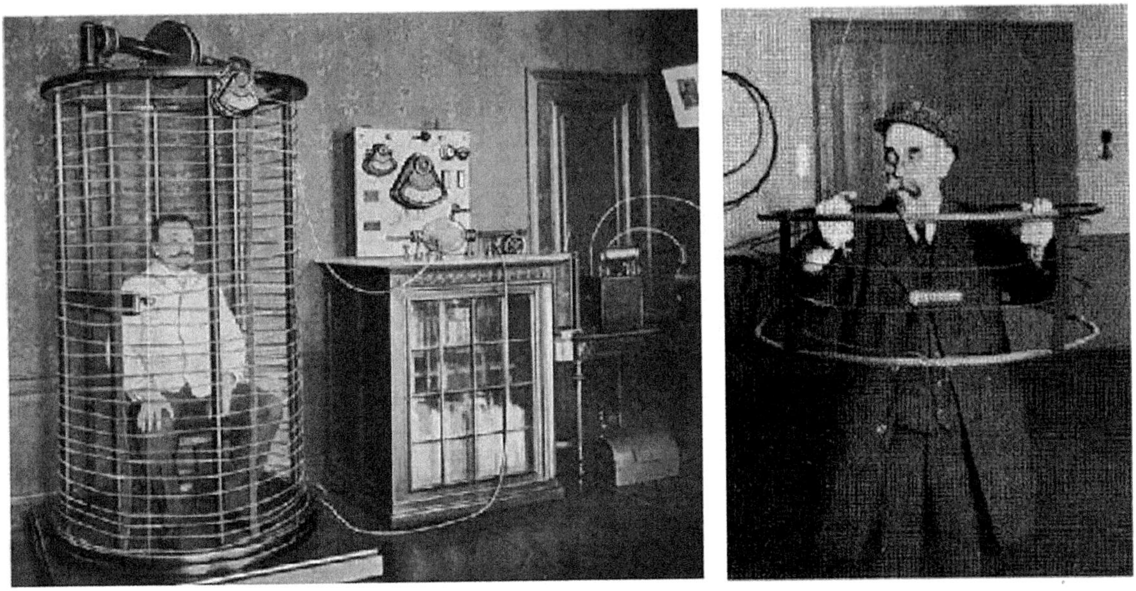

Figure 5.1. Setups for early magnetostimulation experiments carried out by Jacques Arsene d'Arsonval around 1893

is not generated by direct application of currents via electrodes but induced in conductive tissues by time-varying magnetic fields. This effect was the focus of nineteenth century studies by Jacques Arsene d'Arsonval (Figure 5.1). The use of magnetic field coils to stimulate the peripheral nervous system also has a long history for pain management and has more recently been extended to the central nervous system with transcranial magnetic stimulation (TMS).[4,5] The potential for MRI gradient coils to generate electric fields in the body capable of stimulating the peripheral nerves was recognized early in the development of MRI[6] and observed in commercial systems shortly thereafter.[7–9] Ever since, this unwanted effect has been of growing significance and has been acutely felt by the latest generation of whole-body MRI gradient hardware (reaching up to $300\,\mathrm{mT\,m^{-1}}$ gradient strength at slew rates of over $200\,\mathrm{T\,m^{-1}\,s^{-1}}$).[10,11] PNS can render significant portions of the gradient hardware operational parameter space inaccessible to the user. Here, the operational gradient parameter space for trapezoidal waveforms is defined as the hardware-accessible area under the plot of gradient strength versus slew-period duration (which defines the E-field 'pulse' duration). In practice, the PNS limitation is particularly acute for fast readout techniques such as echo-planar imaging (EPI) and steady-state free precession sequences (SSFP) that employ short gradient rise times.[12–15]

The continued push toward faster sequences has motivated the design of gradient coils that minimize PNS. This has led to general rules of thumb for limiting the electric fields induced in the body, for example, by limiting the linear region of the gradient coil. This both limits exposure to only the imaged body part and reduces the maximum B-field amplitude produced (which in turn limits $\mathrm{d}B/\mathrm{d}t$). Experiments with gradient coils of differing linear field of views (FOVs) have shown that the PNS thresholds scale with the inverse of the linear FOV.[16] Even if this scaling law were the end of the story (a designer would choose the needed FOV and live with the resulting threshold), accurately modeling PNS in gradient coils would be valuable to better understand which nerves were responsible and how effects change with individual body type/habitus and position without the need for extensive human testing. But an additional intriguing possibility exists in the hypothesis that improved understanding of the phenomena might lead to additional methods for limiting PNS, enabling the use of even faster, stronger gradient coils in MRI. This would require the existence of sufficient degrees of freedom in gradient design to allow multiple winding patterns to achieve the needed gradient linearity and shielding but generate different

PNS thresholds. In this case, PNS threshold modeling could uncover these possibilities in the design phase.[17]

There are some reasons to be hopeful. Firstly, the gradient design is largely only dependent on the generated B_z component, since only that component encodes the image (the B_x and B_y 'concomitant' terms contribute only to second order for modulating spin phase). In contrast, all components of the gradient coil's field could lead to PNS, depending on nerve orientation. But, Maxwell equations allow an infinite variety of total magnetic fields which can achieve a given B_z spatial pattern. This was exploited by Hidalgo-Toborn *et al.*[18] who showed that additional coil windings producing a B_x or B_y concomitant field component could partially cancel a gradient coil's existing concomitant field and significantly reduce PNS. Differences in the concomitant field pattern may partially explain the ability to find gradients with similar linear FOVs but a range of PNS thresholds. We show below a study of two head gradients with this behavior. In short, it is likely that a detailed knowledge of the origin of PNS and the ability to predict thresholds for a variety of cases is needed to explore the trade-offs between PNS thresholds and other important gradient performance parameters. If successful, this could enable the incorporation of PNS as an additional metric among many design considerations.

This chapter focuses on the recent (and not so recent) work, which contributes to our understanding and ability to model PNS on a theoretical basis. Modeling the *E*-field distribution in the body is a good start, and considerable advances have been made in detailed body models and computational tools for this purpose. However, knowledge of the electric field alone does not predict PNS. Firstly, nerves with large axon diameters (which are the most excitable) must be present in the *E*-field hotspot. In addition, the relative orientation between the *E*-field and the nerve is also an important determinant of whether an action potential is generated. Thus, the model needs three pieces: a detailed electromagnetic coil and body model, the knowledge of the nerve locations, orientations and type within the body model, and a neurodynamic model to determine if the fields are sufficient to generate an action potential (our definition of stimulation). Recent work has accumulated all of these components and integrated them to form a comprehensive tool to analyze the gradient coil's interaction with the nervous system. This chapter reviews this work from the point of view of its potential uses in MRI.

5.2 SIMULATION OF GRADIENT SWITCHING-INDUCED ELECTRIC FIELDS IN THE HUMAN BODY

PNS arises from the excitation of the largest peripheral nerves in the body due to secondary effects from the switching gradient magnetic field. The time-varying magnetic fields (used for spin encoding) are accompanied by electric fields, which are the driving force behind PNS. Therefore, the first step in predicting PNS is to accurately estimate these electric fields in the body. Early attempts to model the *E*-field distribution used analytical or semi-analytical approaches. For example, Roth *et al.*[19] and Durand *et al.*[20] derived an analytic solution for the *E*-field induced by a simple solenoid coil in a homogeneous cylindrical model of the arm. By considering the two major *E*-field sources, namely the time-varying magnetic field and the resulting charge accumulation at the air-tissue surface, the authors showed that the electric field is strongest close to the loop at the body surface.

As computing power increased, more advanced approaches were proposed that allowed investigation of complex wire patterns[21] and heterogeneous models.[22,23] Bowtell and Bowley[24] analyzed an existing MRI gradient coil wire pattern; however, the EM field calculation was still limited to a homogeneous body model. Use of more detailed models is needed because in humans, the electric fields are heavily shaped by the distribution of tissue conductivities. Correct representation of tissue heterogeneity is important because charge accumulation and electric current bottle-neck effects occur due to the interface between tissue classes. To better represent these effects, numerical approaches were formulated relatively early by Davey *et al.*[25] and Wang and Eisenberg[26] who approximated the body using hexahedral (voxels) or tetrahedral (i.e., pyramids) mesh models and used finite difference time domain (FDTD) methods or finite element methods (FEM) to find approximate solutions for the induced EM fields in the quasi-static regime. Mouchawar *et al.*[27] simulated the electric fields and current densities induced in a simplified dog thorax voxel model consisting of 9035 bricks with six tissue classes. They also performed cardiac stimulation experiments on the dogs, yielding a correspondence between d*B*/d*t* values at the stimulation threshold and the induced current densities in ampere per meter.[28] Others modeled a 2-mm resolution heterogeneous whole body model (~6 M mesh cells) within a realistic MRI gradient coil.[29–31] These authors found that switching the gradient coil at $148\,\mathrm{T\,m^{-1}\,s^{-1}}$ induces a peak electric field of $6.2\,\mathrm{V\,m^{-1}}$ (the threshold suggested at the time by the National Radiological Protection Board). In addition, the authors point out that common stimulation sites correspond to locations where the bone is close to the skin, which underscores the importance of the electric current bottle-neck issue.

This early work on *E*-field distributions arising from gradient coils uncovered a fundamental limitation of this approach. Firstly, an experimental step was still needed to link the simulated *E*-field values to actual PNS thresholds. In addition, as these authors pointed out, the correlation between hotspots of the electric field or electric field gradient and PNS sensations is vague at best. There is some level of agreement, for example, common PNS loci such as the nose, scapula, chest, arms, hands, buttocks, and thighs do correspond to electric field or electric field gradient hotspots.

Thus, using the electric field as a surrogate for PNS poses significant limitations because this approach disregards the role of the nerves themselves. First, the body is only sparsely populated with large diameter nerves. Second, only the electric field component running parallel to the nerve fibers is effective for inducing PNS, meaning that a nerve with a 'lucky' orientation may run through a high *E*-field region without being stimulated. Third, the nerve membrane dynamics (i.e., the temporal dynamics of the ion flow in different nerve sections) play an important role. This added complexity can be addressed by combining the electromagnetic field simulations with explicit models of nerve fiber excitation (with their ion dynamics) and accounting for their relative orientation with respect to the local electric field.

5.3 NEURODYNAMIC MODELING

The use of electrical equivalent circuits to model peripheral nerve fiber dynamics dates back to 1898 when Hoorweg pointed out similarities between nerve fibers and underwater cables[32] for which transmission theories and circuit models had been already developed by William Thomson (Lord Kelvin) in the 1850s.[33,34] These early investigations led to the formulation of linear electrical equivalent circuit models such as those shown in Figure 5.2(a). In this model, the intracellular and extracellular spaces are connected at the nodes of Ranvier via RC circuits that are tuned to match the nerve's membrane conductance G_n and capacitance C_n. The circuits also contain voltage sources V_r that represent the actively maintained transmembrane resting potential (approx. −80 mV for peripheral nerves). The different RC circuits (at each node of Ranvier) are connected via an axial conductance G_{ax}, allowing for an intra-cellular current to flow along the axon. The distance between the nodes of Ranvier scales with the fiber diameter, ranging between 0.5 mm (for 6 μm diameter fibers) and 1.5 mm (for 16 μm diameter fibers). This electrical model of the nerve fiber is represented mathematically by a set of time-dependent differential equations that are solved numerically. The intracellular potentials (V_{int}) are sought given a set of extracellular potentials at the nodes of Ranvier (V_{ext}) and their temporal modulation. In the MRI case, the external potentials follow the temporal rate of change of the gradient waveform.

The linear circuit model of Figure 5.2(a) is capable of modeling sub-threshold stimuli reasonably well (e.g., depolarization and hyperpolarization of the membrane). However, modeling of super-threshold stimuli (where the ion channels come into play) requires a more accurate representation of the voltage-dependent ion permeabilities at the nodes of Ranvier. Figure 5.2(b) shows an electrical circuit, where the nodes of Ranvier are equipped with the Hodgkin–Huxley model[35] of voltage-dependent ion channels. In their famous experiments, Hodgkin and Huxley conducted patch clamp experiments on giant squid nerves to measure the permeability of the sodium and potassium ion channels as a function of the transmembrane potential. Specifically, each ion channel is equipped with a number of so-called *gates*. Sodium channels have three activation gates (*m*-gates) and one inactivation gate (*h*-gate). Potassium channels have four activation gates (*n*-gates) and no inactivation gates. The gates are modeled as connected in series, thus all gates need to be open for an ion to pass through the channel. For each gate, a *gating variable* is defined that determines the probability that the gate is 'closed' or 'open' (value between 0 and 1). Finally, voltage-dependent *transition rate constants* $\alpha(V)$ and $\beta(V)$ are defined for each class of gates that quantify the transition rate from 'close' to 'open' (α) and from 'open' to 'close' (β). For example, the differential

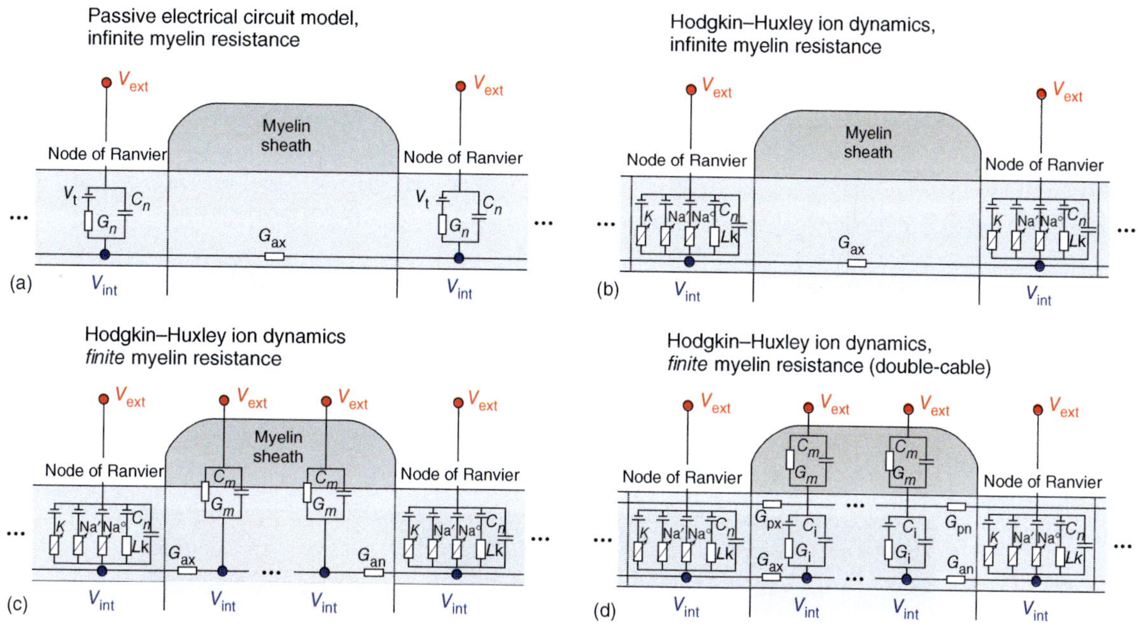

Figure 5.2. Stages of neurodynamic model complexity: (a) passive single-cable model without explicit representation of the voltage-dependent ion conductivity or the finite myelin resistance. This model can be refined by (b) including nonlinear Hodgkin–Huxley ion channel dynamics, (c) representation of the myelin as an imperfect insulator, (d) and using a double-cable model of the inter-nodal space with the myelin and the axon being electrically separated by the periaxonal space

equation for the m-gates is then given by

$$\frac{\mathrm{d}m}{\mathrm{d}t} = \alpha_m(1-m) - \beta_\mathrm{m} m$$

Other gate classes are similarly described. Finally, the ionic currents across the node of Ranvier for sodium and potassium are determined by

$$I_\mathrm{Na} = \hat{g}_\mathrm{Na} m^3 h\,(V - V_\mathrm{Na}) \text{ and } I_\mathrm{K} = \hat{g}_\mathrm{K} n^4\,(V - V_\mathrm{K})$$

where $\hat{g}_\mathrm{Na}/\hat{g}_\mathrm{K}$ is the maximum sodium/potassium conductance, $V_\mathrm{Na}/V_\mathrm{K}$ is the reversal equilibrium sodium/potassium potentials (which can be calculated by the Nernst equation), and m, h, and n are the gating variables introduced above. If the constant transmembrane conductance G_m of Figure 5.2(a) is replaced by the variable ionic conductances, the resulting circuit model (shown in Figure 5.2b) is capable of action potential generation and propagation.[36–40]

An additional refinement to this model comes from modeling the myelin sheath not as a perfect insulator but with finite resistance. This is done by defining additional internodal compartments connecting the internal cell environment to the extracellular space through the myelin sheath, as shown in Figure 5.2(c). This feature is particularly important for sensory nerves, which have thinner myelination layers. The electrical properties of the trans-myelin RC-circuit representations depend on the axon diameter; larger diameter nerves have a thicker myelination (i.e., smaller conductance G_m and capacitance C_m).

The circuit shown in Figure 5.2(d) provides an additional level of model refinement. Here, the nerve is modeled as a double-cable electrical circuit with currents flowing both along the axon (inner cable) and the myelin sheath (outer cable). The currents are isolated by the intermediate layer or periaxonal space. This circuit model is the basis of one of the most advanced models for peripheral nerve fibers: the McIntyre–Richardson–Grill (MRG) model[41–43] of mammalian nerves.

5.4 EXAMPLE: MODEL OF A SINGLE NERVE RESPONSE TO AN EXTERNAL *E*-FIELD

These neurodynamic models are typically used to study the effect of an externally applied, temporally

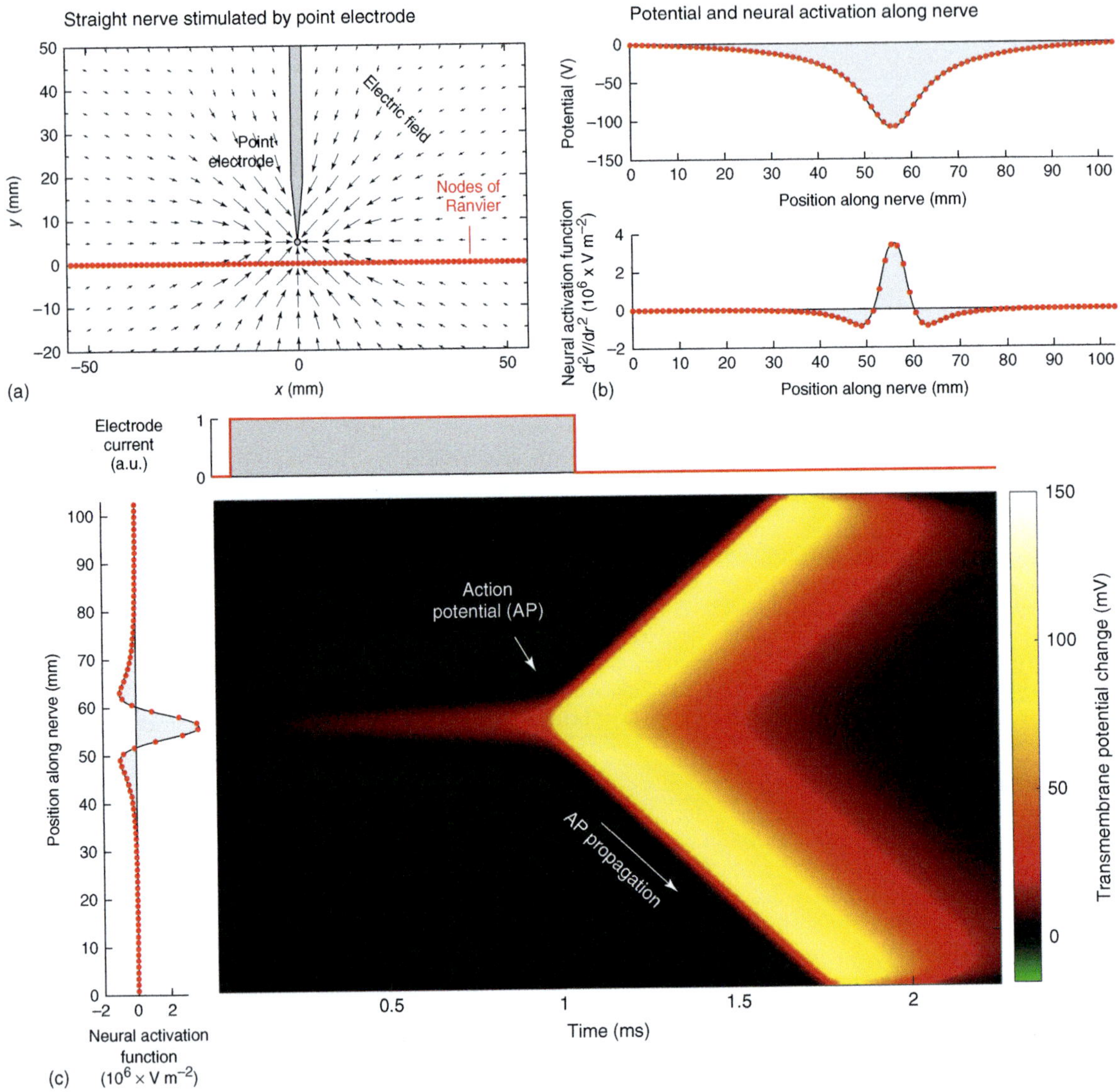

Figure 5.3. (a) Electric field produced by a point electrode, superimposed to a straight nerve fiber. (b) Electric potential and its second spatial derivative (i.e., the neural activation function) plotted against the position r along the nerve. (c) Output of the neurodynamic model, as this nerve is stimulated by the electrode using a 1 ms block pulse. The membrane dynamics is shown as the transmembrane potential change (i.e., relative to the resting potential of −80 mV) as a function of time (x-axis) and position along the nerve (y-axis)

modulated electric potential. Experimentally, the potential is often applied using a point electrode, a configuration used in early (and many recent) experiments on excitability of nerve fibers. Figure 5.3(a) shows an electric field generated by a point electrode applied to a straight MRG nerve fiber (12 μm nerve with 81 nodes of Ranvier). The red dots indicate the positions of the nodes of Ranvier. Projecting the E-field onto the nerve path and integrating the result along the nerve yields the potential (voltage) variation shown in Figure 5.3(b). The second spatial derivative of the potential along the nerve is called the *neural activation function* and is a good predictor of the locus of stimulation along the nerve.[28,44] However, the activation function cannot be used to derive quantitative stimulation thresholds; this requires either assessment of the full neurodynamic model or a more refined version of the activation function.[45]

Figure 5.3(c) shows the nerve's membrane dynamic as determined from the MRG model when the external potential V_{ext} at the nodal and internodal compartments (left sub-panel) is applied for 1 ms and then turned off. The membrane dynamics are obtained by feeding the spatially and temporally varying potential to the MRG neurodynamic model and evaluating the underlying differential equations. The resulting nerve response in Figure 5.3(c) (shown as the transmembrane potential change relative to the resting potential of −80 mV) is plotted as a function of time (*x*-axis) and position along the nerve (*y*-axis). In this case, the stimulus was above threshold and the output of the neurodynamic model shows propagation of two back-to-back action potentials (one propagating left, the other propagating right).

Figure 5.4 shows a more realistic nerve with two kinks (denoted by numbers **1** and **2**), this time excited via magneto-stimulation. In general, the electric fields generated during magneto-stimulation by body-sized coils are less spatially localized than electrode stimulation. In this case, we assumed a homogeneous *E*-field, causing a linear potential change along the straight nerve segments (Figure 5.4b). At the two nerve kinks, however, the potential changes rapidly, yielding two peaks in the neural activation function. Figure 5.4(c) illustrates the membrane dynamic as this nerve fiber is stimulated by a 1 kHz sinusoid. In this case, the external potential V_{ext} is also sinusoidal (locked to dB/dt of the 1 kHz *B*-field). The nerve membrane potential is perturbed from its resting state (hyperpolarization and depolarization) at the two kinks, with the stronger perturbation occurring at the first kink (owing to the higher absolute value of the neural activation function). After 1 ms, an AP is induced at the first kink, which then travels along the nerve in both directions. During the following 3 ms, the fiber is alternately depolarized (red) and hyperpolarized (green); however, no AP is evoked (the fiber is in the absolute refractory period). Note that the two kinks experience opposite effects (hyperpolarization or depolarization) due to the different signs of the neural activation function (Figure 5.4b). After 4 ms, the fiber has partially recovered from the first AP allowing the generation of a second AP, also at the first kink. These examples illustrate two very important aspects about PNS. First, it is the electrical potential, and more precisely its second derivative along the nerve fiber direction, that is a good marker of PNS. Although they both experienced the same electric field strength, the second kink had an insufficient second derivative of the potential (first derivative of the projected *E*-field) to generate an AP. This derivative depends both on the local *E*-field strength and its orientation relative to the nerve path. In fact, the nerve orientation is critical: for example, a nerve perpendicular to a high *E*-field region would experience no PNS. Thus, simulation of PNS thresholds requires both modeling of the induced *E*-field and knowledge of the nerve fiber geometry in the body.

5.5 COUPLED ELECTROMAGNETIC AND NEURODYNAMIC SIMULATIONS

The workflow for coupling electromagnetic (EM) and neurodynamic simulations entails: (i) computing the induced *E*-field in the body (EM simulation), (ii) calculating the resulting electric potential changes along the nerve fibers, and (iii) computing the nerve response by solving a neurodynamic model such as the MRG model along the nerve's path (neurodynamic simulation). The onset PNS is defined as the appearance of the first AP in the simulation. Roth and Basser[46] used linear (Figure 5.2a) and nonlinear (Figure 5.2b and c) neurodynamic models to simulate the response of infinitely long straight nerves (no bends) in a homogeneous volume (no realistic body model) in a solenoid excitation coil. These approaches were extended by examining nerves with finite length (i.e., the nerves may be stimulated at the terminal ends),[47] the current polarity used for point electrode stimulation,[48] extending the type of driving waveform (trapezoidal vs sinusoidal),[49] examining shaped nerve fibers with bents and kinks[1] and accounting for the nerve's refractory period on thresholds created by trains of pulses.[50] Nagarajan and Durand[51,52] used a toroidal coil to stimulate a bundle of multiple fibers including the surrounding perineurium using a simplified cylindrical model.

A limitation of these approaches is that they only modeled isolated nerve and body geometries. Ideally, analysis of an MRI gradient coil would utilize a body model with an anatomically correct geometric representation of all major tissue classes labeled with their relevant electromagnetic tissue properties and an atlas of the largest nerves in the body co-registered to the body anatomy. All nerve segments of the atlas require labeling by their local axon diameter which in

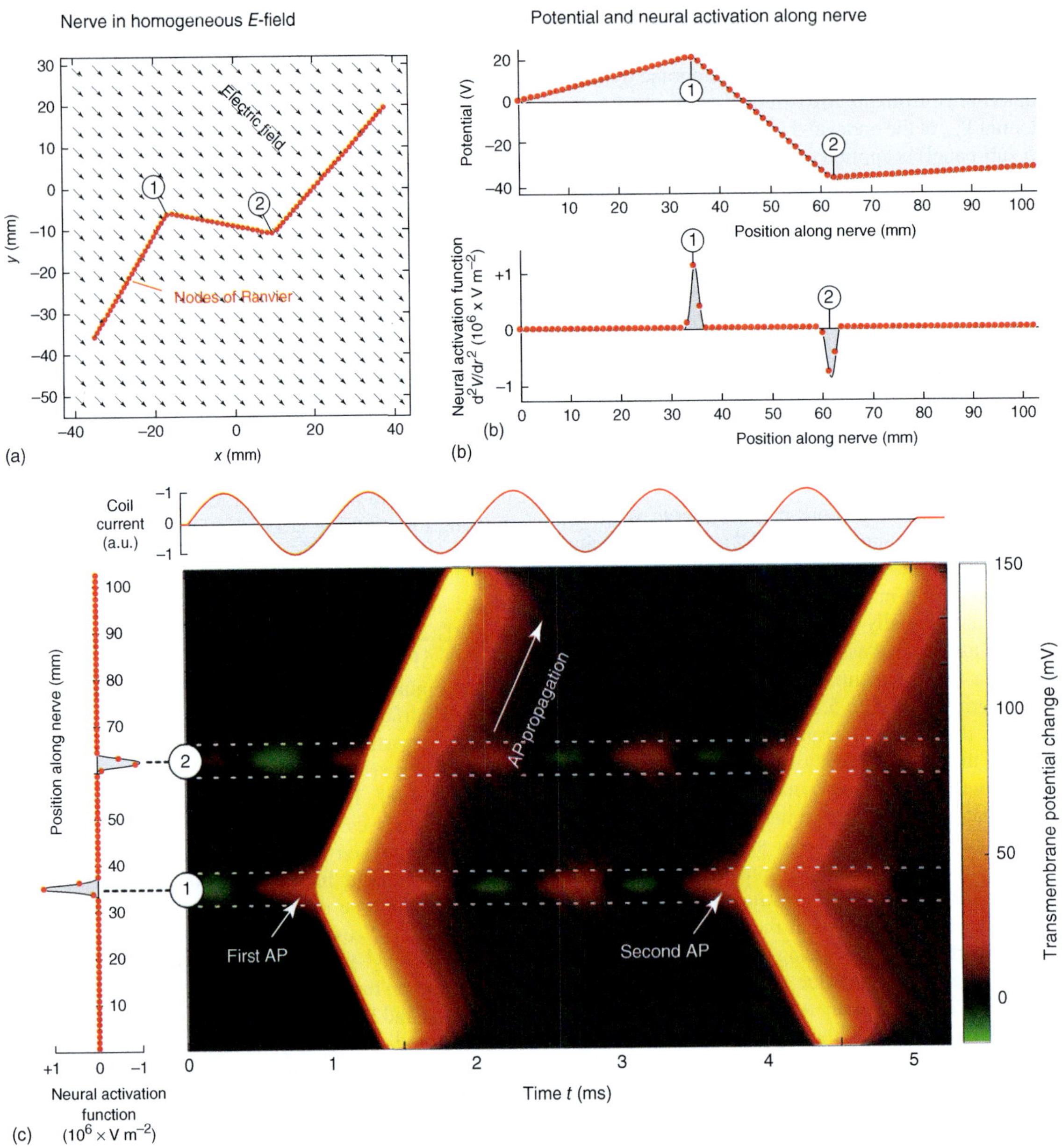

Figure 5.4. (a) Homogeneous electric field (produced by a hypothetical coil), superimposed to a nerve fiber with two kinks (1) and (2). (b) Electric potential and its second spatial derivative (i.e., the neural activation function) plotted against the position r along the nerve. (c) Output of the neurodynamic model, as this nerve is stimulated by a 1 kHz coil current. The membrane dynamics is shown as the transmembrane potential change (i.e., relative to the resting potential of −80 mV) as a function of time (x-axis) and position along the nerve (y-axis)

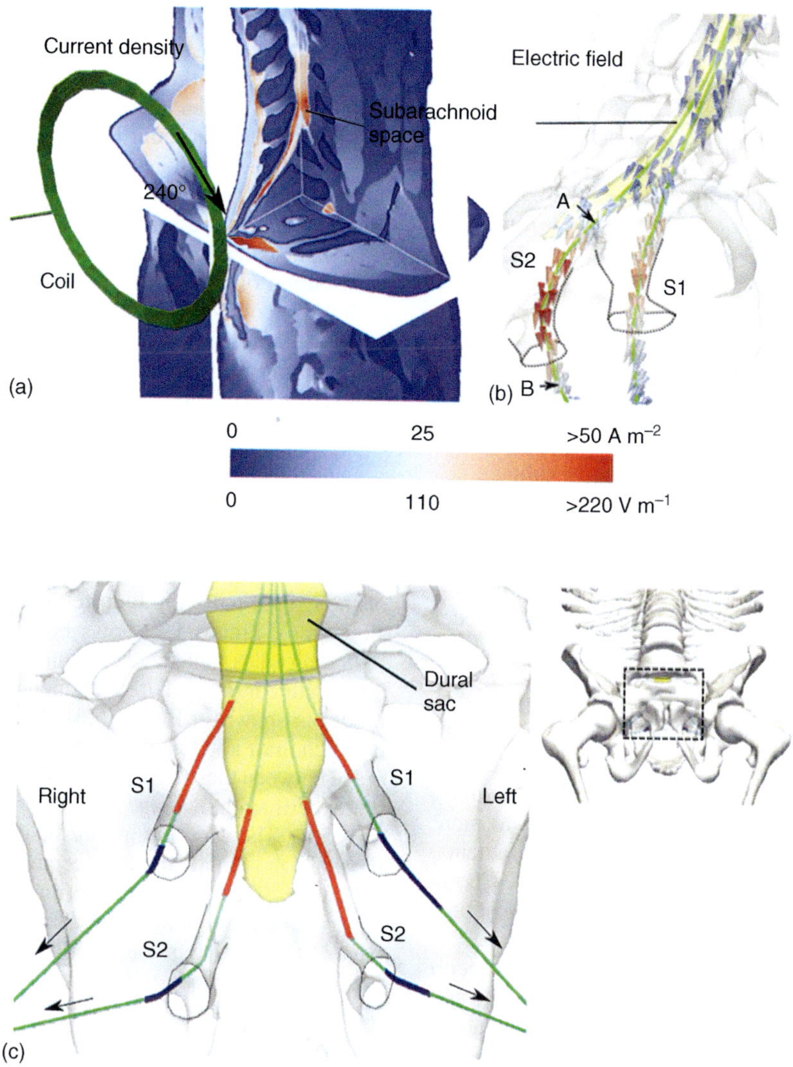

Figure 5.5. Simulation setup used by Laakso *et al.*[54] to model magnetostimulation of the spine. (a) Current density induced in the lower hip region by switching of the solenoid coil. (b) Electric field components running along the spine root pathways (green tracks). (c) Plot of four studied nerve fiber tracks (green) and the stimulation sites (red and blue portions) caused by the imposed electric fields. (Reproduced with permission from Ref. 54. © IOP Publishing, 2014)

turn defines the MRG nerve model parameters such as the internodal spacing.

Ladenbauer *et al.*[53] used a finite element model of the lumbar spine including the spine's nerve roots to simulate transcutaneous spinal cord stimulation by surface electrodes. The authors used an active model of myelinated nerve fibers (similar to one shown in Figure 5.2c) to simulate the response of the spine's nerve roots to the applied electric current.

Laakso *et al.*[54] also modeled the spin's nerve roots and employed a similar active nerve model but used a magnetic coil to induce stimulation. Figure 5.5 summarizes the simulation setup, showing the current density and electric field patterns in the used body model as well as the sections of the analyzed nerve roots that were stimulated by the imposed electric fields. The authors compared the simulated and experimental PNS thresholds (i.e., the smallest coil current for a given coil frequency required to induce an AP) and found good agreement. Other work coupling electromagnetic and neurodynamic simulations analyzed stimulation of the forearm,[55] the ulnar and sciatic nerves,[56,57] the auricular vagus nerve in the ear,[58] and the cervical vagus nerve.[59] These models provide insights into particular body parts or targeted nerves of interest, but more generality (from a full body and nerve model) is needed for situations in which a broad region is exposed and the site of stimulation is unknown.

5.6 WHOLE-BODY PNS SIMULATIONS

The first PNS simulation frameworks including a detailed whole-body EM model with matching nerve atlas have only recently emerged.[60–65] Validation against experimentally determined thresholds was shown first in the arm and leg[62] and later in whole body and head MRI gradient coils.[66] In the latter, the model accurately predicted experimental PNS thresholds of two whole-body gradients and one head gradient (error <10%). The simulations also provided information on the site of activation and which nerves were likely to be the next to fire. This work also assessed the biological variation of PNS thresholds by comparing a male and a female body model. The female was more resilient to PNS induction by whole body gradients, likely due to smaller body size and increased body fat content. The male/female difference was most pronounced for the body gradient systems.

The body models used in the gradient coil simulations[66] had a spatial resolution of 1 mm and include 21 tissue classes. The co-registered nerve atlases have ~1900 individual nerve tracks. The EM fields were simulated using a low-frequency magneto quasi-static FEM solver on a hexahedral mesh (voxels). After computation of the induced *E*-field, the potential change along the nerves was computed by projection of the *E*-field on the nerve tracks and integration. The potential changes (both spatial and temporal as the potential is locked to the gradient waveform) were fed to the MRG model (Figure 5.2d). Finally, PNS thresholds were obtained by increasing the coil's driving amplitude until an action potential was observed (titration process).

Figure 5.6 shows the wire patterns for two body gradient coils (*y*-axis) and their induced *E*-fields. The body gradients induce *E*-fields predominantly in the neck and thorax region. In both cases, the *E*-field is heavily shaped by the conductive body. Figure 5.6 also shows hot-spots of the 'PNS oracle'[45] superimposed to the two nerve atlases. This PNS oracle metric is closely related to the neural activation function but is adjusted to better account for the structure of peripheral nerve fibers such as the nonmyelinated nature of the nodes of Ranvier which positions the largest voltage drop across the node. In addition, the PNS oracle uses a spatial smoothing kernel to account for the contribution of neighboring nodes and is normalized such that it corresponds to the inverse of the predicted PNS threshold. Despite the large number of *E*-field hotspots, only a few nerve tracks experience significant activation (shoulder and upper intercostal nerves), which underscores the importance of proper modeling of the relative orientation between nerve tracks and *E*-field.

The PNS threshold curves for the two body gradients are shown in Figure 5.7. The thresholds are given as the gradient amplitude ΔG_{min} at threshold as a function of the *E*-field pulse duration (equal to the trapezoidal slew-time). Figure 5.7 shows both the experimental PNS thresholds (blue, incl. SD) and the simulated PNS thresholds for the male/female model in red (the male model is shown in Figure 5.6). The PNS thresholds between male and female varied by up to 30%; the average between these two body models agreed well with the experimental average for both gradient coils (error <5%). The variation in thresholds simulated using the male and female models seemed to approximately match the SD seen in the experimental data. Both the experimental and simulation data emphasize the impact of the body type on the PNS threshold. In fact, having multiple body models was crucial to correctly estimate the average PNS threshold of a larger patient cohort, especially for the whole-body gradient coils. The accuracy of the simulated PNS thresholds was accurate enough to correctly rate these two gradient coils with respect to PNS (Figure 5.7, bottom panel), which might be useful to inform the optimization phase of novel MR gradient coils.

5.7 EXAMPLE: PNS-INFORMED DESIGN OF MRI GRADIENTS

In order to further demonstrate the potential of PNS modeling during the design of MRI gradient coils, we show how different head gradient design approaches can have similar gradient efficiencies and linearity but differing PNS thresholds. Given this,

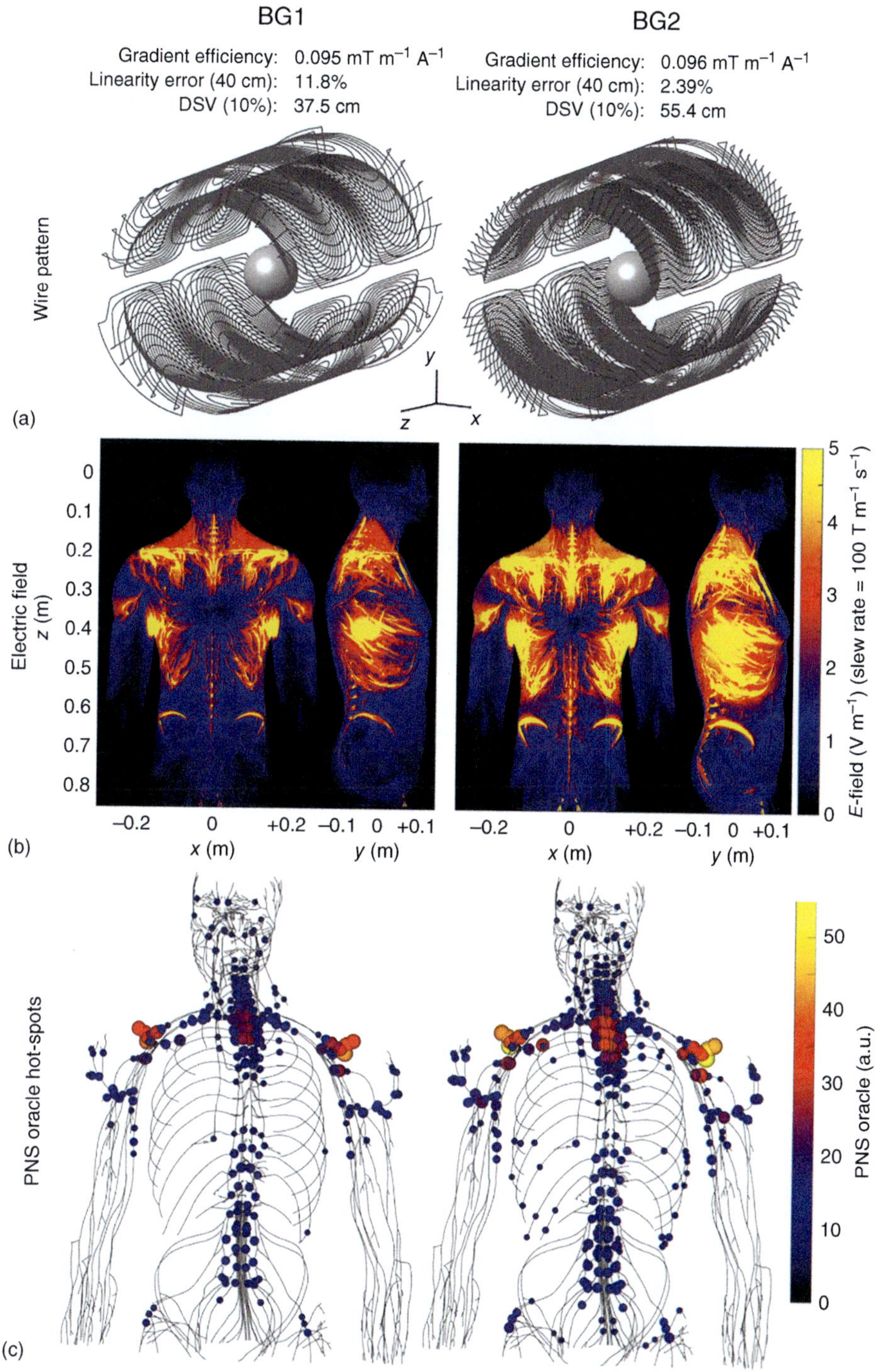

Figure 5.6. PNS simulation results in the male body model of the *Y*-axes of the two body gradients BG1 and BG2 studied in Ref. 66 in terms of the wire patterns (a), the electric field maps as maximum intensity projections (b), and hot spots of the PNS oracle overlaid to the nerve atlas (c). 'DSV' denotes the diameter of the homogeneous spherical volume. PNS threshold curves for these two coils are shown in Figure 5.7

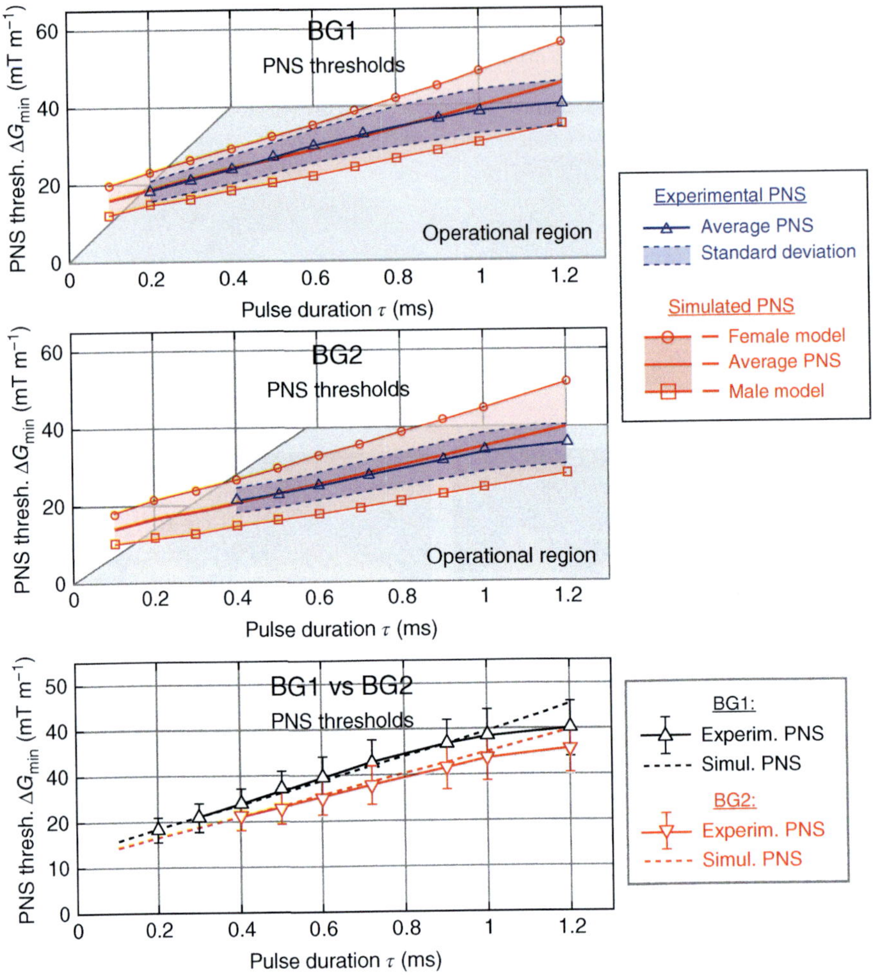

Figure 5.7. Simulated PNS threshold curves for the *Y*-axes of BG1 and BG2 (depicted in Figure 5.6) for both the male and female body model as well as the 'population average' over the male and female model. The PNS threshold is shown as the minimum gradient amplitude ΔG_{min} causing PNS as a function of the *E*-field pulse duration (equal to the trapezoidal slew-time). The experimental data (average and SD) is also shown as solid lines. The bottom panel compares the experimental and simulated average (across sexes) PNS thresholds of the two coils in the same plot

a first use for PNS modeling in gradient design is to simply compare the PNS thresholds of different designs before construction. Figure 5.8 shows the primary windings examined of two different head *x*-gradient designs inspired from the literature. Both gradients are 46 cm inner diameter gradient coils but use different strategies to accommodate the shoulders; HG1 uses a funnel-like opening similar to a published design.[67] The coil HG2 uses a 'folded' design strategy.[68,69] The folded design is shorter in the *z*-direction than HG1, but the folds provide additional DOFs to the design optimizer to create good gradient strength down the base of the neck. Wire patterns were optimized for these three designs using standard Boundary Element Method Stream-Function (BEM-SF)[70–72] so as to maximize gradient linearity while keeping inductance, current density, and power dissipation at reasonable levels. The efficiency of the two designs were 0.323 and 0.264 mT m^{-1} A^{-1} respectively. The deviation from linearity over a 20 cm

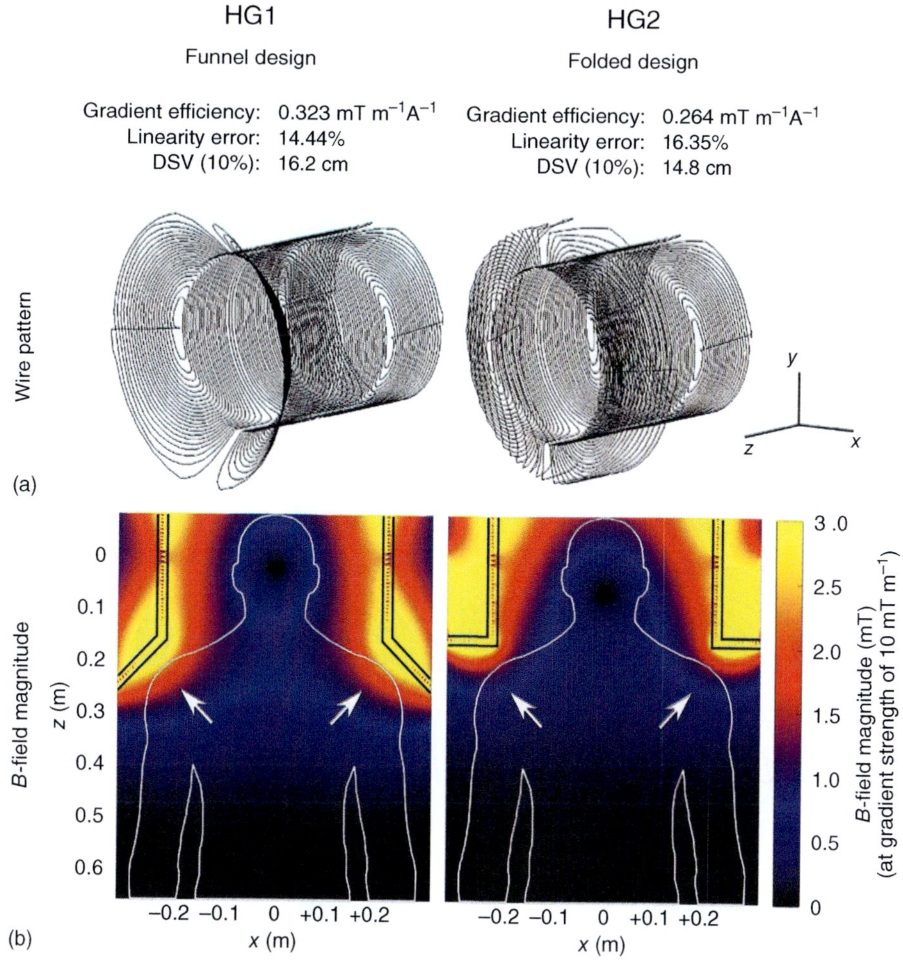

Figure 5.8. (a) Wire patterns of the two generic head gradients (primary windings only). 'DSV' denotes the diameter of the homogeneous spherical volume. HG1 uses a conical funnel-like opening, and HG3 is a folded design. (b) Magnetic field magnitude for a current corresponding to a gradient amplitude of 10 mT m^{-1} applied to the male body model

FOV was 14.44% and 16.35%. For head gradients, the inductance is a relatively minor concern, since their low inductances compared to body gradients allows conventional drivers to slew them at very high rates.

Figure 5.8 also shows the *B*-field magnitude created by HG1 and HG2 for a normalized gradient of 10 mT m^{-1} applied to the male body model (outlined). Both coils induce rather strong concomitant *B*-fields in the upper thorax while keeping the fields in the head facial area small. Note that although both coils apply a 10 mT m^{-1} gradient, the field pattern in the shoulders is very different due to differing concomitant terms. This situation raises different concerns for PNS and it is not clear if and how much the d*B*/d*t* reduction in the shoulders (for HG2) will impact the PNS thresholds. Figure 5.9 shows the *E*-field projection onto the nerves for a 1 kHz sinusoid with a slew rate of 100 T m^{-1} s^{-1} (gradient amplitude of approx. 16 mT m^{-1}). As could be inferred from the *B*-field maps, HG1 and HG2 create *E*-fields mainly in the upper torso, with only weak *E*-fields induced in the facial area. The 'folded' design HG2 produces the lowest *E*-fields of the two studied coils. This is because the *E*-field scales with the *B*-field amplitude and HG2 bends a large fraction of the *B*-fields away from the shoulders. Figure 5.9 also shows the electric

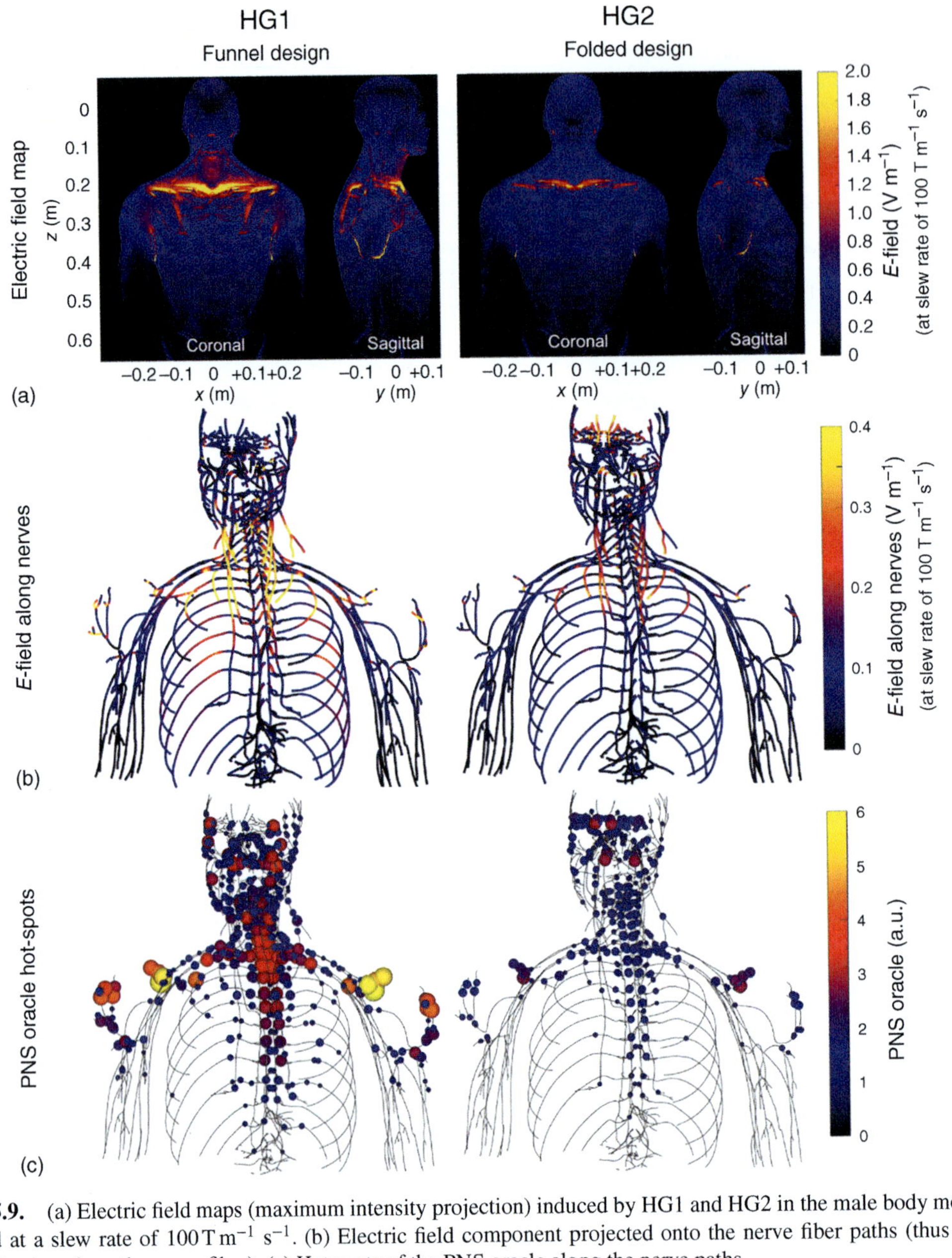

Figure 5.9. (a) Electric field maps (maximum intensity projection) induced by HG1 and HG2 in the male body model when switched at a slew rate of $100\,\mathrm{T\,m^{-1}\,s^{-1}}$. (b) Electric field component projected onto the nerve fiber paths (thus causing a current flowing along the nerve fiber). (c) Hot spots of the PNS oracle along the nerve paths

field projected onto the nerves (the *E*-field component parallel to the nerve fiber paths). This entity determines the amount of current flowing along the axis of the nerve. Finally, Figure 5.9(c) shows the PNS oracle for each design. Electric field and PNS maps clearly show that the design modification in the folded design HG2 allow a reduction of the electric field and the resulting neural activation in the shoulders. For both coils, the nerves in the neck area experience the highest values of projected *E*-fields; however, the highest

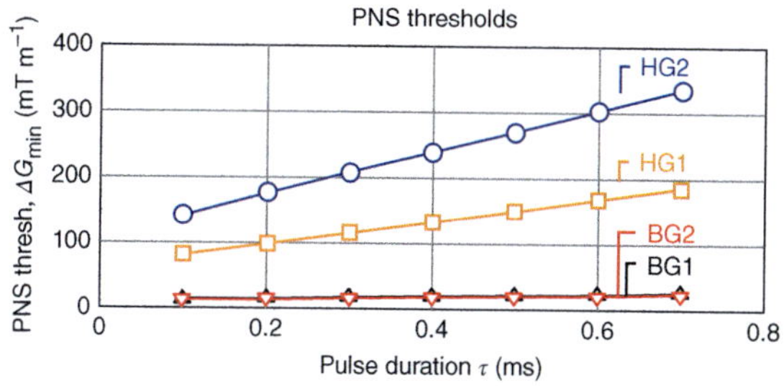

Figure 5.10. Simulated PNS threshold curves in the male body model for the two head gradients HG1 and HG2 (wires shown in Figure 5.8) and the body gradients BG1 and BG2 (wires shown in Figure 5.6) in terms of minimum gradient amplitude ΔG_{min} causing PNS as a function of the *E*-field pulse duration (equal to the trapezoidal slew-time)

neural activation occurs in another body area, i.e., in the shoulder parts. This behavior emphasizes the importance of the relative orientation of nerve fibers and the local *E*-field in PNS. In a sense, the nerve atlas and projection operator act as a filter applied to the induced *E*-field; not all components of the *E*-field matter equally with respect to PNS. This is in contrast to other *E*-field safety issues such as specific absorption rate (SAR), which is dependent only on the magnitude of the *E*-field in an isotropic medium. This orientation dependence, together with the freedom to choose concomitant fields, may open up a design space where winding patterns with similar efficiencies, inductances, and linearity may have differing PNS profiles, as is the case for the two coils shown.

Finally, Figure 5.10 shows simulated PNS threshold curves for HG1 (orange squares) and HG2 (blue circles) for a trapezoidal gradient waveform of differing slew periods (pulse duration). PNS thresholds are given as smallest gradient amplitude ΔG_{min} that induces an action potential in any of the nerves. The threshold is different for each *E*-field pulse duration (slew period of the applied trapezoidal). The simulation predicts a highly desirable 80% increase in PNS thresholds for HG2 (compared to HG1), with only a mild loss of linearity (14.44–16.35%).

This example illustrates the limitations of the scaling laws that have been formulated to relate the size of the linear volume to the PNS thresholds.[16] The authors analyzed PNS thresholds from four different body and head gradient coils and found a linear relationship between the size of the diameter of the homogeneous spherical volume (DSV) and the inverse PNS threshold $1/\Delta G_{\text{min}}$. More specifically, the authors found a slope

$$m = \frac{\Delta(\text{DSV})}{\Delta(1/\Delta G_{\text{rheo}})}$$

of roughly 1.43 (Figure 5.4b in Ref. 16), where ΔG_{rheo} denotes the gradient amplitude stimulation threshold for infinitely small pulse durations. Applying this scaling law to the head coils HG1 and HG2 predicts an increase in PNS thresholds (from HG1 to HG2) of only 15%, which is dramatically lower than the 80% increase observed in the simulated PNS thresholds. This suggests that the scaling laws might work well in coils using similar design strategies but require more complete modeling when different design strategies are compared.

5.8 OTHER USES OF PNS MODELING FOR MITIGATION IN MRI

Beside coil design modifications, accurate PNS modeling can provide a framework to explore other PNS mitigation strategies for MRI. Some ideas found in the literature include segmented gradient coils where the wires are not wound on the surface of a cylindrical former, but on a plate perpendicular to that surface,[73] matrix or 'PatLoc' gradient coils,[74] or multiple-region gradient coils.[75] In addition, Bowtell *et al.*[18] proposed adding additional Helmholtz-like coils to reduce the gradient winding's concomitant *B*-fields, thus reducing the *E*-field and PNS. Although they demonstrated this strategy in a constructed coil, it can be more systematically characterized using PNS modeling. Other strategies for PNS reduction alter the gradient waveform rather than the gradient windings. Recently, we suggested leveraging the different time characteristics of sodium and potassium channels to favorably alter the nerve state during a 'pre-pulse' applied prior to spin excitation.[76] This technique, 'pre-saturation targeting the potassium system' (PRE-TAPS), used a 10 kHz gradient preparation waveform applied in front of the EPI readout to create a nerve membrane state similar to the refractory period, thus lowering the likelihood of the actual EPI readout to generate action potentials.

5.9 LIMITATIONS OF PNS SIMULATION

Like all complex modeling approaches, whole-body PNS modeling is prone to errors and limitations in the body and neurodynamic model. Considerable work is needed to explore the sensitivity of the result to the many model parameters. This effort is in its infancy, but a recent analysis indicates that PNS predictions are reasonably accurate and robust to a wide range of parameters.[57,63,77] In addition, convergence studies have shown that model time-step size and spatial resolution can be chosen for sufficient convergence.[63]

We found that the detailed topology of the tissues together with the electromagnetic properties assigned to the different tissue classes constituted the parameters with the biggest impact on PNS thresholds. Indeed, *E*-field hot spots often occur in converging tissue boundaries that form a bottleneck structure or in thin layers of insulating tissues (like fat) surrounded by well-conducting tissues (e.g., muscle). In order to capture these *E*-field hot spots and their effect on nerve fibers, a spatial resolution of 1 mm (or better) was required for the body model. The degree to which important structures in the body are missing from the model is harder to assess. The endoneurium and perineurium (thin enclosures of the nerve fiber and bundles) are absent in most body models (including those used in the gradient coil simulations in Figures 5.6–5.10) and are likely difficult to fully describe in body models due to their small size.

Another important aspect of the simulation is to correctly couple the simulated electric fields to the neurodynamic model. This requires a high level of consistency between the body model (used for the EM field simulation) and the nerve tracks of the atlas (used for the neurodynamic simulations). For example, a nerve 'invalidly' intersecting a tissue such as bones or air cavities where it does not belong can cause an erroneous sudden change of the electric potential along the nerve, resulting in an artificially low threshold. In addition, the location of the nerve electrical compartments relative to the electric field is important and not accurately known. For example, the exact locations of the nodes of Ranvier are not generally known. To address this, we take a 'worst case' approach by shifting the most active nerve segments to determine the lowest threshold. This is justified given the multiple fibers in a typical nerve bundle; one will likely occupy the worst-case location. Other numerical parameters such as the spatial resolution of the coil discretization can also be assessed by refining the coil model until the *B*-fields (and thus the *E*-fields) converge.

The degree to which the existing models span the space of the important individual variations in the human species is a major issue for all body model-based simulations. The experimental data shows significant variation in the threshold histograms across individuals.[16,78] To this end, it is likely valuable to continue to add more body models to the repertoire available for PNS simulations.

5.10 CONCLUSION

In this chapter, we reviewed the recent work to develop computational approaches for prediction of PNS in MRI. While the integration of the modeling framework's components is recent, each piece is built on long-standing modeling work such as neurodynamic modeling and the study of electromagnetic fields in body models. The coupling of these two, however, seems well suited to improve our understanding of important safety considerations associated with switching gradient fields in MRI, and ultimately may impact gradient designs. The frameworks reproduce stimulation experiment results with good accuracy, allowing quick comparison of designs. They also allow studies which are not possible experimentally, such as the determination of sites of activation beyond the initial threshold. PNS models can also facilitate the study of other mitigation techniques such as the use of nontraditional coil configurations and MRI gradient encoding methods.

RELATED ARTICLES IN EMAGRES

Radiofrequency Fields: Interactions, Biological Effects, and Safety Issues

Whole Body MRI: Local and Inserted Gradient Coils

Safety Considerations in MRI

Safety and Sensory Aspects of Main and Gradient Fields in MRI

Gradient Coil Systems

REFERENCES

1. V. E. Amassian, E. Larry, P. J. Maccabee, and R. Q. Cracco, *Electroencephalogr. Clin. Neurophysiol. /Evoked Potentials Section*, 1992, **85**, 291.
2. J. R. Daube and D. I. Rubin, in 'Aminoff's Electrodiagnosis in Clinical Neurology', ed M. I. Aminoff, Saunders: Philadelphia, PA, 2012, Vol. 6, p 290.
3. M. R. Popovic, K. Masani, and S. Micera, in 'Neurorehabilitation Technology', Springer: Cham, Switzerland, 2016, p 513.
4. S. Groppa, A. Oliviero, A. Eisen, A. Quartarone, L. G. Cohen, V. Mall, A. Kaelin-Lang, T. Mima, S. Rossi, G. W. Thickbroom, P. M. Rossini, U. Ziemann, J. Valls-Solé, and H. R. Siebner, *Clin. Neurophysiol.*, 2012, **123**, 858.
5. J.-P. Lefaucheur, *Expert. Rev. Neurother.*, 2008, **8**, 799.
6. T. F. Budinger, *IEEE Trans. Nucl. Sci.*, 1979, **26**, 2821.
7. M. S. Cohen, R. M. Weisskoff, R. R. Rzedzian, and H. L. Kantor, *Magn. Reson. Med.*, 1990, **14**, 409.
8. M. S. Cohen, R. Weisskoff, and H. Kantor, In *Proceedings of the 75th Anniversary Scientific Assembly and Annual Meeting Radiological Society of North America (Abstracts)*, 1989.
9. W. Irnich and F. Schmitt, *Magn. Reson. Med.*, 1995, **33**, 619.
10. J. A. McNab, B. L. Edlow, T. Witzel, S. Y. Huang, H. Bhat, K. Heberlein, T. Feiweier, K. Liu, B. Keil, J. Cohen-Adad, M. D. Tisdall, R. D. Folkerth, H. C. Kinney, and L. L. Wald, *NeuroImage*, 2013, **80**, 234. Mapping the Connectome.
11. K. Setsompop, R. Kimmlingen, E. Eberlein, T. Witzel, J. Cohen-Adad, J. A. McNab, B. Keil, M. D. Tisdall, P. Hoecht, P. Dietz, S. F. Cauley, V. Tountcheva, V. Matschl, V. H. Lenz, K. Heberlein, A. Potthast, H. Thein, J. Van Horn, A. Toga, F. Schmitt, D. Lehne, B. R. Rosen, V. Wedeen, and L. L. Wald, *NeuroImage*, 2013, **80**, 220 Mapping the Connectome.
12. X. Feng, A. Deistung, and J. R. Reichenbach, *Zeitschrift für Medizinische Physik*, 2018, **28**, 36.
13. C. L. G. Ham, J. M. L. Engels, G. T. van de Wiel, and A. Machielsen, *J. Magn. Reson. Imaging*, 1997, **7**, 933.
14. P. R. Harvey and P. Mansfield, *Magn. Res. Med.*, 1994, **32**, 236.
15. P. Mansfield and P. R. Harvey, *Magn. Reson. Med.*, 1993, **29**, 746.
16. B. Zhang, Y.-F. Yen, B. A. Chronik, G. C. McKinnon, D. J. Schaefer, and B. K. Rutt, *Magn. Reson. Med.*, 2003, **50**, 50.
17. M. Davids, B. Guérin, L. R. Schad, and L. L. Wald, In *Proceedings of the 27th Annual Meeting of ISMRM, Montreal, Canada*, 2019.
18. S. S. Hidalgo-Tobon, M. Bencsik, and R. Bowtell, *Magn. Res. Med.*, 2011, **66**, 1498.
19. B. J. Roth, L. G. Cohen, M. Hallett, W. Friauf, and P. J. Basser, *Muscle Nerve*, 1990, **13**, 734.
20. D. Durand, A. S. Ferguson, and T. Dalbasti, *IEEE Trans. Biomed. Eng.*, 1992, **39**, 58.
21. K. P. Zimmermann and R. K. Simpson, In *Engineering in Medicine and Biology Society, 1995. IEEE 17th Annual Conference*, IEEE, Vol. 2, p 1115, 1995.
22. P. Ravazzani, J. Ruohonen, and F. Grandori, *Adv. Eng. Softw.*, 1995, **22**, 29.
23. P. Ravazzani, J. Ruohonen, F. Grandori, and G. Tognola, *Ann. Biomed. Eng.*, 1996, **24**, 606.
24. R. Bowtell and R. M. Bowley, *Magn. Reson. Med.*, 2000, **44**, 782.
25. K. R. Davey, C. H. Cheng, and C. M. Epstein, *IEEE Trans. Biomed. Eng.*, 1991, **38**, 418.
26. W. Wang and S. R. Eisenberg, *IEEE Trans. Mag.*, 1994, **30**, 5015.
27. G. A. Mouchawar, J. A. Nyenhuis, J. D. Bourland, L. A. Geddes, D. J. Schaefer, and M. E. Riehl, *IEEE Trans. Magn.*, 1993, **29**, 3355.
28. P. J. Basser, R. S. Wijesinghe, and B. J. Roth, *IEEE Trans. Biomed. Eng.*, 1992, **39**, 1207.
29. F. Liu, S. Crozier, H. Zhao, and B. Lawrence, *Concepts Magn. Reson.*, 2002, **15**, 26.
30. F. Liu, H. Zhao, and S. Crozier, *IEEE Trans. Biomed. Eng.*, 2003, **50**, 804.
31. H. Zhao, S. Crozier, and F. Liu, *Magn. Reson. Med.*, 2002, **48**, 1037.
32. J. L. Hoorweg, *Archiv für die gesamte Physiologie des Menschen und der Tiere*, 1898, **71**, 128.
33. W. Thomson, *Proc. R. Soc. Lond.*, 1856, **7**, 382.
34. W. Thomson, On Peristaltic Induction of Electric Currents in Submarine Telegraph Wires'. British Association Report, 1855.
35. A. L. Hodgkin and A. F. Huxley, *J. Physiol.*, 1952, **117**, 500.
36. D. R. McNeal, *Biomed. Eng., IEEE Trans. BME*, 1976, **23**, 329.

37. J. P. Reilly, *Med. Biol. Eng. Comput.*, **27**, 101.
38. J. P. Reilly, V. T. Freeman, and W. D. Larkin, *Biomed. Eng. IEEE Trans. BME*, 1985, **32**, 1001.
39. J. D. Sweeney, K. Deng, E. Warman, and J. T. Mortimer, In *Images of the Twenty-First Century. Proceedings of the Annual International Engineering in Medicine and Biology Society*, Vol. 4, p 1281, 1989.
40. J. D. Sweeney, J. T. Mortimer, and D. Durand, In *IEEE/Engineering in Medicine and Biology Society Annual Conference. IEEE*, 1987.
41. C. Cameron McIntyre and M. Warren Grill, *Biol. Cybern.*, 1998, **79**, 29.
42. C. C. McIntyre, A. G. Richardson, and W. M. Grill, *J. Neurophysiol.*, 2002, **87**, 995.
43. A. G. Richardson, C. C. McIntyre, and W. M. Grill, *Med. Biol. Eng. Comput.*, 2000, **38**, 438.
44. F. Rattay, *IEEE Trans. Biomed. Eng.*, 1986, **BME-33**, 974.
45. M. Davids, B. Guérin, V. Klein, L. R. Schad, and L. L. Wald, In *Proceedings of the 27th Annual Meeting of ISMRM, Montreal, Canada*, 2019.
46. B. J. Roth and P. J. Basser, *IEEE Trans. Biomed. Eng.*, 1990, **37**, 588.
47. S. S. Nagarajan, D. M. Durand, and E. N. Warman, *IEEE Trans. Biomed. Eng.*, 1993, **40**, 1175.
48. R. Plonsey and R. C. Barr, *IEEE Trans. Biomed. Eng.*, 1995, **42**, 329.
49. O. Hiwaki and S. Ueno, *IEEE Trans. J. Mag. Jpn.*, 1994, **9**, 148.
50. A. Hyodo, A. Kyura, and S. Ueno, In *Engineering in Medicine and Biology Society, Proceedings of the 16th Annual International Conference of the IEEE, IEEE*, Vol. 1, p 323, 1994.
51. S. S. Nagarajan and D. M. Durand, *IEEE Trans. Biomed. Eng.*, 1995, **42**, 926.
52. S. S. Nagarajan, D. M. Durand, B. J. Roth, and R. S. Wijesinghe, *Ann. Biomed. Eng.*, 1995, **23**, 116.
53. J. Ladenbauer, K. Minassian, U. S. Hofstoetter, M. R. Dimitrijevic, and F. Rattay, *IEEE Trans. Neural Syst. Rehabil. Eng.*, 2010, **18**, 637.
54. I. Laakso, H. Matsumoto, A. Hirata, Y. Terao, R. Hanajima, and Y. Ugawa, *J. Neural Eng.*, 2014, **11**, 056013.
55. S. Pisa, *Open Biomed. Eng. J.*, 2014, **8**.
56. E. Neufeld, A. M. Cassará, H. Montanaro, N. Kuster, and W. Kainz, *Phys. Med. Biol.*, 2016, **61**, 4390.
57. E. Neufeld, I. V. Oikonomidis, M. I. Iacono, L. M. Angelone, W. Kainz, and N. Kuster, *Phys. Med. Biol.*, 2016, **61**, 4466.
58. A. M. Samoudi, S. Kampusch, E. Tanghe, J. C. Széles, L. Martens, E. Kaniusas, and W. Joseph, *Med. Biol. Eng. Comput.*, 2017, **55**, 1763.
59. A. P. Mourdoukoutas, D. Q. Truong, D. K. Adair, B. J. Simon, and M. Bikson, *Neuromodulation: Technol. Neural Interface*, 2018, **21**, 261.
60. M. Davids, B. Guérin, V. Klein, L. R. Schad, and L. L. Wald, In *Proceedings of the 26th Annual Meeting of ISMRM, Paris, France*, 2018.
61. M. Davids, B. Guérin, L. R. Schad, and L. L. Wald, In *Proceedings of the World Molecular Imaging Congress, New York, NY, USA*, 2016.
62. M. Davids, B. Guérin, L. R. Schad, and L. L. Wald, *Sci. Rep.*, 2017, **7**, 5316.
63. V. Klein, M. Davids, L. L. Wald, L. R. Schad, and B. Guérin, *Phys. Med. Biol.*, 2018, **64**, 015005.
64. E. Neufeld, B. Lloyd, W. Kainz, and N. Kuster, *Front. Physiol.*, 2018, **9**, 1594.
65. Sim4Life, Sim4life is ready for Yoon-Sun, Website, 2018. https://zmt.swiss/news-and-events/news/sim4life/sim4life-is-ready-for-yoon-sun-v4-0/#current (accessed 31 January 2019).
66. M. Davids, B. Guérin, A. v. Endt, L. R. Schad, and L. L. Wald, *Mag. Res. Med.*, 2019, **81**, 686.
67. M. Weiger, J. Overweg, M. B. Rösler, R. Froidevaux, F. Hennel, B. J. Wilm, A. Penn, U. Sturzenegger, W. Schuth, M. Mathlener, M. Borgo, P. Börnert, C. Leussler, R. Luechinger, B. E. Dietrich, J. Reber, D. O. Brunner, T. Schmid, L. Vionnet, and K. P. Pruessmann, *Mag. Res. Med.*, **79**, 3256.
68. T. P. Wade, A. Alejski, C. A. McKenzie, and B. K. Rutt, In *Proceedings of the 24th Annual Meeting of ISMRM, Singapore*, 2016.
69. S. A. Winkler, A. Alejski, T. Wade, C. A. McKenzie, and B. K. Rutt, *Magn. Reson. Med.*, 2017, **78**, 1635.
70. R. A. Lemdiasov and R. Ludwig, *Concepts Magn. Reson.*, 2005, **26B**, 67.
71. G. N. Peeren, *J. Comput. Phys.*, 2003, **191**, 305.
72. M. Poole and R. Bowtell, *Concepts Magn. Reson.*, 2007, **31B**, 162.
73. P. Mansfield and B. Haywood, *Phys. Med. Biol.*, 2008, **53**, 1811.
74. S. Littin, F. Jia, K. J. Layton, S. Kroboth, H. Yu, J. Hennig, and M. Zaitsev, *Magn. Reson. Med.*, 2018, **79**, 1181.

75. D. L. Parker and J. R. Hadley, *Mag. Res. Med.*, 2006, **56**, 1251.

76. M. Davids, B. Guérin, M. Schmelz, L. R. Schad, and L. L. Wald, In *Proceedings of the 26th Annual Meeting of ISMRM, Paris, France*, 2018.

77. P. P. M. So, M. A. Stuchly, and J. A. Nyenhuis, *IEEE Trans. Biomed. Eng.*, 2004, **51**, 1907.

78. E. U. Saritas, P. W. Goodwill, G. Z. Zhang, and S. M. Conolly, *Med. Imaging, IEEE Trans.*, 2013, **32**, 1600.

Chapter 6

Magnetically Induced Force and Torque on Medical Devices

Terry O. Woods

Office of Science and Engineering Laboratories, Center for Devices and Radiological Health, Silver Spring, MD, USA

6.1 INTRODUCTION

Since its introduction in 1984, the use of MRI (magnetic resonance imaging) has continued to increase, with more than 30 million scans performed each year in the United States. Every year, more patients receive MR (magnetic resonance) exams, and though MRI is generally a safe imaging modality that does not use ionizing radiation to create images, there are some inherent hazards created by the electric and magnetic fields produced by the MR system. At the same time, more patients are receiving MR exams and increasing numbers have one or more implanted devices, both passive implanted medical devices (PIMDs) like coronary stents and hip implants and electrically active implantable medical devices (AIMDs) like pacemakers and neurostimulators that rely on a source of electrical energy or other source of power external to the human body (excluding gravity) to achieve their intended function. The presence of implants introduces additional hazards during MRI examinations. These hazards must be addressed by implant manufacturers as they work with the Food and Drug Administration (FDA) and other regulatory bodies to develop MRI safety labeling that indicates if a patient with a specific implant may safely receive an MR examination, and if so, provides the conditions for which scanning may be safely performed. A list of general hazards to patients with AIMDs are given in Table 1 of ISO TS 10974.[1] This chapter considers the effects of magnetically induced force and torque produced by the MR system's static magnetic field, B_0, on implants and other devices.

Magnetically induced force and torque are the hazards that are most familiar to anyone who has used a magnet to fasten a piece of artwork to a refrigerator or seen a compass needle move. However, these seemingly innocuous effects have contributed to fatal accidents involving both implants and nonimplanted devices in and near MR systems where the magnetic fields are tens of thousands of times greater than the Earth's magnetic field and are always present, even

Safety and Biological Effects in MRI.
Edited by Devashish Shrivastava and J. Thomas Vaughan

ISBN: 978-1-118-82130-5
Also published in eMagRes (online edition)
DOI: 10.1002/9780470034590.emrstm1579

when the MR system is not actively scanning. In 1992, a woman with an intracranial aneurysm clip that had been misidentified as safe for exposure to MRI died when the MR system's magnetic field caused the implanted clip to move, tearing the clipped artery and resulting in a fatal hemorrhage.[2] Though rare, these B_0 field-related accidents, also referred to as projectile accidents, continue to happen. A 6-year-old boy was killed in 2001 after being struck in the head by a ferromagnetic oxygen cylinder,[3] and in 2018 a man died after being trapped against an MR system by an oxygen cylinder.[4] The 1992 fatality was the impetus that led to the development of standards committees that continue to work to develop standards for assessing the safety of implants and other devices in the MR environment.[5]

Magnetically induced force is a function of the applied magnetic field and the magnetic properties of the device. The MR system magnet attracts paramagnetic and ferromagnetic materials and repels diamagnetic materials. If the magnetically induced force exceeds the weight of the object, the object will be rapidly moved toward the MR system magnet. Ferromagnetic objects are magnetically saturated in the MR system's magnetic field and the displacement force is proportional to the spatial field gradient (SFG) of the magnetic field.[6] For paramagnetic materials which include most metallic implants, the magnetically induced displacement force is a function of the static magnetic field strength, the SFG of the static magnetic field, and the magnetic susceptibility of the material.[7] The maximum magnetically induced force occurs in regions of high SFG near the entrance to the MR system bore.

The Lenz effect induces a magnetic force on conductive objects that opposes the movement of the object through the magnetic field.[8] This effect may be easily observed by vertically positioning a metal plate (composed of a paramagnetic material like aluminum) in the scanner bore so the small dimension of the plate is aligned with the B_0 field, then tipping the plate over. The plate will fall slowly to the patient table, its motion opposed by the force created by its motion through the B_0 field. Heart valves are the medical device for which the most concern exists about the potential impacts of the force created by the Lenz effect.[8] Investigation of nine different heart valve prostheses advanced through the B_0 field at 1.5 T showed irregularities in pressure profiles of four valves indicating resistance of the occluder to the B_0 field.[9] The irregularities were relatively small and no adverse events have been reported for patients with heart valves, but it is important to be aware of the potential for the Lenz Effect to impact the performance of heart valves and other electrically conductive mechanical devices that are required to move in the large magnetic fields present in or near an MR system.

Magnetically induced torque acts to align the object with the MR system static magnetic field like a compass needle aligns with the Earth's magnetic field. The magnetically induced torque depends on the static magnetic field strength and the magnetic properties, mass distribution, and geometry of the device. The magnetically induced torque is maximum inside the MR system bore. For paramagnetic materials (most implants) and unsaturated ferromagnetic materials, the magnetically induced torque is proportional to the magnetic field strength.[10] For saturated ferromagnetic materials, the magnetically induced torque is insensitive to the value of the static field, and an upper bound may be calculated.[7,11]

Most metals used in implants are paramagnetic, including commercially pure (CP) titanium and titanium alloys, nitinol, some cobalt-chrome alloys, and some stainless steel alloys. Copper, present in electrically active devices, is the most common diamagnetic material. Magnetic susceptibilities for ferromagnetic materials are orders of magnitude greater than those of diamagnetic and paramagnetic materials, leading to magnetically induced forces on ferromagnetic objects that are substantially greater than those acting on paramagnetic objects.[12]

It is important to note that some stainless steels are ferromagnetic and can become dangerous projectiles if brought near an MR system while others are paramagnetic and experience substantially smaller magnetically induced forces. Therefore, it is critical to know the precise type of stainless steel used in a device before attempting to introduce it into the MR environment. Ferritic and martensitic stainless steels including types 303 and 304 as well as the other 300 and 400 series stainless steels specified in ASTM F899 *Standard Specification for Wrought Stainless Steels for Surgical Instruments*[13] are ferromagnetic. The use of these alloys should be avoided for devices that need to be used in and near MR systems. Properly processed nitinol is paramagnetic; however, manufacturing processes like laser cutting can produce ferromagnetic nickel-rich regions that will produce large magnetically induced forces and torques in the MR environment.[14] Fabrication, sterilization, and processing may alter the magnetic properties of a device; therefore, it is critical that the finished device or a specimen that can be demonstrated to represent a worst case for the finished device be assessed for magnetically induced force and torque. Heat treatment and cold work of austenitic stainless steels may produce regions containing martensite or ferrite that would make the device unsafe in or near an MR system. During manufacturing, the magnetic material may be transferred from a ferromagnetic mandrel or other tool to the device during heat treatment or other fabrication steps. It is critical that such transferred material be removed so that its presence does not impact the safety and operation of the device in the MR environment and any MR images acquired near the device.[12] Standards committees have revised specifications for various forms of 316L and 316 stainless steel to require no delta ferrite be present in the alloy to minimize magnetically induced force and torque.[15–20]

6.2 STANDARDS FOR ASSESSING MAGNETICALLY INDUCED FORCE AND TORQUE

ASTM International Committee F04 on Medical and Surgical Materials and Devices developed test methods for assessing magnetically induced force and torque produced by an MR system's static magnetic field. ASTM F2052-15 Standard Test Method for Measurement of Magnetically Induced Displacement Force on Medical Devices in the MR Environment, last revised in 2015, was first published in 2000.[21] ASTM F2213-17 Standard Test Method for Measurement of Magnetically Induced Torque on Medical Devices in the MR Environment, last revised in 2017, was first published in 2002.[22] The scope of both standards is all medical devices. Practical considerations limit F2052 to a device that may be suspended by a string near the entrance to the bore of an MR system and F2213 to a device that will fit within the MR system bore.

F2052 provides a method for measuring the magnetically induced displacement force on an object while suspended from a string at a point in a magnetic field where the displacement force is perpendicular to gravity. Testing is done in a horizontal bore MR system with B_0 oriented horizontally and parallel to the MR system bore. To increase measurement sensitivity, the test location must be on the axis of the bore and at a location where the SFG is within 20% of the maximum value of the SFG on the axis of the bore. The test object is suspended from the test apparatus so that its deflected position is in the prescribed test location where the magnitudes of both the magnetic field strength and the SFG are known. The deflection angle is measured and the magnetically induced deflection force at the test location is calculated. Using the method in F2052 section X3, the test results may be used to calculate a maximum SFG to which the device may safely be exposed.

A deflection angle of 45° at the test location means that *at the test location*, the magnetically induced force is equal to the device weight. A deflection angle of less than 45° at the test location means that *at the test location*, the magnetically induced force is less than the device weight. There is a common misconception that a measured deflection angle of less than 45° means that the magnetic force will be less than the device weight in any location in any MR system. This is absolutely not the case. The deflection angle itself provides no information about the magnetic force that will act on a device and the safety of the device in any MR system. A specific value of deflection angle absent any information about the field conditions at the location where that angle was measured cannot be used to determine the safety of a device at any other location in any other MR system. The maximum SFG should be determined using the measured deflection angle at the test location together with the SFG and magnetic field strength at the test location to calculate a maximum SFG for a given maximum MR system nominal magnetic field strength as outlined in F2052.

F2213 provides methods for measuring the torque experienced by a device inside the MR system bore. It assesses the magneto-static torque due to the interaction of the MR system static field with the magnetization of the test object. It does not address torque induced by currents in lead wires. The MR system static magnetic field produces a torque that acts to align the test object with the magnetic field. All the experimental methods given in F2213 may be used in MR systems with a horizontal magnetic field. Some may be adapted to work with a vertical magnetic field, but different apparatus would need to be developed for use in a vertical magnetic field. The five methods are as follows: the Suspension Method, the Low Friction Surface Method, the Torsional Spring Method, the Pulley Method, and the Calculation Based on Measured Displacement Force Method. The Suspension and Low Friction Surface Methods are not appropriate for objects for which the magnetically induced torque is expected to exceed the torque due to gravity.

The Suspension Method consists of suspending the test sample from a string, positioning it near the MR system isocenter, and observing any motion that aligns the device in a preferential orientation, expected to be parallel to the B_0 field. This method is useful for test samples that are difficult to place on the low friction test plate with principal axes aligned in the required directions. If movement of the device is not observed, the magnetically induced torque is small, and no further evaluation is needed. If magnetically induced torque is observed, then the Low Friction Surface Method, the Torsional Spring Method or the Pulley Method need to be performed.

The Low Friction Surface Method is performed by placing the test object on a low friction, nonmetallic, nonconductive plate positioned near the MR system isocenter. The object is placed on the test plate and rotated in 45° increments through 360°. The process is repeated with each principal axis of the device oriented parallel to B_0. Any motion of the specimen in any orientation is noted. If no motion is observed, the magnetically induced torque is less than the product of the friction force between the test sample and the test plate and the longest dimension of the test specimen. The coefficient of friction between the test plate and the test sample can be determined and used to calculate an upper bound of the magnetically induced torque. If any sample motion is observed, then the magnetically induced torque should be measured using the Torsional Spring Method or the Pulley Method.

The Torsional Spring Method (which was the only method included in the original version of F2213) determines the magnetically induced torque using a torsional spring. The test sample is placed on a holding platform supported by a torsional spring. The frame holding the torsional spring and holding platform is rotated through 360° in 10° increments, and torque as a function of angle is determined by measuring the deflection angle of the holder.

The Pulley Method uses a rotating platform connected to a low-friction, nonmetallic pulley and positioned near the isocenter of the MR system. The test device is fixed on the platform. A lightweight string is wrapped around the pulley and attached to a force gauge. The platform is rotated by pulling the force gauge in a direct line away from the platform. The force is observed as the platform is rotated through 360°. The process is repeated for the device oriented with each principal axis of the device parallel to B_0. The maximum magnetically induced torque is calculated from the maximum observed force.

The Calculation Based on Measured Displacement Force Method provides an upper bound for the magnetically induced torque using magnetically induced displacement force measurements from F2052. This method is most appropriate for devices that are composed of only one material and is not appropriate for implants that contain magnets or ferromagnetic material.

The ASTM work item, tentatively titled Standard Guide for Assessing the Safety of Non-Implanted Items in the MR Environment, addresses the hazards related to the presence and use of items that remain outside the MR system bore. It considers magnetically induced force that might cause the item to become a projectile, the proper functioning of the medical device or other item in the MR environment, and potential interference between the medical device or other item and the MR system (e.g., an electrically active device that creates image artifact or otherwise degrades the MR images or other MR system output).

6.3 LEVERAGING TEST RESULTS AND ACCEPTANCE CRITERIA

In some cases, results for a specimen that has been tested for magnetically induced force may be applied to another item. For instance, if it can be demonstrated that a device is composed of the same alloy, meets the same material specification, and that any differences in processing and/or fabrication between the tested specimen and the device do not affect the magnetic properties of the device, then test results from the test specimen may be generalizable to the device. The FDA Center for Devices and Radiological Health engineering laboratories recently conducted magnetically induced force and torque testing on 11 common implant alloys and reported the test results.[12] For devices composed of the tested alloys, if the above constraints are satisfied, it may be possible to leverage those results to determine an allowable maximum SFG for given nominal field strength MR systems.

A commonly used acceptance criterion for magnetically induced deflection force is that the magnetic force is less than the device weight. The rationale for this criterion is that any magnetic force to which the device is exposed will be no greater than the force acting on it produced by the Earth's gravitational field that would be experienced by a patient with the device during their normal daily activities. Similarly, the worst-case gravitational torque, defined as the product of the maximum linear dimension of the device and the device weight, is commonly used as an acceptance criterion for magnetically induced torque.

Some implants may safely be subjected to magnetically induced forces greater than the implant weight and torques greater than the worst-case gravitational torque. For patients with those implants, a risk-based approach supporting safe exposure of the implant and adjacent tissue to forces greater than the implant weight and torques greater than the worst-case gravitational torque may be developed by considering the mechanical properties of tissues adjacent to the device, its means of fixation in the body, and an assessment of the impact of the maximum magnetic force on the proper functioning of the device, e.g., demonstrating that the magnetically induced force and torque will not dislodge a hemostasis clip and will not injure tissue adjacent to the clip.

Nonimplanted devices subjected to magnetically induced forces greater than their weight should either be excluded from the MRI scan room or prevented from entering the region near the MR system where the magnetically induced force exceeds the device weight and can cause the device to become a projectile. This may be accomplished by one or more of the following: physically securing the device to the MRI scan room so that it cannot be moved toward the MR system, attaching the device to a tether, including a gauss alarm that sounds when the alarm enters a set magnetic field strength, or for devices with wheels, incorporating a dead man brake into the system that leaves the system wheels locked as a default position and requires the user to activate a mechanism that will allow the wheels to move. Extreme care must be taken to avoid projectile accidents when equipment with wheels is present in the MRI scan room.

6.4 MRI SAFETY LABELING

The ultimate goal of MRI safety testing and analyses is to develop labeling that informs patients, MR professionals, and other healthcare providers how a specific device may safely be placed into and used in the MR environment. FDA requests that all implants, external medical devices that are fastened to or carried by a patient (e.g., external insulin pump), and all medical devices that are intended to enter the MR environment be assessed for safety in the MR environment and labeled accordingly. ASTM F2503-20 Standard Practice for Marking Medical Devices and Other Items for Safety in the MR Environment, originally approved in 2005 and published with identical content as ISO 62570, defines terms and icons used for labeling items for safety in the MR environment and recommends information that should be included in the MRI safety labeling.[23]

All medical devices or other items that may enter the MR environment should be labeled MR Safe, MR Unsafe, or MR Conditional, as defined in ASTM F2503:

MR Conditional – 'an item with demonstrated safety in the MR environment within defined conditions including conditions for the static magnetic field, the time varying gradient magnetic fields and the radiofrequency fields. Note: Additional conditions, including specific configurations of the item, may be required.'

MR Safe – 'an item that poses no known hazards resulting from exposure to any MR environment. MR Safe items are composed of materials that are electrically nonconductive, nonmetallic, and nonmagnetic.'

MR Unsafe – 'an item which poses unacceptable risks to the patient, medical staff or other persons within the MR environment.'

The FDA Guidance document, Establishing Safety and Compatibility of Passive Implants in the MR Environment, provides sample MRI safety labeling for passive implants.[24] An example for a fictitious PIMD called the 'star implant' is given below.

6.4.1 MRI Safety Information

Nonclinical testing has demonstrated the star implant is MR Conditional. A patient with this device can be safely scanned in an MR system meeting the following conditions:

- Static magnetic field of 1.5 and 3.0 T
- Maximum spatial field gradient of 3000 gauss cm^{-1} (30 T m^{-1})
- Maximum MR system reported, whole-body averaged specific absorption rate (SAR) of 4 W kg^{-1} (First Level Controlled Operating Mode)

Under the scan conditions defined above, the star implant is expected to produce a maximum temperature rise of less than 2 °C after 15 minutes of continuous scanning.

In nonclinical testing, the image artifact caused by the device extends approximately 2 mm from the star implant when imaged with a gradient echo pulse sequence and a 3.0 T MRI system.

Labeling for passive and electrically nonimplanted devices typically includes a gauss-line restriction that defines where it may safely be placed and used in the MRI scan room. Labeling similar to the following is common for electrically active equipment that must remain outside the MR system bore:

Projectile hazard
Equipment operation may be impacted
Do not exceed 20 mT (200 gauss)

Other examples may be found in the Medicines and Healthcare Products Regulatory Agency Safety Guidelines for MRI Equipment in Clinical Use.[25] Complex passive implants, AIMDS, and nonimplanted devices may require additional information defining the conditions for safe use in the MR environment. For instance, AIMDs may require programming into an MRI mode before scanning and return to non-MRI mode after scanning. Other devices like hydrocephalus shunts may need to be checked to see if device settings were changed by exposure to the MR system and reset if necessary. Some devices require assessments that confirm proper functioning after exposure to an MR system.

The results of magnetically induced force and torque testing for devices that may enter the MR system bore impact the first two bullets in the MRI Safety Information. The allowed static magnetic field strengths are determined based on results of magnetically induced force, torque, and RF-induced heating testing. The maximum SFG value is determined through the magnetically induced force testing and analyses. Similarly, the gauss line restriction for devices not intended to enter the MR system bore is determined by magnetically induced force testing as well as assessments of proper device operation outside the indicated gauss line.

Older MR Conditional labeling for many devices lists an allowable SFG as the value at the test location. For instance, a value of $7.2\,\mathrm{T\,m^{-1}}$ ($720\,\mathrm{gauss\,cm^{-1}}$) is commonly reported. While accurate, because the maximum SFG in patient accessible areas of the MR system is greater than that value for most clinical MR systems, this labeling proved to be problematic as for many implants it needlessly restricts patient access to many clinical MR systems with maximum SFG greater than $7.2\,\mathrm{T\,m^{-1}}$. The 2014 revision to F2052 added the method that uses the measured deflection at the test location together with the SFG and magnetic field strength at the test location to calculate a maximum SFG for a given maximum MR system nominal magnetic field strength. SFG values reported in recent MRI safety labeling were determined using this calculation. Data submitted to FDA and incorporated in MR system compatibility technical specification sheets through 2019 show upper bounds for the maximum SFG for current 1.5, 3.0, and 7.0 T clinical scanners to be 20, 17, and $16\,\mathrm{T\,m^{-1}}$, respectively. It is not anticipated that maximum values for 1.5 and 3.0 T scanners will change significantly in the future; however, 7.0 T systems have only recently been cleared for clinical use and there may be changes in maximum SFG as the system magnet designs continue to evolve.

F2503 is undergoing a major revision at the time of this writing. An ASTM International task group including AIMD and PIMD manufacturers, MR system vendors, the FDA, and other regulatory bodies, representatives of the Society for Magnetic Resonance Radiographers and Technologists (SMRT), physicians, MR test facilities, and university researchers is attempting to clarify and simplify MR Conditional labeling by standardizing the form and content of information included in the labeling. The goal is to develop simpler, more straightforward labeling that can be more easily understood and applied, thereby reducing misinterpretation and improving patient safety.

6.5 SUMMARY

Magnetically induced force and torque can pose hazards to patients and others in the MR environment. This chapter discusses magnetically induced force and torque acting on ferromagnetic, paramagnetic and diamagnetic materials and the standard test methods used to quantify magnetically induced forces and torques. The resulting analysis and interpretation of the standard test results to address magnetically induced force and torque are used to define key elements in the MRI safety labeling used by patients, MRI professionals and other healthcare providers to assure that patients may safely receive needed MR examinations.

REFERENCES

1. ISO/TS 10974, Assessment of the Safety of Magnetic Resonance Imaging for Patients with an Active Implantable Medical Device, International Organization for Standardization: Geneva, Switzerland, 2018.

2. R. P. Klucznik, D. A. Carrier, R. Pyka, and R. W. Haid, *Radiology*, 1993, **187**, 855.
3. D. W. Chen, 'Boy, 6, Dies of Skull Injury During M.R.I', New York Times: New York, 2001, pp B1, B5, https://www.nytimes.com/2001/07/31/nyregion/boy-6-dies-of-skull-injury-during-mri.html (accessed 26 June 2019).
4. V. Doshi, Indian man dies after being trapped in MRI machine, The Washington Post, 2018, http://web.archive.org/web/20190204144703/https://www.washingtonpost.com/news/worldviews/wp/2018/01/29/indian-man-dies-after-being-trapped-in-mri-machine/?utm_term=.66d152ba45b2 (accessed 26 June 2019).
5. T. O. Woods, in 'Wiley Encyclopedia of Biomedical Engineering', ed M. Akay, John Wiley & Sons, Inc.: Hoboken, 2006, p 2360.
6. E. M. Purcell, Electricity and Magnetism, Berkeley Physics Course, McGraw-Hill: New York, 1985, Vol. 2.
7. J. A. Nyenhuis, S.-M. Park, R. Kamondetdacha, A. Amjad, F. G. Shellock, and A. R. Rezai, *IEEE Trans. Device Mater. Rel.*, 2005, **5**, 467.
8. B. Condon and D. M. Hadley, *J. Magn. Reson. Imaging*, 2000, **12**, 171.
9. M.-B. Edwards, J. Mclean, S. Solomonidis, B. Condon, and T. Gourlay, *J. Magn. Reson. Imaging*, 2015, **41**, 74.
10. T. O. Woods, in 'Stainless Steels for Medical and Surgical Applications, ASTM STP 1438', eds G. L. Winters and M. J. Nutt, ASTM International: West Conshohocken, PA, p 82–90, 2003.
11. M. Omatsu, K. Minowa, K. Yokosawa, E. Inagaki, K. Ishizaka, K. Shibayama, and T. Yamamoto, *J. Magn. Reson. Imaging*, 2014, **40**, 1481. DOI: 10.1002/jmri.24500.
12. T. Woods, J. Delfino, and S. Rajan, *J. Test. Eval.*, 2019, **49** (2), https://doi.org/10.1520/JTE20190096.
13. F899-12b, Standard Specification for Wrought Stainless Steels for Surgical Instruments, ASTM International: West Conshohocken, PA, 2012.
14. T. W. Durig and D. E. Tolomeo, 'An Overview of Superelastic Stent Design,' SMST-2000, in *Proceedings of the International Conference on Shape Memory and Superelastic Technologies*, eds S. M. Russell and A. R. Pelton, International Organization on SMST: Pacific Grove, CA, 2001, pp 585–604.
15. F138-13a, Standard Specification for Wrought 18Chromium-14Nickel-2.5Molybdenum Stainless Steel Bar and Wire for Surgical Implants (UNS S31673), ASTM International: West Conshohocken, PA, 2013.
16. ISO 5832-1:2016(E), Implants for surgery – Metallic materials – Part 1: Wrought stainless steel, International Organization for Standardization Organization: Geneva, Switzerland, 2016.
17. F139-12, Standard Specification for Wrought 18Chromium-14Nickel-2.5Molybdenum Stainless Steel Sheet and Strip for Surgical Implants (UNS S31673), ASTM International: West Conshohocken, PA, 2012.
18. F1350-15, Standard Specification for Wrought 18Chromium-14Nickel-2.5Molybdenum Stainless Steel Surgical Fixation Wire (UNS S31673), ASTM International: West Conshohocken, PA, 2015.
19. F2257-14, Standard Specification for Wrought Seamless or Welded and Drawn 18 Chromium-14Nickel-2.5Molybdenum Stainless Steel Small Diameter Tubing for Surgical Implants (UNS S31673), ASTM International: West Conshohocken, PA, 2014.
20. F1586-13e1, Standard Specification for Wrought Nitrogen Strengthened 21Chromium-10Nickel-3Manganese-2.5Molybdenum Stainless Steel Alloy Bar for Surgical Implants (UNS S31675), ASTM International: West Conshohocken, PA, 2013.
21. ASTM F2052-15, Standard Test Method for Measurement of Magnetically Induced Displacement Force on Medical Devices in the Magnetic Resonance Environment, ASTM International: West Conshohocken, PA, 2015.
22. ASTM F2213-17, Standard Test Method for Measurement of Magnetically Induced Torque on Medical Devices in the Magnetic Resonance Environment, ASTM International: West Conshohocken, PA, 2017.
23. ASTM F2503-20, Standard Practice for Marking Medical Devices and Other Items for Safety in the Magnetic Resonance Environment, ASTM International: West Conshohocken, PA, 2020.
24. FDA Guidance for Industry and Food and Drug Administration Staff, 'Establishing Safety and Compatibility of Passive Implants in the Magnetic Resonance (MR) Environment,' dated December 11, 2014, https://www.fda.gov/regulatory-information/search-fda-guidance-documents/establishing-safety-and-compatibility-passive-implants-magnetic-resonance-mr-environment
25. MHRA, Guidelines for Magnetic Resonance Imaging Equipment in Clinical Use, Medicines and Healthcare Products Regulatory Agency, v 4.0, 2014.

Chapter 7

A Review of MRI Acoustic Noise and Its Potential Impact on Patient and Worker Health

Michael C. Steckner
Canon Medical Research USA, Inc., Mayfield Village, OH, USA

7.1 INTRODUCTION

Acoustic noise is an insufficiently recognized hazard of daily life, with a range of health effects.[1] While offensively loud sounds can be partially and quickly blocked by the momentary plugging of ears, the slow and insidious loss of hearing caused by cumulative doses of moderately loud sound is not generally appreciated. Greater attention is required in the MRI environment in order to ensure that the exposure does not contribute to long-term hearing loss and to avoid additional problems for people with known or latent hearing issues. A survey sent to 3250 members of the Japanese Society for Magnetic Resonance in Medicine (JSMRM) (982 deidentified responders)[2] indicated that 11.4% were aware of experiences or episodes suggestive of acoustic trauma (i.e., any indication of hearing loss) to patients. Incidents of acoustic trauma tended to increase with field strength as did usage of hearing protection. Approximately 3% of responders indicated no protection was offered, 17% provided hearing protection on request, 10% indicated a decision was made whether hearing protection was necessary, and 68% indicated the policy was to provide hearing protection in all cases, with no responses from approximately 3% of the responders.

With appropriate protection, it can be shown that patient exposure in an MRI is within regulatory guidelines. Ensuring proper protection is a nontrivial task and a major objective of this chapter. The purpose of this chapter is to improve:

1. The awareness of regulatory guidelines designed to minimize long-term hearing loss.

Safety and Biological Effects in MRI.
Edited by Devashish Shrivastava and J. Thomas Vaughan

ISBN: 978-1-118-82130-5
Also published in eMagRes (online edition)
DOI: 10.1002/9780470034590.emrstm1628

2. The awareness of hearing protection options available, excluding ramifications on communication with the patient.
3. The understanding of the medical consequences of loud sound for the various segments of the patient population and appropriate protection strategies.
4. The understanding of how to properly deploy and check for proper application of hearing protection.
5. The understanding of risks when patients are over-exposed.
6. The technical understanding of noise measurements and the output of MRI scanners.
7. The awareness of reported acoustic incidents.

The dominant cause of routine MRI acoustic noise is gradient activity, the specifics of which are beyond the scope of this chapter.[3,4] There are additional but minor noise contributions from the magnet, cold-head, and ambient room noise (e.g., ventilation systems, etc.). The noise caused by a quenching magnet can be substantial. Characterization of MRI system noise typically includes all sources in the magnet room and is the assumption of this chapter unless stated otherwise. An additional source of perceived acoustic sound is the 'microwave hearing' phenomena caused by the radiofrequency (RF) pulses.[5] All RF pulses produce local heating within the body, which, in turn, produces a tiny thermo-elastic tissue expansion wave that, under ideal conditions, is just audible.

All acoustic noise is delivered by one of three routes:

1. auditory canal;
2. bone conduction; and
3. thermo-elastic expansion wave.

The delivery mechanism is relevant when considering the damping properties of protective mechanisms. Airborne is the most prevalent channel. The bone conduction mechanism operates in all situations where MRI acoustic noise is of concern, but its relative contribution is a function of hearing protection and individual anatomic characteristics, discussed below. If the ear canal is completely plugged (e.g., fetus auditory canal is filled with amniotic fluid) the airborne route is inactive, and bone conduction is the sole transmission channel.[6] If the head is receiving a substantial exposure to RF pulses (e.g., when the head is located at isocenter) there is a possibility the thermo-elastic waves will be heard, if the gradients are not active.

It is useful to identify the possible MRI exposure profiles so that the implications of exposure to MRI acoustic noise for each use case are properly considered, including a determination of whether the necessary assessment tools and protective methods exist. The following categorization is used:

1. The subject within the imaging volume of the scanner.
2. Medical staff using the MRI in an interventional procedure.
3. The medical staff assigned the routine responsibility of operating the scanner.
4. MRI factory workers.
5. MRI volunteers who are scanned for research purposes, training, etc.
6. The medical staff assigned the task of tending to the subject, (not always #3).
7. Nonmedical staff (e.g., family or friends) aiding the subject.
8. Facility staff who may be peripherally exposed to MRI acoustic noise.
9. Public at large transiently near the MRI scanner.
10. Companion animals.

This chapter assumes that categories #8, #9 have no health consequences associated with unprotected exposure to MRI acoustic noise and thus are not considered. The first seven categories, in general, should be candidates for hearing protection and are within the scope of this chapter. Category #4 is not considered in detail because it constitutes a conventional occupational exposure case with known survey tools outside the scope of this chapter. Nominally, categories #3, #6 could also be handled by conventional occupational exposure survey methods and regulations, with the benefit of noise measurements in the proximity of the scanner not presently available, as noted elsewhere in the chapter. On the assumption that category #7 is infrequent, there is the possibility to apply the same considerations as for the patient, assuming the exposure duration is the same. Category #10 is not formally considered in this chapter, although literature is noted below, and custom hearing protection is available for some animals (e.g., 'Mutt Muffs' for dogs). This chapter also does not consider the implications on fMRI studies.

The 'subject within' category #1 requires further division:

(a) the patient who may have normal or sensitive hearing, or using medications with potential to impact sensitivity;
(b) fetus as patient;

(c) expectant mother as patient with fetus (presumed to be equivalent to 'b' with regards to acoustic exposure);
(d) neonates; and
(e) children.

Category #5 is a complex exposure condition that may require case-by-case analysis, as discussed later in the chapter.

The remainder of the introduction discusses:

- quantification and notation of sound measurements;
- pertinent regulations;
- how occupational exposure limits are converted to clinical guidance;
- the estimation of risk due to over-exposure;
- the types of hearing tests;
- the types of hearing protection;
- how hearing protection is characterized;
- an identification of how literature was found for this chapter; and
- a brief review of patient incident reports.

7.1.1 Quantification and Notation of Sound Levels

Sound or acoustic pressure is the deviation from atmospheric pressure and measured in the SI units of Pascal (Pa). The threshold of human detection is generally considered to be $p_0 = 20$ μPa (at 1 kHz, in air) and is used as a standard reference value. Human perception response is approximately logarithmic and thus sound or acoustic pressure levels (SPL) is computed as:

$$\text{SPL (dB)} = 20 \log_{10}\left(\frac{p}{p_0}\right)$$

where p_0 denotes the reference value, p is the measured pressure, SPL is Sound Pressure Level, and dB is decibel, the unit of sound pressure.

The factor of 20 is the result of two factors multiplied: 2*10. The factor of 10 converts from the underlying units of 'bel' (the logarithm of a ratio to a reference value, named after Alexander Graham Bell) to decibel (deci = 0.1). The factor of two relates to decibels computed from 'field' values, such as pressure, versus power values. In most applications, power is a function of the square of the field value. Thus, from the perspective of power, the parameter needed for hearing conservation purposes, a gain of 3 dB doubles acoustic power. From a human perception consideration, a 10 dB increase doubles perceived loudness.

Human acoustic spectral sensitivity is not constant with frequency, or SPL, and may vary with age, gender, and accumulated damage. Equal-loudness contours characterize human spectral sensitivity when exposed to pure, single frequency tones.[7] A series of representative weighting functions standardize human acoustic sensitivity and enable the quantification and characterization of exposure, action or limit values, etc. The weightings used in the MRI literature and this chapter are as follows:

1. characterization of human hearing at low SPL (dBA),
2. characterization of human hearing at high SPL (dBC), and
3. zero (unweighted) SPL (dBZ). Often the Z is not indicated. Also occasionally identified as 'linear'.

Typical notations are, for example, dB(A) or dBA and only 'dB' is assumed to be dB(Z), but cannot be reliably assumed. In general, there is large variability in acoustic notation. This chapter attempts to use what is common in the relevant literature.

As loud sounds cause hearing damage, C weighting would be the more appropriate unit of measure. However, for historical reasons, A-weighted measurements are more commonly used. The MRI literature uses a mix of A and C weightings and when not specified, it is not entirely clear whether it is Z weighting, or accidentally not specified.

Sound levels typically vary with time. There are methods, outside the scope of this chapter, that can reduce the time variations to an equivalent sound energy and those use the following notation: e.g., L_{eq}, or LA_{eq} where L_{eq} denotes 'equivalent level' and if present, the additional letter (e.g., A) denotes the weighing scale. It is also necessary to indicate the period of averaging, and multiple notation variants are found, e.g., $LAeq(8\,h)$, $L_{Aeq,8h}$. Some reports also notate sound exposure levels in dBA with an accompanying statement of time. Rebasing of time exposure requires the use of an 'exchange' rate that defines the number of dB adjustment for halving, or doubling, of the time exposure interval. A consensus seems to be emerging on a 3 dB exchange rate, but some older important documents and organizations use a 5 dB exchange rate.[8] Note that in a few rare instances cited literature values are time rebased (3 dB exchange) to enable comparison to other literature values.

7.1.2 A Primer on the Frequency Response of the Human Auditory System and the Outputs of an MRI

The nominal range of human hearing is 20–20 000 Hz whereas an MRI system is capable of producing sound below 20 Hz and above 20 kHz. Typical lowest human adult voice frequencies are in the 100–250 Hz range with the majority of spectral content below 3500 Hz. Characterizing the acoustic output of an MRI is more complicated. The specific sequence has a significant impact on the output due to the unique characteristics of the (x, y, z) gradient waveforms, in addition to the natural resonance characteristics of the gradient, etc., subassemblies. While an MRI sequence can drive waveforms from around 10 Hz to over 20 kHz, the resonant characteristics contribute substantially to defining the loudest frequencies, which are typically in the 1000–3000 Hz range.

Human hearing sensitivity varies through the frequency range, varies between individuals, generally deteriorates with age, particularly for men and varies with loudness. Spectral sensitivity as a function of loudness is described by Fletcher–Munson curves, and since a 2003 update,[7] equal-loudness contours are used. The dBA and dBC measures noted above use frequency weighting functions, shown in Figure 7.1, derived from the equal-loudness contours. Age-related sensitivity degradation is most significant at the higher frequencies.

The range of dB exposures in daily life varies enormously. A summary[9] is shown in Table 7.1. While understanding the loudness of various daily events is useful, the cumulative dose of noise received is the key factor for hearing conservation purposes, assuming the exposure is not sufficiently loud to cause near-instant damage. The loudest outputs of MRI scanners are reported later in this chapter, and the latest generation of MRI scanners with 'quiet' sequences have an inconsequential output. It is difficult to characterize a noise floor because selecting large field of view (FOV, low gradient amplitudes), etc., typically reduces the noise output. Characterization of sequence families is also difficult because individual scanners, gradient performance options, etc., can cause significant noise output variations. Sample[10] Spin Echo, EPI, and TrueFISP spectra are shown in Figure 7.2. In general terms, fast sequences and smaller FOV are the loudest.

Table 7.1. Selected representative noise levels and various regulatory and recommended limits etc.

dBA average exposure	Example
0	Nominal threshold of human hearing
10	Pin drop
30	Whisper
50	Refrigerator
60	Normal conversation
70 (WHO recommended 24 h limit)	Shower
80 (range of occupational exposure limit)	Heavy traffic
90	Shouted conversation
100 (99 dBA 1 h MRI exposure limit)	Monster truck audience experience
110 (Average worst MRI output, FDA)	Chainsaw
120 (WHO peak limit for children)	Thunderclap
130 (range of loudest reported MRI peak)	Jackhammer
140 (140 dBZ peak limit for adults)	Jet engine at take off

Yellow highlighted entries denote approximate threshold of pain range.
WHO, World Health Organization.

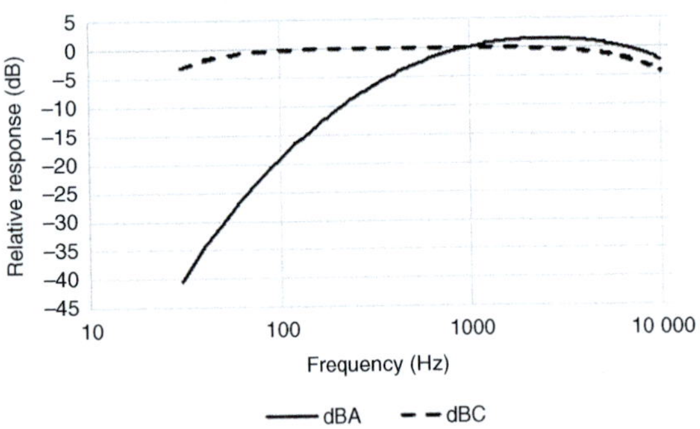

Figure 7.1. dBA, B, C weighting functions

7.1.3 Regulations and Recommendations

There are many different occupational regulatory limits and requirements across the world. Various recognized bodies have also issued recommendations. There may even be different regulations in the same country depending on the industry, such as in the United States. Full coverage of regulations is beyond the scope of this chapter. In general, the more recent regulatory action is converging with the scientific consensus of lower limits and exchange rates. However, it is an additional challenge to extend the occupational exposure limits to an infrequent and short clinical exposure. There does

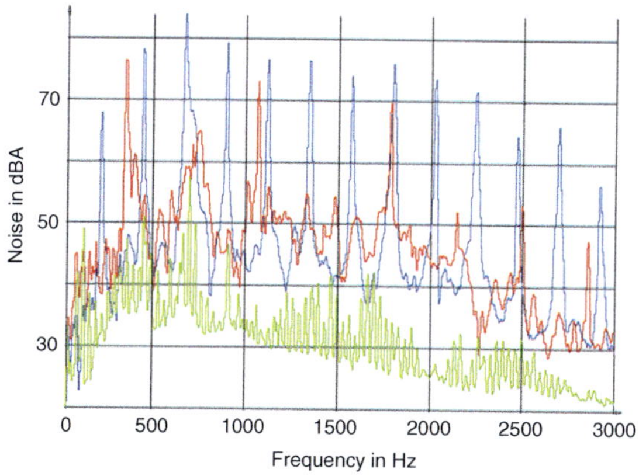

Figure 7.2. Sample sequence spectra of Spin Echo (green), EPI (red), TrueFISP (blue). (Reprinted from Figure A2, NEMA MS-4 (2010) with permission)

not appear to be any data that validates the contribution of infrequent short and loud exposures. The conversion from occupational exposure limits is further compounded by the objectives of occupational limits that according to the World Health Organization (WHO) '… are a product of political and economic compromises and are not intended to protect all workers from any injury or illness.'[11] The UK has developed specific patient acoustic noise guidelines for MRI. These excellent guidelines[12] direct the users to the manufacturer's instruction for use for hearing protection requirements, but additionally require that hearing protection always be provided for patients, volunteers and staff unless it is known the exposure will not exceed 80 dBA.

The European Union (EU) acoustic noise limits[13] are found within the physical agents directive (Directive 89/391/EEC) (European Economic Community) regarding the safety and health of workers. It uses the concept of exposure limits and upper, lower action values, all referenced to 8-h exposures. The exposure limit, after the application of hearing protection, is 87 dBA with a 140 dB peak limit. At the lower exposure action values (80 dBA and 135 dB peak), hearing protection is to be provided and at the upper exposure action values (85 dBA and 137 dB peak) hearing protection shall be used. The exchange rate is not specified in the directive but via reference 14 assumed here to be 3 dB and further corroborated in[11]. The WHO states that '… the more protective occupational exposure limits from … the EU allow for a small, but still significant percentage of workers to develop hearing loss … '[11]

In the United States, the Occupational Safety and Health Administration (OSHA) sets occupational limits. A hearing conservation program is required when the time-weighted average (TWA) exposure is ≥85 dBA in an 8-h exposure. The hearing protection must attenuate the 8-h exposure to at least 90 dBA. A 5 dB exchange rate is used. Peak SPL is not permitted to exceed 140 dB. However, the National Institute for Occupational Safety and Health (NIOSH) recommends an 85 dBA 8-h equivalent occupational exposure limit with a 3 dB exchange rate. Hearing protection is required when the exposure exceeds the 85 dBA level and is required to maintain the exposure to no more than 85 dBA. Confusingly, if the required 85 dBA exposure limit with hearing protection is exceeded, then at 100 dBA, workers should wear double hearing protection (e.g., earplugs and muffs).[8] NIOSH states that with a 40-year lifetime exposure at 85 dBA limits, the excess risk of developing occupational noise-induced hearing loss is 8% versus the 25% excess risk associated with the OSHA and Mine Safety and Health Administration (MSHA) 90 dBA limits. Note that some industry-specific guidelines require double hearing protection, such as the MSHA,[15] when the exposure exceeds an 8-h equivalent exposure to 105 dBA. A 5 dB exchange rate is used.

In the United Kingdom, the Health and Safety Executive (HSE) requires an occupational assessment when the exposure exceeds 80 dBA or peak SPL exceeding 135 dBC. Hearing protection must be provided at 85 dBA (daily or weekly average exposure) or 137 dBC peak, and with protection considered, exposure must not exceed 87 dBA or 140 dBC peak.[16] A 3 dB exchange rate is used. The UK Medicines and Healthcare products Regulatory Agency (MHRA) states that 'hearing protection shall always be provided for [MRI] patients and volunteers unless it can be demonstrated that noise levels will not exceed 80 dBA', with intent to maintain the received noise to below 85 dBA with hearing protection. It also explicitly mentions the consideration of both earplugs and earmuffs for high noise (115 dBA) sequences.[12] They recommend that anesthetized patients should always be given hearing protection and that staff should be trained in the selection and fitting of hearing protection for all patients. The MHRA also requires that sites carry out their own risk assessments related to acoustic noise exposure and that pregnant staff do not remain in the scan room during operations. The Health Protection Agency (HPA) recommendations match the MHRA.[17]

The International Commission on Non-Ionizing Radiation Protection (ICNIRP) recommendations[18] are not regulatory, but often consulted when regulations are developed. The ICNIRP recommendations are the basis for the UK MHRA recommendations: hearing protection offered to the patient if the noise level exceeds 80 dBA, and should be worn by the patients if the noise level exceeds 85 dBA. A reference within the ICNIRP document suggests that for dangerously ill patients a maximum of 67 dBA considered as the hazardous threshold. It does not appear that ICNIRP specifies the exchange rate but assumed here to be 3 dB. In addition, ICNIRP does not specify the time base of the exposure but assumed here to be 8 h.

While standards are typically not regulation, the approval process for medical equipment makes them important. MRI scanners typically claim compliance to the International Electrotechnical Commission (IEC) 60601 series of standards.[19] The general standard states that under normal use, the patient, operator, and other persons shall not be exposed to acoustic energy exceeding 80 dBA over a cumulative 24-h exposure interval using a 3 dBA exchange rate. In addition, it is not permitted to exceed 140 dBC (peak) SPL for impulsive or impact acoustic energy. It is also suggested, based on unreferenced WHO recommendations, that children not be exposed to peak SPL of ≥120 dB. Lastly, it also suggests that if the SPL exceeds 80 dBA, then noise protection measures should be considered. The particular standard for MRI, IEC 60601-2-33,[20] additionally separates the requirements for workers and patients. Since patient exposures are infrequent and typically less than 1 h, hearing protection shall be sufficient to reduce the exposure to 99 dBA. A derivation of this limit is provided elsewhere in this chapter. In addition, the standard stipulates information to be provided in the operators' manual related to vulnerable patients, variations in national requirements, consequences of loud sounds, etc.

The MRI noise measurements required by IEC 60601-2-33 use National Electrical Manufacturers Association/Medical Imaging and Technology Alliance (NEMA/MITA) MS-4.[10] Two measurement methods are provided, Maximum Gradient Acoustic Noise (MGAN) and Maximum Clinical Acoustic Noise (MCAN). MGAN applies a bipolar trapezoidal waveform on all three gradient axes simultaneously, with no dead time, operating at the maximum slew rate, amplitude and duty cycle permitted by the system control software. A search process discovers the physical location and worst-case waveform frequency that produces the maximum MGAN. However, MGAN is not a clinically relevant condition. MCAN is also measured under clinically unrealistic minimum slice thickness, FOV, etc., restrictions. However, given the nearly infinite number of possible sequences and relevant parameters in conjunction with gradient attributes, the measured MCAN may not necessarily be the highest possible clinical exposure. It is then unrealistically assumed that the patient exposure is at the maximum, continuously, for the entire exposure interval. MS-4 requires the MR vendor to provide one of the two measurements. At this time, MS-4 does not quantify acoustic noise levels at locations representative of occupational exposure during an interventional procedure. An update to the test method is considering the quantification of exposure just outside the bore opening. The intent is to provide measurements with equipment known to function safely (e.g., no missile effect issues) in an MRI environment.

Lastly, there are also nonoccupational 24-h recommended limits from both the WHO and Environmental Protection Agency (EPA) of 70 dBA.[21] Deriving MRI scanner limits from nonoccupational exposure recommendations is more difficult given the unknown and varied individual exposure profiles. The WHO also suggests *... that patrons of entertainment venues should not be exposed to sounds levels greater than 100 dBA during a four-hour period ... more than four times a year.*[11]

7.1.4 Translating Occupational Exposure Limits to Patient Limits

Since there are no known regulations or standards regarding appropriate patient acoustic noise exposures, patient limits are derived from the occupational literature. The current IEC 60601-2-33 3.2 edition starts with the 80 dBA limit (24 h) specified in the general standard and uses the 3 dBA exchange factor to derive a 94 dBA limit for a 1-h patient exposure. At this time, the general standard uses the most conservative occupational requirements. Repeating the same analysis, but starting with the ICNIRP/MHRA/NIOSH 85 dBA limit, results in the same 94 dBA 1-h limit since the time base for the exposure limits is different. Based on early acoustic science, a 5 dB forgiveness for a one-time exposure was added to produce the 99 dBA acoustic limit cited in IEC 60601-2-33. Thus, the average limits for MRI exposure are quite similar to exposures measured at US monster truck shows.[22]

Advances in acoustic standards[14] generally confirm the same 5 dB forgiveness for an infrequent one-time exposure lasting approximately 1 h but require assumptions about the patient noise exposure for the remainder of the occupational work week, which is under known regulatory limits. For example, if the patient was subjected to 99 dBA continuously for an hour, then to maintain the 85 dBA limit in a 5 day work week, the patient would need to restrict the average workplace exposure for the remainder of the workweek to under 81 dBA. In the EU, occupational exposure levels above 80 dBA require the availability of hearing protection. If the patient was occupationally subjected to lower noise levels, the MRI acoustic exposure levels could increase. If the scan duration decreases but the exposure is unchanged, the compensation required for the remainder of the work rapidly diminishes. Conversely, slight increases in scan duration at the same exposure levels requires an additional significant reduction in the acoustic noise exposure for the remainder of the week, such that a 1.6 h scan session requires zero occupational noise exposure for the remainder of the workweek. Such a scan session could still be mathematically justified, with more plausible noise exposure levels (e.g., 70 dBA WHO 24-h recommended limit), depending on acoustic exposures outside of the workweek, but those are generally unknown and unregulated.

7.1.5 Risk Estimation

The patient exposure limits in use today are derived from occupational exposure limits. It is an open question about patient risk due to a single, or multiple, acoustic MRI exposures. For occupational purposes, a concept of 'excess risk'has been defined[8]: *Percentage with material impairment of hearing in an occupational-noise-exposed population after subtracting the percentage who would normally incur such impairment from other causes in a population not exposed to occupational noise.* A risk table, identified as NIOSH-1997[8] and shown in Table 7.2, has been computed as a function of age (e.g., an indirect measure of years of occupational exposure), and the average daily exposure level (80, 85, 90 dBA). Note that 85 dBA is the reference value used in IEC 60601-2-33 for computing MRI patient exposure limits. There are other risk assessment tables, but NIOSH-1997 is the most recent. If the MRI exposure was an unlikely constant 85 dBA for the entire 1-h duration of the examination, and coincidentally matched the occupational exposure profile of the patient, then the 85 dBA row in Table 7.2 would identify the excess risk levels for the patient due to both occupational and medical exposures. Presumably, the 1 h MRI exposure would represent an infinitesimal contribution to the occupational excess risk. Conversely, if the occupational exposure was substantially lower (e.g., ≤80 dBA) then it is unknown how much the 1 h 85 dBA exposure to the MRI increases the excess risk estimate at the 80 dBA level in Table 7.2. Furthermore, scan durations greater than 1 h at the maximum 85 dBA exposure represent an unknown additional accumulation of excess risk. However, Table 7.2 may be useful in a clinical risk/benefit analysis with the caveat that the validity of extrapolating occupational risk limits down to infrequent, relatively short MRI examinations is unknown.

It is also instructive to consider the implications of other lifestyle choices on hearing loss risk from infrequent exposures to MRI. Smoking, through its impact on antioxidative mechanisms or the auditory vasculature system, has a major negative impact. One investigation[23] defined hearing loss as: mild, moderate, or marked and compared three population subgroups: nonsmokers, ex-smokers, and current smokers. Analysis showed a statistically significant trend relative to 'pack-years'of smoking. Passive smokers (those who never smoked in their lifetime but were exposed to daily cigarette fumes) also showed hearing loss with a risk level which appear comparable to the 85 dBA row in Table 7.2.[24]

While research has shown that alcohol may have a modest protective effect for hearing,[25] its suspected mechanism relates to how heart health has implications for hearing and thus is not recommended here as a palliative for MRI examinations.

7.1.6 Types of Hearing Tests

For the literature cited in this chapter, three conventional types of hearing tests were used

1. otoacoustic emission (OAE);
2. auditory brain stem response (ABR); and
3. the conventional hearing test (responsive patients only).

Table 7.2. Excess risk estimates for material hearing impairment, by age and duration of exposure

Average daily exposure (dbA)	5–10 years of exposure								>10 years of exposure							
	Age 30		Age 40		Age 50		Age 60		Age 30		Age 40		Age 50		Age 60	
	Risk (%)	95% CI	Risk (%)	95% CI	Risk (%)	95% CI	Risk (%)	95% CI	Risk (%)	95% CI	Risk (%)	95% CI	Risk (%)	95% CI	Risk (%)	95% CI
90	5.4	2.1–9.5	9.7	3.7–16.5	14.3	5.5–24.4	15.9	6.2–26.2	10.3	5.8–16.2	17.5	10.7–25.3	24.1	14.6–33.5	24.7	14.9–34.3
85	1.4	0.3–3.2	2.6	0.6–6.0	4.0	0.9–9.3	4.9	1.0–11.5	2.3	0.7–5.3	4.3	1.3–9.4	6.7	2.0–13.9	7.9	2.3–16.6
80	0.2	0.0–1.1	0.4	0.0–2.2	0.6	0.01–3.6	0.8	0.01–4.7	0.3	0.0–1.8	0.6	0.01–3.3	1.0	0.01–5.2	1.3	0.01–6.8

The normal inner ear will produce faint sounds when responding to a received sound. When hearing loss becomes significant, the inner ear does not produce these sounds. The OAE test measures these responses. It is a particularly useful noninvasive test when the patient is too young to cooperate in a conventional hearing test. OAE use is not restricted to the very young.

ABR, or auditory evoked potential (AEP), records the electrical activity in the brain in response to an auditory stimulus via electrodes positioned on the scalp. Detailed analysis of the electrical activity can identify components associated with the auditory branch of the cranial nerve, the response of the brainstem and signals originating from the auditory nerve.

The conventional hearing test assesses hearing sensitivity at different single (pure) frequencies and is an assessment of air and bone conduction thresholds for each ear.

An attempt to characterize hearing threshold shifts by fMRI was unsuccessful.[26]

7.1.7 Types of Hearing Protection and Usage

There are four general classes of hearing protection discussed in the reviewed literature:

1. earplugs (any protection inserted into or placed on top of the outer ear canal);
2. earmuffs, also referred to as ear defenders in some regions of the world (any external cup-shaped object covering the pinna or auricle either completely 'over the ear' or partially 'on the ear'). It is assumed here all reports of earmuffs are 'over the ear';
3. helmets or acoustic liners (passive foam, or other materials, strategically placed as an acoustic barrier); and
4. Active noise cancellation systems.

An additional hearing protection technique using small passive resonant chambers within the headband is also available but not discussed in the MRI literature.

Any hearing protection with a clamping band over the head is presumably designed for use where nothing else touches the headband. The performance characteristic of such hearing protection when lying down maybe different. In addition, in the author's experience, anything that taps or strokes the headband may be perceived as loud, depending significantly on the isolation provided by the headband design. In the author's experience, the resonant chamber design is very sensitive to any tapping.

Earplugs are probably the most commonly used hearing protection. They can be used in all MRI applications, inexpensive, and can deliver excellent performance if properly applied, as discussed elsewhere in this chapter. Some custom-molded earplugs can provide excellent protection and can be produced in minutes. They are expensive and require a trained technician, thus likely not useful in a busy clinical environment. Others require custom ear molds from an audiologist followed by shipment to a lab for manufacture. Custom molded earplugs and ported musician earplugs are outside the scope of this chapter. Musician earplugs are not appropriate for use in an MRI because they are deliberately designed to only partly attenuate via a filtered port. Earmuffs are in routine use and do not require additional commentary. Note that periodically, earmuffs will also specify performance with the headband below the chin.

Commercial helmets or acoustic liners are not yet widely available for MRI, and there are reports of custom units in the literature with excellent results as discussed in Section 7.4. Within this category are commercially available neonatal MR Conditional incubators that provide acoustic damping.

A full treatment of active noise canceling (ANC) or active noise reducing (ANR) technology is out of scope for this chapter. In short summary,[27] the incoming sound is measured and an opposed phase/equal amplitude output is formed which nulls the sound. This constitutes active noise cancellation because an anti-noise output has been created, as opposed to all other passive methods that only dampen the incoming sound. The challenge for active noise reduction is measuring the incoming sound at one location and predicting the required phase and amplitude necessary to null the sound at the eardrum, the point of sound perception. Active noise cancellation methods demand very high accuracy phase and amplitude prediction nearly instantaneously. Even slight motion can degrade performance. Many successful commercial products are available but very few are designed as MR conditional. One implementation currently requires a special installation and 'training' to identify the MRI noise signal model of specific sequences.

Hearing protection can be applied singly or in specific combinations. All listed methods reduce airborne noise. Bone conduction through the skull is typically attenuated by 40–60 dB relative to the airborne perceived levels.[28] Thus, bone conduction represents a threshold of performance below which any combination of hearing protection typically cannot provide additional protection. Further isolating the head with flight style helmets has been shown to reduce noise levels by an additional 10+ dB[28,29] but are likely not practical for MRI application. Investigations were performed to determine whether the additional vibration of an MRI was of concern.[30] It was concluded that bone conduction is not the dominant mechanism inside the scanner. Further commentary on this bone conduction analysis is found in Section 7.3.

Junior versions of hearing protection are available for both earplugs and earmuffs but may not span the entire range of needs. Junior versions of earmuffs are available for the 5–15-year-old range. Various options exist for younger children: adhesive earmuffs or elasticized headbands with hearing protection cups positioned over the ear. Smaller earplugs do exist but likely do not meet all needs. Silicone earplugs are likely an excellent option where sufficiently small earplugs are not available. Cutting an adult earplug down is not optimal because the earplug may not uniformly expand and leave a small air path. A swallowing or choking hazard has also been identified for very young patients.[31]

The various types of hearing protection are also provided with entertainment systems. It is important to obtain the hearing protection specifications and establish whether it meets MR system manufacturer guidelines. The issues associated with added acoustic energy from the entertainment system, and how to mathematically combine the dB from multiple sources, is out of scope for this chapter. It is presumed here that the maximum acoustic output capabilities of an entertainment system cannot be precisely specified because any patient supplied source (e.g., mp3 file or cd) has an unknown output level.

Ear canal size may not reach adult size until the 20 s. In addition, children's ear canals are firmer than those of an adult, as determined by the difference between high and low viscosity silicone molds of the same ear canals.[31] In addition, mandibular motion has lower impact on children's ear canals, thus if a proper earplug fit is achieved, the level of protection may be higher than an adult.

A compendium of hearing protector device specifications, for units available in the United States for which the manufacturer has voluntarily provided data, is available from NIOSH.[32]

Hearing protection, or more generally 'personal protective equipment (PPE)', is only one of three possible standard tools when attempting to reduce exposure to noise in the occupational context. The other two controls are 'administrative' and 'engineering'. Engineering controls are those measures that reduce noise at the source. The considerable investigations on how to make MRI scanners quieter is outside the scope of this chapter and is an area of active development for the MRI vendors.[33] Administrative controls are those employment measures to reduce worker exposure to a hazard. Such measures are part of an occupational assessment and are outside the scope of this chapter. OSHA considers PPE measures the last line of defense.

7.1.8 The Quantitative Characterization of Hearing Protection

There are multiple ways to quantify hearing protectors. Note that these tests are conducted with volunteers positioned upright and with the head otherwise unencumbered. Some of the common methods are as follows:

1. Noise reduction rating (NRR) used in the United States.
2. Single-number rating (SNR) used in the EU.
3. High-middle-low rating (HML) used in the EU, but not seen in the MRI literature reviewed.

4. Sound level conversion (SLC_{80}) used in Australia and New Zealand, but not seen in the MRI literature reviewed.

Typically, the metrics are derived with approximately eight one-third-octave band noise exposure measurements at one octave spacing spanning from 63 Hz up to 8000 Hz. Several listeners' hearing thresholds are tested with and without the protection and the mean and standard deviation of attenuations are computed for each test band. The standard deviation explicitly acknowledges the distribution of individual noise protection factors and that a decreasing number of subjects achieve a lower (or higher) noise protection factor, following a normal distribution. The degree of supervision of the listeners' preparing for the experiments and the precise details of the experimental protocol vary by design.[34]

NRR is a SNR method developed by the EPA[35] that nominally covers 98% of end uses (two standard deviations). Because of the 98% coverage factor claim and the experimental design of the measurement, NRR is considered to overestimate protection.[36] NRR also has the potential to be misapplied. The NRR is to be subtracted from dBC exposure measurements. If the exposure is measured in dBA, then the NRR must first be reduced by 7 dB.[34] The confusion relates to how to correctly compute an NRR derate factor, as discussed below.

While SNR[37] has a calculation process similar to NRR, the SNR value subtracted from an exposure measurement in dBA or dBC always produces an equivalent noise exposure result in dBA. It is nominally designed to cover 84% of the end uses (one standard deviation) and is formally indicated as SNR_{84}, but additional factors can be introduced to convert to other coverage percentages.[32]

HML[37] produces a SNR but requires three factors and two exposure measurements (dBA and dBC). A more complex calculation is required to reduce the five values to the final SNR. It is not used in the MRI literature and is not needed for this chapter. It is only noted here because it is frequently seen in hearing protection labeling and may be used in some regulatory jurisdictions.

SLC_{80}[38] is designed to more realistically assess the exposure realized in 80% of the hearing protection applications (nearly one standard deviation). Protection is rated both with regards to dB attenuation and a numeric class designation which indicates, in 3 dB increments starting at 10 dB, its suitability for the anticipated exposure level for communication. This explicitly acknowledges that high levels of hearing protection can actually impede communication. This is a challenge in the MRI environment where the communication typically occurs between scans and thus the hearing protection may be excessive for any communications. Also like SNR, the SLC_{80} value subtracted from an exposure measurement in dBA or dBC always produces an equivalent noise exposure result in dBA. While not used in the MRI literature, it is useful to note here for its regulatory implications in some jurisdictions.

The underlying measurements for the various metrics are an average of multiple measurements, providing an estimate of the protection to a population, not an individual, under laboratory testing conditions. Various heuristics have been developed that adjust the hearing protection specification to reflect likely outcomes in practice. This is particularly relevant for NRR measurements because they are considered optimistic. For example, OSHA strongly recommends derating NRR by 50% (after exposure measurement conversion to dBC) for all hearing protection. NIOSH derates earmuffs by 25%, formable earplugs by 50% and all other earplugs by 70%.[39] It is important to clarify that the 7 dB subtraction for dBA to dBC conversion is frequently mistaken as part of the derate system. It is exclusively a unit conversion. While the need and logic of a derate factor are clear, some caution that such approaches are not reliable.[40]

As previously noted, hearing protection performance is strongly dependent on their proper application. It is not known how the standard patient supine position alters hearing protection performance, specifically for earmuffs and resonant chamber devices. There is also the possibility of mechanical coupling between some headband designs and the pillow that transmits sound to the ear. For some specific designs, it may be possible to position the headband on the chest, under the chin. As the patient is typically relatively motionless, the implications of body motion on hearing protection performance are ignored.[41]

Lastly, hearing protection devices are occasionally combined, e.g., foam earplugs with earmuffs and often referred to as 'double hearing protection'. Some dual combinations are not possible either for obvious physical conflicts (e.g., passive resonant chambers with earmuffs) or conflicting attenuation principles (e.g., earplugs conflict with passive resonant chamber operations). In addition, some head coils are closely fitting and may not have sufficient space to accommodate earmuffs. Investigations have demonstrated the benefits of combined protection and how to assess the combined protection.[42] Another simple heuristic developed by OSHA[43] establishes which of the two NRRs is higher then adds an additional 5 dB to account for the second, lower performing, hearing protection device. It is reported that this 5 dB benefit is conservative, and reliably achieved.[44]

Selection of good hearing protection is critical. High-quality hearing protection typically includes detailed package inserts with hearing protection ratings and often the octave band protection values, in addition to application instructions. In the United States, the package and package insert contents are regulated, but some hearing protection may not provide all information. Provision of all the protection information in an approved label is a good indication of a fully evaluated product. The MR vendors typically provide recommended hearing protection specifications for certain exposure conditions.

7.1.9 Identification of the Literature

The literature review (PubMed, [Cumulative Index to Nursing and Allied Health Literature (CINAHLplus)] August 2018) used the following search logic:

1. (((mri) OR magnetic resonance) AND noise AND hearing), 258 items, [CINAHLplus: 75],
2. (((mri) OR magnetic resonance) AND acoustic noise), 648 items, [CINAHLplus: 65],
3. thermoelastic magnetic resonance acoustic, 3 items, [CINAHLplus: 0],
4. thermoelastic mri acoustic, 3 items (matching #3), [CINAHLplus: 0].

Search patterns #1, #2 were then manually sorted for relevant literature. The intent was a wide search to over-capture potentially relevant literature rather than multiple narrow searches that potentially missed relevant literature. However, as this chapter shows, much of the important literature does not involve MRI. All International Society for Magnetic Resonance in Medicine (ISMRM), and predecessor organizations, abstracts were searched and safety-related acoustic abstracts included. ESMRMB congresses since 2012, excluding the joint conferences with ISMRM already searched, produced one additional safety-related acoustic abstract, referenced within this chapter.

Literature related to animals in MRI was not reviewed.[45,46] Literature related to the clinical use of MRI ear imaging, or fMRI, or techniques (hardware or software) to reduce acoustic noise levels were also not reviewed. Note that much of the literature cited in this chapter is not found from the above searches because it does not directly pertain to MRI.

7.1.10 Patient Incident Reports

It is instructive to understand the range of issues experienced by patients. Many countries in the world maintain databases of incidents. For example, the FDA maintains a publicly available post-market surveillance database 'Manufacturer and User Facility Device Experience Database' (MAUDE) for the reporting of adverse events characterized as serious injury, up to and including death. The FDA defines 'serious injury' in 21 CFR 803.3 (w):

Serious injury means an injury or illness that:

1. is life-threatening;
2. results in permanent impairment of a body function or permanent damage to a body structure; or
3. necessitates medical or surgical intervention to preclude permanent impairment of a body function or permanent damage to a body structure. Permanent means irreversible impairment or damage to a body structure or function, excluding trivial impairment or damage.

Hearing loss and tinnitus reports potentially qualify as serious because professional medical care may be required, and many of the reports note professional care. Note that MAUDE includes reports from around the world. If the MR vendor becomes aware of an incident involving a scanner model sold in the United States, they are obligated to file a report with the FDA, if it meets reporting guideline requirements. Therefore, statistical analysis premised on US-only procedures is not valid. Sites and patients may also submit reports to MAUDE.

Approximately 80 cases related to hearing loss, or tinnitus, or noise complaints were found. The search (MAUDE code LNH) included reports back to 1992 and up to July 2018, but the first hearing loss report considered here was in 1999. The LNI (nuclear magnetic resonance spectroscopic system), MOS (magnetic resonance specialty coil) and OIM (MRI disposable kit) MAUDE codes were not searched. There is a small possibility of double counting when a specific event had both an initial and follow-up report. It is widely assumed that MAUDE significantly under reports incidents, but the under-report ratio is unknown. The summary provided here is based on the publicly available information. Additional confidential information is available only to FDA and is presumed to not change any of the general statements made here. Note that the accuracy or completeness of these reports cannot be verified and critical reading is required, but clear broad trends do emerge that provide helpful insights and suggest opportunities for patient care improvement.

It is assumed that tinnitus reports are an ongoing condition, in the time frame of the report. Reports of 'ringing' are presumed to be tinnitus. In some reports, prior history of tinnitus and/or hearing issues are noted. There may be other instances of preexisting hearing issues, but that information is not available. It is also unclear if the technologist/radiographer was aware of such preexisting conditions prior to scanning. Reports of head fullness are interpreted as a temporary hearing threshold shift versus claimed permanent hearing threshold shifts. A few reports note vertigo symptoms, which loud sounds can cause, and discussed elsewhere in this chapter. Many reports indicate the patient sought professional medical help and statements of hearing loss are confirmed. Several reports note hearing tests, a few mention hearing loss against prior hearing results. It is not always clear whether the MRI examination was the proximate cause. In multiple reports, it is claimed the patient did not complain during or after the scans, but only complained days after the scanning. Several reports indicate system testing, sometimes acoustic testing, with no reported system deficiencies. Such tests ensure the equipment was functioning as expected.

Many reports clearly indicate no hearing protection provided. In one case, the patient supplied their own hearing protection for the second MRI session. It is not always clear whether hearing protection was offered but refused. In some cases, scanning started with no hearing protection, but hearing protection provided when the patient complained. In one instance, the patient elected to use only one earplug. In one instance, the patient, with earplugs, complained and was offered an additional set of earplugs, which provides no additional benefit. There are also reports of earplugs falling out. There are several reports of double hearing protection. One report claims that double hearing protection is a standard operating procedure. There are no reports of patient hearing protection training but that does not imply training not provided. One report claimed the earplugs inserted correctly. Without knowing how earplug insertion was checked, the claim cannot be verified, nor can a hearing plug insertion check be definitive. In several reports, the patient stated the hearing protection did not work, which could indicate improper application, or potentially inadequate hearing protection with respect to the MR vendor requirements. One report claimed the earplugs did not meet the MR vendor performance requirements. There are several reports with no indication of hearing protection but that is impossible to interpret. When hearing protection was noted, typically earplugs were specified, sometimes headphones, occasionally only nonspecific 'hearing protection'. There are several reports with audio entertainment systems (vendor typically not specified), but insufficient detail regarding hearing protection or the volume level of patient exposure. In one instance the examination started with the audio system headphones but converted to earplugs. The shortest reported examination resulting in a claimed hearing loss, using hearing protection, is 'approx 12 min'. There is a report of a radiographer with hearing loss from a spontaneous quench. One reported a medical diagnosis of unspecified 'high-frequency hearing loss', but MRI acoustic noise is not typically characterized as 'high frequency'. The author was not able to determine if a frequency of exposure versus deficit mismatch is possible. One investigation tested for MRI-induced threshold shifts at 8–14 kHz but did not test low frequencies.[47] Therefore, it is unknown if the patients had any threshold shift.

While it is assumed here that all systems with $B0 > 1.0\,T$ are capable of exceeding the threshold at which hearing protection is required, there are a few instances of lower field units that may be incapable of reaching the hearing protection requirement threshold apparently inducing hearing loss and/or tinnitus.[48] As noted elsewhere in this chapter, some patients are more sensitive to loud sounds.

None of the reports noted the use of any medications that maybe ototoxic, or with potential to predispose a patient to tinnitus.[49] Note that the ototoxicity of drugs may be permanent, or limited to the treatment period. A few reports noted the patient was receiving steroids to treat the claimed MRI induced hearing loss, but the treatment benefits have been debated.[50] Some of the reports indicated hearing improvement, which might have occurred with the unaided passage of time, the other reports indicated no improvement.

Other English language databases were investigated. The Australian Database of Adverse Event Notifications (DAEN) for medical devices, instituted in 2012, presented one case of temporary hearing loss. A similar investigation of the Canadian MedEffect 'Canada Vigilance Adverse Reaction Online Database', instituted in 1965, produced no reports. While the New Zealand MedSafe and the United Kingdom 'Yellow Card' databases receive incident reports, public searching is not permitted. England also has an unsearchable National Reporting and Learning System (NRLS), and a precursor, which also captures incident reports, some of which are also cross-filed in the 'Yellow Card' system. A request to 'Yellow Card' was filed and the MHRA delivered 15 de-identified reports for noise-related incidents since 1990. The first 'Yellow Card' acoustic incident report was in 2000, close to the first MAUDE report in 1999. Given the similar ages of the United Kingdom and United States incident databases, this 5.3 : 1 incident ratio is remarkably close to the average 4.8 : 1 population ratio since 1990, implications of relative procedure volume, etc., not considered. This ratio alignment may be coincidental because otherwise the UK reporting rate (incidents per million scans) is higher. The incident experiences are generally similar to the MAUDE reports. In addition, one 0.5T scanner report of severe unrelenting headaches, ear pains, and dizziness from a 15-min scanner session with an estimated 90 dB exposure. Another incident highlighted the challenges of hearing protection versus the ability to communicate. While lowering the scanner table at the end of the session, the patient did not hear the instruction to remain on the patient table and the right leg caught in the table lowering mechanism, with apparently no serious consequences. There is an additional database maintained by ECRI Institute (formerly known as Emergency Care Research Institute) on behalf of the state of Pennsylvania where reporting of incidents is required of all medical facilities. However, the database is not publicly searchable. Appropriately anonymized, publicly searchable databases would enable educational investigations. We must learn from prior incidents. The publicly available and anonymized incident reports via the Federal Aviation Administration's (FAAs) Aviation Safety Reporting System (ASRS) are widely recognized as contributing to the improvements in aviation safety.

In summary, the database analysis suggests that there may be insufficient guidance for patients on the proper insertion of earplugs and the need for quick checks of hearing protection applications. While some scanners, some protocols may not exceed standard threshold levels for hearing protection, always providing hearing protection for all patients, and double protection where possible would be beneficial and improve patient comfort. Minimizing the risk for sensitive patients would lower incident rates and imply a general improvement in noise exposure reduction. Use of hearing protection that meets minimum requirements as specified by the MR manufacturer is essential.

7.2 CHARACTERIZATIONS OF MRI ACOUSTIC NOISE OUTPUT

There is an extensive literature on the characterization of MRI acoustic noise output. The literature serves multiple purposes:

1. for safety purposes;
2. for designing quieter sequences;
3. for gradient design and mounting purposes; and
4. for other system component design optimization purposes.

The main focus of this chapter is safety, the other elements only briefly noted, thus an emphasis on the measurement technique and worst-case reported results. Note that the reported values are a mixture of dB, dBA, peak, and average (sometimes noted as root mean square (RMS)) values of varying length, not always specified. Some reports seek loudest possible scanner outputs, others analyze a specific sequence[51] for particular clinical applications (e.g., fMRI).

The earliest paper[52] noted that scanning patients without hearing protection are capable of producing temporary hearing loss and that proper hearing protection can nearly eliminate temporary hearing loss. The difficulty in finding measuring equipment that worked correctly in strong magnetic fields was also reported. Subsequent papers resolved measuring equipment problems and identified that given short exposure times, higher sound level exposures without hearing protection was probably acceptable, except in the case of vulnerable patients[53] where others strongly recommend hearing protection.[54] Early work also demonstrated that active anti-noise methods could reduce noise levels and improve patient communications.[55] Other research investigated the contribution of ambient noise levels from various sources and concluded that with a maximum measured noise of 93 dBA from five different systems, the threat of permanent hearing loss was minimal.[56] With the development of more powerful gradients and faster sequences, MR scanners became capable of exceeding 100 dBA[57] and peaks of up to 108 dBA were measured using tubes to duct noise from isocenter to measurement equipment removed from the magnetic fields (measurement error estimated at ±4 dB).[58,59] Subsequent papers with more powerful gradient systems produced acoustic noise levels up to 115 dBA, averaged over 30 s.[60] Peak measurements on recently emerging 3 T systems reached 138 dB,[61] 132 dBA average,[62] 131/116 dB peak and average.[63] Measurements on a research 4.7 T system reported 130/118 dBA peak and RMS.[64] A recently developed compact (37 cm patient aperture) system with fast gradients (700 $T\,m^{-1}\,s^{-1}$) reported peak/average sound levels of approximately 120/110 dBA, as only slightly louder than a typical clinical system in a per sequence comparison.[65] Systematic techniques for assessing microphones for magnetic field interference and assessing the transfer function characteristics of a conducting tube were developed, in addition to the first demonstration of the benefits of acoustic damping materials inside the magnet covers.[66] A classic analysis paper[3] provided further insights on microphone testing methods, the spatial variation of noise along the scanner axis due to gradient operations, the minimal contribution of background noise (if <10 dB below MRI noise contributions), and how the presence of the patient could increase noise measurements by up to 3 dB. The paper introduced acoustic transfer functions and reported how the different gradient axes produce different signatures, but that the sequence gradient waveform spectrum substantially dominated the output noise spectrum. The companion seminal paper[4] was a thorough review of the engineering options toward mitigating MRI noise. Another paper of note[67] is the result of a systematic effort by the defunct MHRA MagNET group to characterize commercially available MRI scanners, from seven different vendors, to assist in purchasing decisions in the United Kingdom. Field strengths from 0.2 T up to 3 T, both open and cylindrical systems of contemporary vintage but tested in different rooms, were tested with a consistent protocol using well-tested equipment and procedures. Note that this chapter does not methodically investigate the acoustic noise differences between cylindrical versus open systems and focusses only on output levels. The results generally confirmed the expected positive linear relationship between B0 static field strength and acoustic noise, which was systematically proven elsewhere,[68] that the presence of a patient may increase noise levels, the significant contribution of pulse sequence parameters, and the variation of noise as a function of position on the patient table. The measurements used a clinically relevant 'worst-case' sequence, thus the results do not necessarily match with other reports. Initial investigations regarding the acoustic noise signature of 7 T scanners theoretically predicted 140 dB exposures, but was not measured for reasons attributed to peripheral nerve stimulation constraints.[69] However, high acoustic noise levels have also been reported at lower field strengths. One report claimed that the 'average Leq levels were 129 dB SPL for 20 min' in a 0.5 T system with measured 'noise levels in the scanning room' averaged across a range of protocols.[70] It is not clear whether the patients, who were screened to eliminate those with ear pathology and ontological damage, received hearing protection, but a temporary hearing loss was reported, particularly at higher frequencies (4, 8 kHz) beyond the typical output range of an MRI (not provided, but presumed <4 kHz).

The above-cited literature is relatively old and gradient technology has continued to advance. An anonymized survey of recent 510(k) cylindrical 1.5 and 3 T system submissions to the FDA[71] suggests that acoustic noise output has held approximately constant relative to the older published literature. Peak acoustic outputs are well below the 140 dB limit and comparable to the exposures measured at US monster truck shows.[22] Average acoustic output levels were either MGAN or MCAN measurements, as specified by NEMA/MITA MS-4, provided to the FDA. Typically, MCAN information is provided in 510(k) submissions. The results showed that all systems captured in the limited survey require hearing protection. Commercial hearing protection products are available that meet all adult needs, assuming proper fit and positioning. However, not all commercially available hearing protection products may have a rating sufficient for specific systems, particularly for neonates when considering the claimed WHO 120 dB peak limit. Users are directed to their operators' manuals to find the specific make and model recommendations from the MR manufacturer.

The first paper[72] to analyze MRI acoustic noise from the interventional perspective recommended the use of hearing protection because the noise levels at the 5 gauss line exceeded 110/99 dBA peak/average. Other research[73] has shown a ~5 dB improvement in noise levels 80 cm from the magnet bore entrance by placing

7.5 cm sound-absorbing fiberglass on the outer magnet shroud, ~3 dB when placed on the wall of the room, ~1 dB when placed inside on the bore liner, and ~7 dB when wall and shroud padding applied simultaneously. From the patients' perspective, assuming the patient could fit in with a 15 cm aperture reduction, bore lining reduced the noise by ~13 dB, but the additional shroud padding actually increased noise by ~0.5 dB. Additional wall padding had negligible impact on patient exposures.

Recent developments of MRI guided linacs (linear accelerators) for radiation oncology treatment purposes have considered split gradient tube configurations. Recent simulation work suggests the configuration may produce SPLs exceeding 140 dB at certain frequencies.[74]

No literature related to the acoustic signature of a quenching magnet was found. It is expected that the signature will vary as a function of cryostat and venting design. In addition, in the personal experience of the author, how the burst disk fails has a significant impact on the acoustic signature. Those familiar with quenches can attest to the variety of sounds produced and that quenches can be very loud. While the duration of the magnetic field collapse is measured as a fraction of a minute, the escape of helium and associated noise can take many minutes. Presumably, there would be no reason to stay in close proximity to the magnet during a vent and the acoustic noise dose would be short.

7.3 SCANNING THE FETUS

The cochlea starts developing at around 10–12 weeks gestation and is substantially mature by 30–35 weeks[75] gestation. The middle ear is basically formed before the last trimester and the ossicles are adult-sized by the 8th month.[76] The hearing threshold at 27–29 weeks is approximately 40 dB and decreases to near-adult levels (13.5 dB) by 42 weeks gestation.[77] It has been observed that the fetus first responds to sound at around 19 weeks.[75] To date, there has been no reproducible demonstration of harmful acoustic effects on the fetus from 1.5 T MRI exposure. There is even less information available regarding higher field exposures.[78] It has also been stated that 'After four decades of research, the effects of excessive noise on the developing fetal ear are still debated and uncertain.'[79] However, a recent major investigation of maternal occupational noise exposure demonstrated an association between occupational noise exposure during pregnancy and hearing dysfunction in children.[80] Dysfunction was broadly categorized as any threshold shift, tinnitus, diseases of the inner ear or other unspecified disorders of the ear, as determined from an analysis of the register of specialized medical care. Job titles were recorded during pregnancy and assessed against a validated job-exposure matrix specifying the annual average daily 8-h exposure levels into one of three exposure categories (<75, 75–84, >=85 dBA). While shown that the loudest but unknown occupational exposures may result in hearing dysfunction in children, it is presently believed that short and known MRI exposures do not cause hearing dysfunction, as reported in the literature.

The fetus is exposed to both the acoustic MRI noise and vibrations originating from the patient table.[6] The acoustic noise undergoes an impedance mismatch at the air versus skin/fluid interface and is attenuated. In addition, since there is fluid on either side of the fetal eardrum, that mechanism does not function in utero. A simple mathematical model suggests a ~30 dB attenuation in water,[6] consistent with young patients suffering 'glue ear' (Otitis media with effusion). Research in a 0.5 T MRI with a male volunteer, practiced in swallowing intragastric tubes, who received a small hydrophone and an initial 1000 ml of water confirmed the model predictions[6] when lying on a foam mattress for mechanical isolation. Removing the foam mattress decreased the attenuation by approximately 10 dB at lower frequencies. The measurements also suggest that the attenuation below 2000 Hz may not be as large as the higher frequency attenuation, but in general, the attenuation is approximately 10 dB higher than earmuffs. This work is in general agreement with research on pregnant women where microphones were introduced at the beginning of labor, after amniotomy[76] and other more complex modeling and measurements.[81] There is concern that in cases of oligohydramnios (low amniotic fluid levels) the attenuation levels may be lower.[82] Other research[30] is potentially contradictory. In the first phase of investigation bone conduction inside and outside the scanner suggested that the vibration experienced inside the scanner did not result in an increased bone conduction contribution. These results would be consistent with other papers if the volunteers were lying on a pad. However, it is not clear from the study design if standard padding was used. The second phase of the investigation used extra padding to ensure isolation.

There have also been several studies investigating the outcomes of fetus exposed to the noise of an MRI.[82–85] While these papers provide some scan protocol details, the associated acoustic noise levels produced are not reported. Generally, scanning the fetus requires fast, and consequently loud, sequences to minimize motion artifacts, especially in the more recent papers using modern fast gradients. In general, all of the papers report no abnormal findings when compared to the expected rate of hearing deficits in the relevant target population. Early studies used small sample sizes because of the reluctance to scan expectant mothers, unless essential, given the unknown risks associated with the MRI exposure of the fetus. In addition, scanning of the fetus is an indication of some medical concern and hearing dysfunction could be associated with the concern. One paper assessed approximately 100 babies on delivery as either well, or neonatal intensive care unit (NICU) graduates requiring more than 48 h in a NICU.[82] The study size was designed to demonstrate an increased prevalence of hearing impairment of 5% or more, a level well above general population prevalence but only slightly higher than the known excess risk associated with a prolonged NICU stay. The gestational age, birth weight and time between delivery and OAE testing were recorded. None of the well babies presented with OAE measurements outside the range of results expected from a large reference database. One of the NICU graduates had a bilateral hearing impairment, which was within the expected prevalence. When all results were pooled, a significant difference was found in one of the four tested frequency bands (4 kHz). However, the paper considered the difference small when compared to the normal variation in OAE measurements.

At present, there are no standards or regulations setting limits for expectant mothers. The American Academy of Pediatrics encourages further research on the implications of noise and recommends screening for noise-induced hearing loss in babies for when occupational noise sources required the mother to wear of hearing protection.[77] The Committee on Hearing, Bioacoustics, and Biomechanics recommended in their report that until better information was available, it would be 'prudent for pregnant women to avoid exposures of long duration (several hours per day) to sounds of 90 dB SPL and above, the maximum level currently suggested by the U.S. Department of Labor for unprotected ears.'[81]

7.4 SCANNING NEONATES

The preparations necessary to scan neonates are extensive. In addition to hearing protection products already noted, and their limitations for small patients, additional noise level reduction methods have been investigated. It is reported that an incubator fitted with additional acoustic foam pads reduced external noise by approximately 6 dB.[86] The noise reduction properties of the incubator alone are not specified. One incubator website claims an additional 10–15 dB of protection with an undocumented 'acoustic protection option'. An abstract reported LA_{eq} reductions for several different sequences ranging from approximately 2–8 dB.[87] Another incubator company reports A-weighted noise reductions of 12 dB and up (R. Srinivasan, personal communication). Note that there are no formal test methods for measuring the acoustic noise reduction of an incubator.

A specialty system with reduced bore size and other design features claim acoustic noise output of <77 dBA. Specially designed gradient coils have also reported 6–10 dBA noise reductions.[88]

As noted elsewhere, commercially available earplugs are still too large for the smallest ear canals. One novel solution uses a two-component moldable dental putty fitted directly into the ear canal.[89] Analysis with adult volunteers suggests a 20 dBA attenuation.

In addition, experiments with a passive acoustic hood or shield 1 m long, formed to the curvature of the bore and approximately 10 cm thick provided an additional 6 dBA attenuation. One MRI vendor provides a pediatric acoustic hood solution with up to 14 dB of protection. In essence, a thick pad custom fitted to the radius of the bore, and supported by the patient table, is positioned around the patient as an additional sound barrier. Additional thick padding may also be positioned around the coil, on top of the patient table.

Given the difficulties noted, additional layers of hearing protection are recommended since the quality of earplug insertion cannot be reliably determined, unlike most other forms of hearing protection noted here.

7.5 SCANNING CHILDREN

The health implications of excessive noise on children have been extensively studied, as described in a WHO training package.[90] However, the focus of this chapter is the avoidance of hearing damage. There are two major concerns regarding noise-induced hearing loss for children: (i) children's ears are likely more sensitive to loud sounds and therefore more easily damaged than the adult ear, (ii) children do not necessarily have the autonomy to take the steps required to protect themselves. Therefore, it is necessary to consider measures to properly protect and potentially reduce exposures where needed.

So far as the author is aware, there are no regulations that limit noise exposures for children and thus no starting point for developing MRI guidance, but recommendations are available. As previously noted, the author has not been able to discover the source of the IEC 60601-1 WHO-based recommendation of a 120 dB limit. Recently, the WHO issued recommendations for recreational noise exposure limits.[11] The report recommends a conservative 8 h 80 dBA exposure limit based on the statistical objective of protecting 99% of children from a 5 dB hearing loss (the level considered to be generally not noticeable) after 18 years of noise exposure. This is 5 dBA lower than the EU occupational action level for adults. There is also a claimed 8 h 75 dBA EPA recommendation[91] but incorrectly referenced. This correlates with the WHO recommendation at which levels risk of hearing loss is believed to be completely eliminated.[11] As the objectives of the recreational exposure recommendations are different than the occupational regulations, it is difficult to compare exposures and make recommendations. As also noted elsewhere, it is not known whether adjusting a long-term limit to a short-term equivalent limit is practical.

Hearing protection issues identified elsewhere for neonates and people with small ear canals are also applicable to the scanning of children.

Given the challenges noted, double hearing protection is recommended wherever possible since the quality of earplug insertion cannot be reliably determined whereas external hearing protection can be inspected.

7.6 SCANNING VOLUNTEERS

The scanning of volunteers may be the most complex use case given the wide range of scanning frequency and the type of scanning volunteers experience. The frequency of scanning can vary (e.g., once a year to several times a day) and the scanning could be representative of what a patient experiences or the testing of one specific sequence. Typical volunteering could represent training staff on a new system or new protocol, in which case there might be large time gaps between scans as lecturing occurs at the console. Protocol or sequence development could repeat the same scan with minor parameter variations to seek the optimum. The gap between scans could be minimal, or lengthy depending on the MR operator's development process. In addition, experienced and inexperienced volunteers may not be adept at the proper application of hearing protection. It is known that many frequent users of hearing protection in the industrial setting are not properly applying the hearing protection.[92]

Thus, the only recommendations possible at this time are as follows:

1. ensure the scanning volunteer is properly trained and supervised in the use of hearing protection; and
2. consider the noise level of the scan sessions and accordingly schedule the frequency and duration of exposure. Standard ISO 1999[14] demonstrates how to make the relevant computations.

7.7 ADDITIONAL CLINICAL IMPLICATIONS OF MRI ACOUSTIC NOISE

The additional clinical implications of MRI acoustic noise can be divided into two broad categories:

1. implications for the collection of diagnostic information; and
2. implications for the health of the patient.

It has been reported that MRI acoustic noise may have a slight impact on positron emission tomography (PET) tracer uptake rates when compared to PET-only investigations. The investigation concluded the artifact is 'without concern'.[93,94] Otherwise, no additional literature was found detailing other implications of MRI acoustic noise on collecting diagnostic information.

The frustration of MRI acoustic noise on the communication channel between patient and operator and implications for image acquisition is well understood and not discussed here. The author is not aware of any practical solutions.

The implications of scanner noise on fMRI have been extensively studied and well documented. Search string #2, with the additional limiter 'AND functional' produced 348 results in PubMed (August 2018). It is out of the scope for this chapter.

One investigation on an MRI scanner with test sequences operating in the 80–87 dBA range and peaks up to 120 dB did not produce statistically significant threshold shifts but reported a significant increase in distortion product optoacoustic emission amplitude variability.[95] A theory is provided to explain the findings, but it is concluded that MRI noise does not impose a risk of hearing function.

The FDA MAUDE reports frequently make note of the following patient complaints in addition to hearing loss:

1. tinnitus; and
2. dizziness.

The correlation between tinnitus and loud sounds is well known but less so for dizziness.

Tinnitus is the hearing of sound when there is none. The descriptions of sounds heard are quite varied: ringing, hissing, pulsatile sound, etc. Prevalence is estimated at approximately 10% in adults of either gender, at least in the USA and Europe, but other studies suggest similar rates in other countries. Approximately 3% consider it annoying, 2% severely annoying and 1% claim it severely impacts the ability to lead a normal life. Prevalence increases with age up to around 70 years old with conflicting prevalence reports above 70-year old. Prevalence in children is believed to be similar but perhaps less distressing.[96] It is reported that in North America it may afflict one-third of those 55 or older.[97] The main risk factor for developing tinnitus could be incompletely listed as hearing loss but is also associated with many other specific diseases or conditions. In addition, various medications are known to potentially trigger tinnitus.[49] In most cases, the onset is slow but can be abrupt due to loud sound. The author was not able to find literature that provided any indication of how loud and long the sound needs to be to trigger tinnitus, likely because it is a highly variable and personal factor. Furthermore, 40% of those with tinnitus report an aversion to loud sounds (hyperacusis) and 86% of those with hyperacusis also report tinnitus. Whereas it is reported that the normal threshold to loudness discomfort is in the 100–105 dB range those with hyperacusis report a threshold 20–25 dB lower, or 75–80 dB with standard deviations of approximately 15+ dB, with a few patients reporting thresholds of approximately <50 dB.[98] Prevalence of hyperacusis seems to be in the 10% range, may be more prevalent in women, and increases with age.[99] Together, those suffering tinnitus or hyperacusis may need additional considerations beyond the acoustic noise dose measures presented here. In the absence of more scientific data, limit recommendations are not possible and in the case of hyperacusis, may be impractical given the highly variable individual threshold levels. Ideally, screening would identify such conditions in advance so that appropriate measures could be taken. It is vital that those patients apply hearing protection correctly, and double protection where possible.

Mechanisms for noise-induced dizziness are reported in the literature. The Tullio phenomenon is a low frequency, sound-induced dizziness that may also cause vertigo, nausea or eye movement.[100] A couple of possible mechanisms have been suggested. Those suffering superior semicircular canal dehiscence (SSCD) syndrome may also report Tullio phenomenon symptoms in addition to autophony and pulsatile tinnitus. It is believed that the thinning, or complete absence, of the temporal bone by the superior semicircular canal permits noise-induced pressure changes in the superior semicircular canal. Torsional nystagmus has also been induced in dogs with a fistula involving the superior semicircular canal where the otolith apparatus was directly observed to be vibrating due to sound. It has also been reported that people with SSCD may perceive sound below 1 kHz more strongly via bone conduction versus air conduction by 10–15 dB. While properly applied conventional hearing protection will function as expected, the bone conduction pathway contribution is then larger than normally expected. Typically, direct bone conduction, exclusive of the bone/air impedance difference, is perceived at approximately 5–10 dB lower than air conduction in the 1–4 kHz frequency range.[101] Note that there is a significant impedance mismatch between bone and air such that most sound is reflected from the body and thus most perceived noise is airborne. Therefore, the confluence of patient-reported symptoms appears plausible. Identifying those patients with such susceptibilities (e.g., tinnitus) in advance of the MRI and applying extra precautions may help ensure better patient outcomes. The prevalence of SSCD appears to be on the order of 1%.

7.8 TRAINING ON THE USE OF HEARING PROTECTION

The patient's achieved hearing protection is entirely dependent on how well the hearing protection is applied. The application of earplugs is the focus of this section. One investigation showed that the average naïve volunteer with no training, with one specific earplug model, achieved 8 dB (SLC_{80}) of protection. Given the package insert training material, the same volunteers achieved an average additional 16 dB improvement in hearing protection.[102] According to another report, one-on-one training achieved comparable results[103] but the definition of one-on-one training was not provided. Other research investigated the consequences of no training, group training, and one-on-one (gloved assistants inserted the earplugs). Those results showed improvements in hearing protection at each level.[104] It has also been reported that the application of oto-ease lubricant to the earplug during the insertion process can also improve hearing protection by up to 5 dB[105] or higher.[106] Understandably, patients may be concerned about 'putting something in their ear' and causing damage. The adult ear canal is approximately 35 mm long, ending at the eardrum, whereas earplugs are shorter. However, there are sensitive structures near the eardrum that will cause a normal startle reaction.

In addition, a quick visual inspection may possibly indicate if the earplugs were properly applied (e.g., deeply inserted). Note that a deeply inserted earplug is not a guarantee of proper function. Earplugs can crease and leave a small air path for sound. A re-insertion of the earplug may be necessary if creased, but it is impossible to know if the insertion was crease-free without removing the earplug. Sometimes, the crease is visible in the earplug immediately after removal and before the earplug fully expands. The patient can also test their protection by cupping their hands over the ears and listen for an obvious sound level reduction (indicative of potentially incorrectly installed hearing protection) or minimal sound level reduction (indicative of potentially correctly installed hearing protection) while they or someone else speaks.

There are other ways to check the level of hearing protection relatively inexpensively. QuickFixWeb (https://www.cdc.gov/niosh/mining/content/quickfit web.html) provides a noise track that can be played by a computer. After adjusting the computer volume so that the reference soundtrack is barely audible without hearing protection, the secondary track plays at a +15 dB level, with hearing protection. If the secondary track is inaudible the hearing protection is likely providing at least 15 dB of protection. A hardware prototype of the same concept has also been reported, but unknown if commercially available.[107] This test may not be practical in a busy MRI workflow environment. Whispering in the ear of the patient being positioned for the scan and checking for a response may be a fast and practical means of attempting to assess the level of hearing attenuation present with inserted earplugs (E. Kanal, personal communication).

7.9 FUTURE INVESTIGATIONS

The health concerns of loud acoustic sound continue to be an active area of research. Future consensus opinions, ideally in the form of a standard, may have implications for MRI safety limits. The following topics pertaining specifically to the qualities of MRI noise may merit continued watch.

MRI acoustic noise can be characterized as both a narrow band emission and impulsive. Narrowband denotes the spectral width of the sound (the majority of MRI noise typically in the 0–4000 Hz range) and impulsive because the sound creating events are in the millisecond range and not necessarily continuous, although can be nearly so. The implications of both factors for hearing conservation is under active research. Presently, both the OSHA and EU regulations capture impulsive noise under the existing daily noise exposure limits and are automatically controlled by peak exposure limits as well. Whether additional considerations may be needed is an area of current investigation. Presently, much of the investigation focuses on military needs where peak levels can easily exceed occupational peak exposure limits.[108] Research on the implications of narrowband noise exposure does not appear to be as advanced and has apparently not yet reached a level of consensus for a revision to an existing acoustic standard.

MRI acoustic noise is concerning for those suffering from tinnitus and hyperacusis. No set limits can be given for hyperacusis as there is significant variability in personal tolerance thresholds. It also appears to be presently unclear at what lower bounds acoustic noise levels may trigger tinnitus. Such information may be helpful guidance to avoid triggering onset, but could only be impractically implemented if the patient's preexisting condition, and tolerance, was known.

With the increasing number of interventional MRI procedures, it is likely necessary to update MRI standards to measure acoustic noise levels near the bore opening in order to estimate the acoustic exposure profile of workers. This would then provide the necessary information to adequately assess exposure categories

#2, #3, #4, and #6 as listed in the introduction (Interventional procedure staff, MR operators, MR factory workers, and those tending to the patient). Conventional acoustic noise measuring equipment may not function properly near an MRI system and may also pose a missile risk. Measurements provided by the MR vendor with known functioning equipment would support standard occupational exposure assessments.

During the course of this investigation, the author was not able to find any definitive material on the following questions, which may be directly relevant to MRI acoustic noise safety concerns:

1. While the IEC 60601-1 general standard makes optional note of a 120 dB peak recommended limit for children, no reference is given. Supplemental investigations did not discover such recommendations in the official WHO reports. The basis of this recommendation, the age range, etc., is not known. Should specific limits be instituted for children?
2. The limits presented here are time-scaled occupational limits, with provisions for infrequent exposures. It is not clear whether occupational exposure limits can be scaled down to an infrequent 1-h exposure.
3. The performance of hearing protection is not measured in the typical supine patient position. What are the implications, if any?
4. There are statements in the MAUDE database of patients reporting higher frequency band hearing deficits as a result of exposure to lower frequency band MRI noise exposures. What is the mechanism for this frequency band shift?

Lastly, two possible operational needs:

1. A solution to the conflicting requirements for adequate hearing protection with simultaneous ease of communication.
2. It may be helpful to update screening forms to include a question on hearing sensitivities and issues.

There is an additional topic that does not pertain specifically to the qualities of MRI noise that may merit continued watch. The widely cited work of Kujawa[109] reports, using a mouse model, that recovery of temporary hearing threshold shifts may not be indicative of a full hearing recovery. Results suggest that permanent nerve damage may occur. These findings could have significant impact on the understanding of noise-induced damage.

7.10 CONCLUSIONS

There is an ongoing effort to reduce MRI protocol times and reduce noise levels. However, there are many loud and long protocols. It is essential that hearing protection, double where possible, always be applied and that the application of hearing protection be quickly checked by the technologist/radiographer to ensure proper usage. This hearing protection must also be size appropriate for the needs of the particular patient. Based on the derivation of patient exposure limits from occupational exposure limits, this will minimize the risk of an MRI contribution to long-term hearing loss. The methodical use of hearing protection properly applied should reduce the number of adverse events reported and would particularly benefit the noise-sensitive patient.

Presently, acoustic noise limits are considered from the perspective of dose: exposure for a given length of time. While some MRI scanners and protocols are not capable of producing sound levels over approximately 85 dBA and thus no hearing protection is strictly required, patients will benefit from properly applied hearing protection, both from a comfort and health perspective. A potentially significant number of patients may have hearing sensitivities, known or unknown, and would benefit from hearing protection because the concerns may not be a function of dose, but possibly the exposure level.

Earplugs are the dominant form of hearing protection due to their small size and theoretically high performance but are difficult for infrequent users to apply properly. Therefore, training on the proper application of earplugs followed by inspection and/or testing is important for patient comfort and health. Patients may

Table 7.3. Selected acoustic exposure limits and recommendations

dB limit	Purpose
70 dBA	24-h Cumulative general population exposure limit (WHO, EPA recommendation)
80 dBA	8-h Cumulative child exposure limit (WHO recommendation)
85 dBA	8-h Cumulative worker exposure limit (regulation, various countries)
99 dBA	Patient exposure limit, after protection, IEC 60601-2-33 requirement
120 dB	Recommended peak limit for children (WHO)
140 dB	Peak limit for workers and patients (regulation, various countries)

also benefit from the use of double hearing protection, where possible. Additional consideration for the more sensitive ears of children may also be necessary.

In summary, aggregated selected limits and recommendations from various sources shown in Table 7.3.

ACKNOWLEDGMENTS

The author thanks Jana Delfino, Daniel Kraniak and Sunder Rajan of the FDA, Vera Kimbrell of Brigham and Women's Hospital, Maureen Hood of USUHS, William Murphy of NIOSH, David Grainger of MHRA and the ''Yellow Card'' team, and IEC MT40 committee colleagues for their thoughtful insights.

REFERENCES

1. G. Jansen, in 'Handbook of Acoustical Measurements and Noise Control', ed C. M. Harris, McGraw-Hill: New York, 1991.
2. T. Nakai, N. Kamiya, M. Sone, H. Muranaka, T. Tsuchihashi, N. Yamada, and S. Yamaguchi, *Magn. Reson. Med. Sci.*, 2012, **11**, 253.
3. R. A. Hedeen and W. A. Edelstein, *Magn. Reson. Med.*, 1997, **37**, 7.
4. W. A. Edelstein, R. A. Hedeen, R. P. Mallozzi, S. A. El-Hamamsy, R. A. Ackermann, and T. J. Havens, *Magn. Reson. Imaging.*, 2002, **20**, 155.
5. P. Roschmann, *Magn. Reson. Med.*, 1991, **21**, 197.
6. P. Glover, J. Hykin, P. Gowland, J. Wright, I. Johnson, and P. Mansfield, *Br. J. Radiol.*, 1995, **68**, 1090.
7. ISO 226, Acoustics – Normal equal-loudness-level contours, 2003.
8. NIOSH, Occupational noise exposure revised criteria, 1998.
9. E. Berger, R. Neitzel, and C. A. Kladden, Noise navigator sound level database, E-A-R 88-34/HP.
10. NEMA MS 4, Acoustic noise measurement procedure for diagnostic magnetic resonance imaging devices, 2010.
11. B. Roberts and R. Neitzel, Noise exposure limit for children in recreational settings: Review of available evidence, 2018. http://www.who.int/deafness/make-listening-safe/Monograph-on-noise-exposure-limit-for-children-in-recreational-settings.pdf
12. MHRA. Safety Guidelines for Magnetic Resonance Imaging Equipment in Clinical Use, Medicines & Healthcare products Regulatory Agency: UK 2015.
13. EU. DIRECTIVE 2003/10/EC, 2003.
14. ISO 1999:2013 Acoustics – Estimation of Noise-Induced Hearing Loss, International Standards Organization: Geneva, Switzerland, 2013.
15. MSHA, VOLUME III - 30 CFR PARTS 40 THROUGH 50 AND PARTS 62 and 100 Interpretation and Guidelines on Enforcement of the 1977 Act, 1996. https://www.msha.gov/volume-iii-30-cfr-parts-40-through-50-and-parts-62-and-100
16. UK law 2005 No.1643, Health and safety: the control of noise at work regulations, 2005. http://www.legislation.gov.uk/uksi/2005/1643/pdfs/uksi_20051643_en.pdf
17. HPA, MRI procedures: protection of patients and volunteers, 2008. https://www.gov.uk/government/publications/magnetic-resonance-imaging-mri-protecting-patients
18. ICNIRP, *Health Phys.*, 2004, **87**, 197.
19. IEC, IEC 60601-1 – Medical electrical equipment – Part 1: General requirements for basic safety and essential performance, 2012.
20. IEC, IEC 60601-2-33 – Medical electrical equipment – Part 2-33: Particular requirements for the basic safety and essential performance of magnetic resonance equipment for medical diagnosis, 2015.
21. R. Neitzel, E. Svensson, S. Sayler, and J. Ann-Christin, *Noise Health*, 2014, **16**, 270.
22. J. C. Morley, T. Seitz, and R. Tubbs, *Appl. Occup. Environ. Hyg.*, 1999, **14**, 645.
23. K. J. Cruickshanks, R. Klein, B. E. Klein, T. L. Wiley, D. M. Nondahl, and T. S. Tweed, *JAMA*, 1998, **279**, 1715.
24. J. Chang, N. Ryou, H. J. Jun, S. Y. Hwang, J. J. Song, and S. W. Chae, *PLoS One*, 2016, **11**, e0146608.
25. P. Dawes, K. J. Cruickshanks, D. R. Moore, M. Edmondson-Jones, A. McCormack, H. Fortnum, and K. J. Munro, *J. Assoc. Res. Otolaryngol.*, 2014, **15**, 663.
26. P. Bogorodzki, T. Wolak, K. Kochanek, E. Piatkowska-Janko, P. Skarzynski, A. Pilka, J. Kotus, and A. Czyzewski, A fMRI study of Temporary Hearing Threshold Shift. Paper presented at: ISMRM, 2010.

27. C. K. Chen, T.-D. Chiueh, and J.-H. Chen, *IEEE Trans. Biomed. Eng.*, 1999, **46**, 186.
28. E. H. Berger, R. W. Kieper, and D. Gauger, *J. Acoust. Soc. Am.*, 2003, **114**, 1955.
29. M. E. Ravicz and J. R. Melcher, *J. Acoust. Soc. Am.*, 2001, **109**, 216.
30. A. Moelker, R. A. Maas, M. W. Vogel, M. Ouhlous, and P. M. Pattynama, *J. Magn. Reson. Imaging.*, 2005, **22**, 163.
31. E. Berger, Children and hearing protection: what is available and is it used?, 2006.
32. NIOSH, Hearing protector device compendium, https://www.cdc.gov/niosh/topics/noise/hpdcomp/
33. A. Katsunuma, H. Takamori, Y. Sakakura, Y. Hamamura, Y. Ogo, and R. Katayama, *MAGMA.*, 2002, **13**, 139.
34. S. Gerges, Hearing protectors. Paper presented at: Fifth International Congress on Sound and Vibration, 1997.
35. EPA, Product noise labeling. Paper presented at: CFR Part 211, 2002.
36. A. Behar, *Am. Ind. Hyg. Assoc. J.*, 1990, **51**, 659.
37. ISO, ISO 4869-2:1994 Acoustics – Hearing protectors – Part 2: Estimation of effective A-weighted sound pressure levels when hearing protectors are worn.
38. AS/NZS, AS/NZS 1270:R2014 Australian/New Zealand Standard Acoustics—Hearing protectors.
39. A. Biabani, M. Aliabadi, R. Golmohammadi, and M. Farhadian, *Saf. Health Work.*, 2017, **8**, 364.
40. E. Berger, The naked truth about NRRs, 1993. http://multimedia.3m.com/mws/media/600634O/e-a-r-log-20-truth-about-nrr.pdf
41. J. G. Casali and M. Y. Park, *Hum. Factors*, 1990, **32**, 9.
42. E. H. Berger, *Am. Ind. Hyg. Assoc. J.*, 1983, **44**, 321.
43. OSHA, OSHA Technical Manual. Section III: Health Hazards. Chapter 5. Noise, 2013. http://https://www.osha.gov/dts/osta/otm/new_noise/index.html
44. D. C. Byrne and W. J. Murphy,. Double hearing protection: 5 dB or not to be? 2016. http://https://www.researchgate.net/publication/299784651_Double_Hearing_Protection_5_dB_or_Not_to_be
45. A. M. Lauer, A. M. El-Sharkawy, D. L. Kraitchman, and W. A. Edelstein, *J. Magn. Reson. Imaging.*, 2012, **36**, 743.
46. R. Krimins, L. Gainsburg, A. Lauer, M. Solaiyappan, and D. Kraitchman. Hearing loss in dogs after routine neurological MRIs. Paper presented at: ISMRM, 2015.
47. E. Y. Lim, I. P. Tang, M. Peyman, N. Ramli, P. Narayanan, and R. Rajagopalan, *Eur. Arch. Otorhinolaryngol.*, 2015, **272**, 3109.
48. D. G. J. P. De Wilde and C. D. L. Price, *Prog. Nucl. Magn. Reson. Spectrosc.*, 2007, **51**, 37.
49. C. Lanvers-Kaminsky, A. A. Zehnhoff-Dinnesen, R. Parfitt, and G. Ciarimboli, *Clin. Pharmacol. Ther.*, 2017, **101**, 491.
50. D. R. Trune and B. Canlon, *Anat. Rec. (Hoboken)*, 2012, **295**, 1928.
51. T. Miyati, T. Banno, H. Fujita, M. Mase, H. Narita, M. Imazawa, S. Sanada, K. Koshida, and T. Kasuga, *Front. Med. Biol. Eng.*, 2001, **10**, 345.
52. R. E. Brummett, J. M. Talbot, and P. Charuhas, *Radiology*, 1988, **169**, 539.
53. J. H. Langkowski, F. Thiele, R. Maas, and H. Kooijman, *Rofo.*, 1989, **151**, 483.
54. E. Zwicker, K. Schorn, and T. Vogl, *Laryngorhinootologie*, 1990, **69**, 413.
55. A. M. Goldman, W. E. Gossman, and P. C. Friedlander, *Radiology*, 1989, **173**, 549.
56. R. Hurwitz, S. R. Lane, R. A. Bell, and M. N. Brant-Zawadzki, *Radiology*, 1989, **173**, 545.
57. F. G. Shellock, S. M. Morisoli, and M. Ziarati, *Radiology*, 1994, **191**, 91.
58. M. McJury, A. Blug, C. Joerger, B. Condon, and D. Wyper, *Br. J. Radiol.*, 1994, **67**, 413.
59. M. J. McJury, *Clin. Radiol.*, 1995, **50**, 331.
60. F. G. Shellock, M. Ziarati, D. Atkinson, and D. Y. Chen, *J. Magn. Reson. Imaging.*, 1998, **8**, 1154.
61. M. E. Ravicz, J. R. Melcher, and N. Y. Kiang, *J. Acoust. Soc. Am.*, 2000, **108**, 1683.
62. J. R. Foster, D. A. Hall, A. Q. Summerfield, A. R. Palmer, and R. W. Bowtell, *J. Magn. Reson. Imaging*, 2000, **12**, 157.
63. Y. Hattori, H. Fukatsu, and T. Ishigaki, *Nagoya J. Med. Sci.*, 2007, **69**, 23.
64. S. A. Counter, A. Olofsson, E. Borg, B. Bjelke, A. Haggstrom, and H. F. Grahn, *Acta Otolaryngol.*, 2000, **120**, 739.

65. P. T. Weavers, Y. Shu, S. Tao, J. Huston, S.-K. Lee, D. Graziani, J.-B. Mathieu, J.-D. Trzasko, T. K. F. Foo, and M. A. Bernstein, *Med. Phys.*, 2016, **43**, 1259.

66. S. A. Counter, A. Olofsson, H. F. Grahn, and E. Borg, *J. Magn. Reson. Imaging*, 1997, **7**, 606.

67. D. L. Price, J. P. De Wilde, A. M. Papadaki, J. S. Curran, and R. I. Kitney, Acoustic noise on 1.5T MRI systems: worst case and comparative measurements. Paper presented at: ISMRM, 2001.

68. A. Moelker, P. A. Wielopolski, and P. M. Pattynama, *MAGMA.*, 2003, **16**, 52.

69. S. Schmitter, M. Mueller, W. Semmler, and M. Bock, Maximum sound pressure levels at 7 Tesla – what's all this fuss about? Paper presented at: ISMRM, 2009.

70. S. Sasheendran, M. Kumar, Y. Krishna, and B. Rajashekhar, *JAIISH*, 2010, **29**, 248.

71. FDA. FDA Scanner Acoustic Noise Survey data presented to MT40 standards Committee 2018 (private communication).

72. A. Moelker, R. A. Maas, F. Lethimonnier, and P. M. Pattynama, *Radiology.*, 2002, **224**, 889.

73. A. Moelker, M. W. Vogel, and P. M. Pattynama, *J. Magn. Reson. Imaging.*, 2003, **17**, 270.

74. Y. Wang, F. Liu, E. Weber, and S. Crozier, Investigation of acoustic noise reduction method for MRI-LINAC hybrid system. Paper presented at: ISMRM, 2015.

75. P. G. Hepper and B. S. Shahidullah, *Arch. Dis. Child.*, 1994, **71**, F81.

76. D. Querleu, X. Renard, F. Versyp, L. Paris-Delrue, and G. Crepin, *Eur. J. Obstet. Gynecol. Reprod. Biol.*, 1988, **28**, 191.

77. Noise: a hazard for the fetus and newborn. American Academy of Pediatrics. Committee on Environmental Health. *Pediatrics*, 1997, **100**, 724.

78. ACR. ACR–SPR practice parameters for the safe and optimal performance of fetal magnetic resonance imaging (MRI), 2015.

79. F. E. Thurston, Is external noise a risk to fetal hearing development? a review. Paper presented at: Seminars in Hearing, 2008.

80. J. Selander, M. Albin, U. Rosenhall, L. Rylander, M. Lewne, and P. Gustavsson, *Environ. Health Perspect.*, 2016, **124**, 855.

81. Prenatal Effects of Exposure to High-Level Noise Committee on Hearing Bioacoustics and Biomechanics. Defense Technical Information Center Technical Report ADA113724, 1982.

82. M. J. Reeves, M. Brandreth, E. H. Whitby, A. R. Hart, M. N. J. Paley, P. D. Griffiths, and J. C. Stevens, *Radiology*, 2010, **257**, 802.

83. P. N. Baker, I. R. Johnson, P. R. Harvey, P. A. Gowland, and P. Mansfield, *Am. J. Obstet. Gynecol.*, 1994, **170**, 32.

84. H. Clements, K. R. Duncan, K. Fielding, P. A. Gowland, I. R. Johnson, and P. N. Baker, *Br. J. Radiol.*, 2000, **73**, 190.

85. B. Strizek, J. C. Jani, E. Mucyo, F. De Keyzer, I. Pauwels, S. Ziane, A. L. Mansbach, P. Deltenre, T. Cos, and M. M. Cannie, *Radiology*, 2015, **275**, 530.

86. M. N. Paley, A. R. Hart, M. Lait, and P. D. Griffiths, *Br. J. Radiol.*, 2012, **85**, 952.

87. D. Price, T. Burrows, G. Kendall, E. Cady, and N. Robertson, Acoustic noise levels in an MR-conditional neonatal incubator during 3T MRI. Paper presented at: ESMRMB, 2012.

88. C. Ireland, R. Giaquinto, J. Tkach, R. Pratt, and C. Dumoulin, A novel acoustic quiet coil for neonatal MRI system. Paper presented at: ISMRM, 2015.

89. A. Nordell, M. Lundh, S. Horsch, B. Hallberg, U. Aden, B. Nordell, and M. Blennow, *Acta Paediatr.*, 2009, **98**, 1278.

90. WHO, Children and noise, 2004. http://www.who.int/ceh/capacity/noise.pdf

91. Council on Environmental Health AAoP, Pediatric Environmental Health, 3rd edn, American Academy of Pediatrics, 2011.

92. W. J. Murphy, C. L. Themann, and T. K. Murata, *Int. J. Audiol.*, 2016, **55**, 688. https://www.tandfonline.com/doi/full/10.1080/14992027.2016.1204470

93. D. B. Chonde, N. Abolmaali, A. G. Sorensen, and C. Catana, The effect of MR acoustic noise on FDG-PET uptake in a simultaneous MR/PET system. Paper presented at: ISMRM, 2011.

94. D. B. Chonde, N. Abolmaali, G. Arabasz, A. R. Guimaraes, and C. Catana, *Invest. Radiol.*, 2013, **48**, 302.

95. W. Wagner, I. Staud, G. Frank, F. Dammann, S. Plontke, and P. K. Plinkert, *Laryngoscope.*, 2003, **113**, 1216.

96. D. Baguley, D. McFerran, and H. D. Tinnitus, *Lancet.*, 2013, **382**, 1600.

97. T. G. Sanchez and C. B. Rocha, *Clinics (Sao Paulo)*, 2011, **66**, 1089.

98. J. Sheldrake, P. U. Diehl, and R. Schaette, *Front Neurol.*, 2015, **6**, 105. DOI: 10.3389/fneur.2015.00105.

99. J. Paulin, L. Andersson, and S. Nordin, *Noise Health*, 2016, **18**, 178.

100. D. Kaski, R. Davies, L. Luxon, A. M. Bronstein, and P. Rudge, *J. Neurol.*, 2012, **259**, 4.

101. S. Stenfelt and B. Hakansson, *Hear. Res.*, 2002, **167**, 1.

102. W. Williams, *Noise Health*, 2004, **7**, 41.

103. A. M. Smith, *Aviat. Space Environ. Med.*, 2010, **81**, 696.

104. A. Joseph, J. Punch, M. Stephenson, N. Paneth, E. Wolfe, and W. Murphy, *Int. J. Audiol.*, 2007, **46**, 609.

105. T. J. Ryan, R. S. Meier, and A. Tatarka, *J. Occup. Environ. Hyg.*, 2017, **14**, 931.

106. R. F. Randolph and F.N. Kissell, The effect of an insertion lubricant on the noise attenuation of foam earplugs. Paper presented at: NOISE-CON, 2008.

107. R. Randolph, QuickFit Earplug Test Device. Paper presented at: CDC NIOSH Technology News, 2008.

108. HFM-147 TG. Hearing Protection – Needs, Technologies and Performance 2010.

109. S. G. Kujawa and M. C. Liberman, *J. Neurosci.*, 2009, **29**, 14077.

Chapter 8
Modeling Blood Flow

Michael Keith Sharp
University of Louisville, Louisville, KY, USA

Several entire books have been written on the flow of blood in the human circulatory system. The scope of a book chapter on the same topic must obviously be limited. The approach that was adopted is to focus on laminar flow, which applies to most of the vasculature, particularly under sedentary conditions. Turbulent flow is encountered in the largest arteries and in more locations under exercise conditions, as well as in some cardiovascular devices. Anatomy and physiology is also largely neglected in favor of presenting fluid dynamic phenomena. For more details, it is recommended that the reader consult monographs and texts such as those by McDonald,[1] Pedley,[2] Fung,[3] Waite and Fine,[4] Caro *et al.*,[5] Chandran *et al.*[6] and Rubenstein *et al.*[7]

Safety and Biological Effects in MRI.
Edited by Devashish Shrivastava and J. Thomas Vaughan

ISBN: 978-1-118-82130-5
Also published in eMagRes (online edition)
DOI: 10.1002/9780470034590.emrstm1589

8.1 BLOOD CELLS

8.1.1 Erythrocytes

The fluid dynamic behavior of blood is dominated by erythrocytes (red blood cells), which typically comprise 40–45% of whole blood volume in adults. The volume percentage of erythrocytes, called hematocrit, is slightly lower in females than in males. Newborns sometimes have elevated hematocrit, as high as 75%. Erythrocytes have a rounded biconcave disk shape (Figure 8.1), with diameter of about 7.65 ± 0.67 μm, maximum thickness of 2.84 ± 0.46 μm, and minimum thickness of 1.44 ± 0.47 μm.[8] This shape allows the cell to readily deform so that it can squeeze through capillaries smaller than the diameter of the cell. Erythrocytes lack a nucleus and are largely filled with hemoglobin, which is the primary transporter of oxygen in the blood stream. Because erythrocytes have a density ($1.11\ \mathrm{g\,cc^{-1}}$) that is greater than plasma, hematocrit can be measured by centrifugation.

8.1.2 Leukocytes

Leukocytes, or white blood cells, are involved in immune response, either by directly attacking foreign bodies or by producing antibodies. Six types of leukocytes, including neutrophils, lymphocytes, monocytes, eosinophils, basophils, and plasma cells, serve specialized functions. Leukocytes are typically spherical, with diameters ranging from 20 to 100 μm. Leukocytes have a density ($1.08\ \mathrm{g\,cc^{-1}}$) intermediate between that

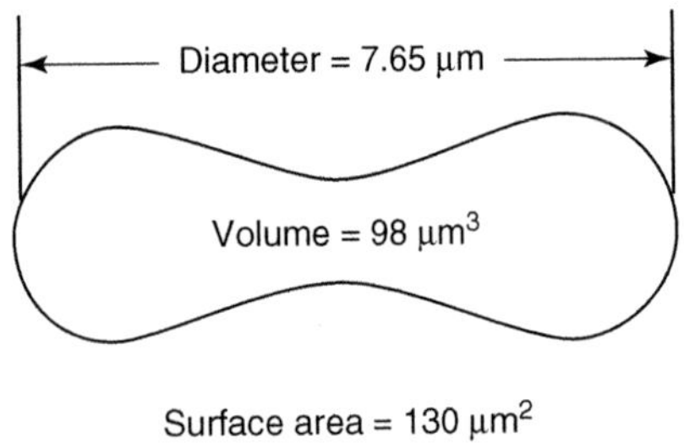

Figure 8.1. Erythrocyte shape.[22] (Reproduced with permission from Springer Science Business Media New York. © 1993)

of plasma and erythrocytes; thus, during centrifugation they are consolidated into a thin layer, called the buffy coat, between the two. The volume fraction of leukocytes in whole blood is less than 1%, so their impact on flow, at least in large vessels, is minimal.

8.1.3 Platelets

Platelets, or thrombocytes, serve to cover wounds in the walls of the circulatory system and, therefore, prevent blood loss. While unactivated platelets are ellipsoidal with major diameter of about 4 μm and minor diameter of about 1.5 μm, when activated they rapidly spread into thin layers, attaching to endothelial cells and other platelets, and signaling a coagulation cascade that results in a fibrin mesh (thrombus) that blocks bleeding. Platelets also have density (1.06 g cc^{-1}) between plasma and erythrocytes; thus, during centrifugation they migrate to the buffy coat. Platelets comprise less than 1% of the volume of whole blood, so in their unactivated state do not influence flow significantly.

8.1.4 Plasma

Erythrocytes, leukocytes, and platelets are suspended in plasma, which is 92% water. Plasma proteins, including albumin, globulins, and fibrinogen, regulate fluid balance, immune response, and coagulation, respectively. The density of plasma (1.03 g cc^{-1}) is slightly higher than that of water (1.0 g cc^{-1}). While variability and non-Newtonian response has been identified, for many purposes, plasma has been treated as Newtonian with viscosity of 1.2 cP at body temperature (37 °C). For comparison, the viscosity of water at the same temperature is 0.69 cP.

8.2 BLOOD RHEOLOGY

Fibrinogen is involved in aggregation of erythrocytes into columnar stacks of cells called rouleaux. At low shear rate, the structure of the aggregates grows over the course of minutes to branching networks that require a threshold (yield) stress before blood flow can occur. At intermediate shear rate, the rouleaux are broken up into single cells that retain their characteristic biconcave disk shape, and at high shear rate, the cells are deformed and elongated within fractions of a second into spindle-like shapes aligned with the direction of flow. Blood, therefore, is not only non-Newtonian, but is also viscoelastic (Figures 8.2 and 8.3). In Figures 8.2 and 8.3, blood rheology is quantified by the real (viscous) and imaginary (elastic) components of complex viscosity in oscillatory flow at 2 Hz

$$\eta = \eta_v + i\eta_e \tag{8.1}$$

Psuedoplasticity (shear thinning) is evident in the viscous component, but the shear rate for these measurements was too high to show a yield stress. Thixotropy (time-dependent 'shear thinning' due to deformation and alignment of cells) is similarly evident in the elastic component. The effects of strain, hematocrit, and age have been curve fit as[9]

$$\begin{aligned}\log(\eta_v - 0.00692) &= -3.2978 - 0.0904\,S \\ &+ 0.0272(H - 37.25) + 0.0023\,A \\ &- 0.0024\,S(H - 37.25) - 0.0005\,SA\end{aligned} \tag{8.2}$$

$$\begin{aligned}\log(\eta_e) &= -5.0641 - 0.5898\,S - 00354\,S^2 \\ &+ 0.0544(H - 37.25) + 0.0043\,S(H - 37.25) \\ &- 0.0028\,S^2(H - 37.25)\end{aligned} \tag{8.3}$$

where S is strain, H is (percent) hematocrit, and A is age in years.

8.3 FLOW IN A STRAIGHT, RIGID TUBE

Solutions for steady flow with several models of blood rheology will be presented in the following sections, in the order of increasing complexity. Steady flow is strictly more applicable to venous flow than to arterial flow, because the pressure gradient driving flow is nearly constant. However, pulsatile arterial flow also has a nonzero mean component that is sufficient for simplified modeling purposes.

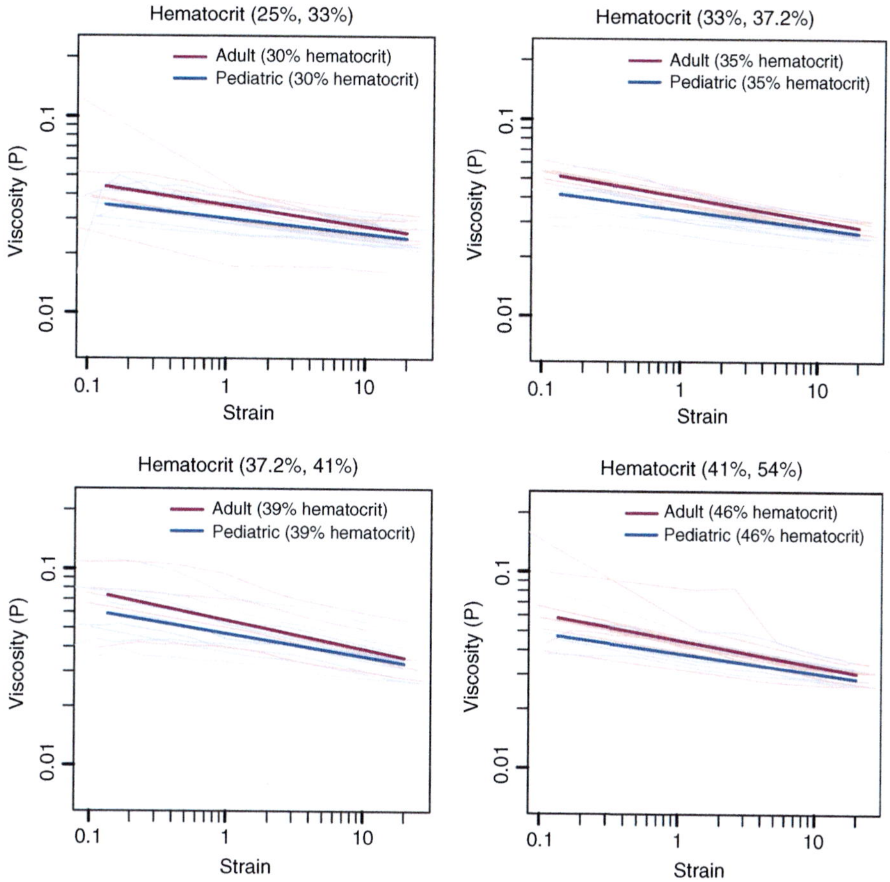

Figure 8.2. Viscosity for pediatric and adult subjects in four hematocrit quartiles. For hematocrit intervals, round brackets indicate exclusion of the endpoint in that interval, whereas square brackets are inclusive of the endpoint. The bold lines represent the model at the midpoint hematocrit of each quartile. Light lines denote the subject data. The conditional R^2 for the model (indicating the proportional reduction in residual variance by including age and hematrocrit relative to a model without those terms) was 0.411.[9] (Reproduced with permission from Biomedical Engineering Society. © 2017)

8.3.1 Newtonian

A Newtonian fluid has a simple, proportional relationship between shear stress and rate of strain

$$\tau = -\mu \frac{\partial w}{\partial r} \tag{8.4}$$

for fully developed flow in a straight tube, where τ is the shear stress, $\mu = 3.5$ cP is the viscosity,[6] w is the axial velocity, and r is the radial coordinate. Note that forward flow corresponds to a negative velocity gradient, thus the minus sign on the right-hand side of equation (8.4). The shear stress exerted on the wall (where shear stress is maximum) is given by

$$\tau_{\mathrm{w}} = -\frac{a}{2}\frac{\partial p}{\partial z} \tag{8.5}$$

where a is the radius of the tube, and $\partial p/\partial z$ is the axial pressure gradient, which is negative for forward flow, giving a positive wall shear stress. The velocity profile is given by

$$w = -\frac{1}{4\mu}\frac{\partial p}{\partial z}(a^2 - r^2) \tag{8.6}$$

Integrating over the cross section of the tube to find the flow rate gives

$$Q = -\frac{\pi a^4}{8\mu}\frac{\partial p}{\partial z} \tag{8.7}$$

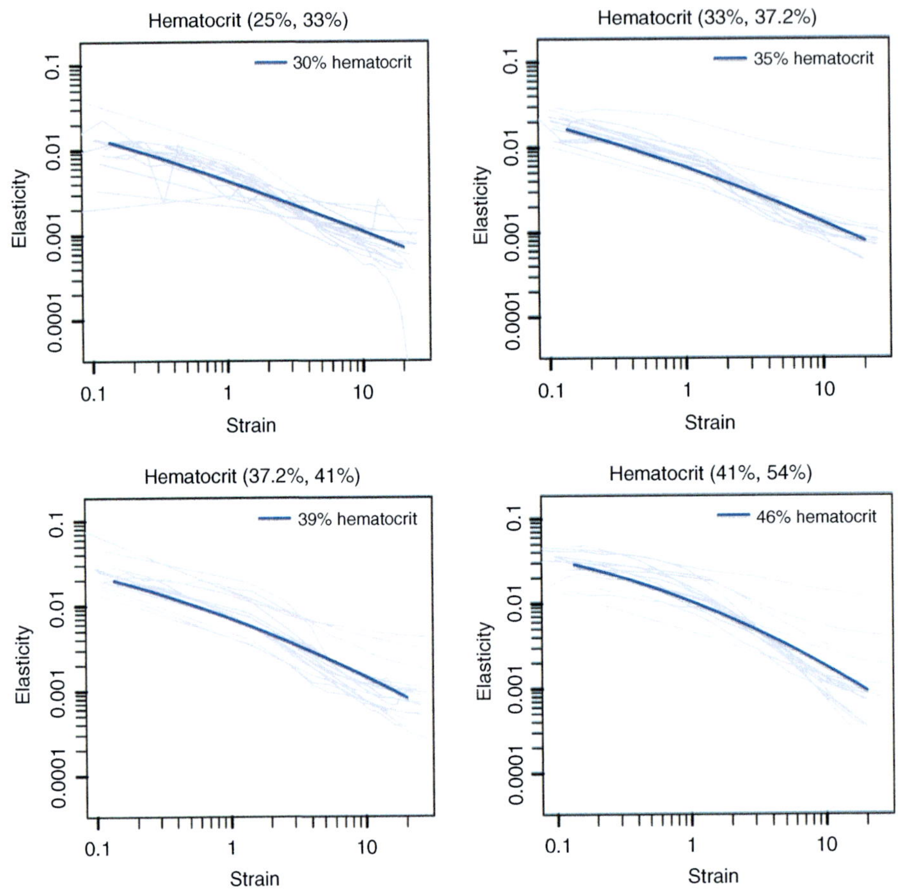

Figure 8.3. Elasticity in four hematocrit percentiles. Differences between pediatric and adult subjects were not found to be significant. For hematocrit intervals, round brackets indicate exclusion of the endpoint in that interval, whereas square brackets are inclusive of the endpoint. The bold lines represent the model at the midpoint hematocrit value of each quartile. Light lines denote the subject data. The conditional R^2 for the model (indicating the proportional reduction in residual variance by including hematrocrit relative to a model without those terms) was 0.204.[9] (Reproduced with permission from Biomedical Engineering Society. © 2017)

8.3.2 Bingham

The Bingham model adds a yield stress to the Newtonian relationship

$$\tau = \tau_{yB} - \mu_B \frac{\partial w}{\partial r} \tag{8.8}$$

where $\tau_{yB} = 7$ mPa is the yield stress, and $\mu_B = 3.31$ cP is the Bingham viscosity.[6] No flow occurs if the wall shear stress [equation (8.5)] does not exceed the yield stress. For greater wall shear stress, a constant-velocity core exists, in which the shear stress is less than the yield stress. The radius of the core is found where the fluid stress equals the yield stress

$$r_c = \frac{2\tau_{yB}}{-\partial p/\partial z} \tag{8.9}$$

The core velocity is given by

$$w_c = -\frac{1}{2\mu_B}\frac{\partial p}{\partial z}\left[\frac{1}{2}\left(a^2 - r_c^2\right) - r_c(a - r_c)\right] \tag{8.10}$$

and the velocity in the periphery is

$$w = -\frac{1}{2\mu_B}\frac{\partial p}{\partial z}\left[\frac{1}{2}\left(a^2 - r^2\right) - r_c(a-r)\right] \quad (8.11)$$

Integrating over the cross section of the tube to find the flow rate gives

$$Q = -\frac{\pi a^4}{8\mu_B}\frac{\partial p}{\partial x}\left[1 - \frac{4}{3}\frac{r_c}{a} + \frac{1}{3}\left(\frac{r_c}{a}\right)^4\right] \quad (8.12)$$

Note that as r_c becomes small compared to a, or equivalently, as τ_{yB} becomes small compared to τ_w, the flow rate reduces to the Poiseuille value for a Newtonian fluid [equation (8.7)].

8.3.3 Casson

The Casson model has a yield stress and a psuedoplastic response for higher shear stress

$$\sqrt{\tau} = \sqrt{\tau_{yC}} + \mu_C\sqrt{-\frac{\partial w}{\partial r}} \quad (8.13)$$

where $\mu_C = 3.29$ cP is the Casson viscosity, and $\tau_{yC} = 13.8$ mPa is the yield stress.[10] The radius of the constant-velocity core is again given by equation (8.9). The velocity of the core is

$$w_c = -\frac{1}{4\mu_C^2}\frac{\partial p}{\partial z}\left[a^2 - r_c^2 + 2r_c\left(a - r_c\right)\right.$$
$$\left.-\frac{8}{3}r_c^{1/2}\left(a^{3/2} - r_c^{3/2}\right)\right] \quad (8.14)$$

and for the periphery

$$w = -\frac{1}{4\mu_C^2}\frac{\partial p}{\partial z}\left[a^2 - r^2 + 2r_c\left(a - r\right)\right.$$
$$\left.-\frac{8}{3}r_c^{1/2}\left(a^{3/2} - r^{3/2}\right)\right] \quad (8.15)$$

Integrating over the cross section gives

$$Q = -\frac{\pi a^4}{8\mu_C^2}\frac{\partial p}{\partial z}\left[1 - \frac{16}{7}\sqrt{\frac{r_c}{a}} + \frac{4}{3}\frac{r_c}{a} - \frac{1}{21}\left(\frac{r_c}{a}\right)^4\right]$$
$$(8.16)$$

Again, the flow rate reduces to the Poiseuille value for a Newtonian fluid [equation (8.7)] for $r_c \ll a$ (or $\tau_{yC} \ll \tau_w$).

8.3.4 Power Law

The power-law model does not have a yield stress, but does have psuedoplastic behavior

$$\tau = \mu_P\left(-\frac{\partial w}{\partial r}\right)^n \quad (8.17)$$

where $\mu_P = 12.17$ is the power-law viscosity, and $n = 0.799$ is an empirical exponent.[10] The velocity profile is continuous without a constant-velocity core:

$$u = \frac{n}{n+1}\left(-\frac{1}{2\mu_P}\frac{\partial p}{\partial x}\right)^{\frac{1}{n}}\left(a^{\frac{n+1}{n}} - r^{\frac{n+1}{n}}\right) \quad (8.18)$$

and the flow rate becomes

$$Q = \frac{n\pi a^3}{3n+1}\left(-\frac{a}{2\mu_P}\frac{\partial p}{\partial z}\right)^{\frac{1}{n}} \quad (8.19)$$

This flow rate reduces to Newtonian [equation (8.7)] for $n = 1$.

8.3.5 Herschel–Bulkley

This model adds a yield stress to the power-law model

$$\tau = \tau_{yHB} + \mu_{HB}\left(-\frac{\partial w}{\partial r}\right)^n \quad (8.20)$$

where $\mu_{HB} = 8.97$ is the Herschel–Bulkley viscosity, $n = 0.860$ is the exponent, and $\tau_{yHB} = 17.5$ mPa is the yield stress.[10] The radius of the constant-velocity core is again given by equation (8.9). The velocity of the core is

$$w_c = \left(-\frac{1}{2\mu_{HB}}\frac{\partial p}{\partial z}\right)^{1/n}\frac{n}{n+1}(a - r_c)^{\frac{n+1}{n}} \quad (8.21)$$

and for the periphery

$$w_c = \left(-\frac{1}{2\mu_{HB}}\frac{\partial p}{\partial z}\right)^{1/n}\frac{n}{n+1}\left[(a - r_c)^{\frac{n+1}{n}} - (r - r_c)^{\frac{n+1}{n}}\right]$$
$$(8.22)$$

Integrating over the cross section gives

$$Q = 2\pi\left(-\frac{1}{2\mu_{HB}}\frac{\partial p}{\partial z}\right)^{1/n}\frac{n}{n+1}\left[-\frac{n}{3n+1}(a - r_c)^{\frac{3n+1}{n}}\right.$$
$$\left.-\frac{n}{2n+1}r_c(r - r_c)^{\frac{2n+1}{n}} + \frac{a^2}{2}(a - r_c)^{\frac{n+1}{n}}\right]$$
$$(8.23)$$

The flow rate reduces to the Poiseuille value for a Newtonian fluid [equation (8.7)] for $r_c \ll a$ (or $\tau_y \ll \tau_w$) and $n = 1$.

8.3.6 Entrance Length for Steady Flow

The solutions in the previous sections are for fully developed flow, which tends to apply to vessels that are long compared to their radii. A limitation of this assumption is that typical blood vessels have frequent branches, each of which disrupts the velocity profile, forcing it to converge toward the fully developed shape all over again. The entrance length for steady, laminar flow of a Newtonian fluid is

$$\frac{L_e}{D} \approx \frac{\overline{w}a}{8\mathrm{v}} = \frac{\mathrm{Re}}{16} \quad (8.24)$$

where for circular tubes $\mathrm{Re} \equiv \frac{D\overline{w}}{\mathrm{v}}$ is the Reynolds number, $D = 2a$ is the diameter of the tube, $\overline{w}$ is the mean velocity over the cross section, $\mathrm{v} = \mu/\rho$ is the kinematic viscosity, and ρ is the density.

8.3.7 Pulsatile Flow in a Straight, Rigid Tube

Pressure in blood vessels, especially arteries, fluctuates as the heart beats. Therefore, flow in arteries is pulsatile and depends on the Womersley number

$$\alpha = \sqrt{\frac{a^2\omega}{\mathrm{v}}} \quad (8.25)$$

where ω is the heart beat frequency. For a periodic pressure gradient given by

$$-\frac{\partial p}{\partial z} \equiv \sum_{n=0}^{\infty} A_n e^{in\omega t} \quad (8.26)$$

where A_n is the amplitude of the pressure gradient for each harmonic n and t is time. The velocity becomes

$$w = -\frac{1}{4\mu}A_0(a^2 - r^2) - \sum_{n=1}^{\infty} \frac{iA_n}{n}\left(1 - \frac{J_0(r\lambda)}{J_0(a\lambda)}\right)e^{in\omega t} \quad (8.27)$$

where J_0 is Bessel's function of the first kind and order zero and $\lambda = \sqrt{\frac{n\omega}{\mathrm{v}}}$. The first term for the zeroth (steady) component is the same as for Poiseuille flow [equation (8.6)]. Because the higher order terms are oscillatory (with zero mean), the cycle-averaged flow rate is the same as for Poiseuille flow [equation (8.7)].

8.3.8 Entrance Length for Pulsatile Flow

Two boundary layer growth phenomena occur when oscillatory flow is superimposed on a steady entrance flow. First, a viscous boundary layer attempts to regrow each time the flow reverses. The thickness of this boundary layer scales as

$$\delta_1 \sim \sqrt{\frac{\mathrm{v}}{\omega}} \quad (8.28)$$

Notice that this thickness does not depend on the location in the tube. A second viscous boundary layer grows with the distance from the entrance of the tube, the same as for steady flow, which leads to a Reynolds number-dependent entrance length (Section 8.3.6). The thickness of this boundary layer scales as

$$\delta_2 \sim \sqrt{\frac{\mathrm{v}x}{\overline{w}}} \quad (8.29)$$

For large Womersley number, the oscillatory boundary layer never reaches the center of the tube, $\delta_1 < a$. Therefore, the steady boundary layer needs to only grow to the same thickness as the oscillatory boundary for the flow to be fully developed, $\delta_1 = \delta_2$. Equating the two thicknesses gives $L_e \sim \overline{w}/\omega$. More detailed analysis[11,12] adds a constant coefficient to the scaling

$$L_e = 2.64\frac{\overline{w}}{\omega} \quad (8.30)$$

8.4 FLOW IN CURVED TUBES

Flow in curved tubes has been reviewed by Berger *et al.*[13] Several of the basic effects of curvature for which analytical solutions are available are described in the following sections.

8.4.1 Steady Flow in Curved Tubes

Some blood vessels are curved. For instance, the ascending aorta curves approximately 180° over a short distance. For strongly curved vessels such as the aorta, analytical solutions are unavailable, but for mild curvature $\delta = \frac{a}{R} \ll 1$, where R is the radius of curvature of the tube, A perturbation solution[14,15] gives

$$w/\overline{w} = w_0 + \mathrm{Dn}^2 w_1 + \cdots, \quad \psi = \mathrm{Dn}\psi_1 + \cdots \quad (8.31)$$

where $\overline{w}$ is the average axial velocity, $\mathrm{Dn} \equiv \sqrt{\delta}\mathrm{Re}$ is the Dean number, and ψ is the stream function in the plane perpendicular to the axis of the tube. The first term of the axial velocity is the same as for Poiseuille flow

$$w_0 = 2\left[1 - \left(\frac{r}{a}\right)^2\right] \quad (8.32)$$

and the remaining terms skew the profile

$$w_1 = \frac{\cos\phi}{144}\left[\frac{19r}{40a} - \left(\frac{r}{a}\right)^3 + \frac{3}{4}\left(\frac{r}{a}\right)^5 - \frac{1}{4}\left(\frac{r}{a}\right)^7 + \frac{1}{40}\left(\frac{r}{a}\right)^9\right] - \frac{3a}{2R\mathrm{Dn}^2}\frac{r}{a}\left(1 - \left(\frac{r}{a}\right)^2\right)\cos\phi \tag{8.33}$$

where r and ϕ are the radial and angular coordinates in the cross section of the tube. The peak velocity is shifted toward the outside of the curve to location:

$$r/a = 8.4\times10^{-4}\mathrm{Dn}^2,\ \phi = 0 \tag{8.34}$$

The flow rate in the curved tube becomes

$$\frac{Q}{\pi a^2\overline{w}} = 1 - 0.0306\left(\frac{\mathrm{Dn}^2}{288}\right)^2 + 0.0120\left(\frac{\mathrm{Dn}^2}{288}\right)^4 + O\left[\left(\frac{\mathrm{Dn}^2}{288}\right)^4\right] \tag{8.35}$$

Secondary flow is characterized by two counter-rotating vortices with centers at $r/a = 0.43$ (Figure 8.4). Velocities in the cross section are obtained from the stream function as

$$\frac{u}{\sqrt{\delta\overline{w}}} = \frac{\mathrm{Dn}^2\cos\phi}{72}\frac{r}{a}\left[1 - \left(\frac{r}{a}\right)^2\right]^2\left[1 - \frac{1}{4}\left(\frac{r}{a}\right)^2\right] \tag{8.36}$$

$$\frac{v}{\sqrt{\delta\overline{w}}} = \frac{\mathrm{Dn}^2\sin\phi}{72}\left[1 - \left(\frac{r}{a}\right)^2\right]\left[1 - \frac{23}{4}\left(\frac{r}{a}\right)^2 + \frac{7}{4}\left(\frac{r}{a}\right)^4\right] \tag{8.37}$$

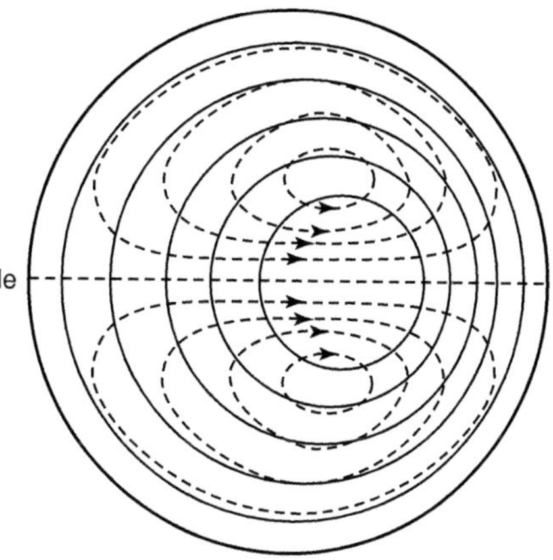

Figure 8.4. Axial velocity contours (solid lines) and secondary flow streamlines (dashed lines) for low Dean Number. (From Berger *et al.*[13])

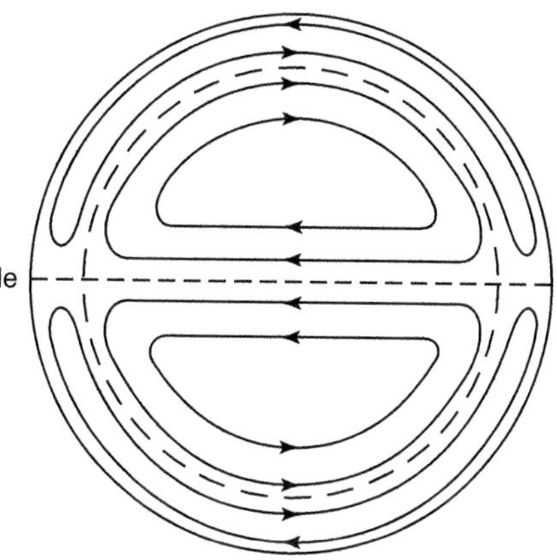

Figure 8.5. Secondary-flow streamlines for high Womersley number and low Dean number.[16] (Reproduced with permission from Cambridge University Press. © 1970)

8.4.2 Pulsatile Flow in Curved Tubes

For pulsatile flow in a curved tube, the same axial- and secondary-velocity profiles apply instantaneously so long as unsteadiness is small compared to viscous effects $\frac{\text{unsteady}}{\text{viscous}} \approx \alpha^2 \ll 1$ and to centrifugally driven convective effects $\frac{\text{unsteady}}{\text{convective}} \approx \frac{\alpha^4}{\mathrm{Dn}^2} \ll 1$. If unsteadiness dominates, $\alpha^2 \gg 1$ and $\frac{\alpha^4}{\mathrm{Dn}^2} \gg 1$, a pair of secondary-flow vortices circulates around the viscous boundary layer near the wall of the tube, and another pair circulates across the inertial core (Figure 8.5). For these conditions, a solution is available for purely oscillatory flow (with zero mean).[16] In the boundary layer, the normalized axial velocity is

$$w = w_0(t,\eta,\phi,\mathrm{Re_s}) + \frac{\sqrt{2}}{\alpha}w_1(t,\eta,\phi,\mathrm{Re_s}) + \cdots \tag{8.38}$$

where

$$w_0 = \sin t - e^{-\eta}\sin(t-\eta) \tag{8.39}$$

$$w_1 = \frac{1}{2}\eta e^{-\eta}\sin(t-\eta) \tag{8.40}$$

where $\eta = \frac{\alpha}{\sqrt{2}}\left(1 - \frac{r}{a}\right)$, and $\mathrm{Re_s} = \frac{W^2 a}{R\omega \nu}$ is the secondary-flow Reynolds number, and W is the amplitude of the core velocity. The rescaled $\left(\Psi = \frac{\alpha}{\sqrt{2}}\psi\right)$ stream function in the boundary layer

$$\Psi = \Psi_0(t, \eta, \phi, \mathrm{Re_s}) + \frac{\sqrt{2}}{\alpha}\Psi_1(t, \eta, \phi, \mathrm{Re_s}) + \cdots \tag{8.41}$$

has the solution

$$\Psi_0 = \left\{ \begin{array}{l} -\frac{\eta}{4} + \frac{5}{8} - \frac{e^{-2\eta}}{8} - \frac{e^{-\eta}}{\sqrt{2}}\cos\left(\frac{\pi}{4} - \eta\right) \\ +\frac{5}{8}e^{-\sqrt{2}\eta}\cos\left(\frac{\pi}{4} + 2t - \sqrt{2}\eta\right) \\ -\frac{\sqrt{2}}{16}e^{-2\eta}\cos\left(\frac{\pi}{4} + 2t - 2\eta\right) - \frac{e^{-\eta}}{\sqrt{2}}\cos\left(\frac{\pi}{4} + 2t - \eta\right) \\ +\frac{1}{16}(9\sqrt{2} - 10)\cos\left(\frac{\pi}{4} + 2t\right) \end{array} \right\} \sin\phi \tag{8.42}$$

and for $\eta \to \infty$

$$\Psi_1 = \left\{ \frac{\eta}{2} - \frac{3}{16} - \frac{9\sqrt{2} - 10}{16}\eta\cos\left(\frac{\pi}{4} + 2t\right) + \frac{16\sqrt{2} - 21}{32}\cos 2t \right\} \sin\phi + A(\phi)\eta^2 \tag{8.43}$$

where

$$A(\phi) = \frac{3}{8}\sin\phi - \frac{\mathrm{Re_s}}{768}\sin 2\phi + \frac{\mathrm{Re_s^2}}{737280}\sin\phi \tag{8.44}$$

For the core

$$w = \sin t \tag{8.45}$$

$$\psi = \psi_0(t, \eta, \phi, R_s) + \frac{\sqrt{2}}{\alpha}\psi_1(t, \eta, \phi, R_s) + \cdots \tag{8.46}$$

For low $\mathrm{Re_s}$, the stream function is expanded as

$$\psi_0 = \psi_{00}(t, \phi) + \mathrm{Re_s}\psi_{01}(t, \phi) + \mathrm{Re_s^2}\psi_{02}(t, \phi) + \cdots \tag{8.47}$$

where

$$\psi_{00} = -\frac{r}{8}(1 - r^2)\sin\phi \tag{8.48}$$

$$\psi_{01} = -\frac{r^2}{3072}(1 - r^2)^2\sin 2\phi \tag{8.49}$$

$$\psi_{02} = -\frac{1}{1474560}\left[\frac{r}{2}\left(1 - r^2\right)^2(2 - 7r^2 + 4r^4)\sin\phi + r^3\left(1 - r^2\right)^3\sin 3\phi\right] \tag{8.50}$$

The second term becomes

$$\begin{aligned} \psi_1 &= \frac{r}{16}(19 - 9r^2)\sin\phi \\ &+ \frac{9}{3072}\mathrm{Re_s} r^2(1 - r^2)^2\sin 2\phi + \frac{\mathrm{Re_s}^2}{3072} \\ &\times \left[\begin{array}{l} \frac{1}{1920}\left(154r - 597r^3 + 840r^5 - 505r^7 + 108r^9\right)\sin\phi \\ +\frac{1}{320}(-r^3 - 7r^5 + 17r^7 - 9r^9)\sin 3\phi \end{array} \right] \end{aligned} \tag{8.51}$$

8.4.3 Regimes of Oscillatory Flow in a Curved Tube

Oscillatory flow in a curved tube provides an example of the power of order-of-magnitude analysis to understand a wide range of fluid flows. To perform the analysis, we begin with conservation of momentum in spherical coordinates (r, θ, ϕ)

$$\frac{\partial u}{\partial t} + u\frac{\partial u}{\partial r} + \frac{v}{r}\frac{\partial u}{\partial \phi} - \frac{v^2}{r} - \frac{w^2\cos\phi}{R} = -\frac{1}{\rho}\frac{\partial p}{\partial r} - \frac{\mathbf{v}}{r}\frac{\partial}{\partial \phi}\left(\frac{\partial v}{\partial r} + \frac{v}{r} - \frac{1}{r}\frac{\partial u}{\partial \phi}\right) \tag{8.52}$$

$$\frac{\partial v}{\partial t} + u\frac{\partial v}{\partial r} + \frac{v}{r}\frac{\partial v}{\partial \phi} + \frac{uv}{r} + \frac{w^2\cos\phi}{R} = -\frac{1}{\rho r}\frac{\partial p}{\partial \phi} + \mathbf{v}\frac{\partial}{\partial r}\left(\frac{\partial v}{\partial r} + \frac{v}{r} - \frac{1}{r}\frac{\partial u}{\partial \phi}\right) \tag{8.53}$$

$$\frac{\partial w}{\partial t} + u\frac{\partial w}{\partial r} + \frac{v}{r}\frac{\partial w}{\partial \phi} = -\frac{1}{\rho}\frac{\partial p}{R\partial \theta} + \mathbf{v}\left[\left(\frac{\partial}{\partial r} + \frac{1}{r}\right)\frac{\partial w}{\partial r} + \frac{1}{r^2}\frac{\partial^2 w}{\partial \phi^2}\right] \tag{8.54}$$

These equations are limited to fully developed flow, since axial derivatives have been discarded, except for pressure. In addition, mild curvature is assumed, so that terms of $O[\delta]$ and higher are neglected in the axial momentum equation. In the cross-sectional momentum equations, however, there are no terms larger than $O[\delta]$ because, while the axial pressure gradient drives the axial flow, it is the centrifugal terms (the w^2/R terms) that drive the secondary flow in the cross section. In each equation, all the other terms can be no larger than the driving term. In this analysis, the pressure terms are ignored. The axial pressure term can be thought of as the independent variable that produces the dependent velocities in the axial momentum equation. But in the cross-sectional momentum equations, since the centrifugal term is the driving term, the pressure terms are dependent variables that for our purposes are simply less interesting than the velocity terms.

At least one of the other terms in each of equations (8.52)–(8.54) must be as large as the driving term for the equation to balance. In the order-of-magnitude analysis, all the possibilities for large (dominant) terms will be identified. Cross-sectional velocities u and v have the same maximum scale, which is designated as the secondary-velocity scale v_s. This scale depends on the dominant character of the flow. The fundamental scales used for this analysis are:

$$r \sim a;\ t \sim \frac{1}{\omega};\ (u, v) \sim v_s;\ w \sim \overline{W};\ (\phi, \sin\phi, \cos\phi) \sim 1 \tag{8.55}$$

where $\overline{W}$ is the amplitude of the average axial velocity. With these scales, the orders of magnitude of the terms become:

cross-sectional unsteady terms $\left(\frac{\partial u}{\partial t}, \frac{\partial v}{\partial t}\right) = O[v_s\omega]$ (8.56)

cross-sectional convective terms

$$\left(u\frac{\partial u}{\partial r}, \frac{v}{r}\frac{\partial u}{\partial \phi}, \frac{v^2}{r}, u\frac{\partial v}{\partial r}, \frac{v}{r}\frac{\partial v}{\partial \phi}, \frac{uv}{r}\right) = O\left[\frac{v_s^2}{a}\right] \tag{8.57}$$

cross-sectional centrifugal terms

$$\left(\frac{w^2 \sin\phi}{R}, \frac{w^2\cos\phi}{R}\right) = O\left[\frac{\overline{W}^2}{R}\right] \tag{8.58}$$

cross-sectional viscous terms

$$\left[\frac{\mathrm{v}}{r}\frac{\partial}{\partial\phi}\left(\frac{\partial v}{\partial r}, \frac{v}{r}, \frac{1}{r}\frac{\partial u}{\partial \phi}\right),\ \mathrm{v}\frac{\partial}{\partial r}\left(\frac{\partial v}{\partial r}, \frac{v}{r}, \frac{1}{r}\frac{\partial u}{\partial \phi}\right)\right] = O\left[\mathrm{v}\frac{v_s}{a^2}\right] \tag{8.59}$$

axial unsteady term $\left(\frac{\partial w}{\partial t}\right) = O[\overline{W}\omega]$ (8.60)

axial convective terms $\left(u\frac{\partial w}{\partial r}, \frac{v}{r}\frac{\partial w}{\partial \phi}\right) = O\left[\frac{v_s\overline{W}}{a}\right]$ (8.61)

axial viscous terms

$$\left[\mathrm{v}\left(\frac{\partial}{\partial r}, \frac{1}{r}\right)\frac{\partial w}{\partial r}, \mathrm{v}\frac{1}{r^2}\frac{\partial^2 w}{\partial \phi^2}\right] = O\left[\mathrm{v}\frac{\overline{W}}{a^2}\right] \tag{8.62}$$

Some of the term-dominance criteria involve v_s. Because this scale depends on which term in the cross-sectional momentum equations is dominant, it will be solved first. For unsteadiness-dominated flow, the unsteady term balances the centrifugal term and

$$v_s\omega \approx \frac{\overline{W}^2}{R} \quad \text{or} \quad v_s \approx \frac{\overline{W}^2}{R\omega} \tag{8.63}$$

For convective-dominated flow in the cross section:

$$\frac{v_s^2}{a} \approx \frac{\overline{W}^2}{R} \quad \text{or} \quad v_s \approx \sqrt{\frac{a}{R}}\,\overline{W} \tag{8.64}$$

For viscous-dominated flow in the cross section:

$$\mathrm{v}\frac{v_s}{a^2} \approx \frac{\overline{W}^2}{R} \quad \text{or} \quad v_s \approx \frac{a^2\overline{W}^2}{\mathrm{v}R} \tag{8.65}$$

Starting with the axial terms, the conditions under which each of the three terms is dominant are determined by forming ratios of the term with each of the other two. Axial flow is dominated by unsteadiness when

$$\frac{\text{unsteady}}{\text{convective}} \approx \frac{\overline{W}\omega}{\frac{v_s\overline{W}}{a}} = \frac{a\omega}{v_s} \gg 1 \quad \text{and} \quad \frac{\text{unsteady}}{\text{viscous}} \approx \frac{\overline{W}\omega}{\frac{\mathrm{v}\overline{W}}{a^2}} = \frac{a^2\omega}{\mathrm{v}} = \alpha^2 \gg 1 \tag{8.66}$$

By inserting the appropriate relationship for v_s [equation (8.63)], these conditions become

$$\frac{a\omega}{v_s} \approx \frac{aR\omega^2}{\overline{W}^2} \approx \frac{\alpha^4}{\mathrm{Dn}^2} \gg 1 \quad \text{and} \quad \alpha^2 \gg 1 \tag{8.67}$$

Axial flow is convective-dominated when

$$\frac{\text{convective}}{\text{unsteady}} \approx \frac{\frac{v_s\overline{W}}{a}}{\overline{W}\omega} = \frac{v_s}{a\omega} \approx \frac{\sqrt{\frac{a}{R}}\overline{W}}{a\omega} \approx \frac{\mathrm{Dn}}{\alpha^2} \gg 1$$

and

$$\frac{\text{convective}}{\text{viscous}} \approx \frac{\frac{v_s\overline{W}}{a}}{\frac{\mathrm{v}\overline{W}}{a^2}} = \frac{v_s a}{\mathrm{v}} \approx \frac{\sqrt{\frac{a}{R}}\overline{W}a}{\mathrm{v}} \approx Dn \gg 1 \tag{8.68}$$

Axial flow is viscous-dominated when

$$\frac{\text{viscous}}{\text{unsteady}} \approx \frac{\mathrm{v}\frac{\overline{W}}{a^2}}{\overline{W}\omega} = \frac{1}{\alpha^2} \gg 1$$

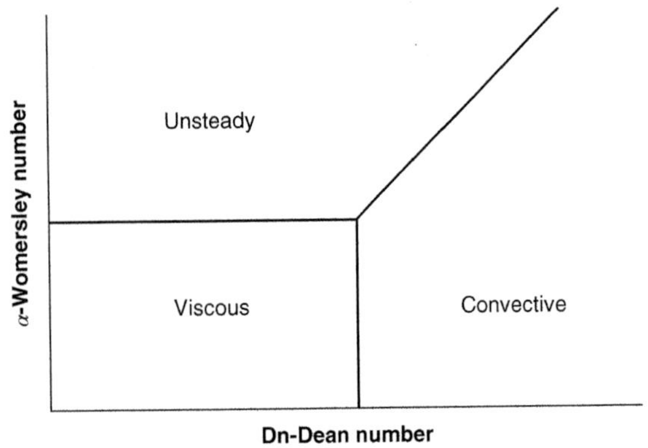

Figure 8.6. Regimes of oscillatory flow in a curved tube

and

$$\frac{\text{viscous}}{\text{convective}} \approx \frac{\frac{\nu \overline{W}}{a^2}}{\frac{v_s \overline{W}}{a}} = \frac{\nu}{v_s a} \approx \frac{\nu}{\frac{a^2 \overline{W}^2}{\nu R} a} = \frac{1}{\mathrm{Dn}^2} \gg 1 \tag{8.69}$$

The term-dominance criteria for the cross-sectional momentum equations are conveniently the same as for the axial momentum equation.

The resulting flow regimes are shown in Figure 8.6. The boundaries between regimes are derived from the relationships between terms in equations (8.67) and (8.68). α determines the transition of the flow from viscous to unsteady, Dn from viscous to convective, and $\frac{\alpha^2}{\mathrm{Dn}}$ from convective to unsteady. Order-of-magnitude analysis does not specify the values of these parameters at the transition boundaries. These must be supplied by more exact experiments or analytical or numerical solutions. But simply identifying the regimes is a valuable step in characterizing the types of flow that can occur in a given problem. Also not identified are the transition regimes where two or more terms are roughly equal. More details on these regimes and numerical results for $15 < \mathrm{Dn} < 150$ and $2.8 < \alpha < 30.2$ are given by Yamane *et al.*[17] Results for $3.25 < \mathrm{Dn} < 364$ and $0.0115 < \mathrm{Dn}^2/\alpha^4 < 10.8$ are given by Sharp *et al.*[18]

8.4.4 Entrance Flow in Curved Tubes

For a uniform, steady velocity profile entering a curved tube, the axial flow initially accelerates on the inside of the curve (Figure 8.7). This phenomenon occurs while the viscous boundary layer is small. Because pressure

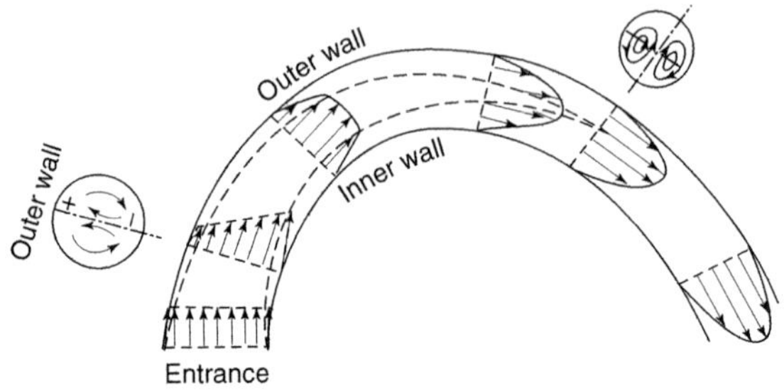

Figure 8.7. Steady entrance flow in a curved tube.[3] (Reproduced with permission from Springer Science Business Media New York. © 1997)

decreases on the inside of the tube relative to the outside due to streamline curvature, the Bernoulli effect in the inviscid core dictates a higher velocity. The higher pressure on the outside also drives secondary flow in the boundary layer symmetrically from outside to inside. Conservation of mass causes flow from inside to outside across the inviscid core to complete the pair of secondary-flow vortices. As the boundary layer grows to fill the tube, the peak axial velocity moves to the outside, as described in Section 8.4.1, while the secondary-flow vortices remain similar.

8.5 FLOW IN BRANCHES

Many of the same phenomena described in the previous sections for flow in a single tube, as well as some new ones, are exhibited in branched tubes. In the arteries, flow predominately occurs from a large parent branch to two daughter branches, while venous flow occurs in the opposite direction. The details of the velocity fields depend not only on the flow waveform and Reynolds and Womersley numbers but also on branch geometry. Geometric parameters include the diameters of branches, the branching angles, and the smoothness (radius of curvature) of the junction. The flow divider (the junction between the two daughter branches) is typically located in the high-velocity region of the flow from the parent branch; thus, velocities at the entrance to the daughter branches are often highest on the flow divider side (Figure 8.8). Boundary layers grow on this side similar to that described in Section 8.3.6 for steady flow. On the opposite sides, however, the walls of the parent and daughter branches form a diverging angle that characteristically leads to an unfavorable, increasing pressure gradient, causing flow separation

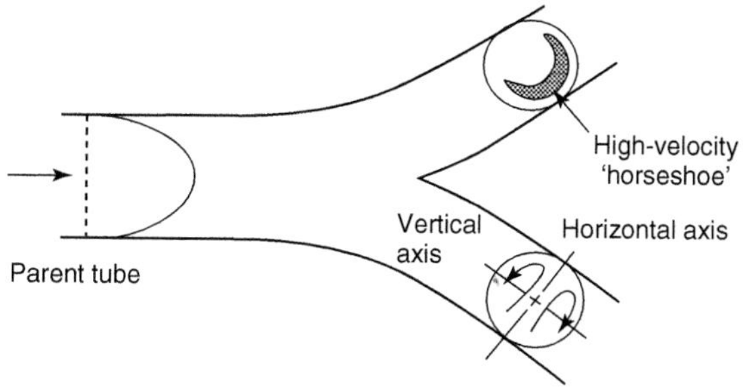

Figure 8.8. Flow from parent to daughter branches (typical of arteries). A parabolic velocity profile in the parent tube is shown on the left. The two-cell secondary-flow pattern is shown on the lower right. Horizontal designates the plane of the branch, and vertical means perpendicular to the plane of the branch. The axial velocity profile is shown on the upper right, with the region of high velocity shaded in gray.[19] (Reproduced with permission from Massachusetts Institute of Technology. © 1986)

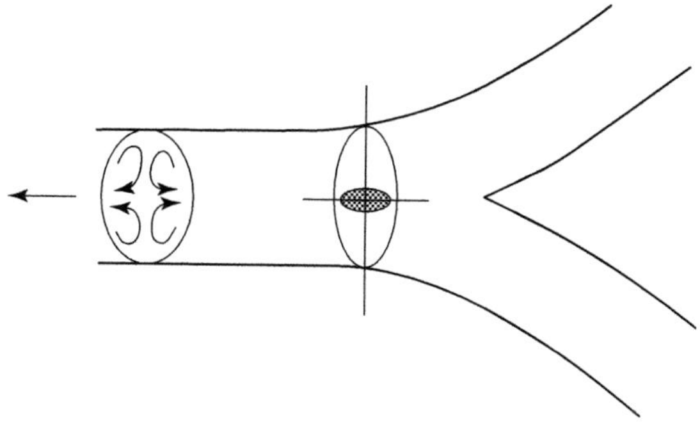

Figure 8.9. Flow from two daughter branches to parent branch (typical of veins). The four-cell secondary-flow vortex pattern is shown on the left. In the middle is the axial velocity pattern, with the region of high velocity shaded in gray.[19] (Reproduced with permission from Massachusetts Institute of Technology. © 1986)

and recirculation. This behavior is familiar from visualization studies of flows in axisymmetric expansions and in external flow around bluff bodies.

The curvature of the streamlines exiting the parent branch and entering each daughter branch causes high pressure on the flow divider side and low pressure on the opposite side. For uniform velocity entering a single curved tube, this pressure gradient caused low velocity on the high-pressure side. However, in a branch, the high velocity at the flow divider typically precludes the appearance of this effect. In fact, the velocity is typically highest on the flow divider side in the daughter branches (Figure 8.8). The other effect of the pressure gradient mentioned for a single curved tube is the initiation of a two-vortex secondary flow. Similar secondary flow is typically exhibited in the daughter branches. This secondary flow spreads the high-velocity region of the flow into a crescent shape, as shown in Figure 8.8. If the daughter branches are straight and long enough, the skewed axial velocity decays to parabolic for steady flow, separated flow reattaches, and secondary flow dissipates to zero.

Flow from daughter branches to a parent branch (typical of veins) includes some similar and some different characteristics (Figure 8.9). Boundary layers in the downstream flow regrow, similar to flow in the opposite direction. Curvature of streamlines is again associated with high pressure on the outside of the curvature. However, for daughters-to-parent flow, the high-pressure sides are not separated by a flow divider, but rather are located next to each other in the middle of the parent branch. The pressure gradient again causes secondary flow, but in this case from the middle of the cross section in both the directions along the walls (through the boundary layer) to the opposite sides. By having high pressure in the middle of the branch and low pressure on opposite sides, the two vortices that are initially formed in the exit of each daughter branch are compressed into half (for a symmetrical branch) of the parent tube. The resulting secondary-flow pattern exhibits four vortices circulating in the same direction as they did in the daughter branches, but with each occupying only one quarter of the parent tube cross section. Secondary flow spreads the region of high velocity into an elliptical shape with long axis perpendicular to the plane of the branch. Recirculation can again occur downstream of the junction, depending on the branching angle and the radius of curvature.

Pulsatile flow in branches introduces the potential for even more complex flow behavior, particularly if the flow waveform involves flow reversal.[19]

8.6 FLOW IN COMPLIANT VESSELS

For locally fully developed, steady, laminar flow in a tube, at each location z the velocity profile is parabolic [equation (8.6)], and the pressure gradient versus flow rate relationship is given by equation (8.7). Conservation of mass dictates that the flow rate is constant all along the tube, but the pressure gradient increases as the tube radius decreases with increasing z (the tube radius decreases because the transmural pressure decreases with increasing z). Therefore, the radius versus transmural pressure property of the vessel wall is required to determine the relationship between flow rate and the total pressure difference from the beginning to the end of the tube. For a thin-walled Hookean vessel, the circumferential strain is approximately proportional to the circumferential stress (neglecting the contribution of Poisson's ratio for the thin wall), and the local radius is

$$a(z) = a_0\left[1 - \frac{a_0}{Eh}p(z)\right]^{-1} \tag{8.70}$$

where a_0 is the vessel radius when transmural pressure is zero, E is Young's modulus, and h is the thickness of the wall. Rearranging equation (8.7) and integrating to solve for pressure difference

$$p(z) - p(0) = \frac{8\mu Q}{\pi}\int_0^z \frac{1}{[a(z)]^4}\mathrm{d}z \tag{8.71}$$

Inserting equation (8.70) into (8.71) and solving for a tube of length L

$$\frac{Eh}{3a_0}\left\{\left[1 - \frac{a_0}{Eh}p(L)\right]^{-3} - \left[1 - \frac{a_0}{Eh}p(0)\right]^{-3}\right\} = \frac{8\mu LQ}{\pi a_0^4} \tag{8.72}$$

Because most blood vessels do not exhibit Hookean response, an alternative linear model is useful

$$a(z) = a_0 + \frac{b}{2}p(z) \tag{8.73}$$

where b is a vessel compliance constant. By replacing the pressures in equation (8.71) with equation (8.73), a relationship between flow rate and vessel radii is obtained after integration

$$[a(0)]^5 - [a(L)]^5 = \frac{20b\mu LQ}{\pi} \tag{8.74}$$

Because of the fifth powers, the downstream radius can have an insignificant effect on flow rate when the downstream radius is smaller than upstream. For instance, if $a(L)/a(0) = 1/2$, the ratio of the fifth powers is $[a(L)/a(0)]^5 = 0.03$, and the dependence of flow rate on downstream conditions can be neglected. This condition typically prevails in veins that are inflated with low transmural pressures, which allows the vessel to collapse to a much smaller cross section as pressure decreases downstream. (A complication not represented in these equations is that the cross section may no longer be circular when transmural pressure is small. Vessels with elliptical cross section are discussed by Fung.[3]) A pressure difference versus flow rate relationship can be recovered by replacing vessel radii in equation (8.74) with pressures from equation (8.73):

$$\left[a_0 + \frac{b}{2}p(0)\right]^5 - \left[a_0 + \frac{b}{2}p(L)\right]^5 = \frac{20b\mu LQ}{\pi} \tag{8.75}$$

8.7 MICROCIRCULATION

For vessels of diameter much larger than that of red cells, blood can be treated as a continuum, i.e., that properties such as density and variables such as velocity can be approximated to be continuous throughout the vessel. At a microscopic level, this amounts to averaging over values that apply locally to plasma, red cells, and any other particles in the flow. This assumption underlies the solutions of the previous sections. But for smaller vessels, the spatial scale of discontinuities associated with the particulate nature of blood becomes larger with respect to the vessel size, and has a stronger influence on bulk flow. One of these effects can be explained by considering the relative concentration of red cells across the tube. Throughout the core of the flow, red cell centers may be located at any radial position. But near the wall, red cell centers must be at least one red cell radius away from the wall. Therefore, a cell-depleted layer exists near the wall. Reinforcing this effect is that hydrodynamic lift also pulls cells away from the wall. The result of the cell-depleted layer is that for blood entering a small

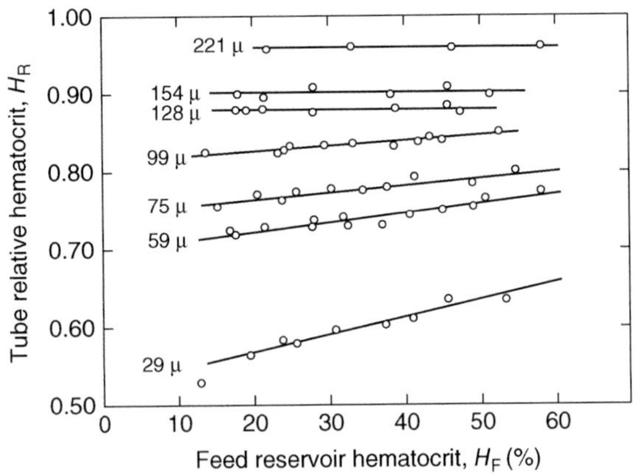

Figure 8.10. The Fahraeus effect. For blood flowing from an upstream reservoir into a small tube, the hematocrit in the tube is reduced relative to that in the reservoir.[23] (Reproduced with permission from Elsevier. © 1971)

tube with feed hematocrit H_F, the hematocrit H_T in the tube is smaller, $H_R = H_T/H_F < 1$ (Figure 8.10). This is called the Fahraeus[20] effect. Because the red cells travel faster through the tube than does the plasma (the plasma in the cell-depleted layer moves particularly slowly), the hematocrit measured in a reservoir downstream of the tube is the same as that upstream. The decreased apparent viscosity in the tube is accurately predicted by the decreased hematocrit in the tube (the Fahraeus–Lindqvist[21] effect).

DISCLAIMER

The subject matter, content, and views presented do not represent the views of the Department of Health and Human Services (HHS), US Food and Drug Administration (FDA), and/or the United States.

RELATED ARTICLES IN EMAGRES

Radiofrequency Heating Models and Measurements

REFERENCES

1. D. A. McDonald, Blood Flow in the Arteries, Williams & Wilkins: Baltimore, MD, 1974.
2. T. J. Pedley, The Fluid Mechanics of Large Blood Vessels, Cambridge University Press: Cambridge, UK, 1980.
3. Y. C. Fung, Biomechanics: Circulation, Springer: New York, 1997.
4. L. Waite and J. Fine, Applied Biofluid Mechanics, McGraw-Hill: New York, NY, 2007.
5. C. G. Caro, T. J. Pedley, R. C. Schroter, and W. A. See, The Mechanics of the Circulation, Cambridge University Press: Cambridge, UK, 2012.
6. K. B. Chandran, S. E. Rittgers, and A. P. Yoganathan, Biofluid Mechanics: The Human Circulation, CRC Press: Boca Raton, FL, 2012.
7. D. A. Rubenstein, W. Yin, and M. D. Frame, Biofluid mechanics: An Introduction to Fluid Mechanics, Macrocirculation and Microcirculation, Academic Press: Waltham, MA, 2012.
8. W. C. O. Tsang, The size and shape of human red blood cells, MS thesis, University of California, San Diego, 1975.
9. M. K. Sharp, M. Gregg, G. Brock, N. Nair, S. Sahetya, E. H. Austin, C. Maascio, M. D. Slaughter, and G. M. Pantalos, *Cardiovasc. Eng. Technol.*, 2017, **8**, 182.
10. S. Kim, B. Namgung, P. K. Ong, Y. I. Cho, K. J. Jin Chun, and D. Lim, *J. Mech. Sci. Technol.*, 2009, **23**, 1718.
11. H. B. Atabek, *Z. Angew. Math. Phys.*, 1962, **13**, 417.
12. H. B. Atabek, in 'Basic Hemodynamics and its Role in Disease Processes', eds D. J. Patel and R. N. Vaishnav, University Park Press: Baltimore, MD, 1980.
13. S. A. Berger, L. Talbot, and L.-S. Yao, *Annu. Rev. Fluid Mech.*, 1983, **15**, 461.
14. W. R. Dean, *Philos. Mag.*, 1927, **4**, 208.
15. W. R. Dean, *Philos. Mag.*, 1928, **5**, 673.
16. W. H. Lyne, *J. Fluid Mech.*, 1970, **45**, 13.
17. R. Yamane, S. Oshima, K. Sudo, M. Sumida, N. Okamoto, and M. Kizaki, *Bull. JSME*, 1985, **28**, 428.
18. M. K. Sharp, R. D. Kamm, A. H. Shapiro, E. Kimmel, and G. E. Karniadakis, *J. Fluid Mech.*, 1991, **223**, 537.
19. D. L. Jan, A study of oscillatory flow through a bronchial bifurcation, PhD thesis, MIT, Cambridge, MA, 1986.
20. R. Fahraeus, *Physiol. Rev.*, 1929, **9**, 241.
21. R. Fahraeus and T. Lindqvist, *Am. J. Physiol.*, 1931, **96**, 562.
22. Y. C. Fung, 'Biomechanics: Mechanical Properties of Living Tissues', 2nd edn, Springer: New York, 1993.
23. J. H. Barbee and G. R. Cokelett, *Microvas. Res.*, 1971, **34**, 6.

Chapter 9
Effect of Magnetic Field on Blood Flow

G.C. Shit and Sreeparna Majee

Jadavpur University, Kolkata, India

9.1 INTRODUCTION

This chapter discusses the models of blood flow in patients with arterial diseases in magnetic field environment. In addition, models of blood flow with magnetic nanoparticles are discussed, as well, for magnetic field-assisted drug delivery. We studied various fluid models, different flow patterns, different arterial conditions, and many internal and external conditions. The models allow to develop significant insights into many cardiovascular problems.

Because of the significant mechanical, geometrical, and structural complexities of modeling blood flow, it is necessary to make a few simplifying assumptions to construct the model, while keeping the problem as close as possible to the physiological aspect. As blood has complex rheological characteristics, different fluid models are needed to model blood flow under different biological and structural conditions.

The study of blood flow through partial occlusion of the arterial passage has attracted the attention of many researchers because of the narrowing of artery (known as stenosis) due to the deposition of cholesterol and other substances in the endothelial of the arterial wall. It involves deposition of low density lipoprotein, cholesterol, and other substances in different-sized arteries.[1] The transport of such lipoproteins from blood into the arterial walls plays an important role in the development of atherosclerotic lesions, which can be detected at one or more locations in the arteries, specifically near the bends, bifurcations, and some other regions where complicated flow patterns of blood can be identified.[2] However, once a mild stenosis is developed, the altered hemodynamics may influence the further development of other stenosis, which may lead to overlapping stenosis. It has been observed that the formation of plaques causes irregular flow rate, boundary layer separation, and high arterial wall shear stress. Several investigators,[3–10] have theoretically and numerically studied the blood flow through arterial segment having stenosis. Some of these studies pointed

Safety and Biological Effects in MRI.
Edited by Devashish Shrivastava and J. Thomas Vaughan

ISBN: 978-1-118-82130-5
Also published in eMagRes (online edition)
DOI: 10.1002/9780470034590.emrstm1635

out that blood exhibits non-Newtonian fluid properties in a diseased condition.

However, in the case of large arteries, blood can be treated as Newtonian fluid at high shear rates. Bandyopadhyay and Layek[11] numerically investigated the pulsatile blood flow through a constricted channel by treating blood as a Newtonian fluid model without considering the effect of magnetic field. They have considered rectangular Cartesian coordinate system to model the problem without taking into account the heat transfer phenomenon. A mathematical model for blood flow has been developed by Ponalagusamy and Selvi[12] through arterial stenosis, in which blood behaves as a Newtonian fluid at the peripheral layer containing plasma and as a non-Newtonian fluid obeying Casson fluid in the core region. They observed that the downstream of the stenotic regions is more important for the diagnosis of arterial diseases. Caro *et al.*[13] and Caro[14] observed that the normal arterial blood flow at high shear-rates blood behaves like a Newtonian fluid. According to Schlichting and Gersten,[15] the steady incompressible, Newtonian, laminar flow described by the Navier–Stokes equations in three-dimensional rigid geometries can be solved mathematically with respect to simple geometries and simple boundary conditions. Deshpande *et al.*[16] have solved the Navier–Stokes equation numerically for steady and laminar flow of Newtonian fluid through axisymmetric, bell-shaped, contoured constrictions in a rigid tube for Reynolds numbers maximum up to 2000 for moderate to severe stenosis. Wille[17] has performed the numerical analysis on the pressure and flow patterns for steady, laminar, Newtonian, and isothermal flow conditions for several models of stenosed vessels with different constriction ratios of 50%, 75%, and 90% with Reynolds numbers of 10, 100, and 200, respectively.

Another significant arterial disease is aneurysm. Duclaux[18] experimentally studied the growth of aneurysms and observed that abdominal aneurysms tend to develop above a critical flow rate, whenever the time-averaged inflow is high enough for the time-averaged diameter of the tissue from its base value. A numerical study has been performed by Finol and Amon[19] on blood flow with double aneurism by treating blood as a Newtonian fluid in a rigid wavy-walled axisymmetric model. They compared their results for steady and pulsatile flow conditions and concluded that hemodynamic stresses are higher in pulsatile flow than in steady flow. The pulsatile flow characteristics in a straight tube with an asymmetric bulge were studied by Yu and Zhao.[20] They found that the center of the vortex was located close to the distal neck. An unsteady flow behavior in a patient-specific abdominal aortic aneurysm (AAA) was experimentally modeled by Stamatopoulos *et al.*[21] The fluctuation of flow disturbances as measured by the r.m.s. (root mean square) of the axial velocity component presents higher values both at the entrance and exit of the aneurysm along the posterior wall at flow peak as well as during the deceleration phase of the cycle. The effect of asymmetry in AAA (abdominal aortic aneurysm) under physiologically realistic pulsatile flow conditions has been explained by Finol *et al.*[22] A numerical simulation of AAA has been performed by Matsuzawa *et al.*[23] They have compared the wall shear stress distribution in nonaneurysm model versus aneurysm model for compose stress and predicted that the wall stress on nonaneurysm model was relatively low and uniformly distributed. The effect of the growth of asymmetric aneurysm and aortic wall thickness has been studied by Scotti *et al.*[24] They concluded that the velocity vector changed dramatically as the aneurysm grew asymmetrically, whereas the vortices in a symmetric aneurysm developed and dissipated within the midsection to the distal end of the aneurysm sac. Salsac *et al.*[25] experimentally studied the symmetric model of AAA and observed that the vortex motions within the dilation induce strong spatial and temporal variations of the wall shear stress. Mukhopadhyay and Layek[26] systematically analyzed the blood flow through a modeled artery with an aneurysm in the presence of hematocrit. They observed that the magnitude of the wall shear stress and the length of the flow separation increase as the hematocrit parameter and the height of aneurysm increase. Rana *et al.*[27] numerically investigated the pulsatile blood flow through AAA and suggested that the pulsatile flow situation is more important for physiological fluid than the steady one. Vergara *et al.*[28] examined the effects of transition to turbulence flow in AAA. They have used a large eddy simulation model on the regions of AAA where the instabilities and fluctuation occur. Khanafer *et al.*[29] numerically analyzed the pulsatile turbulent flow characteristics in an axisymmetric aortic aneurysm model using a simulated physiological waveform. They have estimated the wall shear stress distribution by computational solid stress (CSS) model and the fluid structure interaction (FSI) model that takes into account the flow and solid mechanics.

The application of the principles of magnetohydrodynamics (MHD) is being studied extensively. Haik *et al.*[30] showed that the flow rate of blood can be reduced up to 30% when subjected to a high static magnetic field of strength 10 T. The US FDA has cleared the use of MRI scanners of up to the static magnetic field strength of 7 T. In this regard, Shit [31] has developed a computational model of blood flow under magnetic field environment and estimated the possible hemodynamical effects of the magnetic field. He reported that no clinical disorders are observed in humans when subjected to the magnetic field of strength up to 9 T. The MHD principles are also used in the prevention and the rational therapy of arterial hypertension explored by Vardanyan[32] who reported that a uniform transverse magnetic field alters the blood flow rate under steady-state condition. Sharma *et al.*[33] conducted an experimental study and supported the result that the velocity of blood is appreciably reduced under the influence of magnetic field. Misra and Shit,[34] and Misra *et al.*[35,36] explored the flow behavior of blood in arteries by treating blood as Newtonian/non-Newtonian fluid under normal/pathological conditions in the presence of magnetic field. Misra *et al.*[37–39] have investigated the flow and heat transfer of a viscoelastic electrically conducting fluid under magnetic field effect. They documented that the temperature of the blood alters in the presence of magnetic field, and the results can be used to develop new heating methods. Misra *et al.*[40] have investigated the steady flow simulations of blood flow in an axisymmetric arterial stenosis by treating blood as a non-Newtonian fluid model in the presence of magnetic field. They analyzed the shear thinning behavior of the blood. Further, Sinha and Shit[41] carried out comprehensive theoretical study on the heat transfer characteristics of an electromagnetohydrodynamic flow of the blood through a capillary. They suggested that during surgery the application of magnetic field may be very useful to regulate blood flow temperature.[42,43] Many scientists[44,45] have proposed different applications of studying blood flow in magnetic field such as the development of magnetic devices for cell separation, magnetic particles as drug carriers in the drug-delivery system, magnetic hyperthermia for cancer treatment, and reduction of bleeding during surgery.

A mathematical model was proposed by Furlani and Furlani[46] in which they treated blood to be a Newtonian fluid and studied magnetic targeting of multifunctional carrier particles that deliver therapeutic agents to malignant tissue in vivo. This work was extended by Shaw *et al.*[47] and Shaw and Murthy[48] by considering blood as Herschel–Buckley fluid for both permeable and impermeable microvessels. Mondal and Shit[49] examined the transport phenomena of magnetic nanoparticles during electroosmotic flow in a micro vessel in the presence of external magnetic field and electrokinetic effect. Shaw and Murthy[48] and Shaw *et al.*[50] treated blood as a two-phase Casson's fluid model and studied capture condition for the carrier particle in the noninvasive case. Furthermore, Avilés *et al.*[51] developed a two-dimensional mathematical model for the transport of magnetic particle as drug carrier at the carotid bifurcation region. Larimi *et al.*[52] numerically investigated MDT (magnetic drug targeting) technique by particle tracking in the presence of magnetic field in a bifurcated vessel. They treated blood as a Newtonian fluid and used magnetic iron oxide nanoparticles as drug carrier. Ritter *et al.*[53] simulated drug targeting infused with magnetic carriers by employing high-gradient magnetic separation technique. Computational simulations were also developed by Rotariu and Strachan[54] with an aim to evaluate the flow of magnetic nanoparticles targeted at a tumor site deep inside the body. Boghi *et al.*[55] numerically studied magnetic nanoparticles in drug targeting to a patient-specific coeliac trunk. They used OPENFOAM to perform simulations, focusing on the influence of magnetic probe position and the direction of the circulating electric current. Sharma *et al.*[33,56,57] studied magnetic nanoparticle transportation and its efficiency to capture them in the targeted area under the influence of external magnetic field. Sharma *et al.*[58] mathematically modeled path traces of a cluster of magnetic nanoparticles in a blood vessel under magnetic effect. They also optimized the position of outside magnet for more effective drug targeting at the tumor site. Nacev *et al.*[59] aimed to design and use magnetic drug-delivery system to deal with magnetic nanoparticle transportation in the blood vessel. However, an increase in the thermal conduction was noted in the presence of magnetic field due to the influence of augmented nanoparticles by Sheikholeslami and Shehzad.[60] During theoretical estimation of blood flow, many authors have truncated the nonlinear part of the governing equations. This leads to the overestimation of the rheological phenomenon of blood flow in arteries. To predict the accurate flow behavior of the blood in the diseased arteries, it is necessary to model both linear and nonlinear parts of the governing equations. Such numerical simulation will allow to take into account nonlinearity of the flow phenomenon in the complex geometry of the arteries.

One of the most common methodologies for direct numerical treatment of incompressible fluid flow problems is the adoption of vorticity–stream function formulation. In this direction, Tzirtzilakis[61] has adopted vorticity–stream function formulation and studied blood flow in a channel with stenosis and developed a mathematical model on the basis of the principles of ferrohydrodynamics (FHD) and MHD. Ishikawa *et al.*[62] examined arterial blood flow by taking vorticity-transport equation into account and found that the vortex downstream of stenosis becomes strongest at a certain frequency of pulsation. But their study is restricted in the consideration of heat transfer analysis during blood flow.

9.2 BLOOD FLOW AND HEAT TRANSFER WITH VARIABLE VISCOSITY IN MAGNETIC AND VIBRATION ENVIRONMENT

Let us consider a fully developed, laminar, incompressible and axially symmetric two-dimensional flow through an overlapping constricted artery (cf. Figure 9.1).

Let (r^*,θ^*,x^*) be the cylindrical polar coordinates with x^*-axis along the axis of symmetry of the tube. The velocity components u^* and v^* are, respectively, taken along the axial and radial directions. A magnetic field of strength B_0 is uniformly applied perpendicular to the axial direction of blood flow. Due to the low electrical conductivity of blood, the strength of induced magnetic field is very small in comparison to the applied magnetic field strength. Owing to this assumption, the induced magnetic field has been neglected

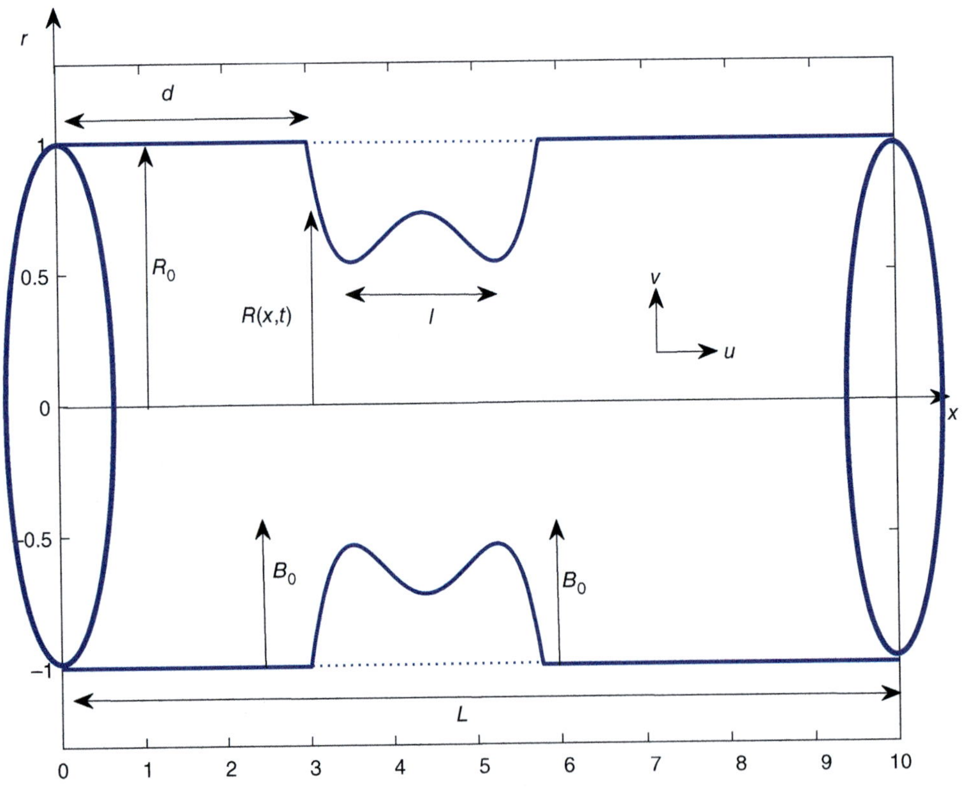

Figure 9.1. Schematic diagram of the model geometry with overlapping stenosis. (Shit and Majee.[63] Reproduced with Permission of Elsevier)

from the present analysis. We have also assumed that the blood flow takes place in a vibration environment in which a human body experiences an acceleration. The effect of heat transfer phenomena during blood flow has also been taken into account. The viscous dissipation due to consideration of temperature-dependent variable viscosity has been introduced in the thermal energy equation. We also assumed that the variation of flow is independent of θ^* due to axisymmetricity of the tube. The governing equations for unsteady two-dimensional fluid flow along with the thermal energy equation are taken as

$$\frac{\partial u^*}{\partial x^*} + \frac{v^*}{r^*} + \frac{\partial v^*}{\partial r^*} = 0 \tag{9.1}$$

$$\begin{aligned}\rho\left(\frac{\partial u^*}{\partial t^*} + u^*\frac{\partial u^*}{\partial x^*} + v^*\frac{\partial u^*}{\partial r^*}\right) &= -\frac{\partial p^*}{\partial x^*} + \mu(T)^*\left(\frac{\partial^2 u^*}{\partial r^{*2}} + \frac{1}{r^*}\frac{\partial u^*}{\partial r^*} + \frac{\partial^2 u^*}{\partial x^{*2}}\right)\\ &\quad + \frac{\partial \mu(T)^*}{\partial T^*}\frac{\partial T^*}{\partial r^*}\frac{\partial u^*}{\partial r^*} + \frac{\partial \mu(T)^*}{\partial T^*}\frac{\partial T^*}{\partial x^*}\frac{\partial u^*}{\partial x^*}\\ &\quad - \sigma B_0^2 u^* + \rho G^*(t^*)\end{aligned} \tag{9.2}$$

$$\begin{aligned}\rho\left(\frac{\partial v^*}{\partial t^*} + u^*\frac{\partial v^*}{\partial x^*} + v^*\frac{\partial v^*}{\partial r^*}\right) &= -\frac{\partial p^*}{\partial r^*} + \mu(T)^*\left(\frac{\partial^2 v^*}{\partial r^{*2}} + \frac{1}{r^*}\frac{\partial v^*}{\partial r^*} + \frac{\partial^2 v^*}{\partial x^{*2}} - \frac{v^*}{r^{*2}}\right)\\ &\quad + \frac{\partial \mu(T)^*}{\partial T^*}\frac{\partial T^*}{\partial r^*}\frac{\partial v^*}{\partial r^*} + \frac{\partial \mu(T)^*}{\partial T^*}\frac{\partial T^*}{\partial x^*}\frac{\partial v^*}{\partial x^*}\end{aligned} \tag{9.3}$$

$$\begin{aligned}\rho C_p\left(\frac{\partial T^*}{\partial t^*} + u^*\frac{\partial T^*}{\partial x^*} + v^*\frac{\partial T^*}{\partial r^*}\right) &= K\left(\frac{\partial^2 T^*}{\partial r^{*2}} + \frac{1}{r^*}\frac{\partial T^*}{\partial r^*} + \frac{\partial^2 T^*}{\partial x^{*2}}\right) + \sigma B_0^2 u^{*2}\\ &\quad + \mu(T)^*\left(\frac{\partial u^*}{\partial r^*}\right)^2\end{aligned} \tag{9.4}$$

where p^* is the blood pressure, $\mu(T)^*$ the temperature-dependent variable viscosity, σ the electrical conductivity, ρ the density of blood, B_0 the applied magnetic field, T^* the temperature, and C_p the specific heat.

The periodic body vibration, for $t^* > 0$, which appears in equation (9.2) has the expression of the form

$$G^*(t^*) = a^* \cos(w_b t^* + \phi_g) \tag{9.5}$$

where a^* denotes the amplitude of body acceleration, w_b the frequency of body acceleration, and ϕ_g the phase difference.

The geometry of the overlapping stenosis can be put mathematically as

$$R(x,t) = \begin{cases} R_0\left[1 - \frac{11}{32}l^3(x-d) + \frac{47}{48}l^2 \right. \\ (x-d)^2 - l(x-d)^3 + \\ \left.\frac{1}{3}(x-d)^4\right] a(t) \\ \qquad\qquad \text{when } d \ll x \ll d + \frac{3l}{2} \\ R_0 a(t); \qquad\qquad \text{elsewhere} \end{cases} \tag{9.6}$$

with $a(t) = 1 + k_r \sin(t + \phi_r)$.

In the above equation, $R(x,t)$ is the radius of the arterial segment in the constricted region, R_0 the radius of the normal artery, d the distance between the inlet and the onset of the stenosis, ℓ representing the distance between two critical heights of the constriction and $\frac{3l}{2}$ measures the length of the overlapping constriction, ϕ_r the phase angle due to arterial wall motion, and k_r the amplitude of the wall motion.

Let us now introduce the following nondimensional variables:

$$x = \frac{x^*}{R_0}, r = \frac{r^*}{R_0}, u = \frac{u^*}{U}, v = \frac{v^*}{U}, p = \frac{p^*}{\rho U^2}, t = \frac{t^* U}{R_0},$$
$$Re = \frac{U R_0}{v}, \theta = \frac{T^* - T_\infty}{T_w - T_\infty}, \mu(\theta) = \frac{\mu(T)^*}{\mu_0} \tag{9.7}$$

where T_w is the temperature of the vessel wall, T_∞ the ambient temperature, and μ_0 the constant value of the coefficient of viscosity.

Using these dimensionless variables, equations (9.1)–(9.4) become

$$\frac{\partial u}{\partial x} + \frac{v}{r} + \frac{\partial v}{\partial r} = 0 \tag{9.8}$$

$$\begin{aligned}\frac{\partial u}{\partial t} + u\frac{\partial u}{\partial x} + v\frac{\partial u}{\partial r} &= -\frac{\partial p}{\partial x} + \frac{1}{\alpha^2}\left[\mu(\theta)\left(\frac{\partial^2 u}{\partial r^2} + \frac{1}{r}\frac{\partial u}{\partial r} + \frac{\partial^2 u}{\partial x^2}\right)\right.\\ &\quad \left. + \frac{\partial \mu(\theta)}{\partial \theta}\frac{\partial \theta}{\partial r}\frac{\partial u}{\partial r} + \frac{\partial \mu(\theta)}{\partial \theta}\frac{\partial \theta}{\partial x}\frac{\partial u}{\partial x} - \mathrm{Ha}^2 u + G(t)\right]\end{aligned} \tag{9.9}$$

$$\begin{aligned}\frac{\partial v}{\partial t} + u\frac{\partial v}{\partial x} + v\frac{\partial v}{\partial r} &= -\frac{\partial p}{\partial r} + \frac{1}{\alpha^2}\left[\mu(\theta)\left(\frac{\partial^2 v}{\partial r^2} + \frac{1}{r}\frac{\partial v}{\partial r} + \frac{\partial^2 v}{\partial x^2} - \frac{v}{r^2}\right)\right.\\ &\quad \left. + \frac{\partial \mu(\theta)}{\partial \theta}\frac{\partial \theta}{\partial r}\frac{\partial v}{\partial r} + \frac{\partial \mu(\theta)}{\partial \theta}\frac{\partial \theta}{\partial x}\frac{\partial v}{\partial x}\right]\end{aligned} \tag{9.10}$$

$$\frac{\partial\theta}{\partial t}+u\frac{\partial\theta}{\partial x}+v\frac{\partial\theta}{\partial r}=\frac{1}{\alpha^2\,\mathrm{Pr}}\left(\frac{\partial^2\theta}{\partial r^2}+\frac{1}{r}\frac{\partial\theta}{\partial r}+\frac{\partial^2\theta}{\partial x^2}\right)+\frac{\mathrm{Ec\,Ha}^2}{\alpha^2}u^2+\frac{\mathrm{Ec}}{\alpha^2}\mu(\theta)\left(\frac{\partial u}{\partial r}\right)^2 \tag{9.11}$$

The nondimensional parameters appearing in equations (9.9)–(9.11) are defined as Womersley parameter $\alpha^2=\frac{UR_0}{\nu}$, Hartmann number $\mathrm{Ha}=B_0R_0\sqrt{\frac{\sigma}{\rho\nu}}$, Prandtl number $\mathrm{Pr}=\frac{\mu C_p}{K}$, and Eckert number $\mathrm{Ec}=\frac{U^2}{C_p(T_w-T_\infty)}$.

The temperature-dependent viscosity in nondimensional form is assumed[64] as

$$\mu(\theta)=e^{-\beta\theta} \tag{9.12}$$

in which the fluid viscosity varies exponentially with temperature, and β is defined as the variable viscosity parameter.

Using the nondimensional quantities, the body acceleration expression defined in equation (9.5) takes in the form

$$G(t)=a_0\cos(bt+\phi_g),\quad t>0 \tag{9.13}$$

The blood is driven by the pumping action of the heart, which in turn produces pulsatile pressure gradient, whose expression in dimensionless form may be taken as

$$\frac{\partial p(t)}{\partial x}=-\bar{k}-k_p\cos(t) \tag{9.14}$$

where $\bar{k}$ and k_p are the constant amplitude of the pressure gradient and the amplitude of the pulsatile component, respectively.

Due to the assumption of long wavelength approximation ($\frac{R}{\lambda}\ll 1$), the axial viscous term can be neglected.[65] Because of the small radial velocity and acceleration, the radial variation of pressure within the artery can also be neglected, and then equation (9.10) simply reduces to $\frac{\partial p}{\partial r}=0$.

Owing to the abovementioned simplifications, equations (9.8), (9.9), and (9.11) reduce to

$$\frac{\partial u}{\partial x}+\frac{v}{r}+\frac{\partial v}{\partial r}=0 \tag{9.15}$$

$$\frac{\partial u}{\partial t}+u\frac{\partial u}{\partial x}+v\frac{\partial u}{\partial r}=-\frac{\partial p}{\partial x}+\frac{1}{\alpha^2}\left[\mu(\theta)\left(\frac{\partial^2 u}{\partial r^2}+\frac{1}{r}\frac{\partial u}{\partial r}\right)+\frac{\partial\mu(\theta)}{\partial\theta}\frac{\partial\theta}{\partial r}\frac{\partial u}{\partial r}+\frac{\partial\mu(\theta)}{\partial\theta}\frac{\partial\theta}{\partial x}\frac{\partial u}{\partial x}-\mathrm{Ha}^2u+G(t)\right] \tag{9.16}$$

$$\frac{\partial\theta}{\partial t}+u\frac{\partial\theta}{\partial x}+v\frac{\partial\theta}{\partial r}=\frac{1}{\alpha^2\,\mathrm{Pr}}\left(\frac{\partial^2\theta}{\partial r^2}+\frac{1}{r}\frac{\partial\theta}{\partial r}\right)+\frac{\mathrm{Ec\,Ha}^2}{\alpha^2}u^2+\frac{\mathrm{Ec}}{\alpha^2}\mu(\theta)\left(\frac{\partial u}{\partial r}\right)^2 \tag{9.17}$$

The boundary conditions in dimensionless form for the present problem are taken as

$$v=\frac{\partial u}{\partial r}=\frac{\partial\theta}{\partial r}=0 \text{ along the central axis of the tube, i.e., at } r=0 \tag{9.18}$$

$$u=0,\quad v=\frac{\partial R}{\partial t},\quad \theta=1 \text{ at the wall } r=R(x) \tag{9.19}$$

The above equations along with appropriate boundary conditions are transformed using

$$\xi=\frac{r}{R(x,t)} \tag{9.20}$$

and discretized by applying finite difference method using Crank–Nicolson scheme. The spatial derivatives are replaced by the central difference and time derivatives as forward difference. We have subdivided the rectangular domain into a network by drawing straight lines parallel to the coordinate axes. The solutions of $u(x,\xi,t)$, $v(x,\xi,t)$, and $\theta(x,\xi,t)$ at any mesh point (i,j) in a computational domain are symbolized as $u^k_{i,j}$, $v^k_{i,j}$, and $\theta^k_{i,j}$, respectively, in which $x_i=i\Delta x, i=0,1,\cdots m;\quad \xi_j=j\Delta\xi, j=0,1,\cdots n;\quad t_k=k\Delta t, k=0,1,2,\cdots$, where m and n are the maximum number of mesh points in the x and ξ directions, respectively.

The numerical computation has been carried out using the data given in Refs 3,65,66, and 67.

Figure 9.2 depicts the variation of axial velocity u for different values of the Hartmann number Ha. From this figure we observe that the axial velocity decreases with the increase in Hartmann number Ha. This happens due to the interaction of magnetic field with blood flow and there arises a resistive force known as Lorentz force, which has a tendency to slow down the motion of blood. In the aorta, we observed that up to 10% blood velocity reduces in the presence of magnetic field of strength 8 T, which corresponds to Ha = 1. It is noticed that the axial velocity is maximum at $\xi=0$, i.e., in the central line of the artery for all the four values of Ha, and hence maximum reduction occurs in the central axis of the tube.

Figure 9.3 illustrates the variation of axial velocity u for different values of the variable viscosity

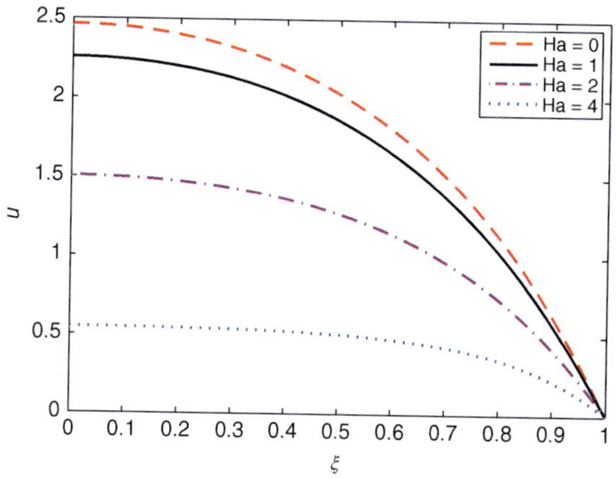

Figure 9.2. Variation of axial velocity u at the middle of the stenosis for different values of Hartmann number Ha in the aorta, when $\alpha = 4$, $\Pr = 25$, $\beta = 0.5$, and $t = 7$. (Shit and Majee.[63] Reproduced with Permission of Elsevier)

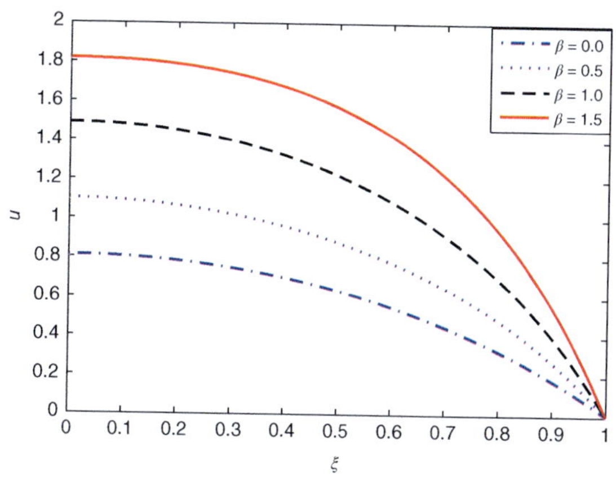

Figure 9.3. Variation of axial velocity u at the middle of the stenosis for different values of coefficient of temperature-dependent viscosity β in the aorta, when $\alpha = 4$, $\Pr = 25$, $\mathrm{Ha} = 2$, and $t = 7$. (Shit and Majee.[63] Reproduced with Permission of Elsevier)

parameter β. When the value of β increases, the axial velocity also increases. The results thus obtained can be depicted as when the viscosity of blood decreases, the axial velocity increases. As the velocity and temperature are coupled together in the governing equations, so when temperature increases, viscosity decreases and thereby velocity increases.

Figure 9.4 marks the variation of axial velocity u with different amplitudes of body acceleration a_0. The

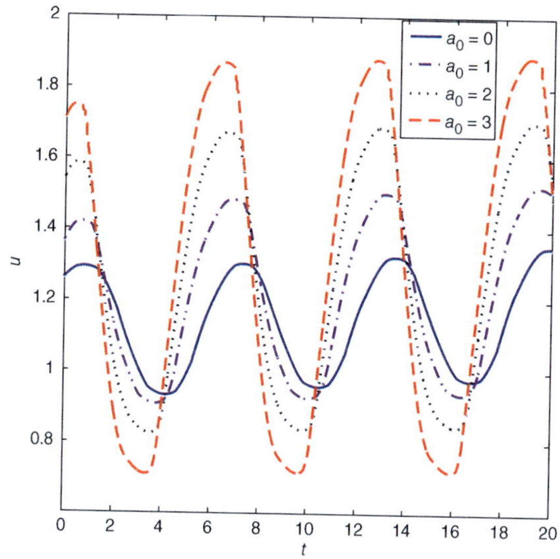

Figure 9.4. Variation of axial velocity u at the middle of the stenosis for different amplitudes of body acceleration a_0 in the aorta, when $\alpha = 4$, $\mathrm{Ha} = 2$, and $\beta = 0.5$. (Shit and Majee.[63] Reproduced with Permission of Elsevier)

axial velocity varies periodically with time t. It is observed that the amplitude of oscillation of axial velocity u has an enhancing effect with increasing body acceleration parameter a_0.

Figure 9.5 shows that the temperature θ increases with the Hartmann number Ha. Therefore, the effect of magnetic field on blood has a therapeutic response.

Figure 9.6 gives the variation of temperature θ for different values of variable viscosity parameter β. It is observed that when the value of β increases, the temperature θ also increases. This result lies in the fact that as the viscosity of blood decreases, the temperature increases.

Figure 9.7 marks the variation of skin friction at the arterial wall along with the dimensionless axial direction x/L. One can observe significant alteration of the skin friction C_{f} in the constricted region. The variation of skin friction is noted with different values of the variable viscosity parameter β. Figure 9.7 depicts that the skin friction C_{f} decreases with increasing β. From Figure 9.6, we have already established the fact that as viscosity increases, temperature decreases, and thereby RBC aggregates become more resistant to hydrodynamic dispersion and the corresponding shear stress increases as does the blood viscosity.[67] From Figure 9.7, we observed that the skin friction is high

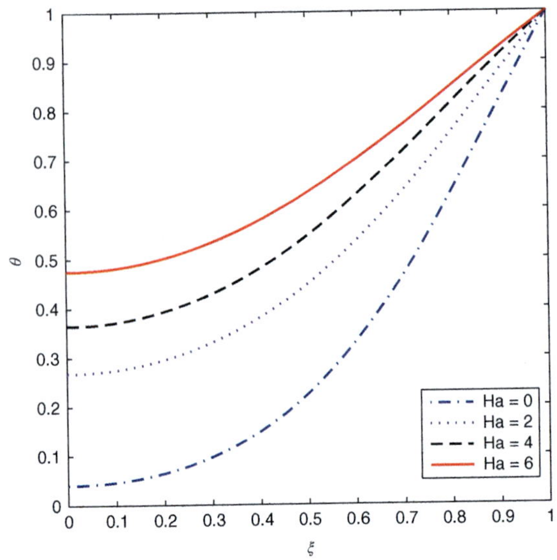

Figure 9.5. Variation of temperature profile θ at the middle of the stenosis for different values of Hartmann number Ha in the aorta, when $\alpha = 4$, $\mathrm{Pr} = 25$, $\beta = 0.5$, and $t = 7$. (Shit and Majee.[63] Reproduced with Permission of Elsevier)

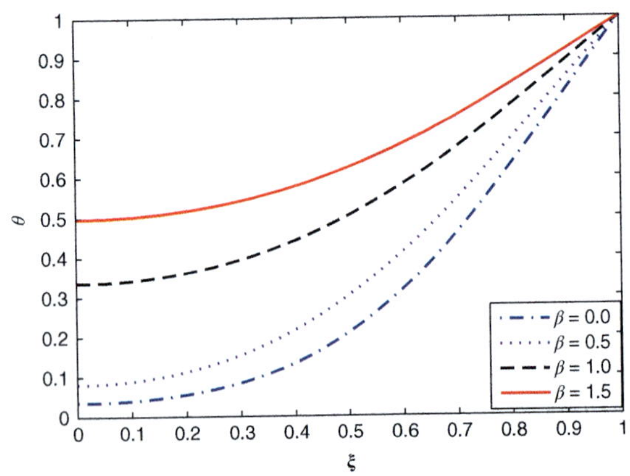

Figure 9.6. Variation of temperature profile θ at the middle of the stenosis for different values of variable viscosity parameter β in the aorta, when $\alpha = 4$, $\mathrm{Pr} = 25$, $\mathrm{Ha} = 2$, and $t = 7$. (Shit and Majee.[63] Reproduced with Permission of Elsevier)

at the throat of the primary stenosis and is low at the middle and the downstream of the stenosis. The lowering positions of the skin friction indicate further deposition.

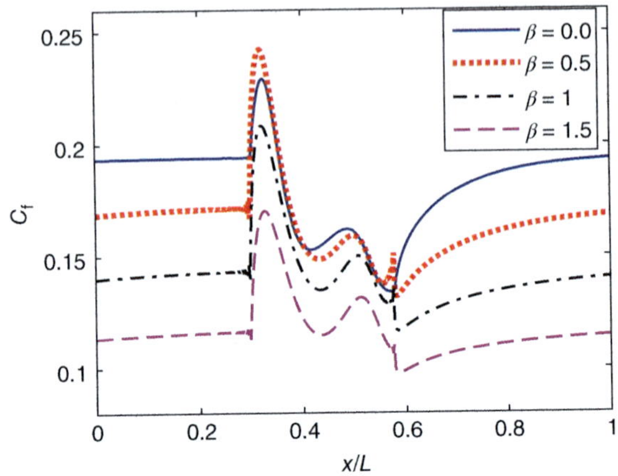

Figure 9.7. Variation of skin friction C_f along the axial direction z in the aorta for different values of variable viscosity parameter β, when $\alpha = 4$, $\mathrm{Ha} = 2$, $\mathrm{Pr} = 25$, and $t = 7$. (Shit and Majee.[63] Reproduced with Permission of Elsevier)

9.3 BLOOD FLOW UNDER STENOTIC CONDITIONS WITH VORTICITY–STREAM FUNCTION FORMULATION APPROACH

In this section, we consider the flow of blood through a single stenosis under magnetic environment.

The governing equations for unsteady two-dimensional fluid flow along with the thermal energy equation are taken as

$$\frac{\partial u^*}{\partial x^*} + \frac{v^*}{r^*} + \frac{\partial v^*}{\partial r^*} = 0 \tag{9.21}$$

$$\rho\left(\frac{\partial u^*}{\partial t^*} + u^*\frac{\partial u^*}{\partial x^*} + v^*\frac{\partial u^*}{\partial r^*}\right) = -\frac{\partial p^*}{\partial x^*} + \mu\left(\frac{\partial^2 u^*}{\partial r^{*2}} + \frac{1}{r^*}\frac{\partial u^*}{\partial r^*} + \frac{\partial^2 u^*}{\partial x^{*2}}\right) - \sigma B_0^2 u^* \tag{9.22}$$

$$\rho\left(\frac{\partial v^*}{\partial t^*} + u^*\frac{\partial v^*}{\partial x^*} + v^*\frac{\partial v^*}{\partial r^*}\right) = -\frac{\partial p^*}{\partial r^*} + \mu\left(\frac{\partial^2 v^*}{\partial r^{*2}} + \frac{1}{r^*}\frac{\partial v^*}{\partial r^*} + \frac{\partial^2 v^*}{\partial x^{*2}} - \frac{v^*}{r^{*2}}\right) \tag{9.23}$$

$$\rho C_p\left(\frac{\partial T^*}{\partial t^*} + u^*\frac{\partial T^*}{\partial x^*} + v^*\frac{\partial T^*}{\partial r^*}\right) = k\left(\frac{\partial^2 T^*}{\partial r^{*2}} + \frac{1}{r^*}\frac{\partial T^*}{\partial r^*} + \frac{\partial^2 T^*}{\partial x^{*2}}\right) + \sigma B_0^2 u^{*2} + \phi^* \tag{9.24}$$

where ϕ^* is the viscous dissipation of energy given by

$$\phi^* = \mu\left[2\left(\frac{\partial v^*}{\partial r^*}\right)^2 + \left(\frac{\partial v^*}{\partial x^*} + \frac{\partial u^*}{\partial r^*}\right)^2 + 2\left(\frac{\partial u^*}{\partial x^*}\right)^2\right] \tag{9.25}$$

where p^* denotes the blood pressure, μ is the coefficient of dynamic viscosity, σ the electrical conductivity, ρ the density of blood, B_0 the applied magnetic field strength, T^* the temperature variable, C_p the specific heat at constant pressure, and k represents the thermal conductivity of blood. The last term of equation (9.22) depicts the magnetic body force ($\vec{J} \times \vec{B}$) per unit volume, in which $\vec{J} = \sigma[\vec{E} + \vec{V} \times \vec{B}]$ is the current density due to ohm's law, $\vec{B}(B_0, 0, 0)$ is the magnetic field vector, and $\vec{E}$ is the induced electric field. The second term on the right-hand side of equation (9.24) is the dissipation of energy due to applied magnetic field.

The boundary conditions are taken as

$$\frac{\partial u^*}{\partial r^*} = v^* = \frac{\partial T^*}{\partial r^*} = 0 \quad \text{at } r^* = 0 \tag{9.26}$$

$$u^* = v^* = 0, \quad T^* = T_w \quad \text{at } r^* = R^*(x^*) \tag{9.27}$$

$$u^* = 2U_0\left[1 - \left(\frac{r^*}{R^*(x^*)}\right)^2\right], \quad v^* = 0,$$
$$T^* = T_w + 2(1 - r^{*2})(T_\infty - T_w) \quad \text{at } x^* = 0 \tag{9.28}$$

and

$$\frac{\partial u^*}{\partial x^*} = \frac{\partial v^*}{\partial x^*} = \frac{\partial T^*}{\partial x^*} = 0 \quad \text{at } x^* = R_0 L \tag{9.29}$$

The geometry of the single stenosis mathematically can be written as

$$R^*(x^*) = R_0\left[1 - \delta e^{-\sigma\left(\frac{x^*}{R_0}\right)^2}\right] \tag{9.30}$$

where R_0 is the radius of the normal artery, δ the depth of the stenosis and σ the shape parameter of the stenosis, T_w the temperature of the arterial wall, T_∞ the ambient temperature, U_0 the characteristic velocity, and the length of the artery is taken as L times the radius of the artery.

The nondimensional stream function ψ_s' is defined by

$$u = \frac{1}{r}\frac{\partial \psi}{\partial r}, \quad v = -\frac{1}{r}\frac{\partial \psi}{\partial x} \tag{9.31}$$

satisfying the continuity equation and the nondimensional vorticity ω,

$$\omega = \frac{\partial v}{\partial x} - \frac{\partial u}{\partial r} \tag{9.32}$$

Eliminating the pressure gradients between the momentum equations, we obtain the vorticity–stream function equations as

$$\frac{\partial \omega}{\partial t} + \left[\frac{1}{r}\frac{\partial \psi}{\partial r}\frac{\partial \omega}{\partial x} - \frac{1}{r}\frac{\partial \psi}{\partial x}\frac{\partial \omega}{\partial r} + \frac{\omega}{r^2}\frac{\partial \psi}{\partial x}\right]$$
$$= \frac{1}{Re}\left(\frac{\partial^2 \omega}{\partial r^2} + \frac{1}{r}\frac{\partial \omega}{\partial r} + \frac{\partial^2 \omega}{\partial x^2} - \frac{\omega}{r^2}\right)$$
$$+ \frac{\mathrm{Ha}^2}{r}\left(\frac{\partial^2 \psi}{\partial r^2} - \frac{1}{r}\frac{\partial \psi}{\partial r}\right) \tag{9.33}$$

and

$$\frac{\partial^2 \psi}{\partial x^2} - \frac{1}{r}\frac{\partial \psi}{\partial r} + \frac{\partial^2 \psi}{\partial r^2} = -\omega r \tag{9.34}$$

In order to convert all the equations including the physical domain into a rectangular domain, we use the following transformation:

$$\eta(x, r) = \frac{r}{R(x)} \tag{9.35}$$

Using equation (9.35) into equations (9.33) and (9.34), one can obtain

$$\frac{\partial \omega}{\partial t} + \left[\frac{\omega}{\eta^2 R^2}\frac{\partial \psi}{\partial x} - \frac{\omega}{\eta R^3}\frac{\partial R}{\partial x}\frac{\partial \psi}{\partial \eta} + \frac{1}{\eta R^2}\frac{\partial \psi}{\partial \eta}\frac{\partial \omega}{\partial x}\right.$$
$$\left. - \frac{1}{\eta R^2}\frac{\partial \psi}{\partial x}\frac{\partial \omega}{\partial \eta}\right] = \frac{1}{Re}\left[\frac{\partial^2 \omega}{\partial x^2} - \frac{\omega}{\eta^2 R^2}\right.$$
$$+ \left(\frac{3\eta}{R^2}\left(\frac{\partial R}{\partial x}\right)^2 - \frac{\eta}{R}\frac{\partial^2 R}{\partial x^2} + \frac{1}{\eta R^2}\right)\frac{\partial \omega}{\partial \eta}$$
$$\left. + \left(\frac{\eta^2}{R^2}\left(\frac{\partial R}{\partial x}\right)^2 + \frac{1}{R^2}\right)\frac{\partial^2 \omega}{\partial \eta^2} - \frac{2\eta}{R}\frac{\partial R}{\partial x}\frac{\partial^2 \omega}{\partial \eta \partial x}\right]$$
$$+ \frac{\mathrm{Ha}^2}{\eta^2 Re R^3}\left(\eta\frac{\partial^2 \psi}{\partial \eta^2} - \frac{\partial \psi}{\partial \eta}\right) \tag{9.36}$$

$$\frac{\partial^2 \psi}{\partial x^2} + \frac{1}{\eta R^2}\left(3\eta^2\left(\frac{\partial R}{\partial x}\right)^2 - \eta^2 R\frac{\partial^2 R}{\partial x^2} - 1\right)\frac{\partial \psi}{\partial \eta}$$
$$+ \left(\frac{\eta^2}{R^2}\left(\frac{\partial R}{\partial x}\right)^2 + \frac{1}{R^2}\right)\frac{\partial^2 \psi}{\partial \eta^2} - \frac{2\eta}{R}\frac{\partial R}{\partial x}\frac{\partial^2 \psi}{\partial \eta \partial x} = -\omega\eta R \tag{9.37}$$

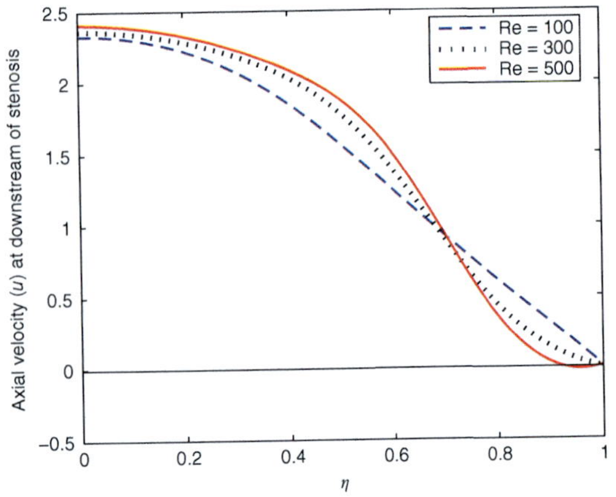

Figure 9.8. Axial velocity u for different values of Reynolds number Re (Ha = 1, Pr = 25, and t = 2). (Majee and Shit.[68] Reproduced with Permission of Elsevier)

and the thermal energy equation gives rise to

$$\frac{\partial\theta}{\partial t}+\left[u\left(\frac{\partial\theta}{\partial x}-\frac{\eta}{R}\frac{\partial R}{\partial x}\frac{\partial\theta}{\partial\eta}\right)+\frac{v}{R}\frac{\partial\theta}{\partial\eta}\right]$$
$$=\frac{1}{RePr}\left[\frac{\partial^2\theta}{\partial x^2}+\left(\frac{3\eta}{R^2}\left(\frac{\partial R}{\partial x}\right)^2-\frac{\eta}{R}\frac{\partial^2 R}{\partial x^2}+\frac{1}{\eta R^2}\right)\frac{\partial\theta}{\partial\eta}\right.$$
$$+\left(\frac{\eta^2}{R^2}\left(\frac{\partial R}{\partial x}\right)^2+\frac{1}{R^2}\right)\frac{\partial^2\theta}{\partial\eta^2}-\frac{2\eta}{R}\frac{\partial R}{\partial x}\frac{\partial^2\theta}{\partial\eta\partial x}$$
$$+\frac{\mathrm{Ha}^2\mathrm{Ec}}{Re}u^2+\frac{\mathrm{Ec}}{Re}\left[2\left(\frac{1}{R^2}\left(\frac{\partial v}{\partial\eta}\right)^2+\left(\frac{\partial u}{\partial x}-\frac{\eta}{R}\frac{\partial R}{\partial x}\frac{\partial u}{\partial\eta}\right)^2\right)\right.$$
$$\left.+\left(\left(\frac{\partial v}{\partial x}-\frac{\eta}{R}\frac{\partial R}{\partial x}\frac{\partial v}{\partial\eta}\right)+\frac{1}{R}\frac{\partial u}{\partial\eta}\right)^2\right] \tag{9.38}$$

For numerical solution of the system of equations (9.36)–(9.38), along with the boundary conditions, finite difference discretization has been performed. Equation (9.37) is a linear equation in ψ and has been

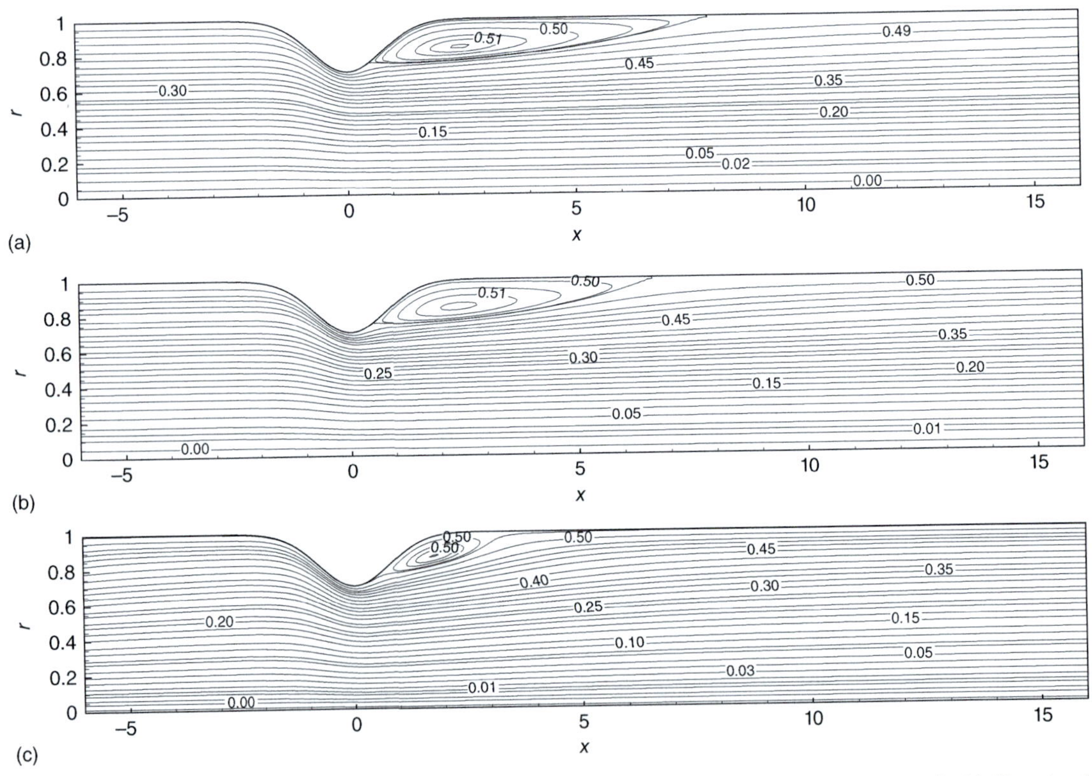

Figure 9.9. Streamline (ψ) contours for different values of Hartmann number: (a) Ha = 0, (b) Ha = 2, (c) Ha = 4, when Re = 300, Pr = 25, and t = 2. (Majee and Shit.[68] Reproduced with Permission of Elsevier)

solved by successive overrelaxation (SOR) method; thereafter, discretizing it explicitly, we obtain $\overline{\psi}_{i,j}^{k+1}$.

For speedy convergence of the numerical schemes, a relaxation parameter α is introduced and modified the solution in the stream function ψ as

$$\psi_{i,j}^{k+1} = \alpha\overline{\psi}_{i,j}^{k+1} + (1-\alpha)\psi_{i,j}^{k} \tag{9.39}$$

In the above equation, by imposing arbitrary values of α, we found that the whole numerical procedure converges faster for SOR scheme with a choice $\alpha = 1.5$.

Finite difference discretization has been carried over in the present problem using alternating direction implicit (ADI) method consisting of two time steps:

Step 1: In the first half time step (kth step to $k + 1/2$ time step), the equations are discretized by considering central difference sweep in the x-direction and leads to the following tridiagonal system to solve.

Step 2: In the second half time step (time step $k + 1/2$ to $k + 1$), the equations are discretized in the η direction in the next half time step from $k + 1/2$ to $k + 1$ to constitute a tridiagonal system.

The variation of axial velocity u with different Reynolds numbers Re is shown in Figure 9.8 at the downstream of the stenosis. We observe that the axial velocity increases with the Reynolds number Re, except in the vicinity of the arterial wall. The reversal trend of the axial velocity near the arterial wall with increasing Re is observed because of the existence of stenosis. More plug flow with increasing Re causes more disorders in blood velocity near the downstream of the area of plaque deposition. This result is very harmful to the patient having hypertension.

Figure 9.9–(c) represents the streamline contours with different Hartmann numbers Ha. These figures illustrate the flow patterns of blood in the arterial segment having stenosis. We can observe the formation of vortices in the immediate downstream of the stenosis. The extent and density of vortices gets reduced with an increase in the magnetic field strength. The streamline contours confirm that the flow reversal takes place at the downstream of the stenosis near the arterial wall. These plots give a clear picture of the flow circulation zone. Moreover, these figures provide a clear idea to find flow separation and reattachment points.

Figure 9.10(a)–(c) exhibits the flow patterns of blood through the streamline contours for different Reynolds numbers Re. We observe that the region of flow circulation is small at $Re = 100$, while it is large at $Re = 500$. However, we can claim that our numerical model captures flow circulation zone at 30% constriction of artery when $Re = 100$. Previous numerical study by Ikbal *et al.*[69] found a small circulation zone at the downstream of the constricted artery having 64% area reduction for $Re = 350$. From the streamline contours presented in these study, one can observe that the streamlines are parallel in the central region of the artery. This may be caused due to the axisymmetricity of the artery. But for higher Reynolds number and more than 50% area constriction, the symmetric condition may violate. However, in a physiological system, the flow is laminar when $100 \leq Re \leq 500$ for large arteries and up to 50% area reduction. In this situation, flow through stenosed artery, the axisymmetric condition is valid. It is expected that at high Reynolds number and around 75% area blockage of the artery, flow circulation can be observed at the upstream. This enables us to attempt further studies in this direction.

Figure 9.11(a)–(c) illustrates the isothermal lines (measure of the temperature disturbances) in the downstream of the stenosis for 30% and 50% blockage while considering Ha = 1. We observe that the isothermal lines are generated near the arterial wall at the downstream of the stenosis due to interaction between the shear effect and thermal energy transport. As the blockage of the artery increases, the temperature contours strongly gets distorted at the downstream, and thereby temperature enhances. Figure 9.11(c) gives the temperature contour for 50% blockage of the stenosis in the arterial wall when Ha = 2. This figure shows that, with an increase in magnetic field strength, the isothermal lines tend to increase near the downstream of the stenosis, which in turn produces therapeutic response.

Figures 9.12 and 9.13 depict the variations of Nusselt number Nu with axial direction x. We have noticed considerable amount of alteration of Nusselt number Nu in the constricted region. It is observed from Figure 9.12 that when Hartmann number Ha increases, the Nusselt number Nu also increases. Figure 9.13 gives the variations of Nusselt number with different Reynolds number Re. The Nusselt number increases with a rise in the Reynolds number Re. The results presented in Figure 9.12 will serve as promising applications in the drug-delivery system with magnetic nanoparticles as carriers. If the location of a tumor in the tissue is observed in the downstream stenotic region, the enhancement of the temperature can be made with drug-delivery system using magnetic nanoparticles.

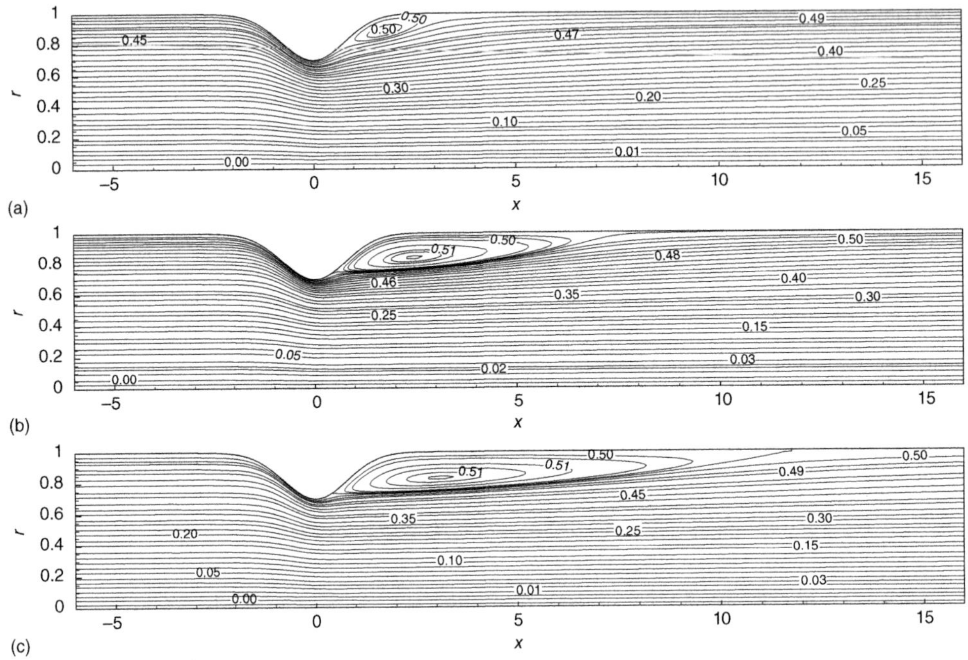

Figure 9.10. Streamline (ψ) contours for different values of Reynolds number: (a) Re = 100, (b) Re = 300, and (c) Re = 500, when Ha = 1, Pr = 25, and t = 2. (Majee and Shit.[68] Reproduced with Permission of Elsevier)

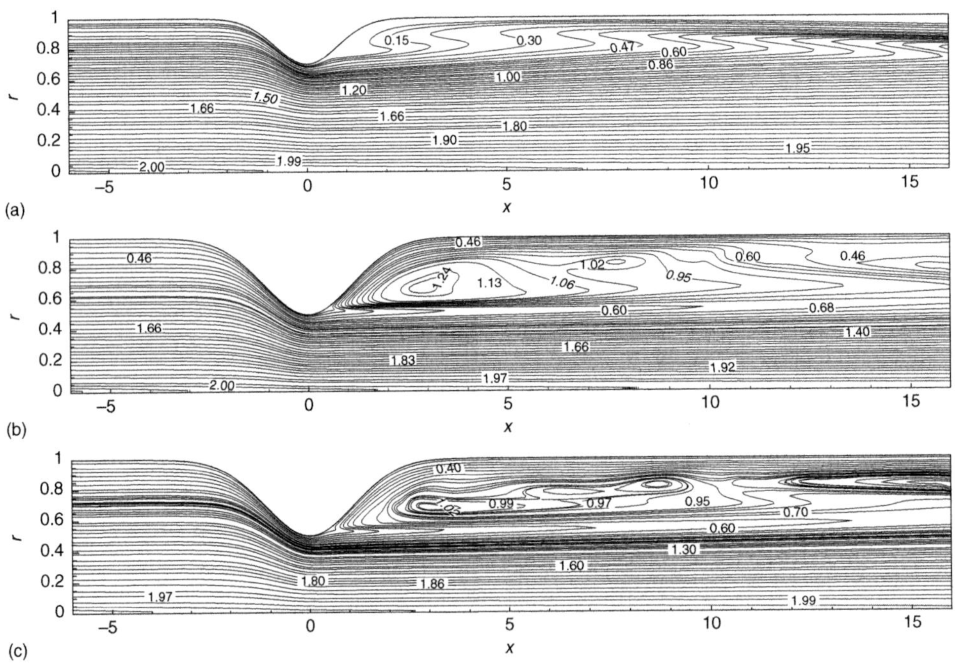

Figure 9.11. Isotherms (temperature contour): (a) 30% stenosis, for Ha = 1, (b) 50% stenosis, for Ha = 1, and (c) 50% stenosis, for Ha = 2, when Re = 300, Pr = 25, and t = 2. (Majee and Shit.[68] Reproduced with Permission of Elsevier)

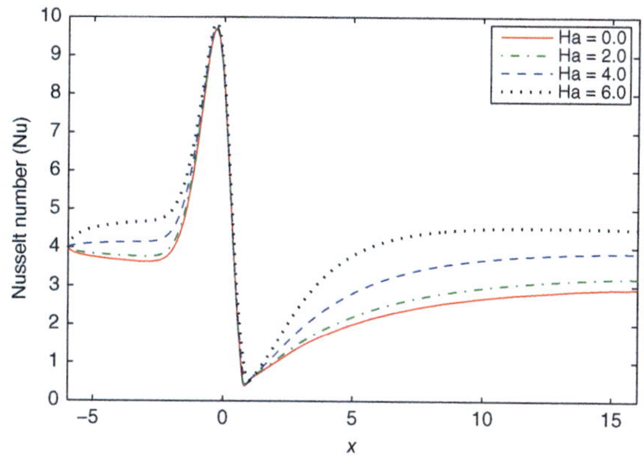

Figure 9.12. Variations of Nusselt number *Nu* for different values of Hartmann number Ha, when Re = 300, Pr = 25, and $t = 2$. (Majee and Shit.[68] Reproduced with Permission of Elsevier)

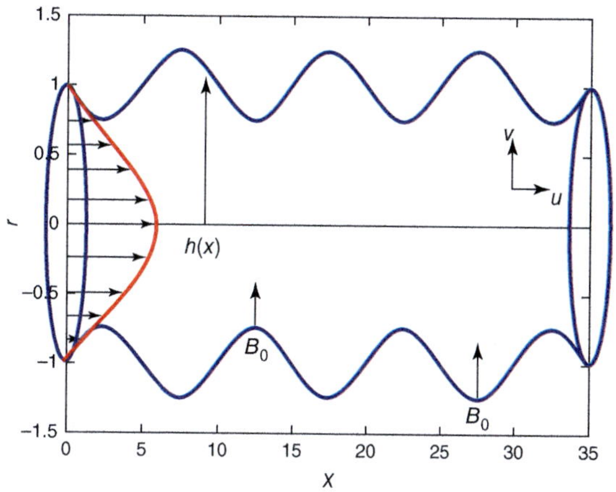

Figure 9.14. Schematic diagram of the model geometry with 25% amplitude of wavy wall. (Shit and Majee.[72] Reproduced with Permission of Elsevier)

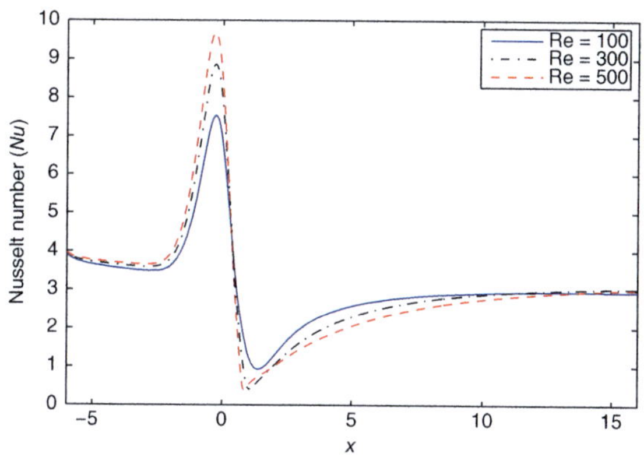

Figure 9.13. Variations of Nusselt number *Nu* for different values of Reynolds number Re, when Ha = 1, Pr = 25, and $t = 2$. (Majee and Shit.[68] Reproduced with Permission of Elsevier)

9.4 MAGNETOHYDRODYNAMIC FLOW OF BLOOD IN A SLOWLY VARYING ARTERIAL SEGMENT

An unsteady, laminar, incompressible, and axially symmetric two-dimensional flow of blood through arterial segment with slowly varying radius $R^*(x^*)$ can be put mathematically as

$$R^*(x^*) = R_0[1 - \alpha \sin(\pi x^*/l_0)] \tag{9.40}$$

where R_0 is the mean radius of the normal artery, α the amplitude of the wavy wall, and $2l_0$ represents the wavelength of the sinusoidally varying tube wall (cf. Figure 9.14).

Under the abovementioned consideration, the governing equations[68,70] for unsteady two-dimensional fluid flow along with the thermal energy equation are taken as in equations (9.21)–(9.25). The boundary conditions are also same as in (9.26)–(9.29).

After nondimensionalizing the above governing equations, we have applied vorticity–stream function formulation and obtained the equations in ω, ψ, and θ.

In order to apply the numerical scheme, the abovementioned equations are transformed and P-R Alternate Direction Implicit method is used to solve them as discussed in the previous section.

Figure 9.15(a) and (b) shows the variation of axial velocity along radial direction η in both systolic and diastolic phases of blood flow, respectively, with different amplitudes of the wavy wall. It can be noted from both the figures that axial velocity increases with an increase in the amplitude of the wavy arterial wall. It is observed that for nonzero values of α, the velocity profiles are ceased to be fully developed during systolic phase. Moreover, Figure 9.15(a) depicts that with an increase in amplitude α, the flow reversal of blood near the wall takes place. However, in the case of diastolic phase as shown in Figure 9.15(b), the flow reversal does not arise.

Figure 9.16(a)–(c) illustrates the streamline contours with different Hartmann numbers Ha. These figures reveal how the flow patterns of blood in the

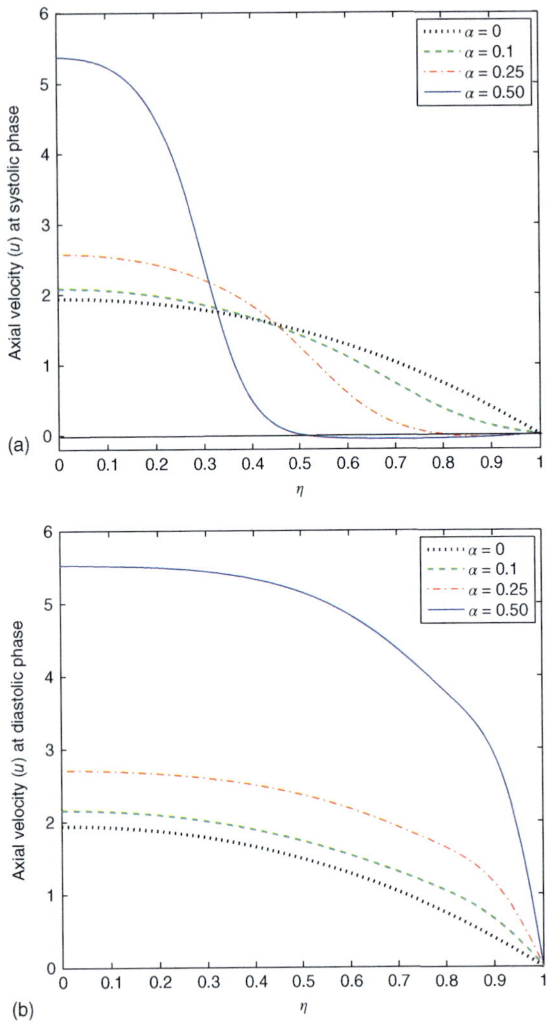

Figure 9.15. Variation of axial velocity u for different values of the amplitude of wavy wall α (a) in systolic phase and (b) in diastolic phase, when Re = 300, Pr = 25, and $t = 2$. (Shit and Majee.[72] Reproduced with Permission of Elsevier)

wavy arterial segment can be visualized. We can observe that the formation of vortices in the converging regions of the arterial wall variation is strong. This is known as primary circulation. In the absence of magnetic field, there also arises a secondary flow circulation with a small eddy structure. For higher values of Ha, the primary flow circulation becomes weak and tend to vanish. However, the secondary circulations completely vanish with Ha ≥ 1. The extent and density of vortices thus formed gets reduced with increase in Hartmann number, which gives the clear idea that by increasing the magnetic field strength, back flow of blood can be removed with a considerable extent. Furthermore, the flow characteristics show negligible changes within the hmodynamical range between Ha = 0 and 1. However, it may be the case that the existence of secondary vortices and its impact in the presence of magnetic field has greater influence in the physiological flow.

Figure 9.17 gives the variation of skin friction in the function of Hartmann number Ha with varying Reynolds number. It is observed that with increase in Reynolds number, the velocity of blood increases, which leads to decrease in skin friction in systolic phase, but shows a opposite trend in diastolic phase up to Ha = 3, beyond which C_f follows its systolic counterpart. It is also noticed that the skin friction tends to have a negative value during the diastolic phases.

Figure 9.18 briefs the variation of skin friction in function of Hartmann number with different amplitudes of wavy wall in both systolic and diastolic phases. It is observed that skin friction gradually increases with increasing Hartmann number as the velocity decreases. Moreover, during systolic flow, skin friction increases with increase in amplitude, but a reverse phenomenon is observed in diastolic phase. When $\alpha = 0$, no variation of C_f is noted for systole and diastole. It means that the skin friction is constant for rigid wall tube, however, showing increasing effect with Ha. The lowering of wall shear stress during diastolic phase is responsible for formation of atherosclerosis.

9.5 MAGNETIC FIELD EFFECT ON BLOOD FLOW THROUGH ABDOMINAL AORTIC ANEURYSM

The two-dimensional flow of blood through a diseased artery having abdominal aortic aneurysm is considered as shown in Figure 9.19.

The cylindrical polar coordinates (r^*, θ^*, and x^*) along x^* as the axis of symmetry of the artery are chosen and assumed that all the flow characteristics are independent of θ^*. The governing equations for unsteady two-dimensional MHD fluid flow along with the thermal energy equation are taken as per equations (9.21)–(9.25).

The geometry of the abdominal aortic aneurysm can be put mathematically as

$$R^*(x^*) = R_0\left[1 + \delta e^{-\alpha\left(\frac{x^*}{R_0}\right)^2}\right] \qquad (9.41)$$

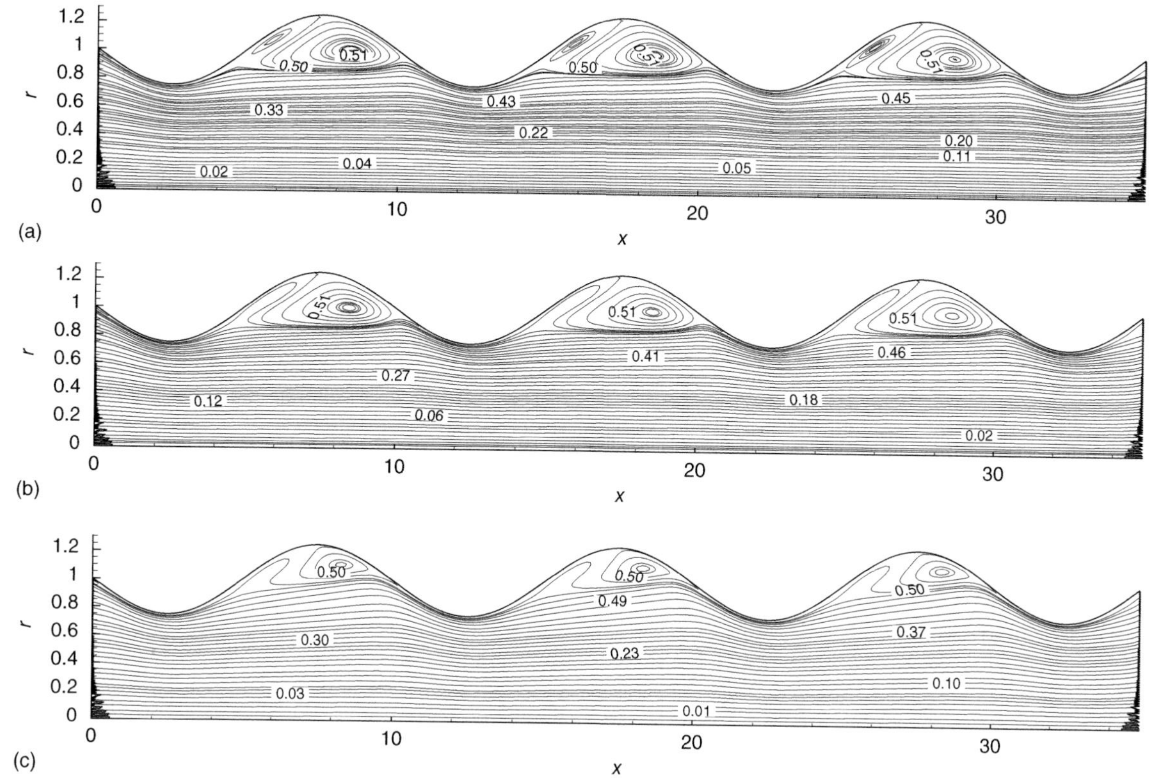

Figure 9.16. Streamline (ψ) contours for different values of Hartmann number: (a) Ha = 0, (b) Ha = 1, and (c) Ha = 4, when Re = 300, Pr = 25, and t = 2. (Shit and Majee.[72] Reproduced with Permission of Elsevier)

The boundary conditions are taken as per equations (9.26)–(9.29).

The above equations are firstly nondimensionalized, and then vorticity–stream function formulation is adapted to solve the equations numerically.

For the purpose of studying specific arterial disease such as aortic abdominal aneurysm, we have developed a numerical model in the present analysis. Using two time step numerical algorithms viz., the standard second-order Peaceman–Rachford ADI method along with implicit finite difference scheme, we have computed the stream function and vorticity contours in a long circular pipe. The resulting approximations are second order in both time and space. Because of the consideration of implicit scheme, the method used in this study is unconditionally stable. We used uniform grids with different mesh sizes along the space and time directions. Our model is confined by a nondimensional arterial length, equal to 22 times the radius of the artery.

Figure 9.20 illustrates the variation of axial velocity with different sizes of AAA. It is observed that as the size of AAA increases, the axial velocity decreases in the downstream of the AAA. However, the maximum velocity at the central line of AAA remains fixed. The reduction of blood velocity with aneurysm size has serious implication in the arterial diseases.

Figure 9.21(a)–(d) exhibits the blood flow pattern via the streamline contours for different Hartmann numbers Ha. From these figures we observe the formation of vortices which detaches from the wall and rolls up into a ring like vortex structure at the throat of the AAA which get reduced and finally vanishes as magnetic field strength is sufficiently increased. This confirms the idea of flow circulation zone and the position of flow reversal that takes place at the bulge of AAA.

Figure 9.22 gives the variation of dimensionless wall shear stress (skin friction) along the length of the arterial segment with different values of Hartmann number Ha. We observe that the skin friction increases with increasing magnetic field strength. It

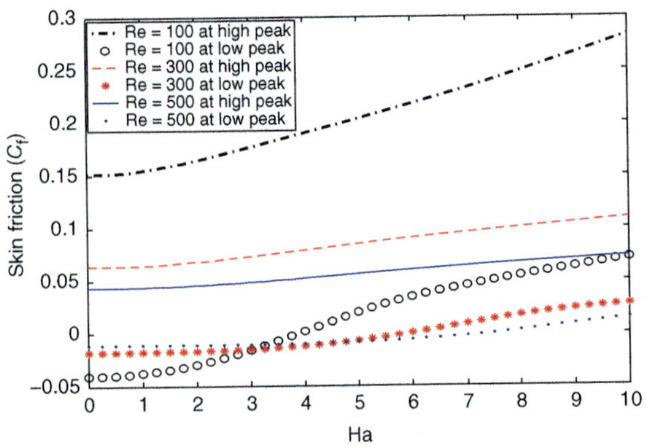

Figure 9.17. Distribution of wall shear stress with Hartmann number Ha for different Reynolds numbers *Re*, when $\alpha = 0.25$, Pr = 25, and $t = 2$. (Shit and Majee.[72] Reproduced with Permission of Elsevier)

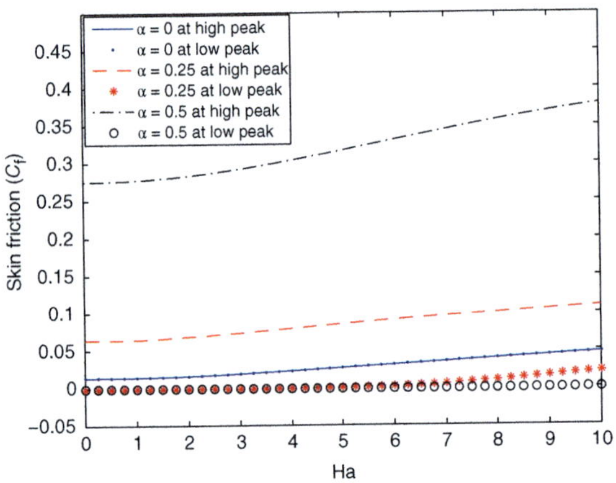

Figure 9.18. Distribution of wall shear stress in function of Hartmann number Ha with different amplitudes of wavy wall α, when Re = 300, Pr = 25, and $t = 2$. (Shit and Majee.[72] Reproduced with Permission of Elsevier)

can also be traced that the wall shear stress sharply falls as the expansion in the arterial segment is reached and grows to the peak in the downstream of AAA. When the blood flows through the aneurysm, WSS patterns alter both quantitatively and qualitatively. When the blood in the aneurysm area becomes stagnant, a slow flow is induced by the wall motion which increases the shear stress on the aneurysmal wall. In the expansion region, wall shear stress becomes negative, which indicates the flow separation region and substantially more predominant than the positive values as very low shear stress results in abnormal metabolic activity in the arterial wall.[71,73] The negative values can be suppressed with a considerable extent by increasing the strength of the magnetic field. However, widespread area low WSS region induces more pathological state[74] which can also be minimized by applying magnetic field strength which abbreviates the low WSS area in the aneurysm region. Separation of boundary layer gives rise to the structure of the flow phenomenon, which is significant in understanding and predicting the flow characteristics. Moreover, the region of negative shear stress gives the idea of the radius of flow circulation eddies. These low shear stress regions have pathological significance and may prolong the residing time of blood constituents that eventually flow into the arterial wall. Thus, these flow controlling parameters can be used in the magnetic drug-delivery system to cure the affected parts in the arterial segment.

Figure 9.23 illustrates the variation of skin friction in the function of Reynolds number *Re* with varying sizes of AAA. In this figure, we observe that the wall shear stress decreases with increasing Reynolds number, whereas it increases with increasing size of the aneurysm. This is due to the fact that increasing of aneurysm size slows down the blood velocity, which in turn increases the wall shear stress. Moreover, in aneurysm artery, WSS is observed to differ in magnitude with a healthy abdominal aorta. WSS at 70% AAA artery increases by 51%, 50% AAA artery increases by 37%, and 10% AAA artery increases by 18% with the value in a healthy aorta, when Reynolds number *Re* = 100. At *Re* = 300, WSS at 70%, 50%, and 10% AAA artery increases by 43%, 14%, and 14%, respectively, with the value in a healthy arterial segment. Again at *Re* = 500, WSS at 70%, 50%, and 10% AAA artery increases by 42%, 14%, and 28%, respectively, with the value in a healthy abdominal aorta. This is an important observation to note that when Reynolds number increases, even a minor AAA of about 10% can cause large pathological impact with WSS change of 28%, which is higher than in cases with low Reynolds number.

Figure 9.24 corresponds to the variation of the magnitude of Nusselt number along with the Hartmann number Ha for different values of Reynolds number *Re*. It is shown that the magnitude of Nusselt number increases with an increase in magnetic strength

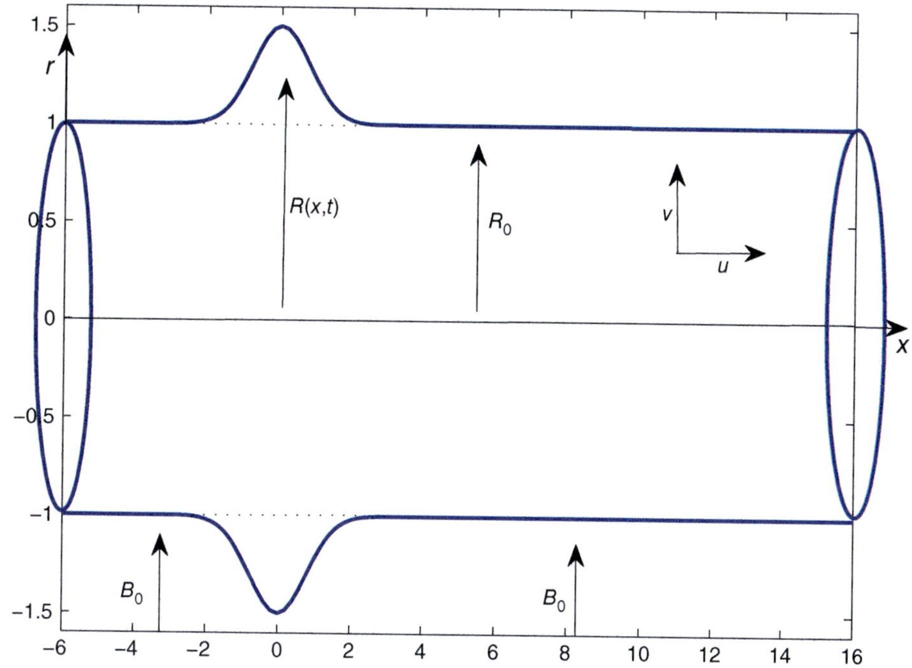

Figure 9.19. Schematic diagram of the model geometry with 50% arterial aneurysm. (Shit and Majee.[75] Reproduced with Permission of Elsevier)

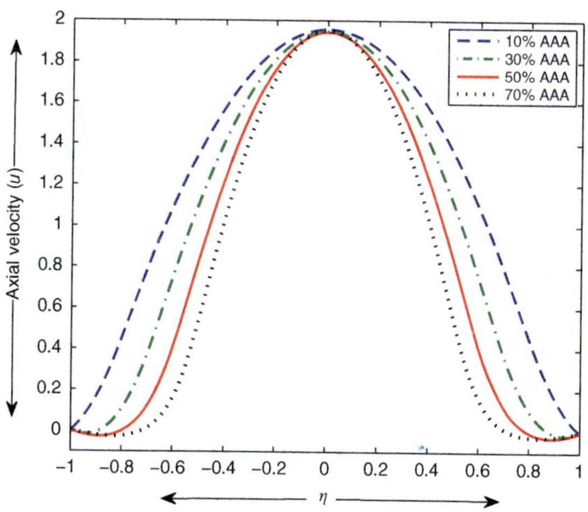

Figure 9.20. Variation of axial velocity u at $x = 0$ for different heights of the aneurysm at the outset, when Ha = 1, Re = 300, Pr = 21, and $t = 2$. (Shit and Majee.[75] Reproduced with Permission of Elsevier)

as well as Reynolds number. When Reynolds number $Re = 500$, the Nusselt number becomes constant from Ha = 0 to Ha = 1, which shows that if we increase the magnetic field strength up to 8 T, no significant physiological changes can be detected.

9.6 TARGETED DRUG DELIVERY WITH MAGNETIC NANOPARTICLES

9.6.1 Mathematical Modeling

In this section, an unsteady two-dimensional and fully developed blood flow (at the entry) through a stenosed artery is considered (cf. Figure 9.25), into which magnetic nanoparticles are injected in the blood stream and captured them at a specific location under the influence of an externally applied magnetic field. The cylindrical polar coordinates (r^*, θ^*, and x^*) along x^* as the axis of symmetry of the artery are chosen and assumed that all the flow characteristics are independent of θ^*. The governing equations for unsteady two-dimensional MHD fluid flow along with the thermal energy equation and magnetic nanoparticle velocity are taken as

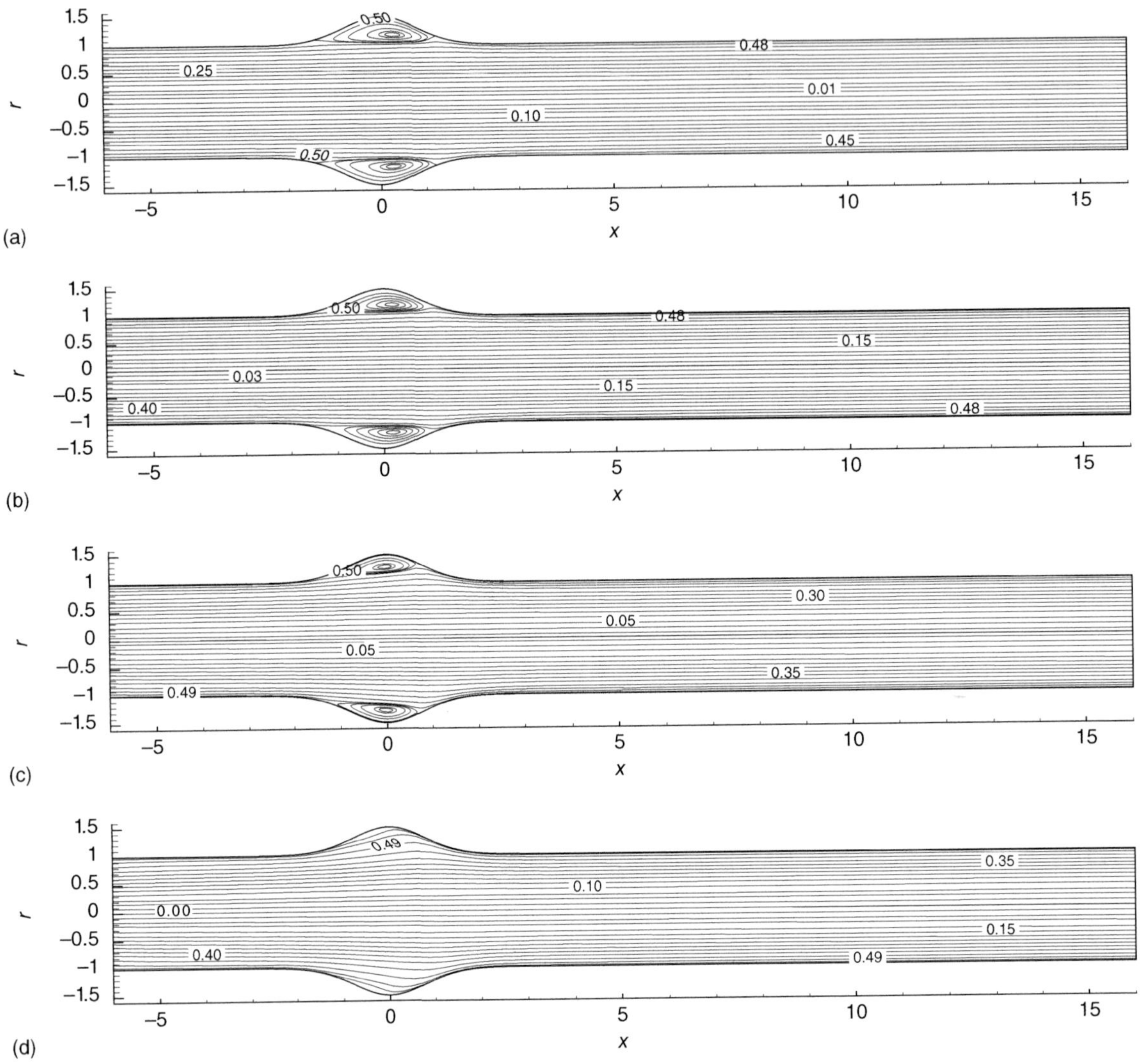

Figure 9.21. Streamline (ψ) contours for different values of Hartmann number: (a) Ha = 0, (b) Ha = 2, (c) Ha = 4, and (d) Ha = 6, when Re = 300, Pr = 21, and t = 2. (Shit and Majee.[75] Reproduced with Permission of Elsevier)

$$\frac{\partial u^*}{\partial x^*} + \frac{v^*}{r^*} + \frac{\partial v^*}{\partial r^*} = 0 \tag{9.42}$$

$$\rho\left(\frac{\partial u^*}{\partial t^*} + u^*\frac{\partial u^*}{\partial x^*} + v^*\frac{\partial u^*}{\partial r^*}\right) = -\frac{\partial p^*}{\partial x^*} + \mu\left(\frac{\partial^2 u^*}{\partial r^{*2}} + \frac{1}{r^*}\frac{\partial u^*}{\partial r^*} + \frac{\partial^2 u^*}{\partial x^{*2}}\right) + K_s N(v_{px}^* - u^*) - \sigma B_0^2 u^* \tag{9.43}$$

$$\rho\left(\frac{\partial v^*}{\partial t^*} + u^*\frac{\partial v^*}{\partial x^*} + v^*\frac{\partial v^*}{\partial r^*}\right) = -\frac{\partial p^*}{\partial r^*} + \mu\left(\frac{\partial^2 v^*}{\partial r^{*2}} + \frac{1}{r^*}\frac{\partial v^*}{\partial r^*} + \frac{\partial^2 v^*}{\partial x^{*2}} - \frac{v^*}{r^{*2}}\right) + K_s N(v_{py}^* - v^*) \tag{9.44}$$

$$\rho C_p\left(\frac{\partial T^*}{\partial t^*} + u^*\frac{\partial T^*}{\partial x^*} + v^*\frac{\partial T^*}{\partial r^*}\right) = k\left(\frac{\partial^2 T^*}{\partial r^{*2}} + \frac{1}{r^*}\frac{\partial T^*}{\partial r^*} + \frac{\partial^2 T^*}{\partial x^{*2}}\right) + \sigma B_0^2 u^{*2} + \phi^* \tag{9.45}$$

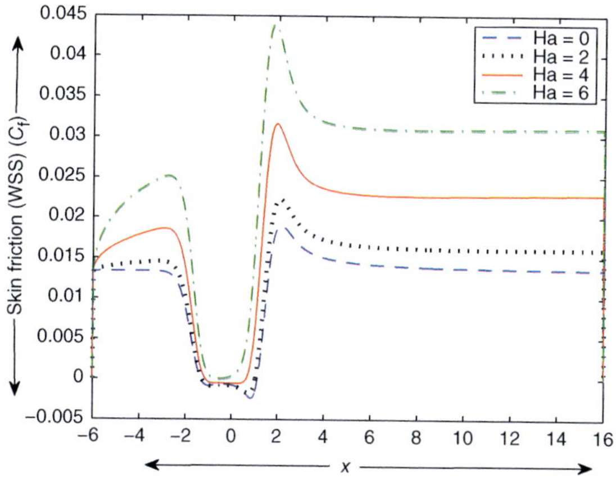

Figure 9.22. Distribution of wall shear stress for different values of Hartmann number Ha, when Re = 300, Pr = 21, and $t = 2$. (Shit and Majee.[75] Reproduced with Permission of Elsevier)

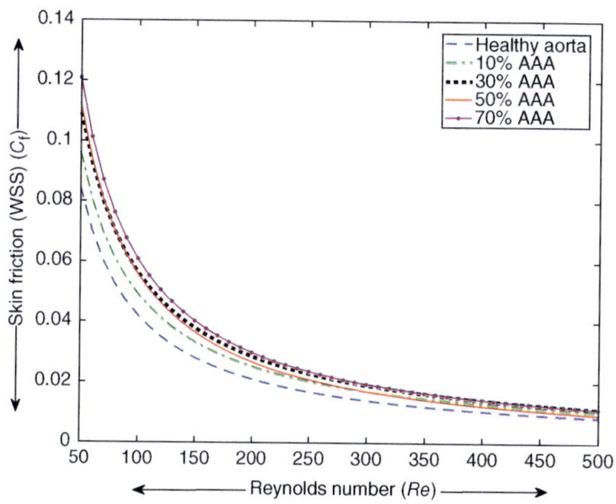

Figure 9.23. Distribution of wall shear stress in function of Reynolds number *Re* for different sizes of aneurysm, when Pr = 21 and $t = 2$. (Shit and Majee.[75] Reproduced with Permission of Elsevier)

where

$$\phi^* = \mu\left[2\left(\frac{\partial v^*}{\partial r^*}\right)^2 + \left(\frac{\partial v^*}{\partial x^*} + \frac{\partial u^*}{\partial r^*}\right)^2 + 2\left(\frac{\partial u^*}{\partial x^*}\right)^2\right]$$

is the viscous dissipation term.

In the above equation, K_s is the Stokes constant, N the number of nanoparticles injected, and v_{px} and v_{py} the velocities of magnetic nanoparticles in the x and y directions, respectively. The motion of a spherical-shaped magnetic nanoparticle is considered

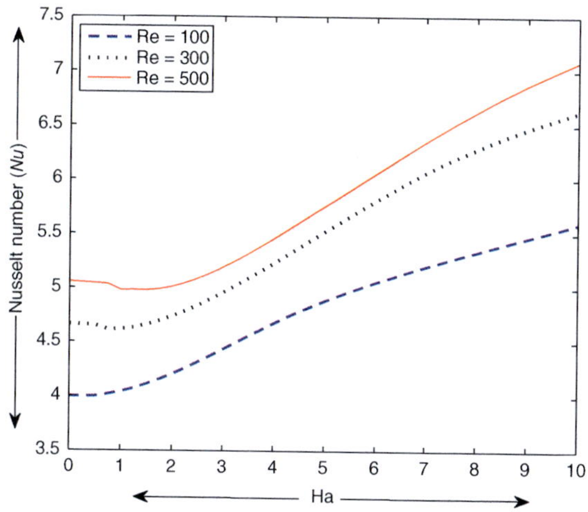

Figure 9.24. Variation of Nusselt number *Nu* along with the Hartmann number Ha for different values of Reynolds number *Re*, when Pr = 21 and $t = 2$. (Shit and Majee.[75] Reproduced with Permission of Elsevier)

in the flow of blood under the influence of applied magnetic field. In this problem, we have neglected the Brownian motion by restricting our attention to low Reynolds number flow regimes where the magnetic and viscous forces are dominated. Therefore, the equations of motion of nanoparticle using the classical Newtonian dynamics can be written as

$$m\frac{\partial v_{px}^*}{\partial t^*} = F_{\rm m} + F_{\rm f} + F_{\rm g} \qquad (9.46)$$

$$m\frac{\partial v_{py}^*}{\partial t^*} = F_{\rm m} + F_{\rm f} + F_{\rm g} \qquad (9.47)$$

where $m = \frac{4}{3}\pi R_{\rm p}^3\rho_{\rm p}$ is the mass of the nanoparticle, ρ_p the density of the nanoparticle, R_p the radius of the nanoparticle, and F_m, F_f, and F_g the magnetic, fluidic, and gravitational forces, respectively.

When the inertial terms $m\frac{\partial v_{px}^*}{\partial t^*}$ and $m\frac{\partial v_{py}^*}{\partial t^*}$ are neglected, the particle motion satisfies the following simple force balance $F_{\rm m} + F_{\rm f} + F_{\rm g} = 0$.

The fluidic force exerted by a nanoparticle is obtained using Stokes' law for the viscous drag on the sphere as

$$F_{\rm f} = -6\pi\mu R_{\rm hyd,p} f_{Dp}(v_{px}^* - u^*) \qquad (9.48)$$

$$F_{\rm f} = -6\pi\mu R_{\rm hyd,p} f_{Dp}(v_{py}^* - v^*) \qquad (9.49)$$

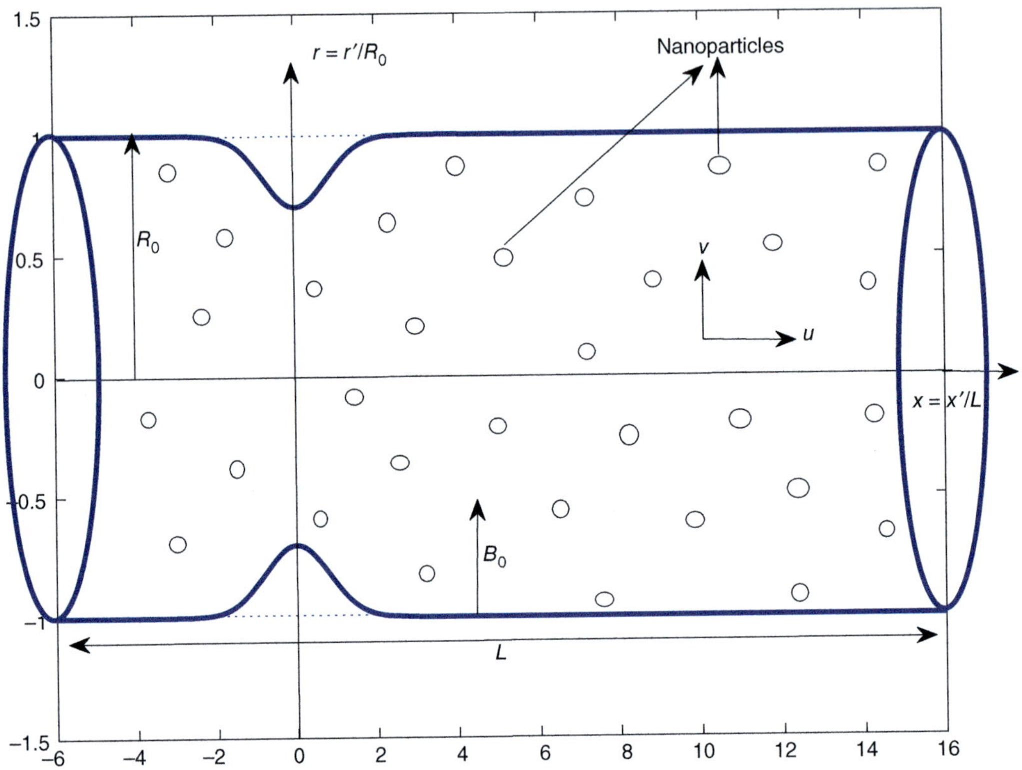

Figure 9.25. Schematic diagram of the model geometry with arterial stenosis. (Majee and Shit.[76] Reproduced with Permission of Elsevier)

When the force on the nanoparticle is fluidic, i.e., F_f, equations (9.46) and (9.47) reduce to

$$m\frac{\partial v_{px}^*}{\partial t^*} = K_s(u^* - v_{px}^*) \tag{9.50}$$

$$m\frac{\partial v_{py}^*}{\partial t^*} = K_s(v^* - v_{py}^*) \tag{9.51}$$

where $K_s = 6\pi\mu R_{\text{hyd,p}} f_{Dp}$ in which $R_{\text{hyd,p}}$ is the effective hydrodynamic radius of the nanoparticle and f_{Dp} the drag coefficient. The boundary conditions for blood flow through a stenosed artery are taken as

$$\frac{\partial u^*}{\partial r^*} = v^* = \frac{\partial T^*}{\partial r^*} = 0 \quad \text{along the central axis of the artery, i.e., at } r^* = 0 \tag{9.52}$$

$$u^* = v^* = 0, \quad T^* = T_w \text{ at the arterial wall, i.e., at } r^* = R^*(x^*) \tag{9.53}$$

$$u^* = 2U_0\left[1 - \left(\frac{r^*}{R^*(x^*)}\right)^2\right], \quad v^* = 0,$$
$$T^* = T_w + 2(1 - r^{*2})(T_\infty - T_w) \text{ at the inlet, i.e., at } x^* = 0 \tag{9.54}$$

and

$$\frac{\partial u^*}{\partial x^*} = \frac{\partial v^*}{\partial x^*} = \frac{\partial T^*}{\partial x^*} = 0 \text{ at the outlet. i.e., at } x^* = R_0 L \tag{9.55}$$

In the above equation, $R^*(x^*)$ represents the geometry of the stenosis which can be put mathematically as

$$R^*(x^*) = R_0\left[1 - \delta e^{-\alpha\left(\frac{x^*}{R_0}\right)^2}\right] \tag{9.56}$$

9.6.2 Mathematical Simplification

Using the dimensionless variables as defined earlier, equations (9.42)–(9.45) become

$$\frac{\partial u}{\partial x} + \frac{v}{r} + \frac{\partial v}{\partial r} = 0 \tag{9.57}$$

$$\frac{\partial u}{\partial t} + \left(u\frac{\partial u}{\partial x} + v\frac{\partial u}{\partial r}\right) = -\frac{\partial p}{\partial x} + \frac{1}{Re} \times \left(\frac{\partial^2 u}{\partial r^2} + \frac{1}{r}\frac{\partial u}{\partial r} + \frac{\partial^2 u}{\partial x^2}\right) + \frac{R_s}{Re}(v_{px} - u) - \frac{\mathrm{Ha}^2}{Re}u \tag{9.58}$$

$$\frac{\partial v}{\partial t} + \left(u\frac{\partial v}{\partial x} + v\frac{\partial v}{\partial r}\right) = -\frac{\partial p}{\partial r} + \frac{1}{Re} \times \left(\frac{\partial^2 v}{\partial r^2} + \frac{1}{r}\frac{\partial v}{\partial r} + \frac{\partial^2 v}{\partial x^2} - \frac{v}{r^2}\right) + \frac{R_s}{Re}(v_{py} - v) \tag{9.59}$$

$$\frac{\partial \theta}{\partial t} + \left(u\frac{\partial \theta}{\partial x} + v\frac{\partial \theta}{\partial r}\right) = \frac{1}{\mathrm{Re\,Pr}} \times \left(\frac{\partial^2 \theta}{\partial r^2} + \frac{1}{r}\frac{\partial \theta}{\partial r} + \frac{\partial^2 \theta}{\partial x^2}\right) + \frac{\mathrm{Ec\,Ha}^2}{Re}u^2 + \frac{Ec}{Re}\phi \tag{9.60}$$

where

$$\phi = 2\left(\left(\frac{\partial v}{\partial r}\right)^2 + \left(\frac{\partial u}{\partial x}\right)^2\right) + \left(\frac{\partial v}{\partial x} + \frac{\partial u}{\partial r}\right)^2$$

The nondimensional parameters appearing in equations (9.58)–(9.60) are defined as the Reynolds number $Re = \frac{U_0 R_0}{\nu}$, Hartmann number $\mathrm{Ha} = B_0 R_0 \sqrt{\frac{\sigma}{\rho \nu}}$, Prandtl number $\mathrm{Pr} = \frac{\mu C_p}{K}$, Eckert number $\mathrm{Ec} = \frac{U_0^2}{C_p(T_\infty - T_w)}$, and particle concentration parameter $R_s = \frac{K_s N R_0^2}{\mu}$.

Moreover, equations (9.50) and (9.51) become

$$G\frac{\partial v_{px}}{\partial t} = (u - v_{px}) \tag{9.61}$$

and

$$G\frac{\partial v_{py}}{\partial t} = (v - v_{py}) \tag{9.62}$$

where $G = \frac{mU_0}{K_s R_0}$ is the particle mass parameter. Employing the stream function–vorticity formulation as discussed in the previous section, we have solved the velocity and temperature field numerically.

Figure 9.26 represents the variation of axial velocity with varying coefficients of nanoparticle concentration R_s. It is observed that as the concentration of nanoparticles increases, velocity also increases. This is due to the fact that, nanoparticles are not uniformly distributed, rather, they are concentrated more in the vicinity of the centerline of the artery than the wall. This causes lack of uniform distribution due to Brownian and thermophoretic forces and makes the velocity field to be stronger.

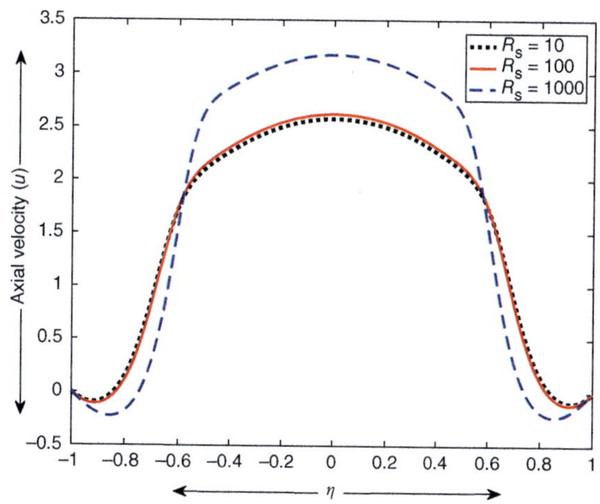

Figure 9.26. Variation of axial velocity u at the downstream of the stenosis for different values of the concentration parameter R_s, when Ha = 1, Re = 300, Pr = 21, and t = 2. (Majee and Shit.[76] Reproduced with Permission of Elsevier)

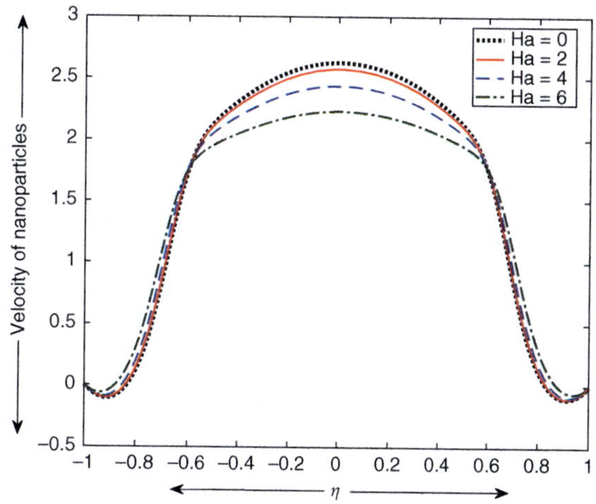

Figure 9.27. Variation of velocity (V_{px}) of nanoparticles at the downstream of the stenosis for different values of the Hartmann number Ha, when Re = 300, Pr = 21, t = 2, and $Rs = O(10^2)$. (Majee and Shit.[76] Reproduced with Permission of Elsevier)

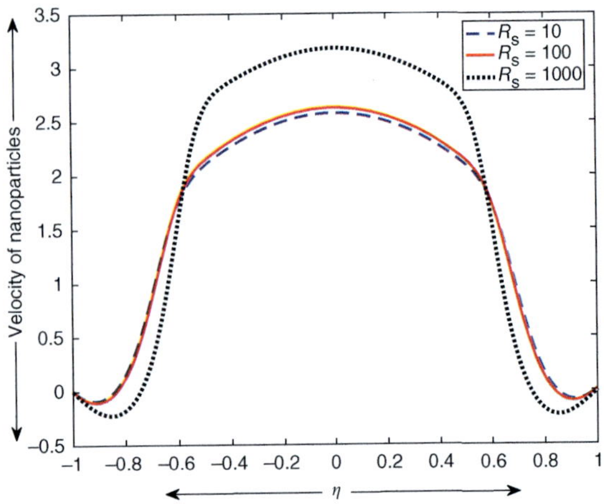

Figure 9.28. Variation of velocity (V_{px}) of nanoparticles at the downstream of the stenosis for different values of the concentration parameter R_s, when Ha = 1, Re = 300, Pr = 21, and t = 2. (Majee and Shit.[76] Reproduced with Permission of Elsevier)

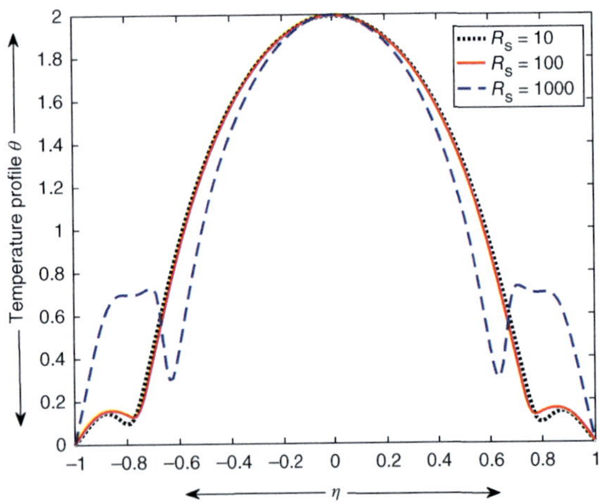

Figure 9.29. Variation of nondimensional temperature θ at the downstream of the stenosis for different values of concentration parameter R_s, when Ha = 1, Re = 300, Pr = 21, and t = 2. (Majee and Shit.[76] Reproduced with Permission of Elsevier)

Figures 9.27 and 9.28 are the axial components of velocity profiles of the magnetic nanoparticles along the radial direction. Both of these profiles show that axial velocity is maximum at the axis. It is observed from Figure 9.27 that the velocity of nanoparticles decreases with a rise in the magnetic field strength. This observation leads to the capturing efficiency of nanoparticles bound with drug at a specific location. Figure 9.28 shows that the velocity of magnetic nanoparticles decreases near the arterial wall with increasing concentration parameter *Rs*. Thus, more augmentation of nanoparticles into the blood stream has more capturing efficiency. Moreover, this defines the flow behavior of the nanoparticles which coincides with the blood flow behavior in macro level.

Figure 9.29 represents the variation of temperature profile with nanoparticle concentration parameter R_s. At the vicinity of the wall, the temperature tends to increase with increasing concentration of the nanoparticles, but as it goes deeper into central line, this phenomenon tends to reverse. This is due to specific loss power (SLP) generation. However, well-dispersed nanoparticles show highest SLP. This is due to increase in magnetic interaction between the nanoparticles which results in certain conditions which decrease the hyperthermia efficiency.

Figure 9.30(a)–(c) depicts the streamline contours with varying nanoparticle concentration parameter R_s. It is observed that as the aggregation of nanoparticles in the blood stream increases, the blood velocity increases, enhancing the intensity of the vortices at the downstream of the stenosis. This may prolong the residing time of the magnetic nanoparticles near the stenosis and increases the capturing efficiency to treat clinically the arterial disease.

Figure 9.31 shows the variation of dimensionless wall shear stress (skin friction) along the length of the arterial segment with varying concentrations of nanoparticles in the blood stream. It is observed that at the throat, wall shear stress increases and grows to a peak and falls sharply at the downstream of the stenosis. At the throat of the stenosis, wall shear stress increases with increasing concentration of nanoparticles, but the opposite trend is followed from the immediate downstream of the stenosis. In this figure, we have compared the shear stress with infused magnetic nanoparticles and without mixing nanoparticles in the blood stream. The shear stresses in both cases have similar profiles, which shows that infusion of magnetic nanoparticles in the arteries does not cause any abnormalities in the flow behavior. Moreover, the region of negative shear stress shows the radius of flow circulation eddies. This low shear stress regions have pathological significance, and increasing concentration prolongs the residing time of the blood constituents that eventually flow alongside the arterial wall, which may cure arterial diseases.

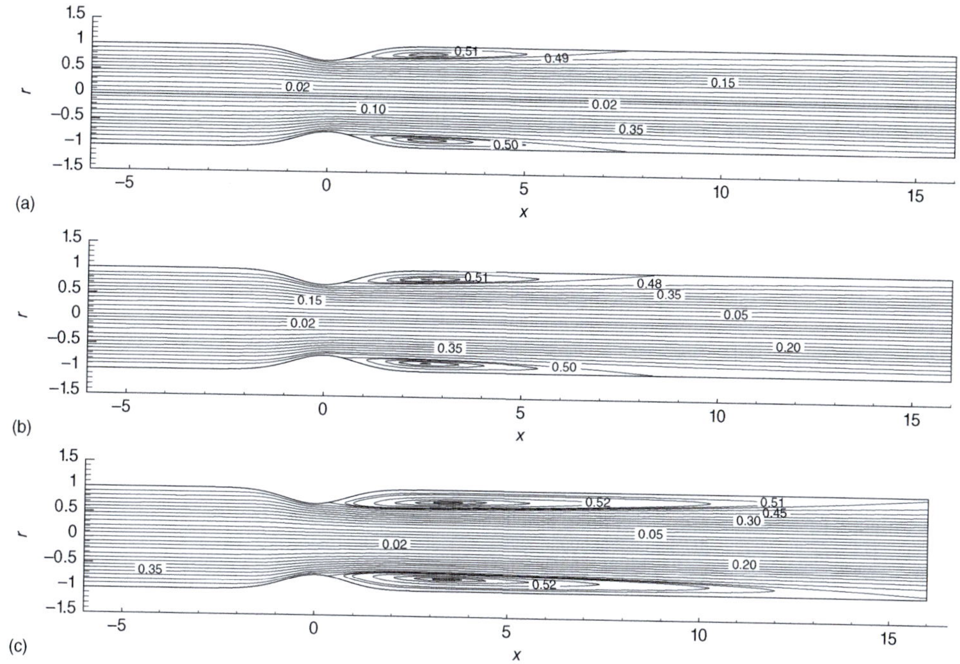

Figure 9.30. Streamline (ψ) contours for different values of concentration parameter: (a) $R_s = 10$, (b) $R_s = 100$, and (c) $R_s = 1000$, when Ha = 1, Pr = 21, and $t = 2$. (Majee and Shit.[76] Reproduced with Permission of Elsevier)

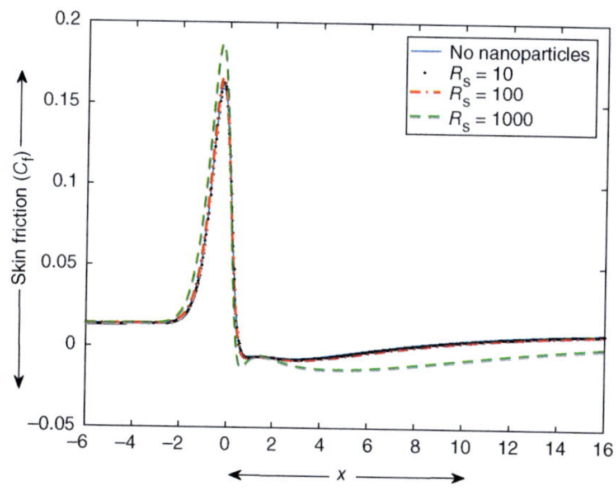

Figure 9.31. Distribution of wall shear stress for different values of concentration parameter R_s, when Ha = 1, Re = 300, Pr = 21, and $t = 2$. (Majee and Shit.[76] Reproduced with Permission of Elsevier)

Figure 9.32 gives the Nusselt number variation with Hartmann number Ha for different concentration parameters. It is observed that as the concentration of particles increases, less magnetic field strength is required to enhance the Nusselt number. The rate of heat transfer at the wall increases with both concentration parameter and higher magnetic strength. Thus, transferring more heat to the surrounding tissues with the injection of magnetic nanoparticles to the blood stream is one of the pioneering results of the present study.

9.7 CONCLUSION

In this chapter, we have derived equations that govern the flow phenomenon of blood in magnetic field environment and solved them numerically for various cardiovascular applications. We have also investigated targeting of the magnetic nanoparticles with the help of external magnetic field toward an area of interest for such applications.

An important property of blood is that it is an electrically conducting fluid. Thus, application of magnetic field induces electric as well as magnetic fields. These fields interact and hence produce a body force per unit volume, known as the Lorentz force, which has a tendency to slow down the motion of fluid. In aorta, we

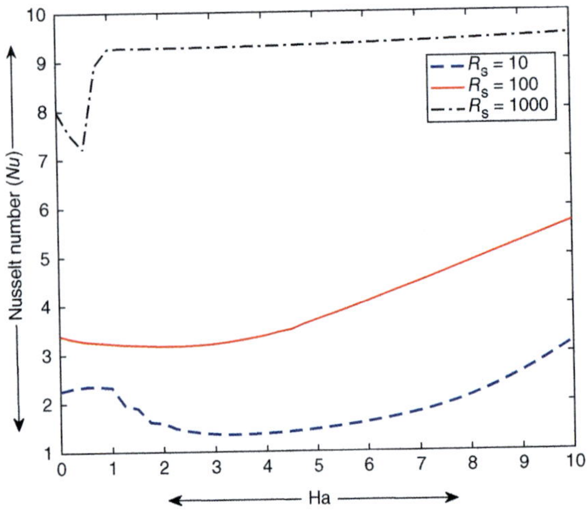

Figure 9.32. Variation of Nusselt number Nu along with the Hartmann number Ha for different values of concentration parameter R_s, when Pr = 21 and $t = 2$. (Majee and Shit.[76] Reproduced with Permission of Elsevier)

observed that up to 10% blood velocity reduces in the presence of magnetic field of strength 8 T, which corresponds to Ha = 1. Moreover, when Reynolds number $Re = 500$, the Nusselt number becomes constant from Ha = 0 to Ha = 1, which suggests that if we increase the magnetic field strength up to 8 T, no significant physiological changes can be detected.

Next, it is shown that the nanoparticles containing drugs form a vortexlike structure which forces the blood to rotate in a circular pattern in the vicinity of the stenosis. This vortex structure increases in intensity as the concentration of the nanoparticles increases in the blood stream. This prolongs the residing time of the blood constituents containing drugs in the vicinity of the stenosis and may enhance the efficiency to treat arterial diseases. The maximum limit of the concentration of the nanoparticles is also calculated, beyond which, increasing the concentration does not appear to have any effect on the body.

Finally, we have noted a significant hyperthermic deficiency in the middle of the artery when concentrations of nanoparticles are increased. This is due to SLP generation because of the interaction between the magnetic nanoparticles, which causes the temperature to decrease.

ACKNOWLEDGMENT

Research support from INSPIRE fellowship (IF140754), Department of Science and Technology, Government of India, is gratefully acknowledged.

REFERENCES

1. R. Ross, *Am. J. Pathol.*, 1993, **143**, 987. https://ci.nii.ac.jp/naid/10017216773/en/
2. D. M. Wootton, and D. N. Ku, *Annu. Rev. Biomed. Eng.*, 1999, **1**, 299.
3. D. Young, *J. Biomech. Eng.*, 1979, **101**, 157.
4. D. MacDonald, *J. Biomech.*, 1979, **12**, 13.
5. D. Sankar, and U. Lee, *Commun. Nonlinear Sci. Numer. Simul.*, 2009, **14**, 2971.
6. G. C. Layek, and C. Midya, *Commun. Nonlinear Sci. Numer. Simul.*, 2007, **12**, 745.
7. J. Misra, and G. Shit, *Int. J. Eng. Sci.*, 2006, **44**, 662.
8. R. Ntchantcho, S. Noubissie, and P. Woafo, *Commun. Nonlinear Sci. Numer. Simul.*, 2007, **12**, 1572.
9. D. Sankar, and U. Lee, *Commun. Nonlinear Sci. Numer. Simul.*, 2011, **16**, 4390.
10. R. Ponalagusamy, R. T. Selvi, and A. Banerjee, *J. Franklin Inst.*, 2012, **349**, 1681.
11. S. Bandyopadhyay, and G. Layek, *Commun. Nonlinear Sci. Numer. Simul.*, 2011, **16**, 252.
12. R. Ponalagusamy, and R. T. Selvi, *J. Franklin Inst.*, 2011, **348**, 2308.
13. C. Caro, T. Pedley, R. Schroter, and W. Seed, in The Mechanics of the Circulation', Oxford University Press, UK, 2012, p 147.
14. C. Caro, *Math. Method Appl. Sci.*, 2001, **24**, 1311.
15. H. Schlichting, and K. Gersten, Boundary-layer Theory', Springer, Germany, 2016.
16. M. Deshpande, D. Giddens, and R. Mabon, *J. Biomech.*, 1976, **9**, 165.
17. S. Ø Wille, *Appl. Math. Model.*, 1980, **4**, 483.
18. V. Duclaux, F. Gallaire, and C. Clanet, *J. Fluid Mech.*, 2010, **664**, 5.
19. E. A. Finol, and C. H. Amon, *J. Biomech. Eng.*, 2001, **123**, 474.
20. S. Yu, and J. Zhao, *Proc. Inst. Mech. Eng. Pt. C J. Mechan. Eng. Sci.*, 2000, **214**, 655.

21. C. Stamatopoulos, D. Mathioulakis, Y. Papaharilaou, and A. Katsamouris, *Exp. Fluids*, 2011, **50**, 1695.
22. E. Finol, K. Keyhani, and C. Amon, *J. Biomech. Eng.*, 2003, **125**, 207.
23. T. Matsuzawa, F. Gao, A. Qiao, O. Ohta, and H. Okada, in Etiology, Pathogenesis and Pathophysiology of Aortic Aneurysms and Aneurysm Rupture', IntechOpen, London, 2011, p 207.
24. C. M. Scotti, J. Jimenez, S. C. Muluk, and E. A. Finol, *Comput. Methods Biomech. Biomed. Eng.*, 2008, **11**, 301.
25. A.-V. Salsac, S. Sparks, J.-M. Chomaz, and J. Lasheras, *J. Fluid Mech.*, 2006, **560**, 19.
26. S. Mukhopadhyay, and G. Layek, *Appl. Math. Comput.*, 2011, **217**, 6792.
27. M. S. Rana, M. F. Rubby, and A. T. Hasan, *Procedia Engineering*, 2015, **105**, 885.
28. C. Vergara, D. Le Van, M. Quadrio, L. Formaggia, and M. Domanin, *Med. Eng. Phys.*, 2017, **47**, 38.
29. K. M. Khanafer, J. L. Bull, and R. Berguer, *Eur. J. Mech. B-Fluid*, 2009, **28**, 88.
30. Y. Haik, V. Pai, and C.-J. Chen, *J. Magn. Magn. Mater.*, 2001, **225**, 180.
31. G. C. Shit, *Model. Simul. Eng.*, 2013, **2013**, 16.
32. V. Vardanyan, *Biofizika*, 1973, **18**, 491.
33. S. Sharma, U. Singh, and V. Katiyar, *J. Magn. Magn. Mater.*, 2015, **377**, 395.
34. J. Misra, and G. Shit, *J. Appl. Mech.*, 2009, **76**, 061006.
35. J. C. Misra, S. D. Adhikary, and G. C. Shit, *Math. Model. Anal.*, 2008, **13**, 401.
36. J. Misra, A. Sinha, and G. Shit, *Int. J. Biomath.*, 2011, **4**, 207.
37. J. Misra, G. Shit, and H. J. Rath, *Comput. Fluids*, 2008, **37**, 1.
38. J. Misra, A. Sinha, and G. Shit, *Appl. Math. Mech. Engl.*, 2010, **31**, 1405.
39. J. Misra, G. Shit, S. Chandra, and P. Kundu, *J. Eng. Math.*, 2011, **69**, 91.
40. A. Alshare, B. Tashtoush, and H. H. El-Khalil, *J. Biomech. Eng.*, 2013, **135**, 114503.
41. A. Sinha, and G. Shit, *J. Magn. Magn. Mater.*, 2015, **378**, 143.
42. A. Ahuja, and W. Hendee, *Phys. Med. Biol.*, 1978, **23**, 937.
43. W.-L. Lin, J.-Y. Yen, Y.-Y. Chen, K.-W. Jin, and M.-J. Shieh, *Med. Phys.*, 1999, **26**, 818.
44. E. Ruuge, and A. Rusetski, *J. Magn. Magn. Mater.*, 1993, **122**, 335.
45. J. Pļaviņš, and M. Lauva, *J. Magn. Magn. Mater.*, 1993, **122**, 349.
46. E. J. Furlani, and E. P. Furlani, *J. Magn. Magn. Mater.*, 2007, **312**, 187.
47. S. Shaw, P. Murthy, and S. Pradhan, *J. Magn. Magn. Mater.*, 2010, **322**, 1037.
48. S. Shaw, and P. Murthy, *J. Nanotechnol. Eng. Med.*, 2010, **1**, 021001.
49. A. Mondal, and G. Shit, *J. Magn. Magn. Mater.*, 2017, **442**, 319.
50. S. Shaw, P. Murthy, and P. Sibanda, *Microvasc. Res.*, 2013, **85**, 77.
51. M. O. Avilés, A. D. Ebner, H. Chen, A. J. Rosengart, M. D. Kaminski, and J. A. Ritter, *J. Magn. Magn. Mater.*, 2005, **293**, 605.
52. M. Larimi, A. Ramiar, and A. Ranjbar, *J. Magn. Magn. Mater.*, 2014, **362**, 58.
53. J. A. Ritter, A. D. Ebner, K. D. Daniel, and K. L. Stewart, *J. Magn. Magn. Mater.*, 2004, **280**, 184.
54. O. Rotariu, and N. J. Strachan, *J. Magn. Magn. Mater.*, 2005, **293**, 639.
55. A. Boghi, F. Russo, and F. Gori, *J. Magn. Magn. Mater.*, 2017, **437**, 86.
56. S. Sharma, A. Gaur, U. Singh, and V. Katiyar, *Procedia Mater. Sci.*, 2015, **10**, 64.
57. S. Sharma, R. Kumar, and A. Gaur, *Procedia Mater. Sci.*, 2015, **10**, 44.
58. S. Sharma, V. Katiyar, and U. Singh, *J. Magn. Magn. Mater.*, 2015, **379**, 102.
59. A. Nacev, C. Beni, O. Bruno, and B. Shapiro, *Nanomedicine*, 2010, **5**, 1459.
60. M. Sheikholeslami, and S. Shehzad, *Int. J. Heat Mass Tran.*, 2017, **106**, 1261.
61. E. Tzirtzilakis, *Physica D*, 2008, **237**, 66.
62. T. Ishikawa, S. Oshima, and R. Yamane, *Fluid Dyn. Res.*, 2000, **26**, 35.
63. G.C. Shit, and S. Majee, *J. Magn. Magn. Mater.*, 2015, **388**, 106–115.
64. S. Nadeem, T. Hayat, N. S. Akbar, and M. Malik, *Int. J. Heat Mass Tran.*, 2009, **52**, 4722.
65. S. Ling, and H. Atabek, *J. Fluid Mech.*, 1972, **55**, 493.
66. K. S. Mekheimer, and M. El Kot, *Int. J. Nonlin. Mech.*, 2012, **47**, 927.

67. Lim, Y.-J. Lee, J.-H. Nam, S. Chung, and S. Shin, *J. Biomech.*, 2010, **43**, 546.

68. S. Majee, and G. Shit, *J. Magn. Magn. Mater.*, 2017, **424**, 137.

69. M. A. Ikbal, S. Chakravarty, and P. Mandal, *Int. J. Numer. Meth. Fl.*, 2011, **67**, 1655.

70. B. K. Holtzman, D. L. Kohlstedt, and J. P. Morgan, *J. Petrol.*, 2005, **46**, 2569.

71. H.-J. Steiger, Pathophysiology of Development and Rupture of Cerebral Aneurysms (Acta Neurochirurgica Supplementum 48), Springer-Verlag, Wien, 1990.

72. G.C. Shit, and S. Majee, *Int. J. Heat Fluid Flow*, 2018, **70**, 237–246.

73. A. M. Malek, S. L. Alper, and S. Izumo, *JAMA*, 1999, **282**, 2035.

74. R. Torii, M. Oshima, T. Kobayashi, K. Takagi, and T. E. Tezduyar, *Comput. Methods Appl. Mech. Eng.*, 2009, **198**, 3613.

75. G.C. Shit, and S. Majee, *Euro. J. Mech.-B Fluids*, 2018, **71**, 1–14.

76. S. Majee, and G.C. Shit, *Euro. J. Mech.-B Fluids*, 2020.

PART B
Radiofrequency Fields

Chapter 10
Safety Standards for MRI

Michael C. Steckner
Canon Medical Research USA, Inc., Mayfield Village, OH, USA

10.1 INTRODUCTION

Standards play a vital role in the development and regulatory approval process of an MRI scanner. While the word 'standard' is routinely and widely used, it has multiple and complex definitions. Additionally, the role by which standards support the range of needs, with the ultimate goal of safe medical equipment, is often unclear to those not involved in the creation, or use, of standards.

This review outlines how:

1. standards are used by equipment manufacturers to develop product that is widely recognized as safe to operate, safe for the patient, and safe for those in the vicinity of the equipment,
2. regulators use the same standards to ensure that product submissions contain information that supports marketing claims, thus ensuring that medical devices are safe and achieve their intended purpose,
3. standards are created, maintained, and updated, by consensus, to ensure appropriateness with respect to the latest widely accepted advances.

For the purposes of this chapter, there are two types of standards: 'documentary' and 'measurement'. The primary focus of this chapter is documentary standards, herein referred to as 'standards', and defined by National Institute of Standards and Technology (NIST) as 'written agreements containing technical specifications or other precise criteria that may contain rules, guidelines, or definitions of characteristics. Standards ensure that materials, products, personnel qualifications, processes, and services are: adequate for their purpose, compatible and/or interchangeable, if necessary; ensure public health and safety; protect the environment; and/or improve economic performance'. (NISTIR 7614, The ABC's of Standards Activities).

Measurement standards relate to devices, procedures, instruments, and other tools to define measurement units. The science of measurement is called metrology. While not the primary focus of this review, measurement standards are also integral to the execution of requirements specified in documentary standards because all quantitative measurements for regulatory purposes require the use of calibrated equipment, which implies traceability of calibration to reference measurement standards. Otherwise, the

Safety and Biological Effects in MRI.
Edited by Devashish Shrivastava and J. Thomas Vaughan
 ISBN: 978-1-118-82130-5
Also published in eMagRes (online edition)
DOI: 10.1002/9780470034590.emrstm1632

topic of measurement standards is out of scope for this chapter.

The purpose of this chapter is the brief summary of key MRI safety standards. However, to place the importance of those standards in context, the remainder of the introduction gives a brief outline of many aspects of standards: the structure of some standards used, the process by which standards are developed, and why standards are beneficial.

There are numerous organizations creating documentary standards. For the purposes of this chapter, it is useful to note that there are both national and international Standards Developing Organizations (SDOs). The details regarding the differences are outside the scope of this chapter. There are also national standards that are adaptations of international standards (e.g., American National Standards Institute/Association for the Advancement of Medical Instrumentation (ANSI/AAMI) 60601-1 derived from IEC 60601-1) and excellent national standards that have been widely adopted and reissued under international auspices (e.g., International Electrotechnical Commission (IEC) 62464-1 derived from several National Electrical Manufacturers Association/Medical Imaging and Technology Alliance (NEMA/MITA) MS standards). There are also instances of different SDOs, reflecting different areas of technical expertise, joining forces to develop a joint standard (e.g., ISO/IEC TS 10974 – *Assessment of the safety of magnetic resonance imaging for patients with an active implantable medical device*, which is not formally a standard at the time of this writing, but a 'technical specification (TS)'). This cursory outline of organizational details will help clarify the naming of some standards discussed in detail later in the chapter.

One example of national MRI standards are the NEMA/MITA 'MS' series. They were created in the early days of MRI to meet regulatory requirements of the US Food and Drug Administration (FDA) in bringing MRI devices to market. The earliest MRI scanners were brought to market by following the FDA's premarket approval (PMA) process (https://www.fda.gov/medical-devices/premarket-submissions/premarket-approval-pma). Later, it was determined that MRI scanners could be introduced to the market by following the comparatively less onerous 510(k) FDA premarket notification process provided, among other requirements, that standards would be available. To accelerate the development process, the already extant Nuclear Medicine NU standard was adapted. Currently, there are 10 active, 2 rescinded, and a new standard which has recently published. The standards define methods for measuring key attributes related to image quality (e.g., slice thickness MS-5) and safety (e.g., whole-body specific absorption rate (SAR) measurement, MS-8). While nominally national standards, they are widely used internationally as they can be or are referenced by IEC 60601-2-33. Significant elements of the MS image quality-related standards are also included in IEC 62464-1. Note that all the MS standards are freely available as pdf download from the NEMA website (www.nema.org), once a free account has been created.

One example of an international MRI standard is IEC 60601-2-33. It is the primary MRI safety standard used by all MR system manufacturers. It is one particular standard in a much larger family of standards discussed in detail below. While it is an international and widely used standard, not all regulators use the same interpretation. For example, the FDA maintains a 'Recognized Consensus Standards' webpage that identifies all standards that have gone through their recognition process. Using IEC 60601-2-33 edition 3.2 as an example, the FDA website, shows it to be a partially recognized standard (i.e., all parts of the standard are recognized except clause 201.12.4.101.3 pertaining to the notification on the user interface regarding normal mode operations, which is not recognized). Note that in the case of the FDA they consider all methods, standards, and different editions of standards, whether recognized or not, to evaluate medical devices. Using recognized standards considerably lowers burden for the submitter and FDA as additional data and/or scientific justification may be required to substantiate claims if unrecognized standards are used. Interpretation of standards by various regulators of the world is not identical; thus, the committee responsible for a given standard attempts to ensure that the intent of the standard is correctly described for those not present during the actual deliberations and writing. Even those present at the time of writing may not always agree on interpretation after publication. As a practical aside, all standards discussed in this chapter were originally written in English, sometimes with British spelling (e.g., IEC and ISO standards), and in all instances by committee with international representation, including the US-based national standards. Some standards organizations (e.g., IEC and ISO) translate the standards into other languages (e.g., French), and in some cases the translations may occur at the national level. For example, in Japan, IEC 60601-2-33 was translated by a member company of the Japan Medical Imaging and Radiological Systems Industries Association (JIRA).

Standards are often described as 'voluntary consensus standards' where the concept of consensus is described below. Not all standards are necessarily voluntary, but the clear majority are. For example, within the context of MRI safety, the author is unaware of any mandated safety standards. However, in the United States, CT scanners are legally mandated to follow the NEMA XR-29 dose reduction standard, by regulation.

A very broad overview of how standards are created and maintained helps the understanding of how standards remain relevant. The following description is a composite of various SDO procedures. It also helps explain how a standard integrates into the MR vendor and regulatory use process. First, a need for a standard for a given issue is established. Need can be established by a variety of paths. As noted above, MITA just published a new standard for assessing the surface temperature heating characteristics of a radio frequency (RF) coil. The need was established by the FDA because they observed a large variance in interpretation of the general guidelines found in the relevant standard (IEC 60601-1). The MR vendors associated with MITA, under MITA auspices, following MITA procedures, code of conduct, and ethics procedures, just completed a comprehensive standard. In other instances, vendors may identify the need for a standard in order to simplify the regulatory process of receiving marketing approval/clearance. One example is the joint effort between the MR manufacturers, as represented by IEC, and active implant manufacturers, as represented by ISO, to develop test methods whereby active implanted devices can be shown to have certain performance attributes. Formally, approval for a new standard is by a 'new work item proposal' (NWIP) process. In the case of ISO and IEC, committee membership is open to experts recognized by their accredited national Technical Advisory Group (TAG) peers and represent their national TAG in the committee. Experts are drawn from industry, regulators, academia, consulting organizations, etc. The output of this collaboration is ISO/IEC TS 10974. Note that TS 10974 is not formally a standard. A TS is a mechanism by which new concepts, potentially worthy of a standard, can be explored and developed. Once sufficient practical experience has been gained, and if the need still exists, a standard may be produced. For example, in the particular case of TS 10974, the committee work to produce a formal standard has recently been started. Once a standard is produced there is a formal review process. The number of stages, and those involved in the review process, is a function of the SDO and their obligations (e.g., World Trade Organization requirements). The review process is a critical stage in the development of the standard. The production of a standard itself assumes some high level of agreement among the committee members. The review process ensures that other experts from within the various national TAGs agree with the output, or are given the formal opportunity to vote on and provide comments that the standards committee must review and respond to. Thus, a standard is often referred to as a consensus document. Once a standard has published it must be maintained via a review/renew/revise/rescind decision cycle process. A schedule is established by which a standard is periodically reviewed (typically 5 years). The standard may be considered as still state of art and renewed, or it is revised, and goes through the comprehensive review process again. Alternatively, it may be determined that the standard is no longer necessary (e.g., no longer being used) and rescinded. A specified review cycle can also identify the interval within which it will not be modified (e.g., stability date).

The TS or standard is not the only mechanism for the release of useful guidance under IEC/ISO auspices. Before introducing the third mechanism, the technical report (TR), it is useful to understand that standards (and a TS) contain 'normative' and 'informative' (also called 'nonmandatory' in some standards) materials. The main value of a standard relates to the normative statements that require adherence to the methodology described within. Thus, the main body of a standard uses 'shall', e.g., must follow, -type instructions. Thus, the claim of voluntary compliance to any given standard is a claim to broadly following the 'shall' statements of the standard. In some situations, the novelty of the product in question may require adaptations of the standard for best application. There also are sections of the standard, typically in the annexes, with additional clarifying and supplemental materials that are intended to only be informative, not mandatory. However, some annexes are labeled as 'normative', and all text in the normative sections that start with 'Note:' are informative. The concept of 'normative' vs 'informative' is also a point of interpretation variation for some regulators. Some regulators tend to view all materials as normative. The TR is considered as only an informative document. For example, the TS 10974 committee could not find consensus, despite significant efforts, on a single method, or methods, for the quantification of uncertainty. The TR mechanism was used to provide general guidance on uncertainty principles (ISO/TR 21900) such that the two generalized methods discussed in committee (the so-called lumpers vs splitters approach where sources or uncertainty are aggregated or separately considered and summed) were both viewed as valid methods. This example also emphasizes the importance of consensus in the standards writing process. The author is aware of other examples, outside the scope of this MRI chapter, where the standards committee was unable to find consensus on important, but contentious, matters, and no guidance was provided in the standard or any other document.

Creating a standard can be a lengthy process. The ISO and IEC standards procedures have mechanisms for the correction of errors (corrigendum) and updates (amendments) to standards. The amendment process is particularly useful for issuing midcourse updates. Amendments are also subject to the review and voting process. Some SDOs issue amendments in either a fully integrated edition or as a standalone document which shows just the clause additions/deletions and alterations. Thus, when purchasing a standard it is important to determine which version to buy by confirming which edition, amendments, and corrigenda are in the file, and whether it is a redline version that shows you the changes with respect to a previous edition.

Standards bring many benefits. One example benefit for regulators worldwide is the ability to cite what is widely held to be the state-of-art appropriate requirements rather than attempt to recreate the necessary guidance at the national level. Adherence to known standards also helps regulators because they are familiar with the requirements and methodology due to their internal recognition process and regular use in submissions. One example benefit for the MR manufacturers is the simplification of the development and manufacture process such that in the ideal case, one product is acceptable by all regulators. In practice, that is not fully achieved because the interpretation of an international standard can vary between national regulators. Additionally, there are some national adaptations of standards, and the MR manufacturer either complies with the national requirements or demonstrates that the product simultaneously meets all requirements. There have also been instances where the adoption rate of an international standard varies across the world, and thus a product must simultaneously meet both old and new requirements for some transition time. In practice, all MR manufacturers likely implement some form of country-specific product because of language and mains (power) supply differences, etc.

Careful reading of standards will reveal instances where requirements are deliberately unspecified. Within the complicated web of standards and regulations, it is possible that another document could claim the authority to define requirements. Two examples follow. First, the MR safety standard IEC 60601-2-33 specifies acoustic noise limits for the patient because there are no regulatory limits. Also, there are no acoustic noise limits defined for the worker in IEC 60601-2-33 because there are other regulations regarding occupational exposure. Thus, there are references to 'local regulation' where appropriate and also to the 'responsible organization', which is defined as the accountable entity for the use and maintenance of the equipment. These concepts attempt to transfer ownership of details as appropriate. This also, in part, explains why some items are not in a standard. The second example relates to ISO/TS 10974. In the hierarchy of active implanted devices, it is a 'horizontal' standard providing generalized testing methods ideally appropriate to a wide range of active implanted devices. However, certain subclasses of active implants (e.g., cardiac versus neurological devices) may have subtle test variations best handled by the appropriate 'vertical' standard. Thus, requirements are likely not generalizable to all active implants, but to a particular implant class or a marketing claim specific to a particular make and model, to be negotiated with the regulators. The TS 10974 example is further complicated by the fact that almost no vertical standards have yet been published and that for certain classes of active implanted devices may never exist if the market segment is too small to sustain the necessary standards development effort.

Note that standards use the International System of Units (SI). In one case related to spatial field gradients (SFG), non-SI units are used for historical reasons. In this case there has been a recent push to publish in both units in order to eliminate any error when converting from one unit set to the other.

Lastly, standards do not exist for all needs such as a newly emerging 'electrical medical equipment' device concept or a new product development (e.g., parallel transmit). In such cases, standards that are similar are used with the necessary adaptations or extensions appropriate for the particular item. In some cases, scientific publications may exist that present methods that are generally accepted as an appropriate measurement procedure. It can be reasonably expected that regulators will require a higher level of justification in these situations. Some regulators may even be available prior to formal submission to discuss what might be appropriate justification regardless of whether a new product development or clarification of how existing standards will be interpreted for the particular application.

10.2 CLARIFYING SOME KEY SAFETY TERMS

In the world of standards there is a vast collection of terms with specific definitions. A few of them are defined in this section, a few are defined later in this document as it is the raison d'être of the particular standard (e.g., F2503 – Standard Practice for Marking Medical Devices and Other Items for Safety in the Magnetic Resonance Environment) being discussed.

It is the purpose of this chapter to discuss the role of standards in patient safety. Thus, it is appropriate to outline key safety-related terms. Note that the actual formal definitions are not all provided here because within some definitions are yet more defined terms. The definitions provided here may not be complete but illustrate the key concepts.

It is first necessary to define safety. Regarding the IEC 60601 family of standards, which is outlined later in this chapter, the start of every standard title is 'Particular requirements for the basic safety and essential performance of… ' Safety is divided into two components: 'basic safety' and 'essential performance'. Consider an MRI scanner as 'medical electrical (ME) equipment'. There is the highly unlikely possibility that the patient or operator could be electrically shocked, like any other piece of electrical equipment, or pinched while the patient table is moving. Those are aspects of basic safety. Additionally, consider a unique aspect of the MRI scanner vital to its clinical operation, such as the RF transmit chain. Consider the patient safety implications if some highly unlikely system failure caused the RF amplifier to apply continuous full power. All MR scanners have mechanisms to detect such faults and stop this unsafe condition nearly instantly. The patient is safe in this so-called single fault condition. Now further speculate that the protective mechanism also failed. An extremely unlikely double fault condition has occurred for which there might not be an additional protective mechanism. At that point, essential performance has been lost because the risk has reached a level determined to be unacceptable by the manufacturer.

Note that the above definition of safety used the concept of risk. An important standard for risk management is ISO 14971 – *Medical devices – Application of risk management to medical devices*. Excerpting some key definitions:

Safety: freedom from unacceptable risk,
Risk: combination of the probability of occurrence of harm and the severity of that harm,
Harm: physical injury or damage to the health of people, or damage to property or the environment.

Thus, it is explicitly recognized that one cannot be perfectly safe. ISO 14971 provides tools by which manufacturers determine the necessary performance levels noted above. It is useful to note here that the role of regulators (and the FDA mission statement specifically) is the 'responsib[ility] for protecting the public health by ensuring the safety, efficacy, and security of human and veterinary drugs, biological products, and medical devices'. With regard to MRI scanners, the so-called 510(k) process is used by the MR system vendors. The FDA does not regulate the practice of medicine. Thus, a physician in consultation with the patient can use medical devices in ways not intended by the MR vendors, with potentially higher levels of risk, but to the benefit of the patient. This is the so-called off-label use of a device, which device vendors cannot support.

10.3 ASTM INTERNATIONAL STANDARDS

There are five published ASTM standards related to MRI safety, four methods addressing hazards plus one regarding MRI safety labeling. An additional new document is under development. The general focus of the ASTM standards pertaining to MRI is the safety of implants when in the MR environment. At the time of this writing, several of the standards are in their regularly scheduled review process. Thus, additional commentary is provided on current progress. A clear distinction is made between what is presently in the standard and what is being debated for the next edition. There is no guarantee that the debate commentary provided here will publish as suggested.

ASTM F2052 – Standard Test Method for Measurement of Magnetically Induced Displacement Force on Medical Devices in the Magnetic Resonance Environment.

ASTM F2213 – Standard Test Method for Measurement of Magnetically Induced Torque on Medical Devices in the Magnetic Resonance Environment.

F2052 and F2213, respectively, measure the displacement force and torque on an implant. A discussion on these two standards is presented elsewhere in this book.

ASTM F2119 – Standard Test Method for Evaluation of MR Image Artifacts from Passive Implants.

F2119 assesses the artifact generated by a device, immersed in a solution that mimics an average, homogenized in vivo electromagnetic environment, beside a reference object known to cause no distortions, with a spin echo (SE) and gradient recalled echo (GRE) sequence. Two images are acquired for each of the three orthogonal directions in both of the read/phase orientations: one with both objects and another image with just the reference object, using the SE sequence. An additional gradient echo image set is acquired in the worst case orientation identified by the SE images. The artifact is quantified by measuring the size of the distortion zone as defined in the standard. This standard is useful for informing users regarding the expected dimensions of artifacts around the device, where the images obtained using an SE and/or GRE-based sequences may be adversely affected.

The present review and revision cycle is considering the introduction of computational analysis, and the experimental component will consider updating the MR sequences used to quantify artifact size.

ASTM F2182 – Standard Test Method for Measurement of Radio Frequency Induced Heating On or Near Passive Implants during Magnetic Resonance Imaging.

The RF fields of an MRI are capable of inducing significant heating on or near conductive implants. This test method provides a way to quantify the heating. The dimensions of a test phantom and the appropriate, body average characteristics of the phantom filling media are specified. An experimental method is described for positioning and instrumenting the device under test. The experimental results may be used together with an appropriate whole-body computational model to scale measured heating to estimate tissue heating.

The intent of the present review and revision cycle is to improve the accuracy of the test and provide guidance on the assessment of uncertainty.

F2503 – Standard Practice for Marking Medical Devices and Other Items for Safety in the Magnetic Resonance Environment.

F2503 is perhaps the most well known of the five standards because it concerns the marking of devices. It is also mirrored internationally via IEC 62570. It is the source of the 'MR Conditional', 'MR Safe', and 'MR Unsafe' definitions, and symbols, and points to other standards used to characterize the item to be labeled.

MR Conditional – 'an item with demonstrated safety in the MR environment within defined conditions. At a minimum, address the conditions of the static magnetic field, the switched gradient magnetic field and the radiofrequency fields. Additional conditions, including specific configurations of the item, may be required.'

MR Safe – 'an item that poses no known hazards resulting from exposure to any MR environment. MR Safe items are composed of materials that are electrically nonconductive, nonmetallic, and nonmagnetic.'

MR Unsafe – 'an item which poses unacceptable risks to the patient, medical staff, or other persons within the MR environment.'

In clinical practice, there is a vast array of MR Conditional labels. Understanding and correctly executing all these labels is turning into a challenge for many implants. In addition to the considerable time required for MRI system operators to identify the specific model of implant, and acquire the correct device documentation, a lot of time is required to thoroughly understand the MR Conditional limits and develop a scanning protocol that meets requirements. There are numerous instances of different labels prescribing the same limits or actions in very different ways because there is no standardization (e.g., gradient slew rate limits). There are also labels that are scientifically and technically accurate but impossible for the operator to act on because the required information to implement such labeling is not provided by the MR manufacturers to the users (e.g., defining gradient slew rate in units of tesla per second).

F2503 is presently undergoing a major revision at the time of this writing. An exceptional effort is underway involving active and passive device implants and MR vendors, the FDA, other regulators, and representatives of Society for MR Radiographers & Technologists (SMRT), physicians, and consultants to improve label interpretation by standardizing the labeling information. By coordinating labeling practices, the confidence in label interpretation is improved with hopefully a simultaneous reduction of misinterpretation.

WK58852 – Standard Guide for Assessing the Safety of Nonimplanted Items in the MR Environment.

This document considers the implications of ancillary passive and active equipment brought into the MR magnet room (e.g., MRI syringe pump, additional monitoring equipment, and IV pole) but outside the bore of the scanner. The basic questions relate to (i) safety of the device with respect to projectile hazard, (ii) the effect of MRI environment on the functioning of the device, and (iii) the impact the presence and functioning of the ancillary equipment on the MRI (e.g., additional noise in image). Closely associated with those questions are the appropriate instructions for use (IFU) with respect to possible restrictions on main magnetic field, permissible closeness to the magnet covers, etc. This working committee is tasked with investigating these items and the possibility of developing test methods.

10.4 IEC STANDARDS

The primary focus of this chapter section is IEC 60601-2-33 *Particular requirements for the basic safety and essential performance of magnetic resonance equipment for medical diagnosis*, often referred to as 'the MR safety standard', presently in edition 3.2. However, proper coverage requires an explanation of the surrounding hierarchy of standards. IEC has promulgated a series of standards based on the 'general' standard IEC 60601-1 *Medical electrical equipment – Part 1: General requirements for basic safety and essential performance*. It is further extended by a series of 'collateral' and 'particular' standards that delve into specific topics in detail. Collateral standards are those that cover an important topic relevant to many different types of ME equipment (e.g., implications of electromagnetic disturbances). Particular standards focus on specific types of ME equipment (e.g., MRI). Collateral standards are coded as IEC 60601-1-X, and particular standards are identified as IEC 60601-2-Y. Presently, there are about 10 collateral and 60 particular standards. Focusing on the particular standards, the structure of the documents tends to parallel the general standard. This enables the 'addition', 'replacement', and 'amendment' of general, or collateral, standard text by the particular standard as necessary. For example, MRI requires its own specific set of terms and definitions and thus constitute an addition to the 'terms and definitions' section of the general standard. An example of a replacement are the unique attributes of MRI 'audible acoustic energy' and how it is managed. Amendment, which also includes deletions, examples relate to limiting the scope of application of some portion (e.g., clause) of the standard or deleting unnecessary normative references, deleting specific elements in a clause etc. Thus, while the MR safety standard reads as a coherent and complete document, in detailed application, the context of the full IEC 60601 family of standards needs to be understood.

Regarding IEC 60601-2-33, a high-level summary of the document would be:

1. the IFU,
2. the technical description of the MR equipment,
3. how to protect against the hazardous outputs,
4. the methods for demonstrating compliance with requirements.

The first two items are the core of the 'accompanying documents' (e.g., manuals) which are considered as part of the ME equipment. Their intent is '...to promote the safe use of medical electrical equipment during its expected service life'. These accompanying documents '... shall specify any special skills, training and knowledge required of the intended operator or the responsible organization and any restrictions on locations or environments in which the medical electrical equipment can be used'. As defined in the general standard, *the 'responsible organization' is the 'entity accountable for the use and maintenance of [the] medical electrical equipment ... '*. Therefore, these are important documents for ensuring that equipment is installed and operated correctly. The last two items are the guidance to the manufacturer on what protection the patient requires and how the manufacturer demonstrates the outputs are functioning properly. Together, these four key items represent a substantial portion of IEC 60601-2-33 and are discussed in greater detail below.

Please note that many of the quotes have been slightly modified from the original text in two ways:

1. defined terms in IEC/ISO standards are capitalized. Those have been removed to improve readability,

2. Some definitions use acronyms (e.g., ME = medical electrical) and are written out here to improve readability.

Also, all comments here relate to edition 3.2 unless otherwise specifically noted as current points of discussion for edition 4.0. In case of edition 4.0 discussion points, the final standard may differ.

10.4.1 The MR System Instructions for Use

The IFU is expected to '... list all system messages, error messages, and fault messages that are generated related to safety concerns unless these messages are self-explanatory'. The MR safety standard itemizes 24 separate items, each with its own set of requirements. They are:

(a) Prescreening of the patient and the MR worker
(b) Medical supervision of patients
(c) Emergency medical procedures
(d) Exposure of the patient and MR worker to excessive acoustic noise
(e) Controlled access area
(f) Liquid and gaseous cryogens
(g) Operating modes
(h) Exposure of the patient and MR worker to the static magnetic field
(i) Exposure of the patient to time-varying magnetic fields
(j) Exposure of the patient to RF magnetic fields
(k) Occupational exposure to electromagnetic fields (EMF)
(l) Auxiliary equipment
(m) Emergency field shut down unit
(n) Fire precautions
(o) Artifacts
(p) Recommended training
(q) Quality assurance
(r) Maintenance
(s) Emergency actions in case of a quench
(t) Scanning of patients with active or passive implants
(u) Scanning of pregnant patients
(v) Scanning of patients with elevated body core temperature
(w) About function
(x) FPO (fixed parameter option)

Space does not permit a summary of all 24 items. Only a few items are discussed here.

10.4.1.1 e) Controlled Access Area

The commonly used terminology for access areas derives from the American College of Radiology (ACR) guidance document: Zone I, II, and III, and were derived from the MR safety standard (IEC 60601-2-33). The controlled access area is approximately equivalent to Zone II and III. It is the '*area around the MR system, to which access is controlled for safety reasons to prevent harm from the magnetic field*'. The controlled access area marks, but does not have to be a hard barrier, the 5 G (0.5 mT) line.

While outside the scope of this section, the reader who is familiar with the ACR Zone concept may be puzzled by the omission of Zone IV in the above explanation. While not a strict equivalent, Zone IV is approximately equivalent to the so-called Special Environment, which is defined in IEC 60601-1-2 '*General requirements for basic safety and essential performance – Collateral Standard: Electromagnetic disturbances – Requirements and tests*'.

10.4.1.2 t) Scanning of Patients with Active or Passive Implants

In the past, the scanning of patients with implants was generally considered unsafe. However, with the emergence of testing methods that characterize interactions between implants and the magnetic field outputs of an MR scanner, and new implant technical developments, a new class of MR Conditional implants has motivated changes in the MR safety standard. At the present time, patients with implants are contraindicated for scanning, unless the implant is labeled as MR Safe or MR Conditional, with the later indication accompanied by instructions to the MR system operator on scanner operating constraints. These changes occurred in 't' and has motivated the new sections 'w' and 'x'.

10.4.1.3 w) About Function

Increasingly, implants are using MR conditions that require knowledge of the particular make and model of scanner. Sub-clause 'w' requires the MR manufacturers to make available, on the user interface, the location of and/or the actual information regarding:

- the nominal B_0 value of the scanner,
- the maximum SFG of the scanner outside the fixed covers,

- the maximum spatial encoding gradient amplitude and slew rate,
- the nominal frequency range per nuclei, and
- the maximum combined gradient output at specific locations.

By making the information more readily available, accuracy and speed of label interpretation should improve.

The use of the word nominal seems to cause some confusion. A nominal 3 T scanner may be exactly 2.9 T in the imaging volume and >3 T elsewhere around the magnet. It is intended that the implant vendors using this value understand the variability across MR systems. This likewise also impacts frequency computations. Part of the confusion relates to how the implant label is written and interpreted, for example the mathematical implied specificity of a statement such as <3 T.

10.4.1.4 x) FPO (Fixed Parameter Option)

The FPO was introduced to enable a simplified approach to the scanning of implants. By negotiation between the MR and active implant vendors, a set of RF pulse (peak and rms) and gradient dB/dt (peak and rms) limit values were selected that represented a compromise on state of implant design and technology and the need to provide a clinically useful scanner performance, which was defined to be approximately equivalent to normal mode scanning. The concept, first introduced at 1.5 T as FPO:B (B = basic), was intended to simplify the interpretation of MR Conditional labels. Implants so labeled would then cause the MR operator to, during the patient registration process, select FPO:B and thereby constrain the scanner outputs to the agreed limits. It would still be necessary for the MR operator to comply with other MR Conditional requirements (e.g., landmark exclusions), but the intent was a simplified process that minimized the likelihood of MR operator error if all the control parameters had been manually entered. The concept as defined has not yet been implemented by any of the MR manufacturers, and only a relatively few implants have been labeled to FPO:B. However, the understanding, definitions, and limit values have been helpful in establishing an alternate solution where the MR operator enters the MR Conditional limits, thus allowing more design flexibility for the implant vendors. It is a topic of current debate whether the static FPO:B should be further enhanced with some form of 'MR Conditional control'.

10.4.2 Technical Description

It is necessary to provide technical details regarding the MR scanner in order to install it and use it safely. There are six subsections to this portion of the standard of which only the most commonly cited section is discussed here.

The 'compatibility technical specification sheet' identifies those elements that must be provided. Well-known examples are the position of the specified isomagnetic contours (e.g., 5 G line) and locations outside the fixed magnet covers of maximum $\boldsymbol{B}_0$, SFG, and the so-called force product $\boldsymbol{B}_0$*SFG.

10.4.3 Protection against Hazardous Outputs

The MR scanner is capable of several hazardous outputs that can be characterized as electrical, mechanical, etc. Within those broad categories are some of the following more commonly discussed MRI hazards:

1. Acoustic noise,
2. Gradient subsystem,
3. RF subsystem,
4. Static magnetic fields ($\boldsymbol{B}_0$).

At the highest level of abstraction are the absolute limits that are deemed appropriate. In some cases these limits are defined in the MR safety standard or are specified elsewhere. There is the additional long-established concept of outputs levels that are considered to be physiologically stress free, or not. The formal definitions from IEC 60601-2-33 are given below and are only used with regard to the field outputs of an MR scanner, not the acoustic noise levels:

NORMAL OPERATING MODE: *mode of operation of the MR equipment in which none of the outputs have a value that can cause physiological stress to patients.*

FIRST-LEVEL-CONTROLLED OPERATING MODE: *mode of operation of the MR equipment in which one or more outputs reach a value that can cause physiological stress to patients, which needs to be controlled by medical supervision.*

SECOND-LEVEL-CONTROLLED OPERATING MODE: *mode of operation of the MR equipment in which one or more outputs reach a value that can produce significant risk for patients, for which explicit ethical approval is required (i.e., a human studies protocol approved to local requirements).*

With regard to gradient field outputs, the first-level mode is defined to start at 80% of the first-level limits and is approximately the likely lowest levels at which the most sensitive patients may perceive peripheral nerve stimulation. The array of limits on RF outputs are categorized by body region and duration of exposure, and full discussion is outside the scope of this chapter. There is no simple explanation of how the normal vs first-level limits are derived, and the reader is directed to IEC 60601-2-33 for the limit tables. Lastly, $\boldsymbol{B}_0$ operations above 3 T, not to exceed 8 T, are considered in the first-level mode.

Note that the definition for first-level operations calls for medical supervision, which is defined as:

> *adequate medical management of patients who can be at risk from some parameters of exposure to the MR equipment, either because of the medical condition of the patient, the levels of exposure or a combination.*

The medical supervision does not always require a physician but does expect risk/benefit analysis and decisions regarding the appropriate level of monitoring.

10.4.4 Demonstrating Compliance with Requirements

Formal methods are required so that users of the standard can demonstrate that they are meeting the output limit requirements. The methods are either within the standard or a reference provided to some other standard (e.g., references to NEMA/MITA standards).

10.5 ISO STANDARDS

There are no ISO MRI safety standards, but there are many ISO standards that are routinely used by the MR system vendors and ISO standards for implantable device manufacturers that directly relate to MRI safety. The previously mentioned ISO 14971 is one example of a standard routinely used by MR system vendors to assist risk management decisions but is not an MRI-specific standard.

Perhaps the most significant ISO document related to MR safety is the previously mentioned TS 10974 – '*Assessment of the safety of magnetic resonance imaging for patients with an active implantable medical device*'. With the advent of new technologies and engineering tools, active implant vendors have developed a new generation of products whose recipients' can be safely scanned in an MRI under a specific set of clearly defined scan conditions (e.g., $\boldsymbol{B}_0$ field strength and acceptable SAR restrictions). TS 10974 provides a series of test methods that can be used to establish appropriate MRI scan conditions in conjunction with risk management analysis, etc. Table 10.1, from Table 1 in TS 10974, identifies the general hazards present in the MR environment when an active implant is present and the test(s) necessary to assess the active implant and the associated test clause.

A final clause 18 also discusses 'Markings and accompanying documentation' to inform the patient,

Table 10.1. Potential patient hazards and corresponding test methods

General hazard	Test method	Clause
Heat	RF field-induced heating of the AIMD	8
	Gradient field-induced device heating	9
Vibration	Gradient field-induced vibration	10
Force	$\boldsymbol{B}_0$-induced force	11
Torque	$\boldsymbol{B}_0$-induced torque	12
Unintended stimulation	Gradient field-induced lead voltage (extrinsic electric potential)	13
	RF field-induced rectified lead voltage	15
Malfunction	$\boldsymbol{B}_0$ field-induced device malfunction	14
	RF field-induced device malfunction	15
	Gradient field-induced device malfunction	16
	Combined fields test	17

implanting physician, radiologist, and technologist/radiographer about their MR Conditional active implant.

The first and second editions of TS 10974 focused exclusively on 1.5 T scanners. Presently, the second edition is being extensively revised to become a full standard and will include updates for evaluating devices in 3 T MRI scanners. Note that several active implant device vendors already have 3 T approved devices on the market using methods adapted from TS 10974. At the present time there are no plans for developing test methods for open MRI or 7 T scanners.

An equivalent document does not exist from any SDO for passive implants, but several of the previously mentioned ASTM standards and elements of TS 10974 are being used.

10.6 NEMA/MITA STANDARDS

This last section presents the NEMA/MITA standards. Of the 11 available standards, 7 are related to image-quality assessments, and the following are related to MR safety:

MS-4 Acoustic Noise Measurement Procedure for Diagnostic Magnetic Resonance Imaging Devices.
MS-8 Characterization of the Specific Absorption Rate for Magnetic Resonance Imaging Systems.
MS-10 Determination of Local Specific Absorption Rate (SAR) in Diagnostic Magnetic Resonance Imaging.
MS-14 Characterization of RF Coil Heating in Magnetic Resonance Imaging Systems.

These standards are discussed below.

10.6.1 MS-4 Acoustic Noise Measurement Procedure for Diagnostic Magnetic Resonance Imaging Devices

MS-4 describes two methods for characterizing the acoustic noise output of an MR scanner. These measurements support analysis requirements found in IEC 60601-2-33 regarding minimum sufficient hearing protection. The two measurement methods are:

MGAN – maximum gradient acoustic noise.
MCAN – maximum clinical acoustic noise.

MGAN provides a method for determining the maximum possible noise output level of the MR scanner when driven with the worst case gradient waveform, inclusive of system-limiting protections. While clinically unachievable in practice, the method should find the maximum possible output. MCAN uses the worst case clinical sequence under worst case sequence parameters permitted by the sequence adjustment software. In practice, it is difficult to know exactly which sequence and parameter set is worst case. Thus, it cannot be claimed with certainty that the measured results are the worst possible clinical exposure but are presumed to be close. The results of one of the measurements are to be reported.

MS-4 is presently being revised. Current discussions focus on three topics:

1. The latest generation of more powerful gradients requires a simple revision to the MGAN search algorithm to ensure finding the worst case condition.
2. There are a profusion of general acoustic measurement standards, nearly 200 from ISO alone, including a standard on drafting test codes (ISO 12001). Given the output of MS-4 is required by an IEC standard, it is important to ensure the standard is correct.
3. There is a growing use of MRI systems for interventional procedures, and thus a need to make measurements suitable for the characterization of occupational exposures close to the scanner covers. One of the challenges will be defining what constitutes an appropriate scanner output for such measurements and likely not MGAN or MCAN.

10.6.2 MS-8 Characterization of the Specific Absorption Rate for Magnetic Resonance Imaging Systems

MS-8 measures whole-body SAR inside volume RF transmit coils assumed to produce relatively homogeneous RF fields by either of a pulse-energy or calorimetric method. MS-8 recently completed a major rewrite that considers the challenges of SAR measurements at 3 T and in large aperture systems where RF field nonuniformity can become significant. Requirements for system loading were preserved for continuity purposes, but additional flexibility on how to demonstrate that the load is equivalent to a 50–90 kg human was included. Additional information was provided to improve the quality of results such as an insulation time constant recommendation for calorimetry and how to make use of flux loops.

10.6.3 MS-10 Determination of Local Specific Absorption Rate (SAR) in Diagnostic Magnetic Resonance Imaging

MS-10 is an infrequently used standard that requires major work to update for advances in MR system technology. An update will be beneficial given the growing realization that local thermal damage is the relevant safety concern. There are numerous reports of local tissue damage, whereas it is believed there are no known cases of systemic thermal overload. Thus, it appears that all the SAR limits are presently acting as some form of local SAR control.

In current configuration, the standard outlines how to make a tissue equivalent phantom and how to measure the results. Temperature probes are then positioned at SAR hotspots, as determined by thermal camera, modeling, etc. SAR is then determined from the initial slope of the temperature curve.

10.6.4 MS-14 Characterization of RF Coil Heating in Magnetic Resonance Imaging Systems

MR manufacturers are obligated to test all coils to confirm that patients are not exposed to contact temperatures above 41 °C, as required by IEC 60601-1. 41 °C is a safe, long duration contact temperature that does not require justification. The temperature is determined under normal worst case operating conditions, at the location of worst case heating, after sufficient time has elapsed to ensure that the temperature has reached near steady state (rate of temperature increase of less than 2 °C over 1 h). Additionally, the FDA requires MR manufacturers to test detachable coils in the 'unplugged' condition to avoid harmful heating. This is a unique example of a codified 'single fault condition'. Typically, medical equipment vendors are expected to define which single fault conditions need to be considered.

The standard focuses the standard coils in clinical use today, both imaging and spectroscopy, but it is recognized that the methods could form the basis for testing other coils presently not in scope. A method is provided for configuring the coil and system for worst case exposure with respect to air flow, pads, coil position, etc. Instructions are also given on how to set the appropriate power levels for testing based on a theory of operation that accounts for B1 shimming. Provision is also made for 'overtesting' the power levels to accelerate a test that can take many hours. A test methodology is also provided for the various types of coils. One of the key features is the necessity of a prescreen procedure for identifying the worst case heating locations and how to determine the thermal time constant of the material for overtesting purposes. A methodology is also provided for analyzing the data and the coil to ensure that the coil meets safety requirements. A coil must not exceed the allowable temperature for the current or next patient and must pass a posttest coil condition inspection. A coil is permitted to fail in order to protect the patient on next use. By these assessments, it can be determined if a coil passes or fails the test. It is beneficial from both the regulatory and manufacturer's perspective if a test method can be reduced to pass/fail criterion.

10.7 CONCLUSION

This brief introduction to selected key standards in MRI safety demonstrates the utility of standards, how they are created and used, and outlines some of the key materials found within various standards. There are significant challenges in writing a standard that can be understood by readers not involved in the writing of a standard. There are additional challenges in writing a standard that covers a wide range of possible hardware platforms yet provides a result that shares recognizably common attributes across all MRI system vendors in order that concepts, training, terminology, etc. can be shared or reused by all MR system operators and thus promote MR safety.

Chapter 11

On the Choice of RF Safety Metric in MRI: Temperature, SAR, or Thermal Dose

Devashish Shrivastava

In Vivo Temperatures, LLC, Burnsville, MN, USA

11.1 INTRODUCTION

Magnetic resonance imaging (MRI) requires depositing radiofrequency (RF) power to the human body. This RF power is absorbed nonuniformly and together with nonuniform thermal properties and blood flow results in nonuniform tissue heating. The possibility of producing hot 'spots' or hot 'regions' of tissue along with systemic heating,[1–7] which, in turn, may induce local, regional, or systemic adverse effects is a safety concern. Therefore, a reliable and robust RF safety metric is needed to avoid or limit RF heating-induced thermogenic hazards in MRI.

Safety and Biological Effects in MRI.
Edited by Devashish Shrivastava and J. Thomas Vaughan
 ISBN: 978-1-118-82130-5
Also published in eMagRes (online edition)
DOI: 10.1002/9780470034590.emrstm1584

Thermogenic hazards are related to the absolute temperature as well as temperature–time history. Specific absorption rate (SAR) is related to the temperature and temperature–time history through thermal properties and a blood flow-related parameter.[7,8] Thus, absolute temperature, SAR, and temperature–time history-based model all three seem appropriate for a choice as a safety metric. This chapter briefly reviews the challenges associated with each of these three approaches in ensuring RF safety and possible solution strategies to overcome the challenges.

11.2 TEMPERATURE AS AN RF SAFETY METRIC

International Commission on Non-Ionizing Radiation Protection (ICNIRP) in its 1998 report[9] attributed '*a large number of physiological effects*' in cellular and animal systems to the rise of body temperature in excess of 1–2 °C. These effects included 'alterations in neural and neuromuscular functions; increased blood–brain barrier permeability; ocular impairment (lens opacities and corneal abnormalities); stress-associated changes in the immune system; hematological changes; reproductive changes (e.g., reduced sperm production); teratogenicity; and changes in cell morphology, water and electrolyte content, and membrane functions'. Such findings became the basis for limiting the local and core body temperature change to less than 0.5 °C in the Normal Mode and less than 1 °C in the First Level during MRI.[10] Limits for the absolute temperature were set to ≤39 °C in the Normal Mode and ≤40 °C in the First Level for local and systemic temperatures, respectively, to allow imaging febrile patients, when needed. Note that the normal core body temperature in humans is ~37 °C.

Determining local and systemic in vivo temperatures noninvasively is challenging. One could envision two possible ways – using endogenous magnetic resonance thermometry (MRT) and using a validated thermal model. Measuring in vivo temperatures reliably and robustly, using endogenous MRT with sufficient accuracy and precision (~0.1–0.2 °C to be able to detect the change of 0.5–1.0 °C), has yet to be realized due to the motion and susceptibility-related artifacts. For more on the endogenous MRT methods and their limitations to measure in vivo temperatures, interested readers are encouraged to refer to the material presented elsewhere in this chapter.[7]

Predicting in vivo temperatures by solving an appropriate thermal model (also called the bioheat transfer model) is another approach. Any such model needs to be developed based on first principles and appropriately validated to predict reliable temperatures. This is so since lack of a rigorous first principles-based development makes it hard to directly relate model parameters to underlying physiology, causing confusion and discontent regarding the interpretation of the results. Lack of an appropriate validation makes the results unreliable. As an example, the two models that were used in the past to determine the current safety thresholds of 10 g average as well as whole-head and -body average SAR (i.e., the two-node model of Adair and Berglund[11,12] and an arbitrarily simplified version of the Pennes' bioheat transfer equation[13]) have been shown to underestimate local and/or systemic tissue heating for a given SAR.[3,4] In addition, the lack of a formal rigorous derivation of the Pennes model has, in the past, made the interpretation of the model parameters and results ambiguous. For more on how to develop an appropriate bioheat model for a given application, interested readers may refer to the material presented in Ref. 7.

First principles-based derivation allows model parameters to be directly correlated to the underlying physiology to develop better, deeper understanding. Appropriate validation using humans or human-relevant animal models (i.e., animal models with thermoregulatory mechanisms and thermal properties comparable to humans) allows the model to predict reliable temperatures. Generic bioheat transfer model (GBHTM) is one such model framework.[7] The GBHTM has been derived from first principles and validated to predict systemic as well as local temperature changes for 3, 7, and 9.4 T MRI applications using human-sized swine (i.e., swine of ~50–100 kg).[3–5,8] The framework has been helpful in reinterpreting Pennes' bioheat transfer equation and relating Pennes' empirical parameters to physiology.[7,8] The GBHTM has also been shown to predict relatively more accurate local and systemic temperature changes compared to the Pennes' equation.[3,4,7] Another example of the GBHTM's ability to predict reliable systemic in vivo temperature changes in humans is presented in Table 11.1. Please note that since exact experimental conditions, in which the following data have been collected, are unknown, the simulations were performed assuming natural convective heat loss.

Table 11.1 presents the mass (M), height (H), whole-body average SAR, heating duration (HD), starting core temperature as measured in the tympanic membrane ($T_{core,start}$), and change in the core temperature after the exposure as measured ($dT_{core,meas}$) and as predicted by the GBHTM ($dT_{core,sim}$) in 11 healthy subjects in 1.5 T. The experimental data (i.e., the first seven columns in Table 11.1) are taken from Table 11.2 of Ref. 14. The parameters such as M, H, SAR, HD, and $T_{core,start}$ were used as inputs to the GBHTM to predict $dT_{core,sim}$. Each simulation took <30 s.

Two main observations are made from Table 11.1. First, in general, the temperature change predicted by the GBHTM is comparable to the measured change (bold). The values predicted by the GBHTM are slightly larger but within the typical standard deviation and/or error of the fluoroptic and infrared (IR)-based thermometry probes (i.e., ~0.1–0.2 °C) and the uncertainty related to the quantification of the 'true' deposited whole-body average SAR (~20%). The exact experimental conditions are unknown to further improve the modeled predictions. For example, the type of temperature probes used and the time when the measurements were taken are unknown. In other words, it is not known if the measurements were taken using fluoroptic probes or IR probes and if the measurements were taken continuously or if the subject was pulled out and the measurements were taken after the subject came out of the bore. If the subject is pulled out, it gives the body some time to cool off before the measurements are taken, possibly explaining the lower measured temperature. Also, details of

Table 11.1. Table 11.1 presents the mass (M), height (H), whole-body average SAR (SAR), heating duration (HD), starting core temperature as measured in the tympanic membrane ($T_{core,start}$), and change in the core temperature after the exposure as measured ($dT_{core,meas}$) and as predicted by the GBHTM ($dT_{core,sim}$) in 11 healthy subjects in 1.5 T. The experimental data (i.e., the first seven columns in Table 11.1) are taken from Table 11.2 of reference 14. The parameters such as M, H, SAR, HD, and $T_{core,start}$ were used as inputs to the GBHTM to predict $dT_{core,sim}$. Each simulation took <30 s

Patient No.	M (kg)	H (m)	SAR (W kg^{-1})	HD (s)	$T_{core,\ start}$ (°C)	$dT_{core,meas}$ (°C)	$dT_{core,sim}$ (°C)
1	76	1.76	4.24	660	37.4	NA[a]	0.7–0.8
2	**80**	**1.8**	**4.28**	**900**	**36.9**	**0.7**	**1.0–1.1**
3	**82**	**1.82**	**4.31**	**900**	**36.2**	**0.9**	**1.0–1.1**
4	**95**	**1.92**	**4.3**	**900**	**36.5**	**0.9**	**1.0–1.1**
5	**90**	**1.7**	**4.24**	**900**	**36.4**	**0.7**	**1.0–1.1**
6	**95**	**1.88**	**4.26**	**900**	**36.8**	**0.9**	**1.0–1.1**
7	106	1.91	4.15	900	36.4	0.5	1.0
8	*96*	*1.97*	*4.26*	*300*	*36.9*	*0.1*	*0.3–0.4*
9	*74*	*1.82*	*4.2*	*300*	*36.9*	*0.7*	*0.3–0.4*
10	79	1.86	4.3	900	37	0.3	1.0–1.1
11	**89**	**1.91**	**3.23**	**900**	**36**	**0.6**	**0.8**

[a]No core temperature measurement is available for patient 1 since patient 1 felt uncomfortable and decided to discontinue the study.

Table 11.2. The relationship between the peak local SAR, averaged SARs, and local temperature

SAR_{peak} (W kg^{-1})	σ (mm)	$SAR_{1\,g}$ (W kg^{-1})	$SAR_{10\,g}$ (W kg^{-1})	$\frac{SAR_{peak}}{SAR_{1\,g}}$	$\frac{SAR_{peak}}{SAR_{10\,g}}$	T_{peak} (°C)
100.0	10.0	91.4	67.9	1.09	1.47	5.85
100.0	5.0	71.1	29.5	1.41	3.39	3.39
100.0	4.0	60.0	19.7	1.67	5.09	2.63
100.0	3.0	43.4	11.2	2.30	8.96	1.88
100.0	2.0	22.4	5.0	4.46	20.14	1.12

the quantification of the 'truly' deposited whole-body average SAR – instead of the 'delivered' whole-body average SAR (which overestimates the SAR absorbed by the body) – are unknown. Using 'delivered' whole-body average SAR in computations, instead of the 'absorbed' whole-body average SAR, is expected to overestimate systemic tissue heating. Finally, it is possible that the above temperature measurements were made under forced convection (i.e., the fan inside the bore was on), resulting in slightly lower temperatures compared to the ones predicted assuming natural convection (i.e., the fan is not turned on).

Second, regarding the other measurements (non-bold), one may note that these measurements seem inconsistent. For example, the deposition of the whole-body average SAR of ~4.0 W kg^{-1} for 300 s resulted in the measured core temperature change of 0.1 and 0.7 °C (italic); also, the deposition of the whole-body average SAR of ~4.0 W kg^{-1} resulted in the temperature change that is lower (underline) than the temperature change measured due to the deposition of the whole-body average SAR of ~3.0 W kg^{-1} for the same 900 s (last row). It is possible that these apparently inconsistent data are the result of altered boundary conditions. Additional information regarding the experimental and boundary conditions may help further improve the predictions.

More such data are needed in humans or human-relevant animals of various shapes and sizes (e.g., short vs tall and lean vs obese) and physiological states (e.g., neonates vs children vs adults, male vs female, pregnant, hypertensive, hypotensive, diabetic, and infarction) to further verify and improve the predictions of models such as the GBHTM to reliably predict and thereby help regulate local and systemic temperatures in real time to improve safety. Some may argue that an appropriately validated temperature model such as the GBHTM can be implemented even today to relatively improve safety since the effect of the physical variables and physiological states has been disregarded historically while developing the current SAR safety thresholds and performing MRI. Yet others may argue that the need to gather appropriate data to systemically study the effect of these physical and physiological variables on the induced temperatures has never been greater to assure safety and harness full potential of the new technologies, such as ultrahigh field MR scanners (>3 T), beam steering, multiband imaging, and parallel imaging. Technologies such as these together with a temperature-based safety metric may very well transform the medical diagnostics of future by providing critical physiologic information to clinicians, scientists, and engineers much faster and at much higher spatial resolution safely.

11.3 SAR AS AN RF SAFETY METRIC

Whole-body average, partial-body average, whole-head average, and 10 g average SAR values are used as safety metrices to keep in vivo temperature changes below 1–2 °C (or absolute in vivo temperature below 40 °C) and avoid thermogenic hazards. Whole-body average, partial-body average, and whole-head average SARs are used (instead of temperatures) since they are relatively easier to compute and control. Values for 10 g average SAR are computed using simple geometries (such as sphere for the head or cylinder for the trunk) and/or human body models and related to the whole-body average, partial-body average, or whole-head average SARs (that are easier to control) to limit local temperature rise.

While relatively easier to compute and control, it should be noted, however, that the choice of SAR as a safety metric unnecessarily constrains the RF power input for short scans and unjustifiably assumes safety for longer scans. This is so because temperature – the real safety-related concern – changes slowly – not instantaneously – for a given SAR and may keep rising (i.e., may not approach a steady-state value) if the power deposition is not interrupted. This is in addition to the fact that the threshold value for SARs is computed using thermal models that are not validated for human MRI applications and tend to underpredict deep tissue heating for a given SAR (e.g., Refs. 1–7, 11).

Since the goal of the SAR thresholds is to limit local temperature rise, it is worth investigating the relationship between the SAR and temperature. The exact relationship between the local SAR and temperature is given by the convective energy equation (CEE).[7]

$$\rho C_{\mathrm{p}} \frac{\partial T}{\partial t} + \nabla \cdot (\rho C_{\mathrm{p}} u T) = \nabla \cdot k \nabla T + \mathrm{SAR}\rho \quad (11.1)$$

where ρ is the density, C_{p} is the specific heat at constant pressure, T is the temperature, t is the time, u is the three-dimensional velocity field, and k is the thermal conductivity. Please note that through equation (11.1) (which is the first principles-based exact thermal model) local temperature is related to the local SAR – and not a volume-averaged SAR (i.e., 1 g, 10 g, partial-body, whole-head, or whole-body). Further, local temperature is affected by the diffusion from the surrounding medium and blood flow. Since thermogenic hazards are related to the local temperature and temperature–time history, expressions are needed that relate 'averaged' SARs to local temperatures to ensure RF safety.

The exact relationship between the whole-body average SAR and the systemic core temperature change can be obtained by whole-body volume averaging of the CEE.[7] The relationship can be simplified significantly if the magnitude of the whole-body average SAR and the SAR deposition duration are such that the effect of (i) the change in the energy transport due to bulk fluid motion, such as respiration and (ii) the change in the difference between the core and skin temperature can be neglected due to the heating. The simplified, albeit somewhat conservative, relationship is presented below.

$$\delta T_{\mathrm{c}} = \frac{\mathrm{SAR}}{C_{\mathrm{p}}\beta}(1 - \mathrm{e}^{-\beta t}) \quad (11.2)$$

where δT_{c} is the change in core temperature over the baseline temperature, SAR is the 'truly' absorbed whole-body average SAR, C_{p} is the whole-body average specific heat at constant pressure, t is the duration of the SAR deposition, h is the convective heat transfer coefficient from surface S, m is the mass of the body, and β is a coefficient defined as $(hS)/(mC_{\mathrm{p}})$.

The relationship between the peak local SAR ($\mathrm{SAR}_{\mathrm{peak}}$), peak 1 g average SAR ($\mathrm{SAR}_{1\,\mathrm{g}}$), peak 10 g average SAR ($\mathrm{SAR}_{10\,\mathrm{g}}$), and peak local temperature change (T_{peak}) can be developed by solving the GBHTM for a representative power distribution and time in the tissue of interest.[7] An example of such relationship is presented in Table 11.2 as a function of the averaged SAR (i.e., 1 g and 10 g) for a symmetrical two-dimensional (2D) power distribution (equation (11.3)) with the peak local SAR (SAR_{peak}) of 100 W kg^{-1} deposited for 15 min in a uniform, normally perfused tissue.

$$SAR_{Local} = SAR_{peak}\left[e^{-\frac{(y-y_0)^2}{2\sigma^2}}\right]\left[e^{-\frac{(z-z_0)^2}{2\sigma^2}}\right] \quad (11.3)$$

where y_0 and z_0 are, respectively, the y and z coordinates of the SAR_{peak}, and σ is the standard deviation.

Table 11.2 can be used to estimate the T_{peak} for a given SAR_{peak} by linearly scaling the T_{peak} with the SAR_{peak} for a given ratio of the peak and averaged SARs (when the local temperature is not expected to adversely affect thermal physiology). Please note that the T_{peak} is computed over the baseline systemic temperature. Thus, to estimate the total peak temperature change, the baseline temperature change (computed per equation (11.1)) should be added to the T_{peak}. Such tables or correlations relating averaged SARs to peak SAR and temperatures are needed for representative power distributions and power deposition times in the tissues of interest to control local tissue heating and use average SARs as efficient RF safety metrices.

11.4 THERMAL DOSE AS AN RF SAFETY METRIC

Adopting a threshold based on a 'weighted' integral of temperature–time history (also referred to as thermal dose) as an RF safety metric allows MR scanners the flexibility of depositing any amount of power as long as the integral stays below the accepted threshold. In principle, this method provides MRI scanners more flexibility compared to the temperature and/or SAR-based criteria and has the potential to make MRIs provide critical physiological information much faster and at much higher spatial resolution, safely. However, implementing such a method is not without challenges. Besides including all complexities of determining local temperatures in vivo (one needs temperatures as a function of time to calculate a weighted temperature–time history!!), the method begs to address the following three challenges that are specific to this approach and nontrivial: (i) choice of a well-accepted 'safe' physiological effect (i.e., safety criterion) that can be related to the chosen threshold; (ii) validation of the chosen model and threshold to predict the safety criterion; and (iii) the effect of repeated exposures on the validity of the model and threshold.

Several thermal dose models exist that may be considered to develop an RF safety metric. Given below is a brief description of two such models that are used frequently to estimate thermal damage. For more information on different ways to compute thermal dose, and the evaluation of those methods, please refer to materials presented in Ref. 7.

11.4.1 Cumulative Equivalent Minutes at 43 °C (CEM43)

Cumulative Equivalent Minutes at 43 °C or CEM43 is represented as follows:

$$\mathrm{CEM43}(x, y, z, t) = \int_0^{\tau} R^{T(x,y,z,t)-43}\,\mathrm{d}t \quad (11.4)$$

where the weighting factor R is independent of the tissue type and is equal to 0.5 for $T \geq 43$ °C and 0.25 for $T < 43$ °C and τ is the total time (includes duration of heating as well as the time it takes for the tissue to return to near baseline temperature).

In 1970s and later, it was noted that when cells, grown in a petri dish, were exposed to a fixed temperature over a fixed duration in ovens, the cell survivability, as determined by clonogenics, was reduced as a function of the temperature and time.[15] Further, it was observed that:

1. the cell survivability reduced by ≥~90% when the cells were exposed to the uniform temperature of ~43 °C for 60 min;
2. for every degree temperature rise over the temperature of ~43 °C, the cell survivability reduced by approximately the same amount in only half the time of the previous temperature exposure (i.e., ~90% reduction in cell survivability when exposed to 43 °C for 60 min, or 44 °C for 30 min, or 45 °C for 15 min, or 46 °C for 7.5 min); and
3. for every degree temperature decay under the temperature of 43 °C, the cell survivability reduced by approximately the same amount in four times the time of the previous temperature exposure (i.e., ~90% reduction in cell survivability when exposed to 43 °C for 60 min or 42 °C for 240 min).
4. The above results (and thus, R) were independent of the cell type.

The observations resulted in the development of the concept of CEM43, as expressed in equation (11.4). Note that the concept:

1. was developed as a 'metric' to predict and/or estimate a given endpoint (i.e., reduction in cell survivability of ~90%) due to a given temperature–time history and
2. assumes, by definition, that the endpoint can be achieved in half the time of the previous temperature exposure for every degree rise in temperature over 43 °C and in four times the time of the previous temperature exposure for every degree decay in temperature below 43 °C.

Thus, to implement the concept of CEM43, in the traditional sense, as a metric to achieve an endpoint, data are needed to show that:

1. the weighting factor R is independent of the tissue type and
2. the endpoint can be achieved in half the time of the previous temperature exposure for every degree rise in temperature over 43 °C and in four times the time of the previous temperature exposure for every degree decay in temperature below 43 °C.

To implement the concept of CEM43, in the general sense, as a metric to achieve an endpoint, data are needed to:

1. determine the weighting factor R for a tissue type and endpoint and
2. show that the endpoint can be achieved as a function of the R-weighted temperature–time history.

11.4.2 Arrhenius Equation-based Thermal Dose Model

Arrhenius equation-based nondimensional thermal dose (Ω) is computed using equation (11.5),

$$\Omega = \int_0^{\tau} A e^{\frac{-E_a}{RT(t)}} \mathrm{d}t \tag{11.5}$$

where T is the absolute temperature (K), t is the time (s), τ is the total time (s), A is the frequency factor (s^{-1}), E_a is an activation energy barrier ($\mathrm{J\,mol^{-1}}$), and R is the universal gas constant ($8.3143\,\mathrm{J\,mol^{-1}\,K^{-1}}$). The Ω, in fact, is the logarithm of the ratio of the original concentration of tissue and the remaining concentration of tissue at time τ exposed to a given temperature–time history.

The values of the frequency factor A and activation energy barrier E_a are chosen as $3.1 \times 10^{98}\,s^{-1}$ and $6.28 \times 10^5\,\mathrm{J\,mol^{-1}}$, respectively. These values were proposed originally in 1947 by Henriques and Moritz in their seminal papers investigating the effect of temperature and time on the induced thermal damage.[16–18] Since then, several values of A and E_a have been published for various tissue types and with significant variation.[7] To explain these variations, it has been shown that A and E_a are, in fact, dependent on each other and not independent.

In summary, both the CEM43 approach and the Arrhenius equation-based approach were developed to predict thermal damage. If 'limited' thermal damage should be one of the safety criterion; or, if there is any other physiological/clinical endpoint that is more relevant; and the relationship between the endpoint and the threshold (based on the Arrhenius Ω or CEM43) for single and repeated exposures are only the examples of some of the questions that the MRI community may need to consider to implement a thermal dose threshold as an RF safety criterion.

In addition, determination of the thermal dose in the tissue of interest requires the knowledge of the complete spatiotemporal temperature distribution (refer to equations (11.4) and (11.5)), which includes heating as well as cooling of the tissue back to near baseline temperatures. Such temperature distribution can be obtained by either direct measurements or computational simulations. For direct measurements, sufficient number of measurements must be made in tissue using calibrated means (e.g., temperature probes and imaging techniques during heating as well as cooling back to near baseline temperature) with appropriate response time and spatiotemporal resolution. For computational simulations, appropriately validated bioheat transfer models must be used. Inappropriate direct temperature measurements (i.e., lack of sufficient number of measurements during heating and cooling, calibration, response time, and spatial and temporal resolution) or the use of the invalidated/inappropriately validated bioheat transfer models (e.g., a bioheat transfer model should be validated in the tissue of interest in vivo for the representative condition of use) is expected to introduce unknown amount of uncertainties in the determination of the temperature distribution and thermal dose. The effect of measurement uncertainties on the development of a validated thermal and thermal dose model should be carefully studied. The role of such uncertainty on the prediction of temperature and thermal dose should be studied to be able to implement a reliable thermal dose-based RF safety metric.

11.5 SUMMARY

The challenges associated with implementing the temperature, SAR, and thermal dose threshold-based RF safety metric are discussed. The potential of a validated bioheat transfer model, such as the GBHTM framework, in improving RF safety is discussed along with the additional considerations and data that would be needed to appropriately implement a thermal dose threshold-based metric to make MRI more flexible, powerful, yet safer.

DISCLAIMER

The subject matter, content, and views presented in this chapter are mine do not represent the views of the Department of Health and Human Services (HHS), US Food and Drug Administration (FDA), and/or the United States.

RELATED ARTICLES IN EMAGRES

Radiofrequency Heating Models and Measurements

REFERENCES

1. W. P. Shuman, D. R. Haynor, A. W. Guy, G. E. Wesbey, D. J. Schaefer, and A. A. Moss, *Radiology*, 1988, **167**, 551.
2. B. J. Barber, D. J. Schaefer, C. J. Gordon, D. C. Zawieja, and J. Hecker, *AJR Am. J. Roentgenol.*, 1990, **155**, 1105.
3. D. Shrivastava, L. Utecht, J. Tian, J. Hughes, and J. T. Vaughan, *Magn. Reson. Med.*, 2014, **72**, 1141.
4. D. Shrivastava, T. Hanson, J. Kulesa, J. Tian, A. Gregor, and J. T. Vaughan, *Magn. Reson. Med.*, 2011, **66**, 255 (PMC3339408).
5. D. Shrivastava, T. Hanson, R. Schlentz, W. Gallagher, C. Snyder, L. DelaBarre, S. Prakash, P. A. Iaizzo, and J. T. Vaughan, *Magn. Reson. Med.*, 2008, **59**, 73 (PMC2754718).
6. D. Shrivastava, T. Hanson, J. Kulesa, L. DelaBarre, G. Adriany, P. A. Iaizzo, and J. T. Vaughan, *Magn. Reson. Med.*, 2009, **62**, 888 (PMC2782895).
7. D. Shrivastava, Theory and Applications of Heat Transfer in Humans, John Wiley & Sons, Inc: Hoboken, NJ, 2018.
8. D. Shrivastava and J. T. Vaughan, *J. Biomech. Eng.*, 2009, **131**, 074506.
9. ICNIRP, *Health Phys.*, 1998, **74**, 494.
10. International Electrotechnical Commission. Medical electrical equipment—part 2–33: particular requirements for the basic safety and essential performance of magnetic resonance equipment for medical diagnosis [60601–2-33 Ed 3.2b], International Electrotechnical Commission: Geneva, 2015.
11. E. R. Adair and L. G. Berglund, *Magn. Reson. Imaging*, 1986, **4**, 321.
12. E. R. Adair and L. G. Berglund, *Ann. N. Y. Acad. Sci.*, 1992, **649**, 188.
13. H. H. Pennes, *J. Appl. Physiol. 1998*, 1948, **85**, 5.
14. J. S. Van Den Brink, *Concepts Magn. Reson. B*, 2019, **2019**, 9618680.
15. S. A. Sapareto, L. E. Hopwood, W. C. Dewey, M. R. Raju, and J. W. Gray, *Cancer Res.*, 1978, **38**, 393.
16. F. C. Henriques and A. R. Moritz, *Am. J. Pathol.*, 1947, **23**, 531.
17. A. R. Moritz and F. C. Henriques, *Am. J. Pathol.*, 1947, **23**, 695.
18. A. R. Moritz, *Am. J. Pathol.*, 1947, **23**, 915.

Chapter 12
RF Coil and MR Safety

J. Thomas Vaughan

Columbia University in the City of New York, New York, NY, USA

12.1 INTRODUCTION

Radio-frequency (RF) coils are the antenna-like devices from which a RF signal is transmitted to stimulate a nuclear magnetic resonant signal response from anatomy.[1] The same coil or another coil is used in turn to receive the signal response which is then used to make an MR image for MRI or an MR spectrum for MRS. Much of the RF energy transmitted from an RF coil is absorbed in the tissues of the anatomy at a specific absorption rate (SAR), resulting in tissue heating. Excessive heating can result in hyperthermia for the patient, or more commonly to local superficial (first and second degree) burns or local internal (third degree) burns. Approximately 60% of all adverse MR safety incidents are related to RF-induced heating from RF coils and devices to which they couple. The objective of this chapter therefore is to bring a better understanding of the kinds of RF coils used in MRI and the way these coils impart RF energy to the body. The hope is that through a better understanding of the coil–tissue system, effective coil application, and consequential heating, we can design and use RF coils in a safer and more effective way.

12.2 SURFACE COIL

The simplest RF coil is the *LC* loop shown in Figure 12.1. The capacitor, *C*, is selected to resonate the wire loop, *L*, at the Larmor frequency, $f = \omega/2\pi$. This is the frequency that couples most efficiently to protons or other nuclear species processing at $\omega = \gamma \boldsymbol{B}_0$ for a given $\boldsymbol{B}_0$ magnet field strength and nuclear species γ. The coil is designed to inductively couple to the field shown by the transaxial and axial profiles (right). This coil is still in common use today and is the unit element for arrays with as many as 128 of these *LC* loops.[1] The high-frequency coil's field propagation and losses in its human tissue load are described by the time-dependent field equations. A time-harmonic magnetic field, $\boldsymbol{B}_1/\mu$, in a lossy, anisotropic, and inhomogeneous coil–tissue system can be described by the Maxwell–Ampere law.[2–4]

$$\nabla \times \boldsymbol{B}_1/\mu = (\boldsymbol{J}_e + \boldsymbol{J}_d)$$

Safety and Biological Effects in MRI.
Edited by Devashish Shrivastava and J. Thomas Vaughan

ISBN: 978-1-118-82130-5
Also published in eMagRes (online edition)
DOI: 10.1002/9780470034590.emrstm1638

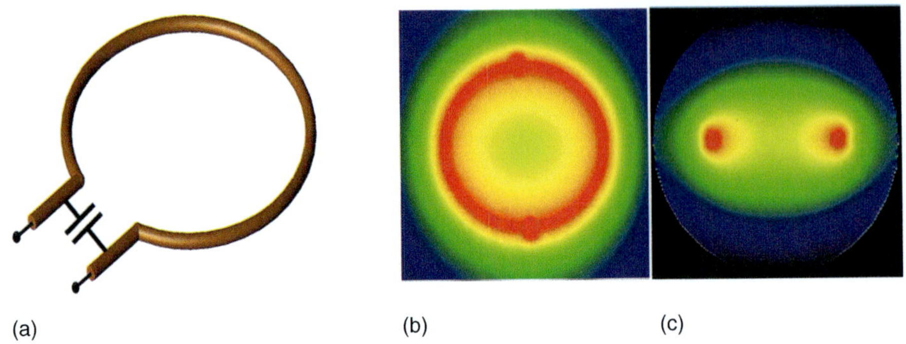

Figure 12.1. RF coil. (a) $\omega = 1/(LC)^{1/2}$. (b) $\boldsymbol{B}_1$ field transaxial. (c) $\boldsymbol{B}_1$ field axial

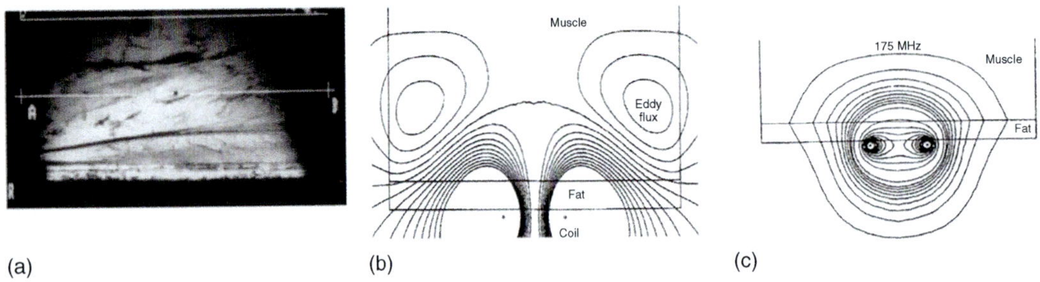

Figure 12.2. MRI and RF magnetic field models of coil + tissue system. (a) Gastrocnemius MRI with coil. (b) $\boldsymbol{B}_1$ vector potential, Webers. (c) $\boldsymbol{B}_1$ flux density, W mm^{-2}

The RF coil plus human calf muscle MRI can be modeled for a clearer understanding of the electromagnetic and thermodynamic mechanisms of this system. The finite element method (FEM) was used to simulate the coil–tissue system depicted in Figure 12.2 as a two-layer cylinder, with the top layer mimicking muscle tissue and the bottom layer skin and subcutaneous fat.[3,4] Frequency-specific table values for permittivity ε and conductivity σ for muscle and fat, respectively, were assigned to the corresponding tissue segments. A cross section of the coil loop is seen below, adjacent to the tissue phantom. The magnetic vector potential or flux lines in webers are seen in the middle figure. The magnetic flux density or $\boldsymbol{B}_1$ field for the coil is shown in the right-hand figure, in two log cycles. This is the field for which we design and apply RF coils. Our design goal is to achieve the inherent field of view (FOV) coverage for a given coil design as efficiently as possible. Maximum $\boldsymbol{B}_1$ field magnitude and penetration are sought for minimum transmit energy, always under the FDA guideline limits to be discussed. Note the refraction (broadening) of the $\boldsymbol{B}_1$ field in the fat dielectric layer and the on-axis attenuation of the field in the more conductive, high-water-content muscle layer, compared to the air beneath the coil.

$\boldsymbol{J}_\mathrm{e} = \sigma\boldsymbol{E} = -j\omega\sigma\boldsymbol{A}$ The conduction current, density A mm^{-2} is described by Ohm's Law.

$\boldsymbol{J}_\mathrm{d} = -j\omega\varepsilon\boldsymbol{E} = \omega^2\varepsilon\boldsymbol{A}$ The displacement current, density A mm^{-2} is described by Euler's Law.

$\boldsymbol{A}$ is the magnetic vector potential in Webers. Note the linear proportion of the frequency of the conduction currents and the quadratic proportionality between the displacement currents and the Larmor frequency. This observation modifies the rule of thumb that SAR increases quadratically with frequency. In fact, eddy current ohmic losses to the tissue conductor will increase linearly with frequency, and displacement current losses to the tissue dielectric will increase quadratically. This is indeed closer to what we observe. Two-cycle axial plots in our simulated phantom are shown for $\boldsymbol{J}_\mathrm{e}$ and $\boldsymbol{J}_\mathrm{d}$ in Figure 12.3. Note the counter (shielding) currents in both plots as well as the dramatic changes at the air and tissue boundaries.

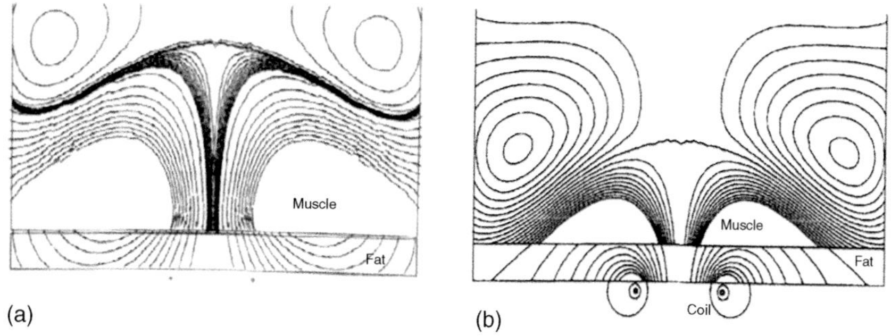

Figure 12.3. Conduction and displacement currents for the coil + tissue model. (a) Conduction currents, $A\,mm^{-2}$. (b) Displacement currents, $A\,mm^{-2}$

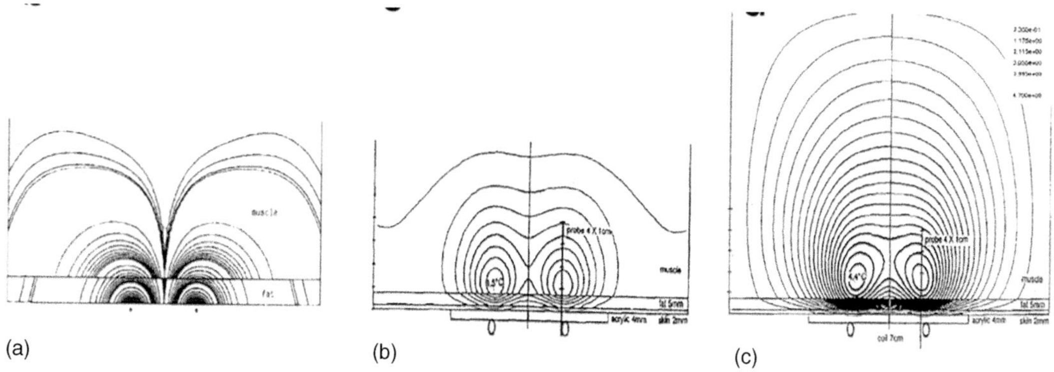

Figure 12.4. SAR and temperature. (a) SAR, $W\,kg^{-1}$. (b) Temperature, perfused. (c) Temperature, nonperfused

The sum of the eddy current and displacement current losses integrated over the tissue volume gives the total power loss density $P_{\text{t loss}}$ or SAR, $W\,kg^{-1}$, as seen plotted in Figure 12.4. Notice that the maximum SAR magnitude for the coil will be at the surface of the phantom or tissue. A slight increase in power loss density is seen as the field transitions from the low-conductivity fat layer to the more conductive muscle layer, muscle being more lossy than fat.

$$P_{\text{t loss}} = 0.5 \int_v (\boldsymbol{J} \cdot \boldsymbol{J}^* / \sigma) \mathrm{d}v, \quad \boldsymbol{J} = \boldsymbol{J}_\mathbf{e} + \boldsymbol{J}_\mathbf{d}$$

$$P_{\text{t loss}} = W[\boldsymbol{T}_\text{b} - \boldsymbol{T}] - \nabla \cdot K \nabla \boldsymbol{T},$$

compact bioheat equation

Equating the power loss density, $P_{\text{t loss}}$, to temperature, $\boldsymbol{T}$, in a bioheat equation gives us the tissue-temperature plots resulting from ohmic and dielectric losses to the tissue of the coil–tissue system. The bioheat equation of which there are several[5] couples electrodynamic losses as calculated and/or measured as SAR to the thermodynamics of heat transfer. This requires assignment of new tissue properties to our model that effect its thermodynamics. These include a perfusion-related parameter W, blood temperature $\boldsymbol{T}_\text{b}$, and thermal conductivity K. Bioheat equations can also include terms for metabolic heating, dynamic heart rates, sweating, dynamic vessel dilation, and other thermoregulatory reflex and environmental factors influencing temperature. A particularly accurate and validated, first principles-derived bioheat equation is found here.[5] In the model of Figure 12.4, we have added a thermally insulting, acrylic coil package layer.[3,4] We see that perfusion-related parameter alone makes a large difference in the temperature profile for equal RF transmit energy input and equal value contour lines. And both perfused and nonperfused models show that the thermal hotspot is deep into the anatomy and not at the surface where the maximum SAR values occur. This points to the real possibility of burns or thermal damage occurring beyond our ability to see or feel them. Given that the largest number of incidents reported to the FDA are superficial first and second degree burns where we can easily detect them, how many more burn lesions occur below the surface, beyond detection? These FEM models were validated by constructing physical phantoms of the models and inserting nonfield perturbing fluoroptic temperature probes through the hotspots indicated in the contour plots. The hotspots were measured to be accurate and precise in their position and magnitude.

It is worth studying these results for several key points of understanding. (i) Temperature or thermal dose is the safety hazard with RF transmit energy, and not SAR by itself. (ii) SAR is an electrodynamic loss term, telling us neither the magnitude nor the spatial profile of our thermal contours. In other words, SAR tells us neither the temperature nor the location of our hotspot. (iii) We must equate SAR to temperature through a bioheat equation to learn this information. (iv) Thermal hotspots are most likely to occur below the surface, beyond our ability to easily detect them. (v) Perfusion is an important factor in excessive heating. Restricted or suppressed perfusion from tight clothes, bandages, edema, strokes, sedation, and anesthesia, diseases such as diabetes or long scans without shifting position should be considered and corrected where possible when imaging.

Given the importance of these results and conclusion to the practice of RF safety, it is equally important to validate these results, not only in phantoms but in vivo. The literature is full of numerical models showing SAR calculated from cartoon models of humans and plastic boxes of aqueous media. Safety-related conclusions from these sources have limited applicability, if any. Literature is also full of tables of widely varying tissue constants for permittivity, conductivity, and thermal properties. There is an equal variety of simulation software available, and less expertise with how to effectively apply it. As a result, not only does reliance on SAR miss the mark, but SAR calculations can be highly inaccurate to meaningless for RF safety applications. We must calculate temperature, and we must validate our models, in vivo.

Other than core temperature, we do not yet have the ability to measure temperature contours within a live human to the 0.2 °C absolute accuracy and precision that we need to monitor and assure safety, but we do have the ability to directly detect temperature to these levels in anesthetized animals. The World Health Organization recommends using farm pigs for several reasons.[5] Farm pigs are inexpensive and widely available. They can be selected for similar thermal mass and surface areas to humans. Like living humans being imaged, pigs have similar heat-regulating reflexes such as perfusion, heart rate, vessel dilation, respiratory rate, and metabolic heating. And of course, their tissue electrical and thermal properties are similar to humans. Importantly, unlike humans, we can anesthetize them, interface them with fluoroptic probes, and measure absolute temperature to the needed degrees of accuracy and precision to validate our models. And we can in turn use our models to guide, predict, and explain our experimental results.[5–17] Figure 12.5 illustrated our methods. Numerical simulations were employed to predict RF heating distribution in the leg muscle of an anesthetized pig.[3,4] The model was used to predict the thermal contours and thereby the placement of our fiber optic probes. The probes were inserted with an 18-gauge needle through the predicted hotspot beneath our coil placed on the pig's leg.

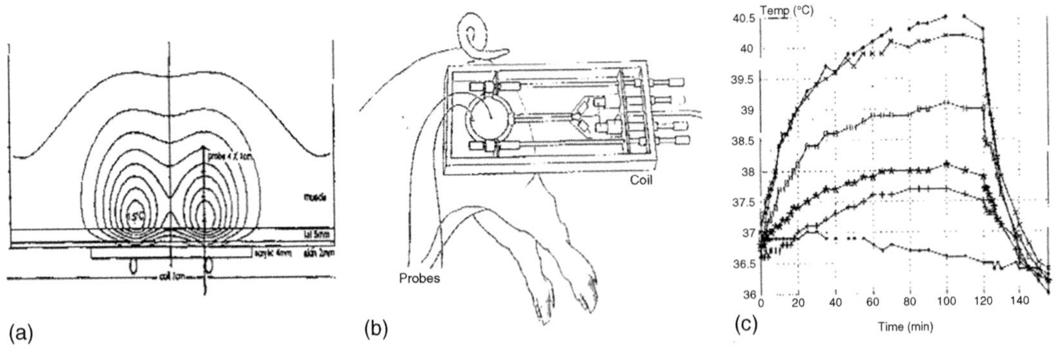

Figure 12.5. Simulations and measurements. (a) Numerical simulation. (b) In vivo model. (c) In vivo measurements

Temperature vs time was then measured at different depths as RF energy was transmitted through the coil at an FDA guideline level. The temperature measurements verified that the highest temperature levels were reached deep under the surface.[3,4]

12.3 VOLUME COIL

To this point, we have explored the basic concepts and mechanisms of RF heating, prediction, and measurement with the most basic coil element, the single loop solenoid. While this element is widely used, it is employed mostly today as a receiver coil element in close fitting arrays for best signal detection sensitivity. The more common transmit coil is a volume coil chosen for best uniform excitation fields. These transmit coils are mostly always rung-type structures of the bird cage or TEM type. Because these are the coils that impart RF transmit RF field energy to the head and body, we must consider these structures as well.

Figure 12.6 shows a very simple model of an eight-element head coil transmitting a linear field to a three-layer head load. The layers are (i) high-water-content, high-conductivity brain, (ii) low-water-content, low-conductivity skull/scalp/fat, and (iii) eyes with aqueous humor properties. Thermal properties corresponding to the tissues named were similarly assigned. While the simplicity of this model derives from its dating to the early 1990s as one of the first 3D FEM simulations for MRI applications, its simplicity lends itself to an easy observation still valid in the most complex models today, and again to empirical validations. In this TEM structure, each rung in (a) is in independent resonant element. Many of the newest body coils today are similarly built for multichannel transmit and $\boldsymbol{B}_1$ shimming applications, making this model highly relevant still. When linear, or in circularly polarized modes, the $\boldsymbol{B}_1$ transmit field of this structure constructively interferes in the center of the head to produce the field contour shown to peak in the head. This effect is more pronounced at higher fields, this model being for 4 T (170 MHz). The SAR profile in (c) is opposite, however, with the SAR being maximum at the surface of the conductive brain layer nearest the transmit coil elements. The thermal profile in (d) is opposite to that predicted for the SAR, with the maximum temperature found in the brain center where SAR is minimum. Why is this? The normal temperature profile of the well-perfused brain is at core temperature, falling off a few degrees at the surface of the skin. When energy is added by a transmit coil operating within guidelines, this curved temperature profile is elevated as when with a fever. SAR may raise the skin and superficial CSF and brain by a larger delta, but the guideline limit of 38 °C may be first reached in the head center where it is already elevated. Again it is important to note that highest temperatures and their potential consequences may be internal and not correlated spatially with SAR contours (e.g., Refs. 5–17).

12.4 BODY COIL

With these basic concepts in mind for simple surface and volume coils, we will now explore more complex coil designs and anatomy models for more realistic results. The RF body coil is shown in the context of a scaled down MRI magnet in Figure 12.7. Minus the magnet, Figure 12.8 shows additional RF coil components. The copper-colored, slotted tube surrounding

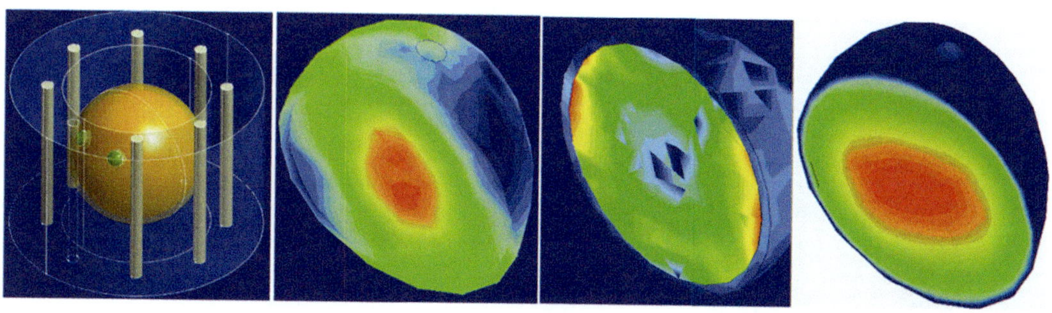

(a) (b) (c) (d)

Figure 12.6. Model of the RF volume coil. (a) Head loaded coil. (b) $\boldsymbol{B}_1$ field. (c) SAR profile. (d) Temperature profile

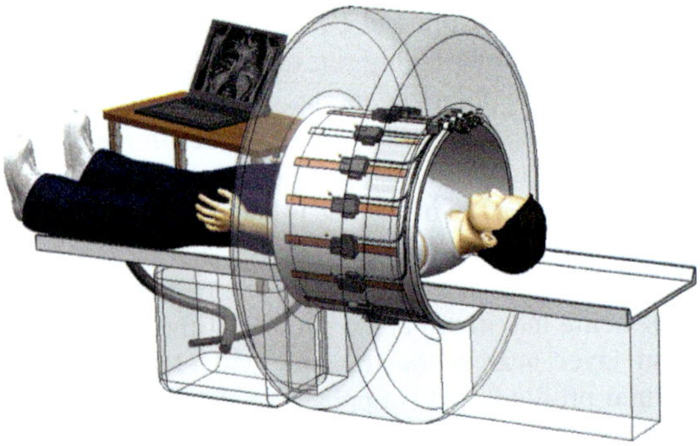

Figure 12.7. Body coil (copper-colored elements) in a short magnet. This body coil is of the multichannel transmit, TEM design

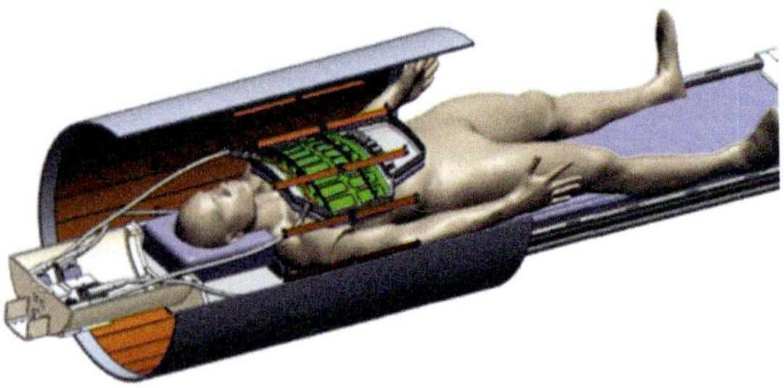

Figure 12.8. TEM body coil with Faraday shield and receiver array

the TEM coil elements serves as both a Faraday cage shielding the RF coils inside from the gradient and magnet coils outside of the shield. In the TEM coil, this shield also serves as a conductor of the TEM elements. A loop array receiver is also shown in place on the body in Figure 12.8. Figure 12.9 shows real examples of the multichannel TEM coil and the loop array receiver. Independent power amplifiers are mounted on the 16-channel transmit coil. Individual, manual tune and match rods are mounted for tuning and matching, and phasing, each element in this experimental coil.

The body coil lines the bore of the magnet, surrounding the patient. It transmits a uniform, nominally circularly polarized, transverse field with the goal of uniform excitation of the protons within the FOV of the coil, typically about a 40 cm dsv. A significant technical challenge of body coil design and application is to build a coil that can generate this FOV field efficiently and homogeneously, especially when loaded with a human body. Figure 12.10 shows a characteristic RF magnetic $\boldsymbol{B}_1$+ field profile in the transaxial and axial planes of the unloaded TEM coil.

In Figure 12.11, however, we see frames of the traveling $\boldsymbol{B}_1$+ (top) and $\boldsymbol{E}$ fields (bottom) of the body-loaded TEM coil within the bore of the magnet. Due to tissue dielectric wavelength shortening, refraction, and attenuation, RF field propagation and loss from multiple coil transmit elements generate wave interference patterns within the body. These interference patterns and the resulting nonuniform $\boldsymbol{B}_1$ and $\boldsymbol{E}$ fields result in nonuniform image signal, losses, and consequential SAR gradient and local heating. Present at all fields, these inhomogeneous image and SAR patterns are more pronounced at higher fields with shorter RF wavelengths. Figure 12.12 shows the image results of a homogeneous, circularly polarized body coil after body loading.

Figure 12.13 provides a useful series of numerical simulations of RF field propagation and losses and resultant heating in the human body positioned in a 45 cm long by 61 cm diameter body coil centered at

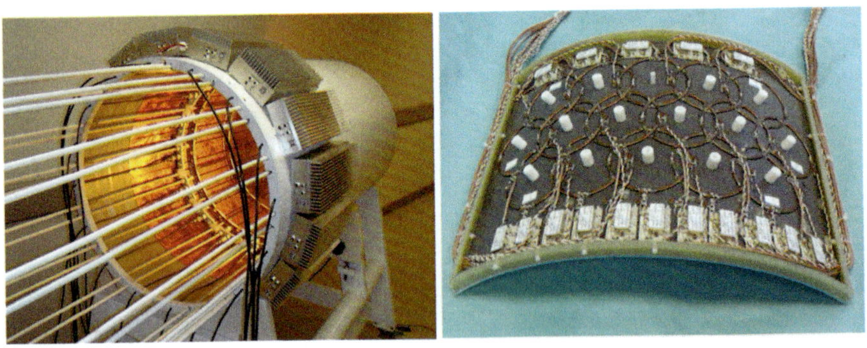

Figure 12.9. Real 16-channel TEM body coil with onboard multichannel transmit and manual channel match and tune and with 16-channel array receiver

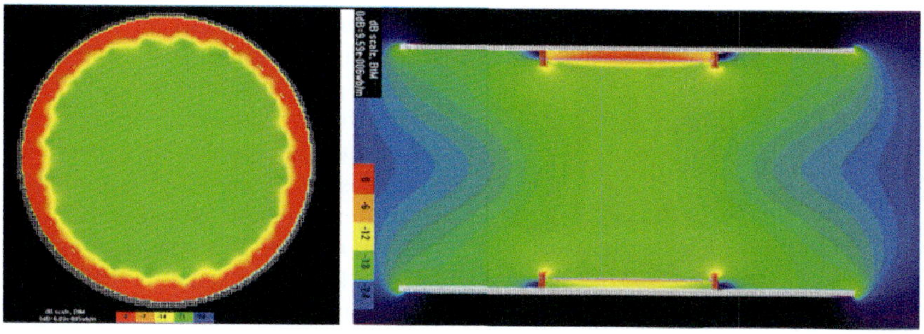

Figure 12.10. Unloaded homogeneous body coil, transaxial and axial views. Field contour lines = 1 dB

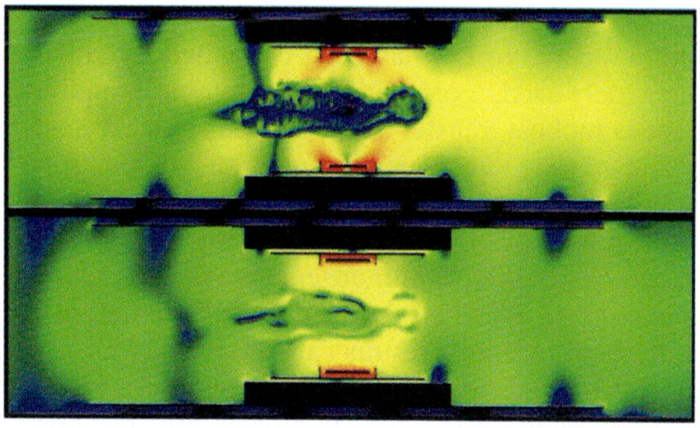

Figure 12.11. Loaded 7 T body coil with $\boldsymbol{B}_1$ field (top) and $\boldsymbol{E}$ field (bottom)

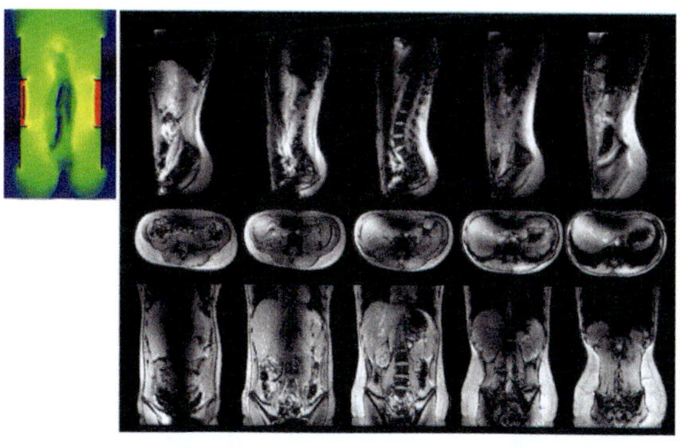

Figure 12.12. 7 T whole-body images. Inhomogeneous images resulting from RF field interference patterns, without $\boldsymbol{B}_1$ shimming

the heart. Efficiently and effectively transmitting the $\boldsymbol{B}_1$ field shown in the first picture is the objective of our MR scan. Even though the body coil and gradients are designed to image only a 40 cm FOV within the center of the MR magnet, we can see that we excite the whole body, head to toe, with our body coil. Viewing the Faraday shield as the outer conductor and the human body as the lossy center conductor of a coaxial segment, the 45 cm energized coil elements simply act to excite this coax system. The same reasoning applies for $\boldsymbol{E}$ field excitation in the second figure. In fact we see field peaks near each end of the coax line composed of body and shield where we would expect to find the voltage nodes. The $\boldsymbol{E}$ field is also high in the arms adjacent to the coil transmit elements. Next in the model series is the SAR plot. As expected, the SAR gradients are highest in the arms adjacent to the transmit coil elements. We also see it peaking in the head and in the lower legs in a pattern similar to the $\boldsymbol{E}$ field, which is also expected. It is important to note that neither the head nor the legs are inside the body coil in this simulation. This observation also calls into question the FDA guidelines specifying 3.2 W kg^{-1} for the head and 4 W kg^{-1} for the body. While these guidelines correctly recommend a lower SAR for the head, they can be easily misinterpreted in practice. If as in this example someone imaging the body sets a power limit of 4 W kg^{-1}, they may be unknowingly delivering 6 W kg^{-1} or more to the head. One will also notice the periphery of the body nearest the transmit coil elements receive the highest SAR. The center of the body away from the transmit coil is exposed to lower SAR, with the spine, pelvis, and major leg bones receiving the least. This is perhaps fortuitous for titanium implants in these regions. Equating SAR to temperature/time gives the heating plot ΔT of Figure 12.13. We expect heating to correlate to SAR as this is the instantaneous thermal response. While useful, temperature presented as a time rate in repose to SAR can mislead to imply that SAR gradients can be used to predict the location if not the magnitude of thermal hotspots. The rate of temperature change slows down as the time progresses in a living system due to diffusion

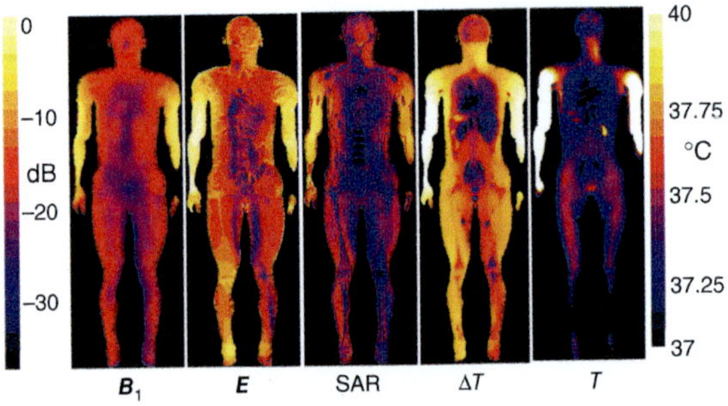

Figure 12.13. EM and thermal fields of body imaging, coronal view

and advection. Further, indigenous thermal gradients near surface may result in the SAR-induced absolute temperatures deep in the body much higher than the temperatures near the surface. The absolute temperature, in °C, of a tissue over a period of time (thermal dose) is what we need to know to best assure RF safety in the MR scan. The final plot of Figure 12.13 shows the absolute temperature for the whole-body model input of 4 W kg^{-1}. Now compare this plot to the SAR plot. While temperature elevation in the arms correlates spatially with the SAR gradients, other regions in the body do not. The lower spine, pelvis, and leg bones where minimum SAR is predicted show elevated temperatures. More importantly, the temperature contour plot, $\boldsymbol{T}$, is the only plot giving us an accurate, absolute temperature magnitude which is the needed safety metric. This temperature, measured or predicted for different time spans, is used to determine the thermal dose. Different tissue types succumb as damage or death at different cell-specific thermal doses.

The safety consequence of SAR is induced RF heating. While SAR is related to heating through an accurate bioheat equation, SAR should not be considered an adequate safety metric by itself. SAR is an electrodynamic loss term, in W kg^{-1}. It does not directly give the location or the magnitude of heating, the thermodynamic loss term. Temperature or the thermal dose for a tissue, organ, or system is the safety hazard for RF transmit fields in MR with which we should be concerned. It is heating that causes pain, burns, and hyperthermia.

In the context of temperature, another point should be made about the current FDA, SAR, and the IEC temperature guidelines. As mentioned earlier, if we excite the torso with a body coil transmitting 4 W kg^{-1}, we will likely be well exceeding the FDA guideline of 3.2 W kg^{-1} for the head. And if we allow the IEC temperature guideline of 39 °C for the torso, we will be heating the head to the same degree, 1 °C above the IEC guideline for the head. This is due to the well-perfused brain remaining at core temperature. It is important to be aware of these possible misinterpretations. It is also interesting if alarming to note the arms in the model below exceed 40 °C. Efforts should always be made to keep the arms away from the body coil (walls of the magnet bore) as much as possible. But do not use strapping or ace bandages to do so as this restrict perfusion to the arms, another important component of the bioheat equations.

Another point to note here (Figure 12.13) is that the temperature change (ΔT) as well as the absolute temperature ($\boldsymbol{T}$) has been computed by solving the widely used, 'gold standard', empirical, simplified Pennes bioheat transfer equation. This bioheat model is known to violate conservation of energy and, if appropriately implemented, underestimate temperatures in deep tissue. In other words, the values for the temperature change and absolute temperature are expected to exceed the numbers presented in the figures at steady state. More accurate results can be obtained by solving the first principles-based, validated generic bioheat transfer model or the generic bioheat transfer model (GBHTM),[5–15] as discussed below.

Figure 12.14 gives a sagittal view of the same models. The same discussion applies.

As noted earlier, numerical simulations must be experimentally validated before conclusions can be drawn. As with the surface coil above, we turn to the WHO porcine model for validating head and body, volume coils. In Figure 12.15 we have created a pig atlas based on image data, assigning the electrical and

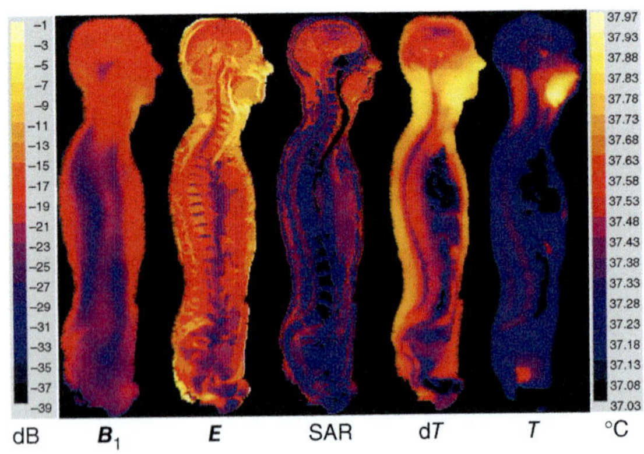

Figure 12.14. EM and thermal fields of body imaging, sagittal view

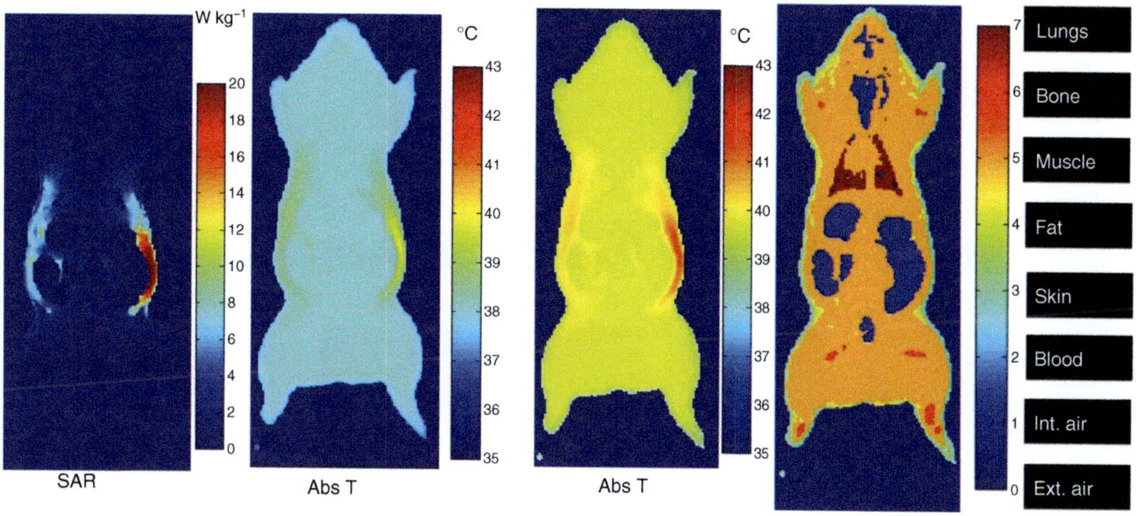

Figure 12.15. Model validation though animal modeling

thermal constants to the tissue segments indicated. By this model a series of human adult-sized farm pigs were placed in a body coil and excited at the FDA and SAR guidelines of 3 and 4 W kg^{-1}. Temperature vs time measurements to 0.2 °C accuracy and precision were used to test and validate (or invalidate) two bioheat transfer models, Pennes and GBHTM.[5–15] The SAR plot is predicted from an EM solver. The first absolute temperature map was produced by solving the empirical 'gold standard' Pennes bioheat equation which our validation with the porcine model in vivo proved inaccurate. The second absolute temperature plot used our GBHTM model, mechanistically derived from first principles and validated on the porcine model to be highly accurate.[5–15] From these results we see that because of perfusion, the pig body thermal contour is fairly uniform in both models, pushing the IEC temperature guideline of 39 °C (for humans) in the more accurate model. In this case there is some excessive heating near the ribs, the part of the body closest to the transmit coil elements.

12.5 SAFETY REMEDIES BY COIL DESIGN

Equipped with conceptual knowledge, what should we do to improve both the safety and the effectiveness of the MR scan? The first step would be through body transmit coil design and application. Exploring different coil designs through finite difference time domain (FDTD) numerical simulation, we have 'tested' dozens of designs. Those shown in Figure 12.16 represent only a small subset. We began this design survey with the specifications of a 32-element, commercial, high-pass, circularly polarized 3 T birdcage design labeled HPBC CP. To this coil we compared a number of different TEM designs and transmit loop array designs, some of which are shown below. All coils were held to 45 cm in axial length and to 61 cm inside diameter.[1]

All coils were tested in circularly polarized mode and with RF shimming. 'RF' shimming is a preferred term to '$\boldsymbol{B}_1$' shimming here to allow more generally for both $\boldsymbol{B}_1$ and $\boldsymbol{E}$ field shimming which will both be employed for safe and effective body coil transmit. Figure 12.17 shows $\boldsymbol{B}_1$ field plots for the best performing test coils of Figure 12.16. The design objective is for a uniform field, as large as achievable. Below each field plot is the mean $\boldsymbol{B}_1$ field strength achieved, a measure of the coil efficiency. The best design will have the largest, most uniform field with the highest transmit efficiency. Center axial, sagittal, and coronal slices are given for best 3D assessment. All coil excitations were the same. By the results below, the 2×16 and the 2×8 TEM coils with $\boldsymbol{B}_1$ shimming are the best designs, giving strong $\boldsymbol{B}_1$ transmit efficiency performance over large, relatively uniform FOVs. To limit the number of parallel transmit channels, the TEM coil with two rings or eight elements each for a total of 16 channels would be the choice for the most effective body transmit coil of those we considered.[1]

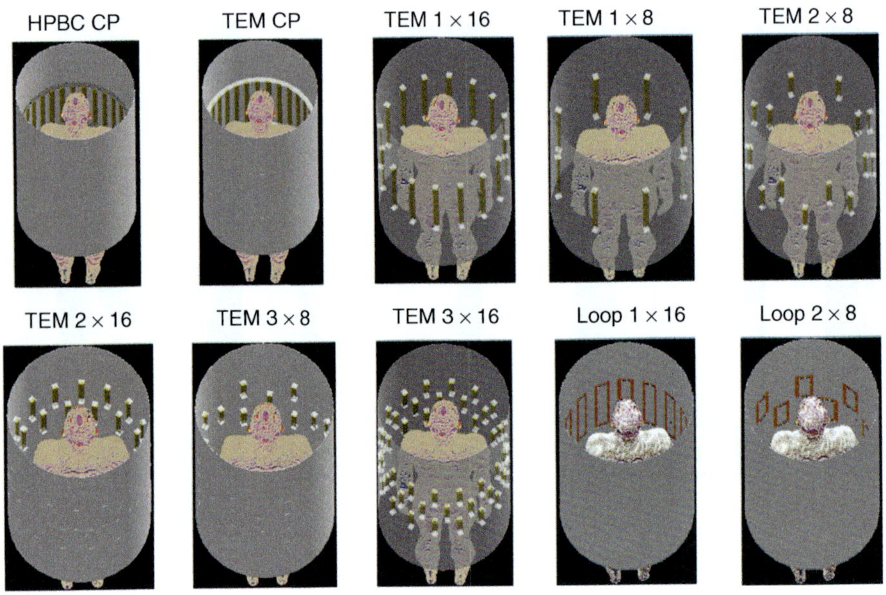

Figure 12.16. Series of potential coils designs. (Based on Ref. 1)

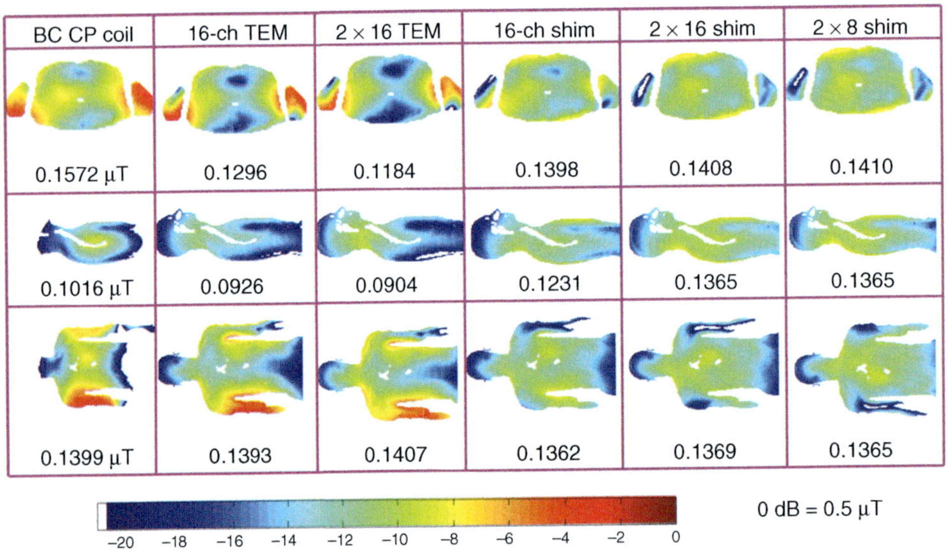

Figure 12.17. Corresponding $\boldsymbol{B}_1$ fields

What about the safest coil? In this case, our design criteria would be the coil with the most uniformly lowest SAR gradients over the largest FOV. Again the input power for all coils was the same. By these criteria, the coils showing the best results were the 2 × 8 and 2 × 16 element, '***E***' field-shimmed coils of Figure 12.18. For the practical reasons of limited transmit channel count above, again the 2 × 8 TEM with ***E*** field shimming is the choice. By these simulations, and experience with many coils of similar design, the 2 × 8 element, 'RF-shimmed' body coil is found to be most safe and effective.[1]

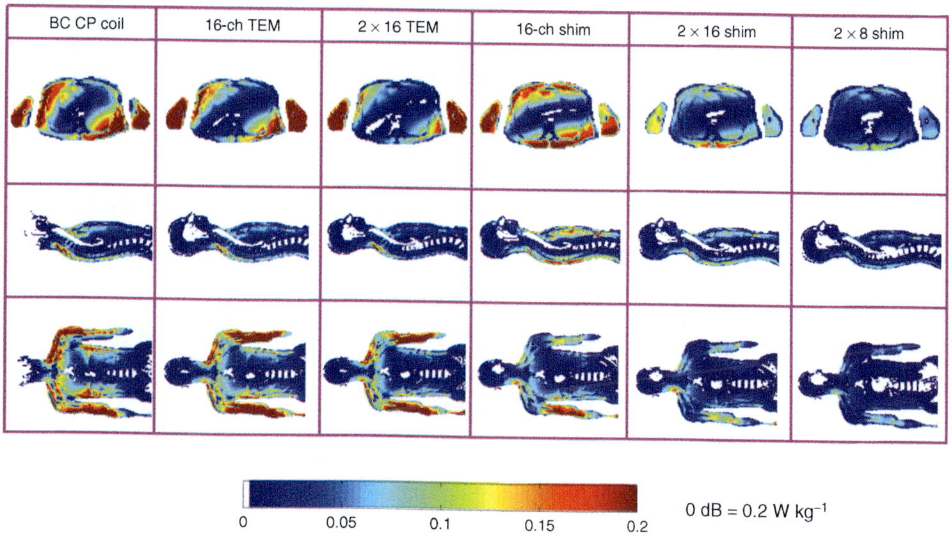

Figure 12.18. Corresponding SAR profiles

12.6 SAFETY REMEDIES BY PRESCAN SAFETY PROTOCOL

In addition to RF coil design, we must apply the RF coil in the safest and most effective way. Electromagnetics and thermodynamics are very specific to coil designs, body geometries and compositions, spatial positions of bodies relative to coils, thermoregulatory physiologies of patients, RF scan protocols and durations, and a host of other factors. Currently, one-or-a-few-sizes-fit-all approaches based on SAR alone is woefully inadequate for RF safety assurance. The considerations above require a precision approach, meaning that we must ideally adjust our safety protocol per patient. And while imaging approaches monitor relative temperature changes of many degrees for therapeutic hyperthermia or cryoablation applications, to meet the IEC guidelines of 1 °C for the head for example, we need absolute accuracy and precision of 0.2 °C in our measurements that can now only be accomplished by the invasive approaches of our pig studies. Therefore, we need another approach. We are developing that precision, predictive approach outlined in Figure 12.19.[15]

Step one is to rapidly, coarsely image the whole human body, head-to-toe (toes not shown). Step two is to create a precision atlas of the specific body by rapidly segmenting this 3D data set into at least three segments, air; high-water-content, high-conductivity tissues; and low-water-content, low-conductivity tissues. Assign these segments appropriate electrical and thermal tissue properties. In step three, we rapidly mesh this model and calculate the power loss density (SAR) as described earlier. In step four, we apply our validated GBHTM bioheat transfer equation together with metadata including heart rate, blood pressure, environmental temperature, RF protocol, RF coil, and patient position, to calculate absolute temperature for the person to be scanned. By this prescan protocol, in less than five minutes we have a predictive temperature contour map of the person with true hotspots flagged and corrective actions suggested. This precision temperature approach will not only improve scan safety but will also improve scan effectiveness by allowing more flexibility with RF power management.

12.7 SUMMARY

The chapter discusses the kinds of RF coils used in MRI and the way these coils impart RF energy to the body. It is shown that the RF heating is related to the SAR through thermodynamic parameters, and significant RF heating, exceeding the current IEC safety guidelines, may occur on the surface as well as deep inside the body, away from the surface and pain/thermal receptors with allowable SAR limits. Since RF heating is subject, RF coil, landmark, and

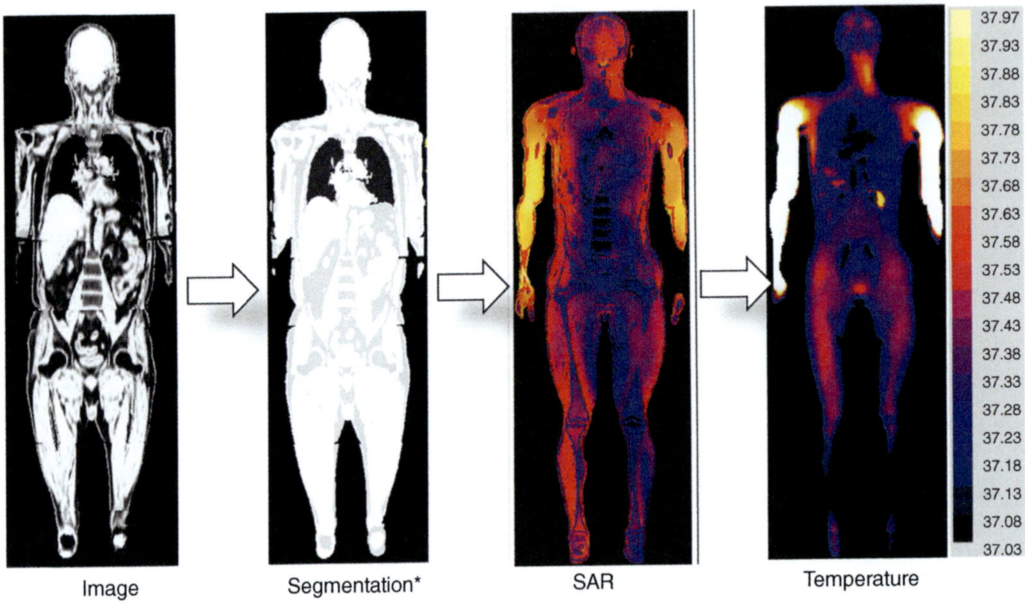

Figure 12.19. Precision temperature profile prediction

pulse sequence dependent, the development and implementation of validated, subject-specific RF safety assessments are needed to ensure safe MRI practices for all patients, for all landmark locations, inside any transmit coil, all the time, while producing the best quality diagnostic images with the highest possible spatial and temporal resolution.

RELATED ARTICLES IN EMAGRES

Birdcage Resonators: Highly Homogeneous Radiofrequency Coils for Magnetic Resonance

Coils for Insertion into the Human Body

Design and Use of Internal Receiver Coils for Magnetic Resonance Imaging

Multifrequency Coils for Whole Body Studies

Radiofrequency Systems and Coils for MRI and MRS

Refrigerated and Superconducting Receiver Coils in Whole Body Magnetic Resonance

Spatial Encoding Using Multiple rf Coils: SMASH Imaging and Parallel MRI

Surface Coil NMR: Detection with Inhomogeneous Radiofrequency Field Antennas

Surface and Other Local Coils for In Vivo Studies

Whole Body Machines: NMR Phased Array Coil Systems

TEM Transceiver Head Array Coils for Ultra High Magnetic Fields

TEM Arrays, Design and Implementation

Quadrature Surface Coils

Double-Tuned Surface Coils

Quadrature Transverse Electromagnetic (TEM) Surface Coils

Radiofrequency Fields and SAR for Transverse Electromagnetic (TEM) Surface Coils

Double-Tuned Birdcage Coils: Construction and Tuning

Radiofrequency Fields and SAR for Bird Cage Coils

TEM Body Coils

Transverse Electromagnetic (TEM) Surface Coils for Extremities

Receiver Loop Arrays

Coil Array Design for Parallel Imaging: Theory and Applications

Millipede Coils

Microcoils

Catheter Coils

Radiofrequency Heating Models and Measurements

Characterization of Multichannel Coil Arrays on the Benchtop

A Standard Procedure for Analyzing Radio Frequency MRI Coils

Litz Coils for High Resolution and Animal Probes, Especially for Double Resonance

RF Field Modeling for Double-Tuned Volume Coils

An Historical Introduction to Surface Coils: The Early Days

Transceiver Loop Arrays

Radiofrequency Coils for NMR: A Peripatetic History of Their Twists and Turns

Nested Surface Coils for Multinuclear NMR

Birdcage Volume Coil Design

Bioeffects and Safety of Radiofrequency Electromagnetic Fields

Radiofrequency Fields: Interactions, Biological Effects, and Safety Issues

RF Device Safety and Compatibility

Safety Considerations in MRI

REFERENCES

1. J. T. Vaughan and J. R. Griffiths, RF Coils for MRI, John Wiley & Sons: Chichester, UK, 2012.
2. J. D. Jackson, Classical Electrodynamics, John Wiley & Sons: Chichester, UK, 1999.
3. J. T. Vaughan, J. Harrison, H. P. Hetherington, W. T. Evanochko, and G. M. Pohost, In *11th Annual Scientific Meeting of the Society for Magnetic Resonance in Medicine*, Berlin, Germany, August 8–14, 1992, Vol. **2**, p 4026.
4. J. Harrison, B. T. Thorn, and G. M. Pohost, In *12th Annual Scientific Meeting of the Society for Magnetic Resonance in Medicine*, New York, August 14–20, 1993, Vol. **3**, p 1369.
5. D. Shrivastava (ed), Theory and Applications of Heat Transfer in Humans, John Wiley & Sons: Chichester, UK, 2018.
6. D. Shrivastava and J. T. Vaughan, *J. Biomech. Eng.*, 2009, **131**, 074506 (PMC2737815).
7. D. Shrivastava, L. Utecht, J. Tian, J. Hughes, and J. T. Vaughan, *Magn. Reson. Med.*, 2014, **72**, 1141.
8. D. Shrivastava, T. Hanson, J. Kulesa, J. Tian, A. Gregor, and J. T. Vaughan, *Magn. Reson. Med.*, 2011, **66**, 255 (PMC3339408).
9. D. Shrivastava, T. Hanson, R. Schlentz, W. Gallagher, C. Snyder, L. DelaBarre, S. Prakash, P. A. Iaizzo, and J. T. Vaughan, *Magn. Reson. Med.*, 2008, **59**, 73 (PMC2754718).
10. D. Shrivastava and J. T. Vaughan, In *ISMRM Workshop: Ultra-high Field Systems and Applications 7T and Beyond*, Lake Louis, Alberta, Canada, 2011.
11. D. Shrivastava, J. Kulesa, J. Tian, G. Adriany, L. DelaBarre, and J. T. Vaughan, In *ISMRM Annual Meeting*, Montreal, Canada, 2011.
12. D. Shrivastava, J. Kulesa, T. Hanson, J. Tian, and J. T. Vaughan, In *8th Biennial 2011 Minnesota Workshops*, Minneapolis, USA, 2011.
13. D. Shrivastava, L. Utecht, J. Tian, T. Hanson, and J. T. Vaughan, In *ISMRM Annual Meeting*, Melbourne, Australia, 2012.
14. D. Shrivastava, J. Hughes, L. Utecht, J. Tian, R. Visaria, and J. T. Vaughan, In *ISMRM Annual Meeting*, Salt Lake City, USA, 2013.
15. D. Shrivastava, J. Tian, J. Hughes, and J. T. Vaughan, In *Proceedings of the ASME/FDA 2013 1st Annual Frontiers in Medical Devices: Applications of Computer Modeling and Simulations*, Washington, DC, USA, 2013.
16. W. P. Shuman, D. R. Haynor, A. W. Guy, G. E. Wesbey, D. J. Schaefer, and A. A. Moss, *Radiology*, 1988, **167**, 551.
17. B. J. Barber, D. J. Schaefer, C. J. Gordon, D. C. Zawieja, and J. Hecker, *AJR Am. J. Roentgenol.*, 1990, **155**, 1105.

Chapter 13

Local SAR Assessment for Multitransmit Systems: A Study on the Peak Local SAR Value as a Function of Magnetic Field Strength

Alexander J.E. Raaijmakers[1,2] and Bart R. Steensma[1]

[1] *University Medical Center Utrecht, Utrecht, The Netherlands*
[2] *Eindhoven University of Technology, Eindhoven, The Netherlands*

13.1 INTRODUCTION

In the classical magnetic resonance imaging (MRI) perspective, the B_1-field is mostly considered perfectly homogeneous, so the resulting tip angle after a radio-frequency (RF) pulse will have the same value everywhere in the excited slab. However, for larger body cross sections and/or larger B_0 values, this perfect homogeneity is not achieved. In fact, for the not-so-moderate cases the B_1-field may show extreme variations from its peak value to almost zero.

This larger B_1-field inhomogeneity with increasing B_0 field strength is caused by wavelength effects. The RF field should be regarded as a (superposition of) propagating electromagnetic waves. These waves have a wavelength that is inversely proportional to their frequency, i.e., the Larmor frequency. If the wavelength is large in comparison to the dimensions of the imaging region, the propagation effects of the RF field are negligible, and the RF field is indeed more or less homogeneous. This is the case at 1.5 T or lower and for head/extremity imaging at 3 T. If the wavelength is comparable to the imaging region, then propagation effects begin to play a role, and minor RF field inhomogeneities become apparent.[1] This is the case for body imaging at 3 T[2] and head imaging at 7 T.[3] If the wavelength is shorter than the dimensions of the imaging region, propagation effects become dominant and the RF field is strongly inhomogeneous. This is the case for body imaging at 7 T (Figure 13.1)[4] and also for head imaging at even larger field strengths.[5]

These inhomogeneities are caused by a standing wave pattern of the electromagnetic RF waves in the patient. A way to address this issue is to use multiple transmit elements.[6] The resulting B_1^+ field distribution will be the superposition of the B_1^+ field of all these transmit elements. Although this sum distribution

Safety and Biological Effects in MRI.
Edited by Devashish Shrivastava and J. Thomas Vaughan
 ISBN: 978-1-118-82130-5
Also published in eMagRes (online edition)
DOI: 10.1002/9780470034590.emrstm1577

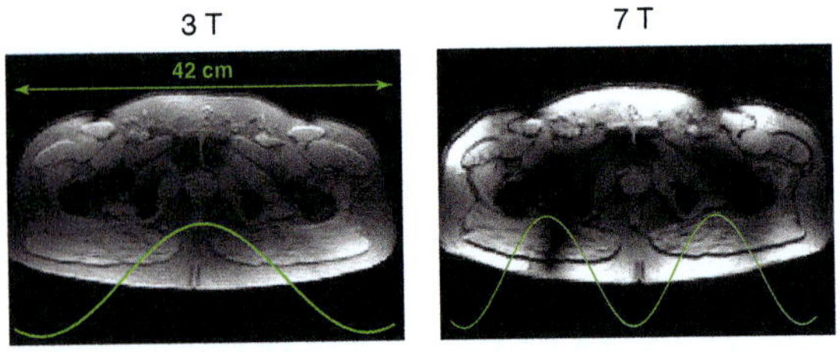

Figure 13.1. Wavelength in tissue at 3 and 7 T and the corresponding signal inhomogeneities for prostate imaging

will likely also contain inhomogeneities, the pattern of these can be steered by adjusting the phases and amplitudes of the individual transmit elements. A system that is capable of this is called a multitransmit system. By optimizing the phases and amplitudes of the transmit channels, the B_1^+ homogeneity in the imaging region can be improved.[7–9]

For 3 T imaging, multitransmit systems are available that have two channels.[10] The transmit coil is a birdcage body coil where the two linear modes can be driven independently with optimized phase and amplitude. The same system is used at 7 T for head imaging. For body imaging at 7 T, the inhomogeneities are too severe to compensate with only two transmit channels. For this purpose, 8- and 16-channel multitransmit systems have been developed. Transmit coils are mostly surface arrays where the elements are placed directly on the body.[11–17]

The specific absorption rate (SAR) exposure in MRI systems is regulated by guidelines published by the IEC[18] and the FDA.[19] According to these guidelines, multitransmit systems need to adhere to limitations on global SAR, regional SAR, and local SAR. Global SAR and regional SAR can easily be measured, but the assessment of local SAR is more challenging. The introduction of considerable degrees of freedom in the RF field distribution of multitransmit systems enables tailoring the B_1^+ field component of this distribution to optimize coverage of the imaging region. However, this also influences the local SAR distribution. The local SAR distribution depends heavily on the actual phase and amplitude settings of the coil array. And therefore the peak local SAR value (which is the value that needs to be constrained by the guidelines) also depends heavily on amplitude and phase settings.

This chapter will present an overview of local SAR considerations for multitransmit systems. The presented methodology to assess local SAR for multitransmit systems will be used to assess the local SAR distribution for prostate imaging at 3, 7, 10.5, and 14 T. A secondary objective of this work is to investigate the dependency of the peak local SAR value on magnetic field strength. In many standard MRI text books and courses, it is claimed that SAR increases quadratically with magnetic field strength (Haake *et al.*, Section 27.4.5[20]). This claim is evaluated here for prostate imaging as was also recently done for head imaging.[21] Since simulations on local SAR simultaneously provide distributions of B_1^+ and B_1^-, transmit efficiency and intrinsic signal-to-noise-ratio (SNR) is also reported for each field strength.

13.2 METHODS

13.2.1 SAR Assessment for Multitransmit Systems

Both global SAR and regional SAR can be determined by measuring the sum of the average powers that are emitted from the coil array to the body. If considerable coupling and/or reflection takes place between/from the coil array elements, the net power toward the coil array can be calculated from the sum of forward powers minus the sum of reflected powers[22,23] [equations (13.1a) and (13.1b)]:

$$\mathrm{SAR_{global}} = \frac{\sum_n |a_n|^2 - |b_n|^2}{m_{\mathrm{patient}}} \tag{13.1a}$$

$$\mathrm{SAR_{regional}} = \frac{\sum_n |a_n|^2 - |b_n|^2}{m_{\mathrm{exposed}}} \tag{13.1b}$$

Here forward and reflected powers are expressed in terms of the forward and reflected wave amplitudes a_n and b_n of channel n. A detailed explanation of the concept of forward and reflected wave amplitudes is provided in many RF text books, for example, by Pozar.[24] m_{patient} is the mass of the patient, and m_{exposed} is the mass of the region in the patient that is exposed to RF fields. Because forward and reflected wave amplitudes a and b can be measured using directional couplers, global and regional SAR can be easily measured to ensure adherence to the guidelines. However, these constraints do not prevent the occurrence of local temperature hotspots. Therefore, local SAR also needs to be constrained.

Local SAR is defined as the deposited power per unit mass. If an infinitesimal amount of power dP is deposited in an infinitesimal amount of tissue with mass dm, then the local SAR at position $\vec{x}$ is defined as:

$$\mathrm{SAR}(\vec{x}) = \frac{\mathrm{d}P(\vec{x})}{\mathrm{d}m(\vec{x})} \tag{13.2}$$

This is equivalent to the amount of power dP deposited in an infinitesimal volume dV divided by the mass dm of that infinitesimal volume dV. The power dP deposited in an infinitesimal volume dV at position $\vec{x}$ is given by:

$$\mathrm{d}P(\vec{x}) = \frac{1}{2}(\vec{J}(\vec{x}))^* \cdot \vec{E}(\vec{x})\,\mathrm{d}V \tag{13.3}$$

In this equation, $\vec{J}(\vec{x})$ and $\vec{E}(\vec{x})$ are the complex amplitudes of the current density and electric field in phasor notation. Assuming reciprocal and isotropic media, the current density is in the same direction as the electric field:

$$\vec{J}(\vec{x}) = \sigma(\vec{x})\vec{E}(\vec{x}) \tag{13.4}$$

Therefore, Ref. 3 simplifies to:

$$\mathrm{d}P(\vec{x}) = \frac{1}{2}(\sigma(\vec{x})\vec{E}(\vec{x}))^* \cdot \vec{E}(\vec{x})\,\mathrm{d}V = \frac{1}{2}\sigma(\vec{x})|\vec{E}(\vec{x})|^2\,\mathrm{d}V \tag{13.5}$$

And considering that

$$\mathrm{d}m(\vec{x}) = \rho(\vec{x})\,\mathrm{d}V \tag{13.6}$$

Equation (13.2) simplifies to

$$\mathrm{SAR}(\vec{x}) = \frac{\mathrm{d}P(\vec{x})}{\mathrm{d}m(\vec{x})} = \frac{\frac{1}{2}\sigma(\vec{x})|\vec{E}(\vec{x})|^2\,\mathrm{d}V}{\rho(\vec{x})\,\mathrm{d}V} = \frac{\sigma(\vec{x})}{2\rho(\vec{x})}|\vec{E}(\vec{x})|^2 \tag{13.7}$$

If all quantities are implicitly assumed to be depending on $\vec{x}$, the expression becomes:

$$\mathrm{SAR} = \frac{\sigma}{2\rho}|\vec{E}|^2 \tag{13.8}$$

Since the guidelines impose restrictions on 10 g-averaged local SAR, expression (13.8) is subsequently averaged accordingly:

$$\mathrm{SAR} = \frac{1}{V_{\mathrm{avg}}}\int_{V_{\mathrm{avg}}} \frac{\sigma}{2\rho}|\vec{E}|^2\mathrm{d}V \tag{13.9}$$

where V_{avg} is the cubical volume of the averaging mass, in this case 10 g.

In a multitransmit system, the electric field is the superposition of the electric fields of all the individual transmit elements. In this superposition, the electric field of each transmit element is related to the current in that transmit element. This can be expressed by a vector multiplication. Here, $E_x^{\prime(n)}$ is the electric field in the x-direction per unit current generated by transmit element n. Again, the dependence of $E_x^{\prime(n)}$ on positional coordinate $\vec{x}$ is implicitly understood. $I^{(n)}$ is the current in transmit element n.

$$\begin{aligned} E_x &= E_x^{\prime(1)}I^{(1)} + E_x^{\prime(2)}I^{(2)} + \ldots + E_x^{\prime(N)}I^{(N)} \\ &= \begin{pmatrix} E_x^{\prime(1)} & E_x^{\prime(2)} & \ldots & E_x^{\prime(N)} \end{pmatrix} \begin{pmatrix} I^{(1)} \\ I^{(2)} \\ \vdots \\ I^{(N)} \end{pmatrix} = \boldsymbol{E}_x^{\prime T}\boldsymbol{I} \end{aligned} \tag{13.10}$$

Similarly:

$$E_x = \boldsymbol{E}_x^{\prime T}\boldsymbol{I},\ E_y = \boldsymbol{E}_y^{\prime T}\boldsymbol{I},\ E_z = \boldsymbol{E}_x^{\prime T}\boldsymbol{I} \tag{13.11}$$

Now the SAR can be calculated by:

$$\mathrm{SAR} = \frac{\sigma}{2\rho}\{|\vec{E}|^2\} = \frac{\sigma}{2\rho}\{|E_x|^2 + |E_y|^2 + |E_z|^2\} \tag{13.12a}$$

$$\mathrm{SAR} = \frac{\sigma}{2\rho}\{\boldsymbol{I}^T\boldsymbol{E}_x^{\prime}\boldsymbol{E}_x^{\prime T}\boldsymbol{I} + \boldsymbol{I}^T\boldsymbol{E}_y^{\prime}\boldsymbol{E}_y^{\prime T}\boldsymbol{I} + \boldsymbol{I}^T\boldsymbol{E}_z^{\prime}\boldsymbol{E}_z^{\prime T}\boldsymbol{I}\} \tag{13.12b}$$

$$\mathrm{SAR} = \boldsymbol{I}^T\left\{\frac{\sigma}{2\rho}\left(\boldsymbol{E}_x^{\prime}\boldsymbol{E}_x^{\prime T} + \boldsymbol{E}_y^{\prime}\boldsymbol{E}_y^{\prime T} + \boldsymbol{E}_z^{\prime}\boldsymbol{E}_z^{\prime T}\right)\right\}\boldsymbol{I} \tag{13.12c}$$

The expression (13.12c) can now be written as:

$$\mathrm{SAR} = \boldsymbol{I}^T\boldsymbol{Q}\boldsymbol{I} \tag{13.13}$$

where $\boldsymbol{Q}$ is the so-called Q-matrix.[25] It is a spatially dependent matrix ($\boldsymbol{Q} = \boldsymbol{Q}(\vec{x})$) that directly relates the currents on the coil array elements to the local SAR at position $\vec{\boldsymbol{x}}$. Its definition follows from equation (13.12c):

$$\boldsymbol{Q} = \frac{\sigma}{2\rho}(\boldsymbol{E}_x^{\prime}\boldsymbol{E}_x^{\prime T} + \boldsymbol{E}_y^{\prime}\boldsymbol{E}_y^{\prime T} + \boldsymbol{E}_z^{\prime}\boldsymbol{E}_z^{\prime T}) \tag{13.14}$$

Since the relevant guidelines have defined their constraints in terms of 10 g-averaged SAR, the following expressions are used to determine this quantity:

$$\mathrm{SAR}_{10\mathrm{g}} = \boldsymbol{I}^T\boldsymbol{Q}_{10\,\mathrm{g}}\boldsymbol{I} \tag{13.15}$$

with

$$\boldsymbol{Q}_{10\,\mathrm{g}} = \frac{1}{V_{\mathrm{avg}}}\int_{V_{\mathrm{avg}}}\frac{\sigma}{2\rho}(\boldsymbol{E}_x^{\prime}\boldsymbol{E}_x^{\prime T} + \boldsymbol{E}_y^{\prime}\boldsymbol{E}_y^{\prime T} + \boldsymbol{E}_z^{\prime}\boldsymbol{E}_z^{\prime T})\mathrm{d}V \tag{13.16}$$

where again V_{avg} is the cubical volume of the averaging mass, in this case 10 g. Since only 10 g-averaged SAR levels are of interest, the 10 g-averaged Q-matrix is quite often also just denoted by $\boldsymbol{Q}$ instead of $\boldsymbol{Q}_{10\,\mathrm{g}}$. Also note that sometimes simulated E-fields are expressed in terms of their rms values. In that case, the factor 1/2 in equation (13.5) and all subsequent equations should be omitted.

13.2.1.1 Practical Example

To illustrate these abstract quantities, an example is presented. Consider an eight-channel multitransmit coil array for prostate imaging at 7 T.[17] It consists of eight transmit elements around the pelvis. Per unit current, each coil array element will generate an electric field distribution. These are indicated in Figure 13.2. The *E*-field vectors $\boldsymbol{E}'_x$, $\boldsymbol{E}'_y$, and $\boldsymbol{E}'_z$ as used in equations (13.10)–(13.16) are created by taking at the same location the values from each of these eight images.

Using the Q-matrices of such an array, the local 10 g-averaged SAR distribution can be determined by performing the quadratic vector–matrix multiplication for every voxel in the simulated model. In this way, the local SAR distribution can be calculated for a given drive vector (phase/amplitude combination) of the transmit array. An example is provided in Figure 13.3.

The *E*-fields as presented in Figure 13.2 are normalized to unit current. However, this is not always the most convenient normalization to work with. Depending on the MRI system vendor and/or the

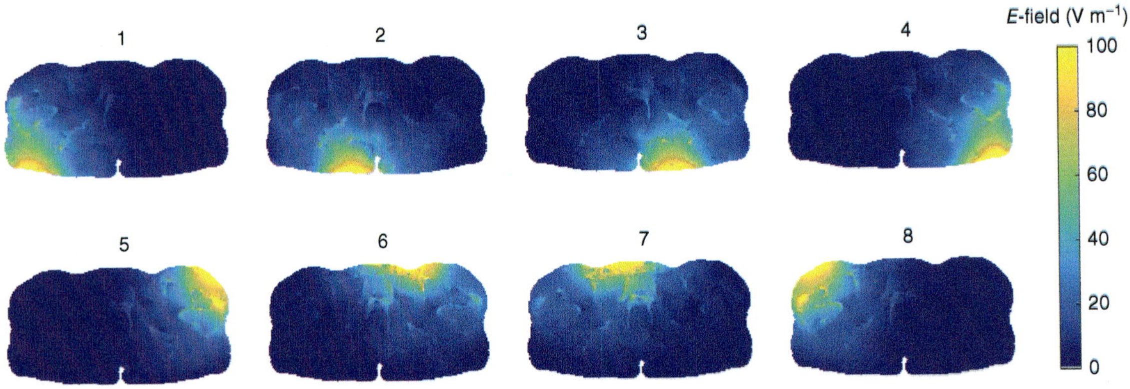

Figure 13.2. *E*-field distributions in the human model Duke using an eight-channel transmit/receive coil array for prostate imaging at 7 T

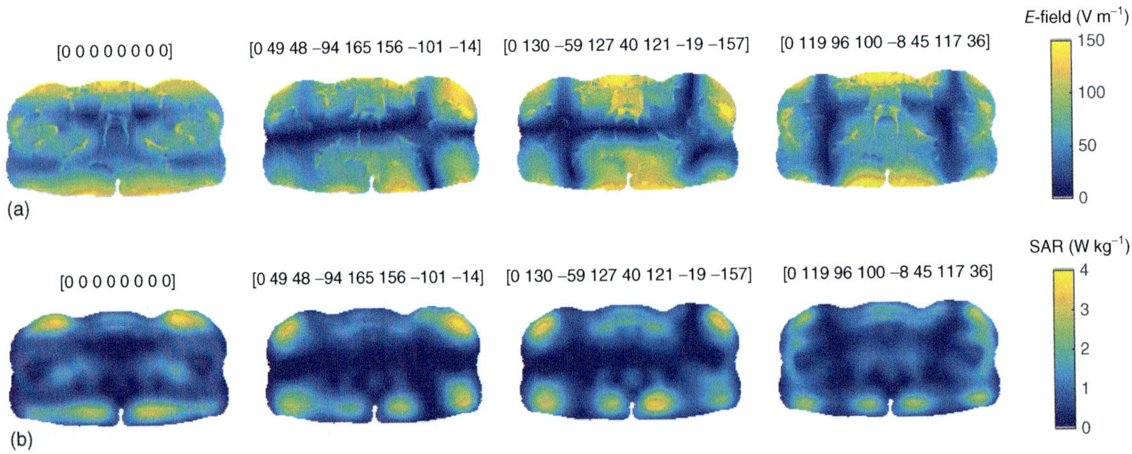

Figure 13.3. Total *E*-field distributions (a) and local 10 g-averaged SAR distributions (b) in the human model Duke using the eight-channel transmit/receive coil array for prostate imaging at 7 T. Presented are distributions for a couple of possible drive vectors. Amplitudes are all equal; phase settings are indicated

simulation software package, E-field distributions may be preferably expressed per unit voltage or per unit forward power to the coil array element. These can be calculated from the E-field distributions per unit current (and vice versa) using the following equation:

$$E_{x,y,z}|_{I=1\mathrm{A}} = Z_{\mathrm{input}} E_{x,y,z}|_{V=1\mathrm{V}} = \sqrt{Z_{\mathrm{input}}} E_{x,y,z}|_{a=1\sqrt{W}} \tag{13.17}$$

Here Z_{input} is the input impedance of the coil array element. Note that only the normalization changes; the spatial distribution of the E-field will stay exactly the same. If an alternative normalization is chosen, the Q-matrix can be constructed with fields normalized to voltage or forward power, and also the input drive vectors are then expressed in terms of voltage or forward power.

13.2.1.2 Domain Reduction

The Q-matrices of each voxel in the simulated model can be stacked into a single array with dimension $[n_{\mathrm{voxels}} * n_{\mathrm{ports}} * n_{\mathrm{ports}}]$. A voxelized model of a coil and human body typically consists of several tens of millions voxels, so the Q-matrices can get very large in size. Storing Q-matrices for multiple human body models or optimizing field distributions with information based on the Q-matrix is too demanding, particularly on a normal PC. Eichfelder and Gebhardt[26] have proposed the use of virtual observation points (VOPs), which is a method that can be used for significant domain reduction of the Q-matrix. The domain reduction comes with a small SAR overestimation where the amount of overestimation is a tradeoff with the amount of domain reduction. The VOP method relies on clustering similar voxel Q-matrices, for voxel locations v, into a single Q-matrix (VOP) such that for each voxel in v, the SAR is equal to the SAR in one particular voxel p plus an additional allowed overestimation factor. The aim is to have as little VOPs as possible, while peak SAR is still estimated reliably. If a cluster is defined around a certain voxel p with Q-matrix Q_p, then all matrices Q_v that are to be included in the cluster need to satisfy a similarity constraint, which is set by allowing a finite overshoot ε. The matrix Q_v is only included in the cluster if $Q_p - Q_v$ is ε-positive semidefinite (psd). This means that for every x, $x^H(Q_p - Q_v)x \geq -\varepsilon$. This guarantees that for a certain normalized excitation vector x, the following holds:

$$x^H Q_p x + \varepsilon \|x\|^2 \geq x^H Q_v x \tag{13.18}$$

In practice, the matrix Q_p is selected by finding the Q-matrix with the largest primary eigenvalue. The voxels that are to be included in the cluster are then selected by comparing the absolute value of the smallest eigenvalue λ_{min} of the difference matrix $Q_p - Q_v$ against ε. If λ_{min} is larger than ε, the criterion $x^H(Q_p - Q_v)x \geq -\varepsilon$ can be guaranteed with a minimal overestimation, by representing the VOP SAR as $\mathrm{SAR_{VOP}} = x^H(Q_p + \varepsilon)x$. In principle, ε defines the maximum allowed overestimation, and in cases where the absolute smallest values of λ_{min} are smaller than ε, SAR in the VOP can also be represented by $\mathrm{SAR_{VOP}} = x^H(Q_p - \lambda_{\mathrm{min}})x$. If all voxel Q-matrices that satisfy this criterion are included in the cluster, the Q-matrix with the largest eigenvalue in the cluster is selected as the Q-matrix Q_p for that VOP. Now the clustering procedure can be repeated to generate a new cluster until all voxels are clustered. Using the method of VOPs can significantly reduce the dimensionality of the Q-matrix array from millions of voxels to hundreds or thousands of VOPs. In general, the number of VOPs can be decreased by choosing a larger overestimation factor ε, which in turn provides less accurate (but never underestimated) SAR values.

13.2.1.3 Intersubject Variability

The methodology presented above is used to assess the peak local SAR for a certain numerical model of a patient. This model will not be the same as the subject inside the scanner. As a result, the peak local SAR may be underestimated, which is a potential safety risk for the patient.

This can be addressed by application of a scaling factor to reach the maximum peak SAR level that can be found in the entire patient population. For head imaging, this scaling factor was found to be 1.4.[27,28] For prostate imaging, the intersubject variability is much larger, resulting in a scaling factor of 2.[29]

An alternative methodology has been presented by Homann *et al.*,[30] where a Dixon scan is used to generate a subject-specific model of the patient inside the scanner. However, this would require a real-time electromagnetic (EM) simulation in between a Dixon scan and subsequent scans. This is currently still out of reach or would require a very considerable investment in general processing unit (GPU) facilities.

A very recent publication has presented an extensive analysis on intersubject variability for prostate imaging at 7 T using 23 models.[31] This approach enables the definition of power limits based on statistics over

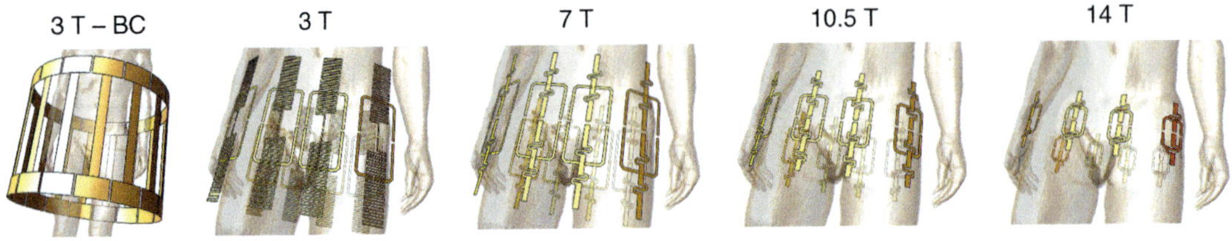

Figure 13.4. Simulation geometries of the investigated transmit arrays for each field strength on human model Duke

many models and many potential phase settings. As a result, these power limits are applicable for any subject in the patient population.

13.2.2 Field Comparison Study

This chapter will present the dependence of local SAR distributions on the magnetic field strength B_0. For this purpose, an eight-channel multitransmit array for prostate imaging is simulated for 3, 7, 10.5, and 14 T using the model Duke of the virtual family.[32] For comparison, the birdcage body coil is also simulated with the model Duke at 3 T. The RF field distributions for the corresponding Larmor frequencies are analyzed by comparing the B_1^+ and local SAR distributions with prostate-shimmed phase settings. In addition, the gamma distributions that correspond to the histogram of peak local SAR values with random phase settings are plotted for each field strength.

The design for the multitransmit array at each investigated field strength is a 16-channel local transceive array consisting of eight dipole antennas and eight loop coil elements. All simulations have been performed using the FDTD simulation package Sim4Life (ZMT, Zurich, Switzerland). The simulation geometries with the design on human model Duke are presented in Figure 13.4. The design for 3 T consists of 8 meandering dipole antennas (30 cm length and 2 meanders per cm[33]) and eight square loop coils with rounded corners (width 8 cm and length 16 cm). For 7 T, the design for the dipole antennas is equivalent to the fractionated dipole antennas as presented by Raaijmakers *et al.*[17] (30 cm length and 30 mm wide meanders per leg) in combination with eight square loop coils with rounded corners (width 8 cm and length 16 cm), which constitutes the same setup as presented by Ertürk *et al.*[34] At 10.5 T, a similar setup was used that was also presented by Ertürk *et al.*[35] Here, all the elements are scaled down to correspond to the reduced wavelength at 450 MHz. The total dipole length is 21 cm, and the loops are 5.2 cm wide and 10 cm long. For 14 T, the same approach has been used where the antennas are reduced in size even further (dipole length 12.6 cm, and loops 4.5 cm wide and 6.5 cm long).

For each setup, the field response of each individual element was simulated separately after which Q-matrices were generated and VOP compression was performed. The phase settings that provide maximum B_1^+ in the prostate were determined, and the corresponding B_1^+ and local SAR distributions were determined. Results are analyzed in terms of peak local SAR per unit power and peak local SAR per unit B_1^+. In addition, the relative SNR values are evaluated for each field strength and array setup.

The SNR for each setup is calculated from the receive sensitivity (B_1^- per unit current), the noise covariance matrix R, and the additional quadratic increase of the signal with B_0-field strength:

$$\mathrm{SNR} \sim (B_0)^2 \sqrt{\boldsymbol{b}^T \boldsymbol{R}^{-1} \boldsymbol{b}} \qquad (13.19)$$

where b is the vector with sensitivities for each receive array element. The expression under the square root is effectively equal to and will therefore be referred to as the B_1^- per unit power. If no different magnetic field strengths are involved and the study aims, e.g., at comparing two different coil array designs at the same field strength, the B_1^- per unit power suffices to evaluate the SNR comparison.

13.3 RESULTS

Figure 13.5 shows the B_1^+ distributions with uniform amplitude and prostate-shimmed phase settings for all investigated field strengths. The B_1^+ magnitude that is achieved in the prostate with 16 × 150 W input power is 26.1, 19.1, 20.0, and 17.4 μT for the local transmit arrays at 3, 7, 10.5, and 14 T, respectively. With the birdcage coil, 19.5 μT is obtained with 2 × 1200 W. The images clearly show the decreasing wavelength,

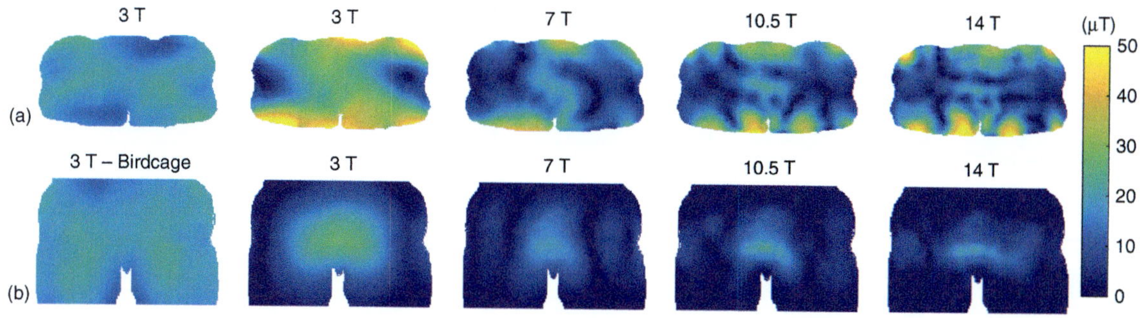

Figure 13.5. Simulated B_1^+ field distributions with uniform amplitude and prostate-shimmed phase settings for the 3 T birdcage body coil and dipole-loop arrays at 3, 7, 10.5, and 14 T. (a) Transverse plane through prostate. (b) Coronal plane through prostate. Distributions are presented for 16 × 150 W input power

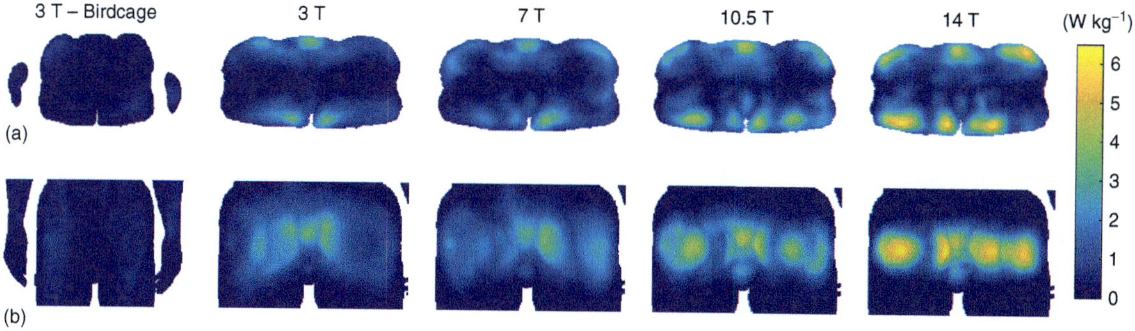

Figure 13.6. Simulated local $SAR_{10\,g}$ distributions for uniform amplitude and prostate-shimmed phase settings for the 3 T birdcage body coil and dipole-loop arrays at 3, 7, 10.5, and 14 T. Maximum intensity projection is shown in axial (a) and coronal (b) orientations. Distributions are presented for 16 × 4 W average input power

which results in a smaller focus area around the prostate for higher field strengths.

Figure 13.6 shows the maximum intensity projection (axial and coronal) of the local SAR distributions that correspond to these prostate-shimmed phase settings. The peak local SAR level that is achieved with 16 × 1 W average input power is 3.6, 3.6, 4.5, and 6.5 W kg^{-1} for the local transmit arrays. With the birdcage, 1.3 W kg^{-1} is obtained with 2 × 8 W average input power.

The simulated field distributions also provide us with the relative intrinsic SNR distributions. These are presented in Figure 13.7 along with the B_1^- per unit power.

The local SAR distributions as presented in Figure 13.6 only provide us the local SAR distributions for prostate-shimmed phase settings. Different phase settings will provide different local SAR distributions, different peak $SAR_{10\,g}$ values, and consequently different power constraints. If, for a particular field strength setup, the peak $SAR_{10\,g}$ levels for a large number of random phase settings (with uniform amplitude) are plotted in a histogram, the result will be a gamma distribution with a particular mean and shape parameter k. Such histograms, with the corresponding fitted gamma distribution, are presented in Figure 13.8. From these distributions, a local $SAR_{10\,g}$ threshold can be identified that is not violated in 99% of the phase settings.[31] In this study, we will define it as $pSAR_{99\%}$. The $SAR_{10\,g}$ could in principle reach higher levels, with the highest level being defined as the worst-case SAR value.[29,31] However, the likelihood of achieving such levels is less than 1% and is therefore not considered relevant for any realistic phase setting or RF pulse sequence.

The results presented above provide a clear picture of the spatial distributions of B_1^+, local $SAR_{10\,g}$, and SNR. However, for B_1^+ and SNR, only the value in

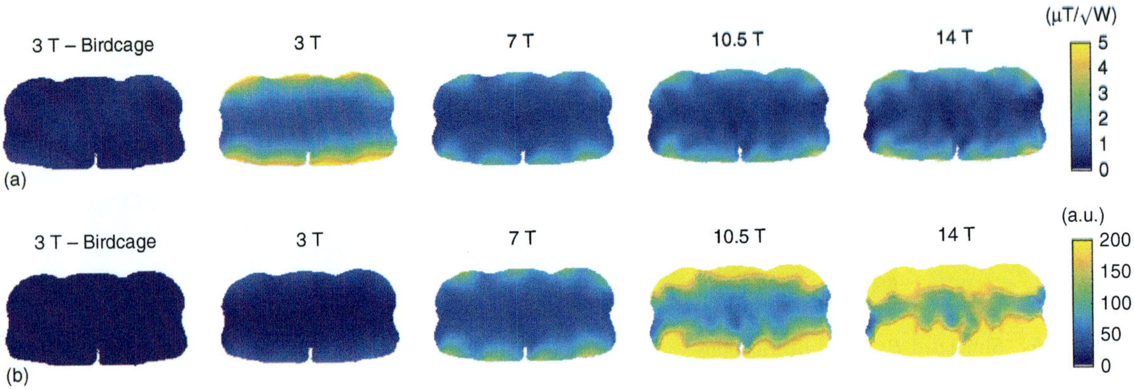

Figure 13.7. Simulated B_1^- per unit power (a) and intrinsic SNR distributions (b) for the birdcage body coil at 3 T and the investigated transmit/receive arrays at 3, 7, 10.5, and 14 T

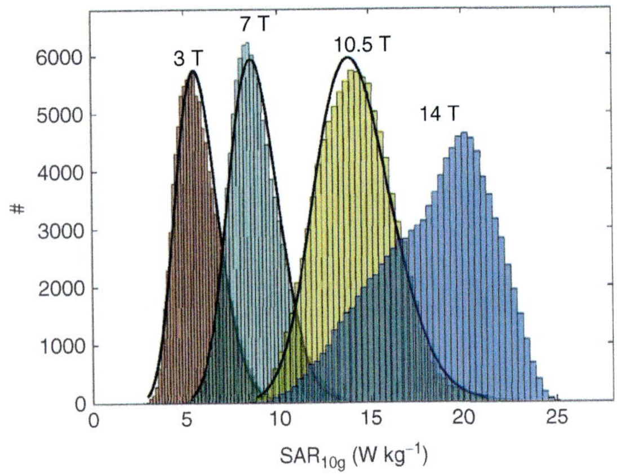

Figure 13.8. Histograms of peak local SAR for the investigated arrays at 3, 7, 10.5, and 14 T. Data consists of peak local SAR values for 100 000 random phase settings

the prostate is important, while for the local $SAR_{10\,g}$, only the peak value is of interest. Figure 13.9 presents a series of graphs to indicate how these quantities depend on the magnetic field strength. Figure 13.9(a) shows the B_1^+ efficiency in the prostate as a function of field strength. In the same diagram, the SAR efficiency as a function of field strength is also plotted against the right axis. Note that SAR efficiency is defined as the B_1^+ per unit peak local $SAR_{10\,g}$ $\left(\frac{B_1^+}{\sqrt{pSAR_{10g}}}\right)$. Figure 13.9(b) shows the peak local SAR per unit power as a function of field strength. In the same graph, the peak local SAR per unit B_1^+ is also plotted against the right axis. This is effectively the reciprocal of the SAR efficiency squared. Finally, Figure 13.9(c) shows the simulated B_1^- per unit power and the intrinsic SNR as a function of field strength.

13.4 DISCUSSION

This chapter has provided a detailed overview of the concepts and methods that are involved in local SAR assessment for multitransmit systems. The maximum allowed exposure levels have been defined for global SAR, regional SAR, and the peak local SAR value. To avoid violation of these guidelines, the input powers to the transmit array elements need to be constrained. The challenge is that the peak SAR level (highest local SAR within the body) cannot be measured. In addition, it depends on the phase and amplitude settings of the array. This is dealt with by calculating the peak local SAR level through *Q*-matrices and domain reduction (VOPs). In this way, the peak local SAR can be calculated online without significant computational effort. However, the obtained peak local SAR value has been calculated for one particular model. At best a couple of models have been evaluated. The subject in the scanner may show different SAR behavior. Therefore, a safety factor is needed to ensure that the peak SAR that has been calculated is indeed the peak SAR for the entire patient population. Much better but more demanding is to perform simulations on a larger set of models. These may be used to assess safe power constraints for the entire patient population.[31] An alternative procedure for subject-specific SAR assessment based on

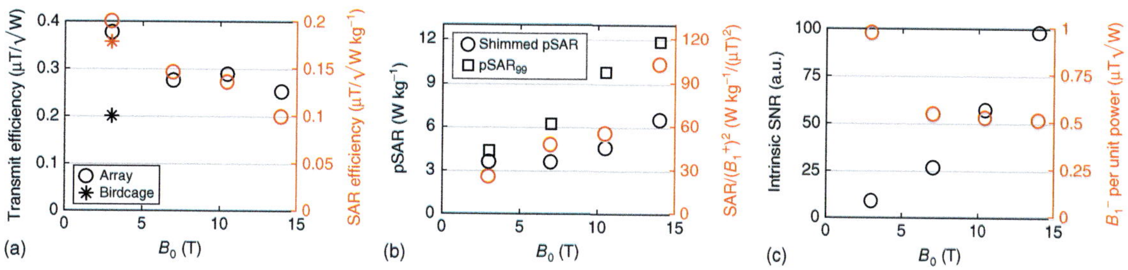

Figure 13.9. (a) B_1^+ and SAR efficiencies in the prostate for the investigated arrays as a function of field strength. The performance of the birdcage body coil at 3 T is also indicated for comparison. (b) $pSAR_{10g}$ with prostate-shimmed phase settings per unit power (left axis) and per unit B_1^+ squared (right axis). In addition, $pSAR_{99\%}$ is plotted for the investigated arrays as a function of field strength (left axis). (c) Simulated B_1^- per unit power (right axis) and intrinsic SNR in the prostate (left axis) for the investigated arrays as a function of field strength

B_1^+ maps and deep learning has recently been presented and shows promising results, but it is not yet used in practice to assess safe power constraints for multitransmit imaging.[36] In addition to the intersubject variability, other sources of error may also be included in the correction factor, e.g., to account for uncertainties in the directional coupler readout.[28]

The presented methodology has been used to investigate the B_1^+ efficiency, local SAR levels, and SNR for the two-channel birdcage body coil at 3 T and eight-channel local transmit arrays at 3, 7, 10.5, and 14 T.

The resulting B_1^+ levels in the prostate as a function of field strength in Figure 13.9(a) show a remarkable pattern. The 3 T body coil is not very efficient as expected, while the local transmit array at 3 T is outperforming all other cases. At 7 T, the transmit efficiency has dropped considerably in comparison to 3 T. This may be caused by the loss of near-field advantage. A more detailed explanation of this perspective is presented further down below. After this, the B_1^+ efficiency does not change much.

The resulting SAR efficiencies (B_1^+ in prostate per square root local SAR) that are plotted in the same figure show a slightly better SAR efficiency for the local transmit array in comparison to the body coil at 3 T. This is quite remarkable: the array with elements directly on the body has a more beneficial B_1^+/peak local SAR ratio than the birdcage body coil. This is achieved by the extremely high efficiency of the local array in comparison to the birdcage coil. For all subsequent field strengths, a gradual reduction in SAR efficiency is shown.

Figure 13.9(b) shows the increase in the peak local SAR value when field strength is increased. Peak SAR levels show a clear increasing trend both normalized to power and normalized to B_1^+. But both trends seem to be approached best by a linear relationship; not quadratic. This, in combination with the work presented by Winter *et al.*,[21] shows that the assumption that SAR increases quadratically with field strength has no foundation in this range of field strengths. In addition, the $SAR_{99\%}$ is plotted, which is the SAR level that may be violated with a 1% probability if random phase settings are used. Also this value is increasing with a similar linear trend.

The peak local SAR value for a multitransmit array depends on the phase settings in a rather unpredictable manner. However, by calculating the peak local SAR for 100 000 random phase settings and plotting the pSAR values in a histogram, some patterns can be observed. Figure 13.8 is showing these histograms for the investigated field strengths. At 3, 7, and 10.5 T, the histograms show a gamma distribution as observed by Meliado *et al.*[31] However, at a field strength of 14 T, the behavior has changed: the distribution has a large tail toward the lower SAR values instead of the other way around with the gamma distribution. An explanation still requires further investigation.

Figure 13.9(c) shows the simulated intrinsic SNR for each field strength together with the B_1^- per unit power. The SNR is by definition the signal in an MRI experiment divided by the noise. Based on the increased magnetization combined with the stronger induction voltage in the receive coil due to the higher frequency, the signal in an MRI experiment increases quadratically with field strength. The noise, on the other hand, is thought to increase linearly with field strength (Haacke and coworkers,[37] par 15.8). Combined, this would provide a linear increase in field strength if the sensitivity of the coil array remained constant. However, the sensitivity of the receive array will also depend on the operating frequency. And in addition, the noise depends on both the field strength and the coil array design while it does not linearly increase anymore for higher field strengths. The combination of this makes the B_1^- per unit power decrease from 3 to 7 T, while it is stable for subsequent field strengths. As a result, the SNR as a function of field strength increases quadratically. This corroborates well with findings by others.[21,38]

The expected quadratic increase of SAR with field strength originates from the following line of thoughts: *E*-fields that are associated with B_1-fields are generated by induction. The amplitude of the *E*-fields is therefore proportional to the time-derivative of B_1 as expressed by equation (13.20a). For time-harmonic signals, this translates into a proportionality with the frequency of the signals [equation (13.20b)]. Since SAR is the square of the *E*-field amplitude, SAR is expected to increase quadratically with field strength [equation (13.20c)]:

$$|\vec{E}| \sim \frac{dB_1}{dt} \quad (13.20a)$$

$$|\vec{E}| \sim \omega B_1 \quad (13.20b)$$

$$\mathrm{SAR} \sim \omega^2 \sim B_0^2 \quad (13.20c)$$

However, from antenna theory, it is known that antennas have a near-field and a far-field. In the far-field, the electric and magnetic field constitute a propagating wave. Propagating electromagnetic waves have a ratio of electric and magnetic field amplitudes (wave impedance) that is determined by the permeability μ and the permittivity ε of the medium in which the wave propagates:

$$Z_{\mathrm{wave}} = \frac{E}{H} = \sqrt{\frac{\mu}{\varepsilon}} \quad (13.21)$$

In this regime, the electric field cannot be increased linearly with the Larmor frequency because a particular amplitude of the B_1-field in microtesla would correspond to a particular electric field amplitude in volts per meter regardless of the frequency (except for much more lenient frequency-dependence of the tissue properties). This does of course not apply to the near-field region. However, as previous studies have emphasized, dipole antennas as transmit elements in MRI should take care to avoid near-field exposure inside the tissue.[11,17] Therefore, some minimum distance is recommended. As a result, the potentially quadratically increasing *E*-fields in the near-field play only a minor role in the resulting relationship of peak local SAR values with magnetic field strength. This may explain the linear rather than quadratic increase in local SAR values (Figure 13.9b).

The near-field region is characterized by strong magnetic or electric fields that are related to the resonance of the coil. It is therefore in fact favorable to use the near-field of RF coils in MRI. However, the size of the near-field region around an antenna is related to the wavelength. This means that for higher field strengths (smaller wavelengths), the near-field may not extend until the imaging target. It is particularly in this regime where dipole antennas are beneficial for use as transmit array elements in MRI.[39] However, until this regime is entered much larger efficiencies can be reached. This may explain the larger transmit efficiency and receive sensitivity at 3 T in comparison to 7 T and higher field strengths (Figure 13.9).

13.5 CONCLUSION

A detailed explanation on local SAR assessment for multitransmit arrays has been presented. With these methods, the peak local SAR, B_1^+ fields, and SNR have been evaluated for prostate imaging at 3, 7, 10.5, and 14 T using loop-dipole transceive arrays. At 3 T, a two-channel birdcage body coil was also included in the comparison. Results show that for these arrays the peak local SAR depends linearly on field strength. The simulated SNR for the investigated setups increases quadratically with field strength.

DISCLAIMER

RELATED ARTICLES IN EMAGRES

Antennas as Surface Array Elements for Body Imaging at Ultrahigh Field Strengths

Quadrature Surface Coils

RF Device Safety and Compatibility

TEM Fields and SAR

Radiofrequency Fields and SAR for Transverse Electromagnetic (TEM) Surface Coils

Radiofrequency Fields and SAR for Bird Cage Coils

Coil Array Design for Parallel Imaging: Theory and Applications

Radiofrequency Coils for NMR: A Peripatetic History of Their Twists and Turns

TEM Transceiver Head Array Coils for Ultra High Magnetic Fields

TEM Arrays, Design and Implementation

TEM Body Coils

Characterization of Multichannel Coil Arrays on the Benchtop

Transceiver Loop Arrays

REFERENCES

1. M. A. Bernstein, J. Huston, and H. A. Ward, *J. Magn. Reson. Imaging*, 2006, **24**, 735.
2. E. M. Merkle and B. M. Dale, *Am. J. Roentgenol.*, 2006, **186**, 1524. DOI: 10.2214/AJR.05.0932.
3. J. T. Vaughan, M. Garwood, C. M. Collins, *et al.*, *Magn. Reson. Med.*, 2001, **46**, 24. DOI: 10.1002/mrm.1156.
4. J. T. Vaughan, C. J. Snyder, L. J. DelaBarre, *et al.*, *Magn. Reson. Med.*, 2009, **61**, 244.
5. T. Vaughan, L. DelaBarre, C. Snyder, *et al.*, *Magn. Reson. Med.*, 2006, **56**, 1274. DOI: 10.1002/mrm.21073.
6. Y. Zhu, *Magn. Reson. Med.*, 2004, **51**. DOI: 10.1002/mrm.20011.
7. B. K. Li, F. Liu, and S. Crozier, *Magn. Reson. Med.*, 2005, **53**, 1251. DOI: 10.1002/mrm.20505.
8. W. Mao, M. B. Smith, and C. M. Collins, *Magn. Reson. Med.*, 2006, **56**, 918. DOI: 10.1002/mrm.21013.
9. G. Adriany, P. F. Van De Moortele, F. Wiesinger, *et al.*, *Magn. Reson. Med.*, 2005, **53**, 434. DOI: 10.1002/mrm.20321.
10. W. A. Willinek, J. Gieseke, G. M. Kukuk, *et al.*, *Radiology*, 2010, **256**, 966.
11. A. J. E. Raaijmakers, O. Ipek, D. W. J. Klomp, *et al.*, *Magn. Reson. Med.*, 2011, **66**, 1488. DOI: 10.1002/mrm.22886.
12. G. J. Metzger, C. Snyder, C. Akgun, *et al.*, *Magn. Reson. Med.*, 2008, **59**, 396.
13. S. Orzada, H. H. Quick, M. E. Ladd, *et al.*, In *Proceedings of the 17th Annual Meeting of ISMRM*, Honolulu, Hawaii, USA, 2009, 2999.
14. C. Thalhammer, W. Renz, L. Winter, *et al.*, *J. Magn. Reson. Imaging*, 2012, **36**, 847. DOI: 10.1002/jmri.23724.
15. L. Winter, C. Özerdem, W. Hoffmann, *et al.*, *PLoS One*, 2013, **8**, e61661.
16. A. B. Rosenkrantz, B. Zhang, N. Ben-Eliezer, *et al.*, *J. Magn. Reson. Imaging*, 2015, **41**, 226. DOI: 10.1002/jmri.24511.
17. A. J. E. Raaijmakers, M. Italiaander, I. J. Voogt, *et al.*, *Magn. Reson. Med.*, 2016, **75**, 1366. DOI: 10.1002/mrm.25596.
18. IEC, Medical Electrical Equipment. Part 2-33: Particular Requirements for the Safety of Magnetic Resonance Equipment for Medical Diagnosis, IEC 60601-2-33, 2010.
19. FDA, 'Guidance for Industry. Guidance for the Submission of Premarket Notifications for Magnetic Resonance Diagnostic Devices', FDA, Rockvile, MD, 2016, 1–30.
20. E. M. Haacke, R. W. Brown, M. R. Thompson, and R Venkatesan, 'Magnetic Resonance Imaging: Physical Principles and Sequence Design', John Wiley & Sons, Inc: Hoboken, NJ, 1999. DOI: 10.1063/1.3554697.
21. L. Winter and T. Niendorf, *Magn. Reson. Mater. Phys. Biol. Med.*, 2016, **29**, 641. DOI: 10.1007/s10334-016-0559-y.
22. Y. Zhu, L. Alon, C. M. Deniz, R. Brown, and D. K. Sodickson, *Magn. Reson. Med.*, 2012, **67**, 1367. DOI: 10.1002/mrm.23126.
23. F. Padormo, A. Beqiri, S. J. Malik, and J. V. Hajnal, *Magn. Reson. Imaging*, 2016, **34**, 690. DOI: 10.1016/j.mri.2015.12.039.
24. D. M. Pozar, 'Microwave Engineering', 3rd edn, John Wiley & Sons, Inc: New York, 2005. DOI: 10.978.0471/448785.
25. F. Bardati, A. Borrani, A. Gerardino, and G. A. Lovisolo, *IEEE Trans. Biomed. Eng.*, 1995, **42**, 1201. DOI: 10.1109/10.476127.

26. G. Eichfelder and M. Gebhardt, *Magn. Reson. Med.*, 2011, **66**, 1468. DOI: 10.1002/mrm.22927.

27. M. De Greef, O. Ipek, A. J. E. Raaijmakers, J. Crezee, and C. A. T. Van Den Berg, *Magn. Reson. Med.*, 2013, **69**, 1476. DOI: 10.1002/mrm.24378.

28. M. Le Garrec, V. Gras, M.-F. Hang, G. Ferrand, M. Luong, and N. Boulant, *Magn. Reson. Med.*, 2016, **78**, 1217. DOI: 10.1002/mrm.26468.

29. Ö. Ipek, A. J. Raaijmakers, J. J. Lagendijk, P. R. Luijten, and C. A. T. Van Den Berg, *Magn. Reson. Med.*, 2014, **71**, 1559. DOI: 10.1002/mrm.24794.

30. H. Homann, P. Börnert, H. Eggers, K. Nehrke, O. Dössel, and I. Graesslin, *Magn. Reson. Med.*, 2011, **66**, 1767. DOI: 10.1002/mrm.22948.

31. E. F. Meliado, A. J. E. Raaijmakers, M. Restivo, M. Maspero, P. R. Luijten, and C. A. T. van den Berg, In *Proceedings of the 24th Scientific Meeting*, International Society for Magnetic Resonance in Medicine: Singapore, 2016, 3660.

32. A. Christ, W. Kainz, E. G. Hahn, K. Honegger, M. Zefferer, E. Neufeld, W. Rascher, R. Janka, W. Bautz, J. Chen, and B. Kiefer, *Phys. Med. Biol.*, 2010, **55**, N23.

33. A. A. Haghnejad, M. Gosselink, I. Voogt, D. W. J. Klomp, P. R. Luijten, and A. J. E. Raaijmakers, In *Proceedings of 26th Annual Meeting ISMRM, Paris, France*, 2018, 1704.

34. M. A. Ertürk, A. J. E. Raaijmakers, G. Adriany, K. Ugurbil, and G. J. Metzger, *Magn. Reson. Med.*, 2016, 1. DOI: 10.1002/mrm.26153.

35. M. A. Ertürk, X. Wu, Y. Eryaman, *et al.*, *Magn. Reson. Med.*, 2016, 1. DOI: 10.1002/mrm.26487.

36. E.F. Meliadò, A.J.E. Raaijmakers, M.H.F. Savenije, A. Sbrizzi, M. Maspero, P.R. Luijten, and C.A.T van den Berg, In *Proceedings of the 26th Annual Meeting ISMRM*, Paris, France, 2018, 0293.

37. R. W. Brown, Y.-C. N. Cheng, E. M. Haacke, M. R. Thompson, and R. Venkatesan, 'Magnetic Resonance Imaging: Physical Principles and Sequence Design', John Wiley & Sons, Inc: Hoboken, NJ, 2014. DOI: 10.1002/9781118633953.

38. O. Ocali and E. Atalar, *Magn. Reson. Med.*, 1998, **39**, 462. DOI: 10.1002/mrm.1910390317.

39. A. J. E. Raaijmakers and C. A. T. Van Den Berg, *Encycl. Magn. Reson.*, 2012.

Chapter 14

Radio Frequency Safety Assessment for Open Source Pulse Sequence Programming

Sairam Geethanath, Julie Kabil, and J. Thomas Vaughan

Columbia Magnetic Resonance Research Center, Columbia University in the City of New York, New York, NY, USA

14.1 INTRODUCTION

A major advantage of Magnetic Resonance Imaging (MRI) is its ability to generate soft tissue contrast.[1,2] In general, this contrast can be tailored to highlight the tissue or pathophysiology of interest.[2,3] This is typically achieved by varying the acquisition parameters through pulse sequence programming. Flexibility in designing such pulse sequences therefore has a direct impact on the development of diverse Magnetic Resonance (MR) techniques and strategies.[1] This flexibility is typically leveraged to achieve novel or improved tissue contrast, shorter acquisition times, and enhanced Signal-to-Noise Ratio (SNR). However, this programming effort requires knowledge of specific programming environments that are MR vendor dependent.[4] Furthermore, these environments are also specific to vendor hardware and software configurations intended for use. This requires considerable human effort and typically impedes the pace of prototyping. Multiple pulse sequence design tools have been developed to enable rapid prototyping and deployment of acquisition strategies and methods. However, it is important to be cognizant of the MR safety risks that are associated with 'custom' or 'open source' pulse sequences. Specifically, assessment of safety issues related to Radio Frequency (RF) heating and Peripheral Nerve Stimulation (PNS) is critical before considering deployment of such sequences.

This chapter describes the fundamentals and implementation details required to assess RF power heating for custom-designed pulse sequences. The chapter is organized as follows: (i) Section 14.2 reviews Specific Absoprtion Rate (SAR) computation theory and focuses on accelerated methods to compute SAR with examples, followed by a brief description of the future direction of body temperature estimation from SAR values or through machine-learning methods; (ii) Section 14.3 describes open source pulse programming features and available tools with a Gradient-Recalled Echo (GRE) example and code; and (iii) Section 14.4 integrates the learning

Safety and Biological Effects in MRI.
Edited by Devashish Shrivastava and J. Thomas Vaughan
 ISBN: 978-1-118-82130-5
Also published in eMagRes (online edition)
DOI: 10.1002/9780470034590.emrstm1633

from the earlier sections to evaluate time-averaged RF power deposition for an open source pulse sequence. For further reading and resources, the interested reader may refer to the Suggested reading' section.

14.2 SAR COMPUTATION

SAR computation as part of pulse sequence design is required at multiple levels. Primarily, a quick SAR computation has to be performed before running a sequence to ensure compliance to IEC standards.[5,6] These are limits specified over a mass of tissue, time, and parts of the body. Rapid SAR calculation is required given the number of user-variable MR acquisition parameters. Secondly, the parameters of flip angle (FA, dependent on B_1^{max}) and repetition time (TR) play a decisive role in the estimation of SAR. These parameters are often changed during an ongoing investigation, and hence SAR computation has to be adapted to these dynamic changes. Subject-specific parameters such as weight, posture, fat distribution, and thermophysiological profile, etc., are derived from highly detailed anatomical, electromagnetic, and biophysical models. Investigating, estimating, and constraining some of these parameters is a prerequisite at higher field strengths ($3T$ and above), owing to the potential MR safety risks related to RF heating.[7–9] The safety risks and system imperfections at such field strengths have been addressed, typically, through the use of parallel RF transmit channels.

The advantages of parallel transmit MRI such as increased radiofrequency (RF/B_1) homogeneity and tailored excitation are well established.[10–14] However, these are limited by the conservative limits on local Specific Absorption Ratio (L-SAR) due to the associated challenges in its evaluation such as subject dependency. The introduction of parallel transmit MR systems requires and simultaneously enables greater control of the transmitted RF power.[14–17] This control is leveraged to mitigate challenges at higher field strengths related to RF inhomogeneity or to achieve accelerated selective excitation pulses. In this chapter, we discuss the formulations for SAR computation in the context of parallel transmit systems with N transmit channels. This is easily reducible and applicable to a single transmit system with $N = 1$.

Consider an electromagnetic (EM) model with conductivity $\sigma(\bar{r})$ and mass density $\rho(\bar{r})$, with $\bar{r}$ denoting the spatial vector. Let $\bar{E}_c(\bar{r},\bar{t})$ represent the electrical field produced by a particular transmit channel c over a space spanned by $\bar{r}$ and a time interval denoted by the array $\bar{t}$. Then, the SAR computed over a volume of tissue V is given by equation (14.1).[18–20] Here, $\|.\|_2^2$ is the Euclidean norm.

$$\mathrm{SAR}(\bar{r},\bar{t}) = \frac{1}{V}\int_V \frac{\sigma(\bar{r})}{2\rho(\bar{r})} \sum_{c=1}^{N} \|\bar{E}_c(\bar{r},\bar{t})\|_2^2 \mathrm{d}V \quad (14.1)$$

14.2.1 Q-matrix Formulation

It is straightforward to observe that the integral presented in equation (14.1) requires increased computational effort, especially in the context of local SAR (L-SAR; 1g or 10g SAR, please refer Dr. Devashish Srivastav's chapter on SAR for a detailed description of L-SAR). In addition, the integral has to be computed over time and space increments for an RF pulse or multiple RF pulses in the case of parallel transmit systems. Therefore, it is important to expedite the calculations by separating the domains of space and time. An approach to compute EM model-based L-SAR and global SAR, known as the Q-matrix formulation, has been proposed by Graesslin *et al.*,[21] briefly described below. Consider a normalization factor for each transmit channel that produces a 1 μT in the isocenter of an empty body coil. The corresponding normalization for the E_c fields would result in a channel-normalized field $\tilde{E}_c$, which can be expressed as a matrix of $N \times 3$, as shown in equation (14.2). The RF waveforms that are played on each of the channels are caused by the complex currents I_c applied on each of the transmit channels. Then, the E_c field can be expressed as in equation (14.2).

$$\begin{aligned}\bar{E}(\bar{r},t_i) &= \sum_{c=1}^{N} \bar{E}_c(\bar{r},t_i) \\ &= \begin{bmatrix} \tilde{E}_{x,1}(\bar{r}) & \cdots & \tilde{E}_{x,N}(\bar{r}) \\ \tilde{E}_{y,1}(\bar{r}) & \cdots & \tilde{E}_{y,N}(\bar{r}) \\ \tilde{E}_{z,1}(\bar{r}) & \cdots & \tilde{E}_{z,N}(\bar{r}) \end{bmatrix} \begin{bmatrix} I_1(t_i) \\ \vdots \\ I_N(t_i) \end{bmatrix}\end{aligned} \quad (14.2)$$

$$\mathrm{SAR}(\bar{r},t_i) = \frac{1}{V}\int_V \frac{\sigma(\bar{r})}{2\rho(\bar{r})} \|\tilde{E}(\bar{r}).I(t_i)\|_2^2 \,\mathrm{d}V \quad (14.3)$$

$$\mathrm{SAR}(\bar{r},t_i) = I^*(t_i).Q(\bar{r}).I(t_i) \quad (14.4)$$

Using equation (14.2) in equation (14.1) and separating the space and time components, we have equation (14.4) with the spatial component termed Q-matrix. Then, the computation of the SAR for a particular RF

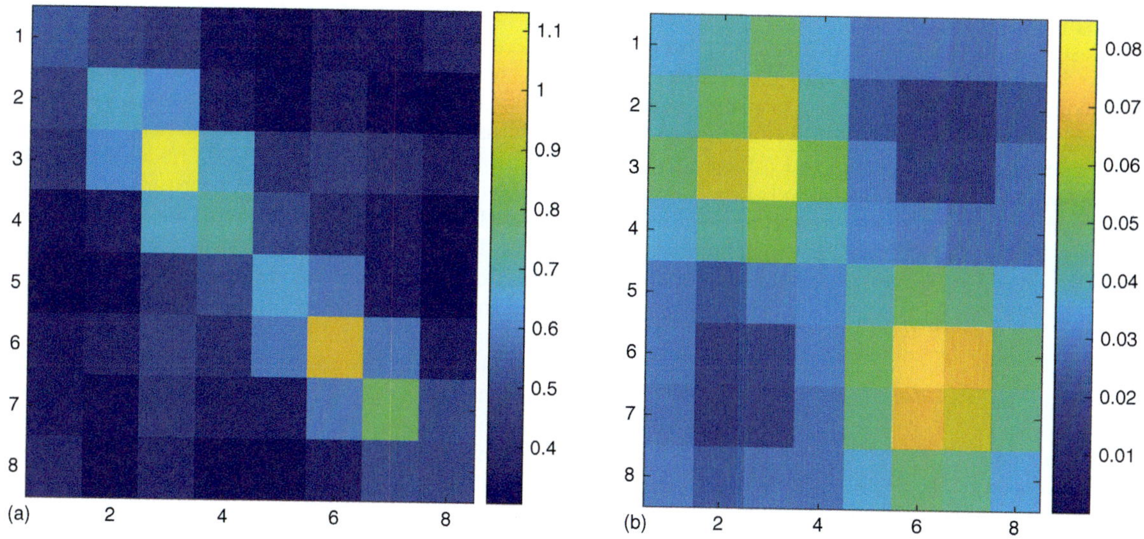

Figure 14.1. Q matrices: (a) The global Q-matrix to compute whole body SAR for an eight-channel transmit system based on the VHM. (b) The corresponding head Q-matrix.

pulse could be done by equation (14.5). This representation speeds up equation (14.5) by precomputing the expected value (average) of the RF pulse over time, resulting in a scalar multiple that is applied to the Q-matrix.

$$\mathrm{SAR}_{\mathrm{pulse}}(\bar{r}) = \sum_{m=1}^{N}\sum_{n=1}^{N} Q_{m,n}(\bar{r}) \cdot \overline{I_m^*(t_i) \cdot I_n(t_i)} \quad (14.5)$$

where,

$$Q(\bar{r}) = \frac{1}{V}\int_V \frac{\sigma(\bar{r})}{2\rho(\bar{r})} \tilde{E}(\bar{r})^{\dagger} \cdot \tilde{E}(\bar{r})\, \mathrm{d}V \quad (14.6)$$

14.2.2 Q-matrix Implementation Example

As an example, Figure 14.1 shows the computed whole body and head only Q matrices for the Visible Human Male (VHM) EM model. This was computed for a 3T MR system with eight transmit channels, using equation (14.4). Q matrices for global and L-SAR were generated for each of the 740 817 cells of the VHM. SAR predictions based on these Q matrices were performed and compared. The predicted and scanner-observed values for quadrature excitation are shown in Table 14.1. Sample MATLAB (The Mathworks Inc, MA) code for computing these matrices are available at Ref. 22. The code also allows computation of 10g local SAR.

Table 14.1. A comparison of Local SAR (L-SAR) and Global SAR (G-SAR) values for quadrature excitation for the implemented method and the scanner observed values

	Implemented	Scanner
L-SAR (W kg^{-1})	2.5995	2.6
G-SAR (W kg^{-1})	0.1670	0.162

14.2.3 Virtual Observation Points

Evaluation of L-SAR based on Q matrices alone, called exhaustive search, is time-consuming due to the large number of *cells* involved in the EM models (order of 700 000 or more) for SAR evaluation. Therefore, the Q-matrix formulation alone cannot be applied for parallel transmit pulse design where SAR has to be computed in near real time. These computational challenges have been addressed by the Virtual Observation Point (VOP) framework.[23] The VOP algorithm is a clustering algorithm which allows estimating peak L-SAR with no underestimation but controlled overestimation (defined by parameter μ). μ can also be tuned to minimize the number of VOPs for faster computation but with a penalty in increased overestimation.

The VOP framework depends on identifying a dominant Q-matrix called B^* that has the highest energy (or norm) in a given cluster of VOPs. Then, for an accepted overestimation percentage μ (say, e.g., 5%), the size of the cluster and membership of Q matrices in that cluster are determined by allowing only those Q matrices that do not exceed a difference of μ once the Q-matrix is rendered positive semidefinite (i.e., there are no negative eigenvalues of the matrix, and if there are, then they are set to 0). This acceptable level of energy (norm of the matrix) is determined by computing the matrix Z such that $||Z|| \leq \mu_{\text{def}}$. To enable potential implementations, the pseudocode used is detailed in the following section.

14.2.3.1 VOP Pseudocode

1. Set μ_{def} in %
2. Set number of observation points N_{VOP}
3. Set the individual observation point $n = 1$
4. While $n \leq N_{\text{VOP}}$ Do

Step 1: Determine B^*

A. Obtain norm of all Q matrices
B. Label the Q matrix with highest norm as B^*
C. Compute Eigen values of remaining Q matrices as Q_E
D. Sort Q_E in descending order

Step 2: Determine Z

E. Set Z = 0
F. Set $A = B^*$
G. Compute $[V, E] = \text{Eigen}(Q)$
H. Set $E < 0$ to 0; to make it *psd*
I. Compute Z_{new} using E and V
J. Compute $Z = Z + Z_{\text{new}}$
K. Compute $\mu_{calc} = ||Z||_2$
L. if $\mu_{\text{calc}} < \mu_{\text{def}}$

Step 2a: Add to cluster
$A = B^* + Z$ $n = n + 1$ else
Step 2b: End of cluster, store A as a VOP
Set VOP = A

14.2.4 VOP Implementation Example

The VOP framework was implemented to enable accelerated calculation of local SAR as detailed in Ref. 23. A 5% overestimation of SAR was chosen to achieve Q-matrix compression and was tested with 1000 tries of random RF shims of unit norm. The implementation of a 5% overestimation bound on SAR values for unit norm shims resulted in 72 VOPs, thereby accomplishing a compression factor of 10 289.125 relative to the total number of Q matrices. To demonstrate the value of the overestimation bound and compression trade-offs, a 10% overestimation experiment was also performed. The resulting VOPS for both cases with their energies (norms) and a correlation with the exhaustive search (described earlier) are shown in Figure 14.2. It is straightforward to note the reduced number of VOPS (higher compression ratio) in the 10% case (Figure 14.2) with a corresponding higher overestimation bound (Figure 14.2).

An intuitive illustration of the VOP is the labeled VHM model shown in Figure 14.3. The figure shows the central axial and coronal slices of the VHM painted with one color per VOP. It is interesting to note the importance of the dominance' of the first VOP (orange color) which covers a significant part of the slices, depicting the compressibility of Q matrices.

14.2.5 Temperature Estimation for RF-induced Heating

Although SAR is the adopted metric for RF safety, the IEC standards' criterion for RF-induced heating is to maintain a less than 1.0°C change in the core body and/or local tissue temperature in the first-level mode. These thermal calculations are typically performed using bioheat transfer models.[9] Briefly, RF-induced heating in the human body is, typically, calculated by implementing a simplified version of the Pennes Bioheat transfer equation (BHTE),[24] which explicitly includes a SAR component. The complete [equation (14.7)] and simplified [equation (14.8)] form of the Pennes BHTE are given below for reference:

$$(\rho.C_p)_T \frac{\mathrm{d}T_T}{\mathrm{d}t} = \nabla \cdot k_T \cdot \nabla \cdot T_T + (1 - \zeta)(w \cdot C_p)_{bl} \times (T_{bl} - T_T) + (\rho\text{SAR})_T + Q'_{\text{met}} \tag{14.7}$$

$$(\rho \cdot C_p)_T \frac{\mathrm{d}T_T}{\mathrm{d}t} = \nabla \cdot k_T \cdot \nabla \cdot T_T + (w.C_p)_{bl}(T_{bl} - T_T) + (\rho\text{SAR})_T + Q'_{\text{met}} \tag{14.8}$$

Here, ρ is the density (kg m^{-3}), C_p is the specific heat (J kg^{-1} K^{-1}), T is the temperature (K), t is the time, ζ is the blood equilibration constant ($0 \leq \zeta \leq 1$), w is blood perfusion (kg m^{-3} s^{-1}), k is the thermal conductivity (W m^{-1} K^{-1}), Q'_{met} is the metabolic heat generation (W m^{-3}), and ρSAR is the RF energy (W m^{-3}). Further, subscripts T and bl refer to tissue and blood, respectively. Please note that the simplified form of the

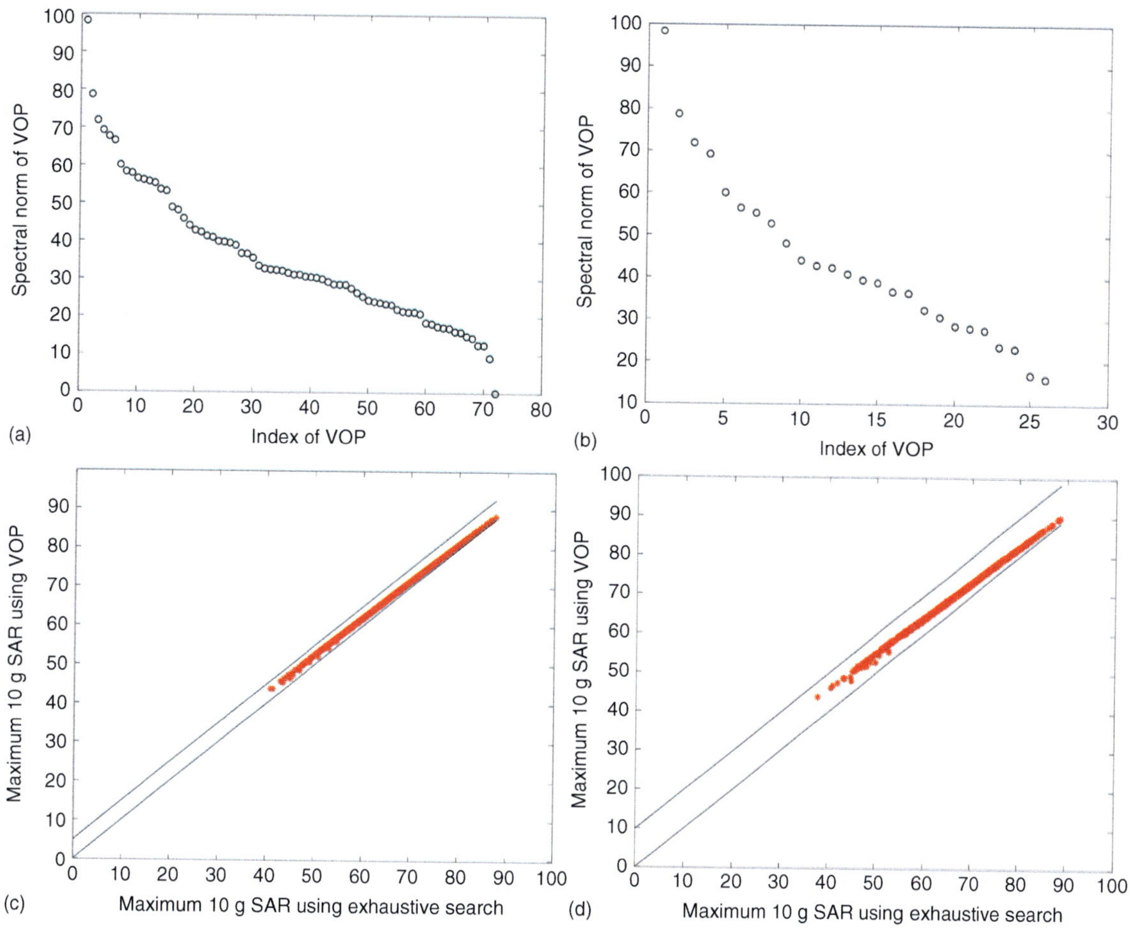

Figure 14.2. Virtual Observation Points: (a) Spectral norm of the 72 VOPs based on a 5% overestimation design; (b) 26 VOPs derived from a 10% design; and (c) and (d) corresponding correlations of the 5% and 10% designs with an exhaustive search using all Q matrices resulting from Section 14.2.2.

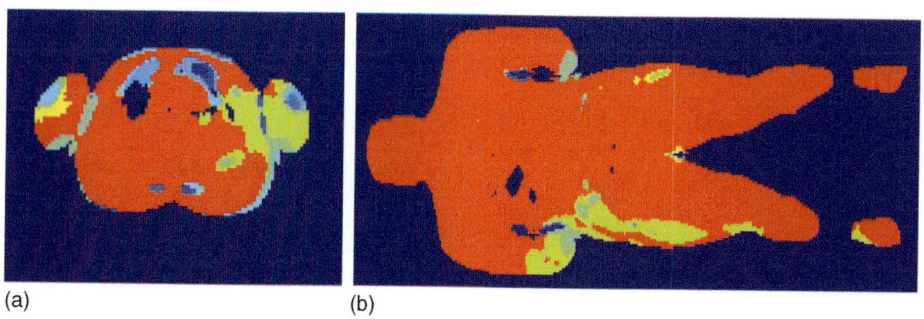

Figure 14.3. VOP labels: (a) The central axial slice of the Visible Human Male model labeled with a color for each VOP and (b) the corresponding coronal slice depicting the spread of the first VOP (orange color).

Pennes BHTE assumes the value of the blood equilibration constant (ζ) as zero. Such an assumption makes the simplified Pennes BHTE overestimate the blood-tissue heat transfer rate, and thus underestimate tissue heating in deep tissue. For more information on the bioheat transfer models in general and Pennes bioheat transfer equation in particular, please refer to Refs. 9,25.

Using machine-learning methods, temperature estimation can be performed from EM and thermal modeling. This approach reduces the lengthy computation times (in the order of hours with graphical processing units) required by conventional EM and thermal solvers to the order of a few seconds to minutes. One such approach called the Noninvasive Temperature Estimation using Machine Learning' (NITE) is capable of estimating temperature hot spots similar to the thermal modeling simulation tool.[26] NITE computes these temperature maps in 3.7 min without GPU parallelization as compared to a proprietary simulation tool that required 10.25 h. These numbers correspond to a phantom that with the height of 174 cm, the total NITE computation time at resolution of 2 mm would result in 870 slices for the whole body. The time per slice computation for NITE is approximately 250 ms for a slice. This rapid calculation of temperature is expected to enable near-real-time temperature monitoring and optimization of MR pulse sequences.

A brief description of the NITE machine-learning algorithm and its components follows.

14.2.5.1 Neural Network Architecture

This was optimized for the desired features of (i) rapid inference, (ii) true multiclass classification, and (iii) limited number of tunable hyperparameters. These features resulted in the choice of an Extreme Learning Machine (ELM).[27] An ELM implementation available at https://github.com/otenim/TensorFlow-OS-ELM implemented on tensorflow (https://www.tensorflow.org/) was utilized for demonstration of the formulation. The only tunable hyperparameter in ELMs is the number of hidden nodes. The number of hidden nodes was 2048, with *sigmoid* as the activation function and *softmax* providing the required probabilities for multiclass classification.

14.2.5.2 Feature Vectors and Training

The input data for training consisted of 6690 examples derived from one slice of the brain temperature simulations (using CST Studio Suite software 2018, CST, Darmstadt, Germany). The validation set was 134 examples corresponding to 2% of the training data. The chosen training data was the slice with the highest temperature range (37.1–39.8°C). This was to be aware of the dynamic range of temperatures the network was likely to see during testing. A ring of surface temperature sensors were assumed to be placed on the phantom. The feature vector consisted of 11 discrete points indicating the distance between a given point and the surface temperature sensors and the corresponding material properties of conductivity, permittivity, and mass cell density. Therefore, each row of the training consisted 35 features (33 thermal properties, norm of the distance, and the actual temperature at the desired location, *P*). Each column of this input data matrix was rescaled to unit range. The data was further augmented by adding random uniform noise with varying levels of intensity (0.1–0.3 in steps of 0.05). Each point *P* had four observations (surface temperature sensors) of these features, with each corresponding to one surface temperature sensor measurement.

14.2.5.3 Training Labels and Testing

A separation of 0.1°C resulted in 28 bins for the temperature range. This vector was stored for translation between actual temperatures and the labels for training.

14.2.5.4 Input Data for Testing

A slice of the brain 5 mm distant from the training slice was utilized for testing. All points in each of the two-dimensional slice along with the corresponding features were flattened and reshaped to the dimensions similar to the ones described for the training data. The resulting labels were converted to temperature bins each of width 0.1°C.

14.2.5.5 Error Quantitation and Statistical Analysis

Training and test results were correlated with CST simulations. The temperatures from CST simulations were binned correspondingly to enable discrete comparisons between the two approaches. NITE reported an accuracy of 82% as compared to the temperature labels generated using CST with a speed up factor of 166.

Table 14.2. Comparison of different open source pulse sequence programming tools that allow sequence simulation, implementation, high level description, and deployment

PSD tool	Simulation	PSD implementation	High-level description	PSD deployment (# vendors)	Citation
ODIN	✓	✓	✓	2	Ref. 28
SIMRI	✓	✓	✓		Ref. 33
JEMRIS	✓	✓	✓	3 (via Pulseq)	Ref. 31
MRI lab	✓	✓	✓		Ref. 34
Sequence tree	✓	✓	✓	1	Ref. 1
Pulseq		✓		3 (via TOPPE)	Ref. 4
TOPPE		✓		3 (via Pulseq)	Ref. 29
Pulseq-GPI /pyPulseq	✓	✓	✓	3	Ref. 30

14.3 OPEN SOURCE PULSE SEQUENCE PROGRAMMING

Custom (in-house tools) pulse sequence programming has been a research augmentation requirement since the early days of MRI acquisition research. More recently, such pulse programming frameworks have been shared publicly.[28] These are typically aimed at rapid prototyping and reproducible research. An advancement of these ideas and implementations has been to provide a standard for describing pulse sequences in a manner that is vendor neutral and human readable. Such a standard is distinguished in its ability to separate the programming from scanner hardware (by including the hardware configuration' as a system variable).[4,29,30] This ability is achieved through the development of interpreters' that translate the pulse sequence standard file format to files interpretable by a specific vendor hardware. Therefore, the open source pulse sequence file standard remains consistent across laboratories and development centers, while deployment on specific vendors would utilize specific interpreters. This allows for both rapid prototyping and a sequence-level reproducibility of results across vendors and magnetic field strengths.

14.3.1 Pulse Sequence Design (PSD) Tools

The MR community has seen a significant number of contributions in this area. These range from open source pulse sequence programming tools dedicated to simulation (Bloch equations, Extended Phase Graphs (EPGs)) as in Refs. 31,32, libraries for designing and visualizing radiofrequency and gradient waveforms,[33,34] and a high-level description of the sequences to modulate acquisition parameters.[34] Some of these packages also provide support for reconstructing data either as part of their simulation pipeline or support to certain standard raw data formats such as the ISMRMRD (International Society of Magnetic Resonance in Medicine Raw Data).[35] A key distinguishing feature is the sequence deployment capability of the package on one or more MRI vendor systems. These tools also benefit non-Cartesian acquisition and reconstruction method development, harmonization of sequences across vendor platforms, and hands-on' teaching tools. Table 14.2 compares some of the tools available as open source libraries for pulse sequence prototyping, development, and deployment. This list is not comprehensive, given the active nature of this research area. The interested reader could visit Ref. 36.

14.3.2 Gradient-recalled Echo example

From the table, it can be noted that the Pulseq (and Pulseq-GPI) standard meets most of the requirements for the standard file format laid out in Section 14.3.1. Also, it provides a human-readable file format that is compatible with three vendor platforms (Siemens Healthineers, GE Healthcare (via TOPPE), and Bruker Corporation). In this example, a GRE pulse sequence will be described. The pulse sequence code is available in MATLAB at (http://pulseq.github.io/) and in Python at (https://github.com/imr-framework/pypulseq).

Briefly, Pulseq relies on a hierarchy of blocks' of time being populated by one or more of a potential six events'. The six events refer to *RF*, the three spatial magnetic field gradients (G_x, G_y, and G_z), the Analog-to-Digital Converter (ADC), and *Delay*. Further, each event has a shape'. Using these three levels of hierarchy, one can concatenate a set of time blocks

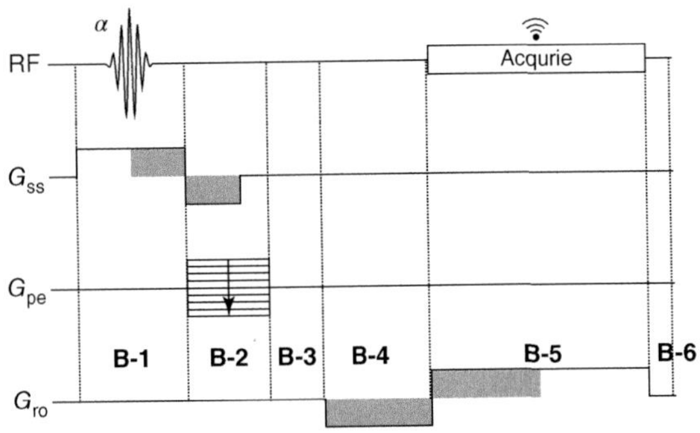

Figure 14.4. The Gradient-Recalled Echo sequence compiled through the concatenation of six blocks (**B-1–B-6**) using the Pulseq library. The blocks include selective excitation, refocusing and prephasing gradients, echo time delay, readout, and repetition time delay.

to play out a desired sequence. For a more detailed description of these hierarchies, please refer Refs. 4, 30.

In this example, we construct a simple GRE sequence by concatenating a series of blocks. The actual code snippet in Python is shown in Section 14.3.2.1 to demonstrate the ease of implementing a sequence using the pyPulseq in Python (or Pulseq for MATLAB). This involves creation of a *seq* object that contains the information of the scanner hardware and related parameters, to which the blocks of events can be appended. For an acquisition with N_{PE} number of phase encodes and a given phase encode index i with $i = (1, 2, \cdots, N_{PE})$, it is possible to define one repetition of the GRE sequence in six blocks of time. This does not include any gradient spoiling that could be used to derive a Spoiled GRE (SPGR) sequence. However, one could use the RF spoiling using the example shown in Figure 14.4.

The first block (**B-1**) accomplishes selective excitation of a slice determined by the *RF* and the slice select gradient (G_{SS}). This is typically performed in the z-direction for trans-axial acquisitions. The value of the phase encoding gradient can then be determined based on the required phase area along a particular axis (e.g., y-direction). The events of the prephasing encoding gradient and the slice refocusing gradient are then played together in block **B-2**. The third block (**B-3**) delays the sequence to accomplish a predetermined echo time (TE) through a wait period of *delayTE*. The prephasing readout gradient played along the x-direction is played in the fourth block (**B-4**). Data acquisition occurs during the fifth block (**B-5**) in the presence of the readout gradient. Any additional delay *delayTR* is then introduced to accomplish the chosen TR in the sixth block (**B-6**).

14.3.2.1 *Python Code for Pulseq GRE Implementation*

1. seq.add_block(rf, gz)
2. gy_pre = make_trapezoid(channel='y', area=phase_areas[i], duration=0.002, system=sys)
3. seq.add_block(gy_pre, gz_reph)
4. seq.add_block(delayTE)
5. seq.add_block(gx_pre)
6. seq.add_block(gx, adc)
7. seq.add_block(delayTR)

14.4 TIME-AVERAGED RF POWER COMPUTATION FOR PULSEQ SEQUENCES

The advent of open source pulse sequence programming detailed above has provided increased opportunities for rapid prototyping of MR acquisition methods. While these opportunities are critical to explore MR acquisition methods, the safety aspects of such implementations are vital. Inadvertent mistakes in the case of RF pulse and sequence design can result in major safety hazards (e.g., in patients with regions of very high local SAR and not sufficient perfusion such as stroke or diabetic patients and in patients with implanted conductive devices). It is therefore critical to evaluate these open source pulse-programmed sequences at multiple stages and levels. The Pulseq interpreters do include a downstream check on SAR, PNS, and other safety aspects before running the sequence. However, it is important to assess certain safety checks before porting the sequence to the scanner. One of the necessary safety checks is the evaluation of SAR (or at least the time-averaged RF power) for the implemented sequence.

For the Pulseq standard, this includes the integration of Sections 14.2 and 14.3. The following paragraphs describe the simple method of determining the time-averaged RF power for a particular Pulseq constructed sequence. Once the pulse sequence has been programmed according to the Pulseq file standard, the *seq* object described earlier can be read block by block similar to the way the sample GRE sequence was constructed. For every *RF* event in these blocks, one could compute the value for the SAR_{pulse} using equation (14.5) or alternatively use the VOP framework outlined in Section 14.2.3.1 to calculate L-SAR in an accelerated but overestimated manner. These SAR values could then be mass normalized to compute the RF power delivered by each pulse. A time average of these power estimates results in a metric shown by the vendors per sequence. The pseudocode for such an implementation is shown in the following section, and the code for validating time-averaged RF power using the Pulseq file standard is available at Ref. 22.

14.4.1 Pseudocode

1. Set *time_elapsed* = 0
2. While *num_events* ≤ *all_events*
3. if *event* has *RF*
   Compute *SAR* and *time_elapsed*
   Store *time_elapsed*
4. Determine *time_elapsed*
5. Compute *RFpower* by mass normalizing *SAR* (using the EM model's mass)
6. Compute time averaged RF power as the ratio of total *RF* power to *time_elapsed*

14.4.2 Time-averaged RF Power Implementation Example

A Turbo Spin Echo (TSE) sequence part of the Pulseq library (writeTSE.m, version 1.2.1) with a $TR/TE = 2000/12$ *ms*, $TE_{\text{eff}} = 60$ ms, slice thickness of 5 mm, field of view 256 × 256 mm^2, and echo train length (ETL) 16 was used to test the implementations described in Sections 14.2 and 14.3. The flip angles for the refocusing pulse were varied in steps of 10° starting from 120° to 180°. Seven separate *.seq* files were generated corresponding to each of the different flip angles. The MATLAB code at Ref. 22 was employed to derive time-averaged RF power values based on the VHM model global *Q*-matrix. The *.seq* files were then ported to a 3T Siemens Prisma Fit scanner and run on a ball of nickel sulfate-doped water, registered with a patient weight of 103.45 kg. The body coil was used for transmission, and a 64-channel head-and-neck coil for signal reception. For each run, the time-averaged RF power was recorded from the vendor's user interface for SAR monitoring. Figure 14.5 shows the time-averaged RF power from the scanner (hollow circles) and the implemented method (filled circles). The

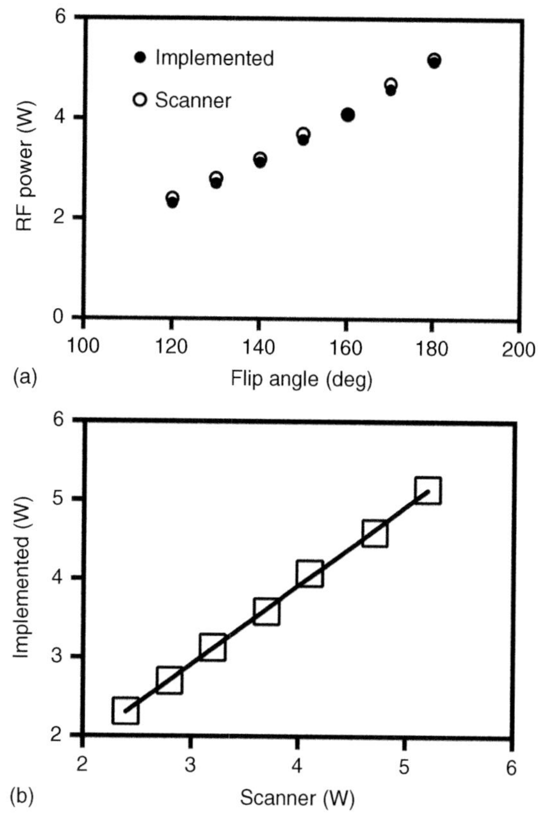

Figure 14.5. Time-averaged RF power: (a) The effect of increasing flip angle from 120° to 180° on the implemented and scanner-observed time-averaged RF power for the Turbo Spin Echo sequence. (b) Correlations between the scanner-observed and implemented methods.

plot shows the correlation plot of the scanner-observed values against the results of the implemented method. The plot shows a high degree of correlation with the linear regression given by $\text{Scanner observed}_{\text{RF\_power}} = 1.007 \times \text{Implemented}_{\text{RF\_power}} - 0.1039$.

ACKNOWLEDGMENTS

The author would like to thank Prof. Joseph V. Hajnal and Prof. Shaihan J. Malik, King's College London, for their inputs and thoughtful discussions on the *Q*-matrix and *VOP* formulations, and the resources at King's College London for testing the implementations. The author would like to thank Dr. Jon Nielsen Fredrick for his inputs on extending the RF safety computation of open source pulse sequences to multiple vendor platforms.

Grant support:

1. Fast Functional MRI with sparse sampling and model-based reconstruction, National Institute of Biomedical Imaging and Bioengineering, 1R01EB023618-01, PI: Noll, Fessler; UM SUBK00009808, PI: Geethanath;
2. Zuckerman Institute Technical Development Grant for MR, Zuckerman Mind Brain Behavior Institute, Grant Number: CU-ZI-MR-T-0002; PI: Geethanath;
3. Zuckerman Institute Seed Grant for MR studies, Zuckerman Mind Brain Behavior Institute, Grant Number:CU-ZI-MR-S-0007; PI: Geethanath.

DISCLAIMER

In no event shall the authors be liable for any claim, damages or other liability, whether in an action of contract, tort or otherwise, arising from, out of or in connection with the Software or the use or other dealings in the Software.

REFERENCES

1. R. W. Brown, E. M. Haacke, Y. C. N. Cheng, and M. R. Thompson, 'Magnetic Resonance Imaging: Physical Principles and Sequence Design', John Wiley & Sons, 2014.
2. I. Ronen and D. Shik Kim, in 'Principles and Advanced Methods in Medical Imaging and Image Analysis', World Scientific, 2008, p 99. DOI: 10.1142/9789812814807_0005.
3. S. Geethanath, *Resonance*, 2015, **20**. ISSN: 0973712X. DOI: 10.1007/s12045-015-0268-2.
4. K. J. Layton, S. Kroboth, F. Jia, S. Littin, H. Yu, J. Leupold, J. Fredrik Nielsen, T. Stöcker, and M. Zaitsev, *Magn. Reson. Med.*, 2017. ISSN: 15222594. DOI: 10.1002/mrm.26235.
5. G. Clarke, In Med. Phys. 2010. DOI: 10.1118/1.3469331.
6. D. Anne Langman, S. Srinivasan, and D. Ennis, In Proceedings of International Society for Magnetic Resonance in Medicine, 2015.
7. J. T. Vaughan and J. R. Griffiths (eds), 'RF Coils for MRI', John Wiley & Sons, 2012. ISBN: 9781119441649.
8. L. Winter, E. Oberacker, C. Özerdem, Y. J., F. Von Knobelsdorff-Brenkenhoff, G. Weidemann, B. Ittermann, F. Seifert, and T. Niendorf, *Magn. Reson. Med.*, 2015. ISSN: 15222594. DOI: 10.1002/mrm.25483.
9. D. Shrivastava (ed), 'Theory and Applications of Heat Transfer in Humans', Wiley Blackwell, 2018.
10. L. L. Wald and E. Adalsteinsson, *MAGNETOM Flash*, 2009, **40**, 124.
11. U. Katscher and P. Börnert, *NMR Biomed.*, 2006, **19**, 393.
12. S. J. Malik, F. Padormo, A. N. Price, and J. V. Hajnal, *Magn. Reson. Med.*, 2012. ISSN: 07403194. DOI: 10.1002/mrm.24153.
13. G. J. Metzger, C. Snyder, C. Akgun, T. Vaughan, K. Ugurbil, and P. Francois Van De Moortele, *Magn. Reson. Med.*, 2008. ISSN: 07403194. DOI: 10.1002/mrm.21476.
14. B. Van Den Bergen, C. A T. Van Den Berg, D. W J. Klomp, and J. J W. Lagendijk, *J. Magn. Reson. Imaging*, 2009. ISSN: 10531807. DOI: 10.1002/jmri.21806.
15. W. Mao, M. B. Smith, and C. M. Collins, *Magn. Reson. Med.*, 2006. ISSN: 07403194. DOI: 10.1002/mrm.21013.
16. H. Homann, I. Graesslin, H. Eggers, K. Nehrke, P. Vernickel, U. Katscher, O. Dössel, and P. Börnert, *Magn. Reson. Mat. Phys. Biol. Med.*, 2012. ISSN: 09685243. DOI: 10.1007/s10334-011-0281-8.
17. C. Akgun, C. Snyder, S. Moeller, P. Bolan, T. Vaughan, K. Ugurbil, P. Van de Moortele, and G. Metzger, In Proceedings 16th Scientific Meeting, International Society for Magnetic Resonance in Medicine, 2008. ISBN: 1545-4428.
18. P. A. Bottomley, R. W. Redington, W. A. Edelstein, and J. F. Schenck, *Magn. Reson. Med.*, 1985. ISSN: 15222594. DOI: 10.1002/mrm.1910020404.
19. P. A. Bottomley and W. A. Edelstein, *Med. Phys.*, 1981, **8**, 510.
20. P. A. Bottomley and E. R. Andrew, *Phys. Med. Biol.*, 1978. ISSN: 00319155. DOI: 10.1088/0031-9155/23/4/006.
21. I. Graesslin, H. Homann, S. Biederer, P. Börnert, K. Nehrke, P. Vernickel, G. Mens, P. Harvey, and U. Katscher, *Magn. Reson. Med.*, 2012. ISSN: 07403194. DOI: 10.1002/mrm.24138.

22. S. Geethanath, sar4seq, 2019, p 1. https://github.com/imr-framework/sar4seq.
23. G. Eichfelder and M. Gebhardt, *Magn. Reson. Med.*, 2011. ISSN 07403194. DOI: 10.1002/mrm.22927.
24. H. H. Pennes, *J. Appl. Physiol.*, 1948, **1**, 93.
25. D. Shrivastava and J. Thomas Vaughan, *J. Biomech. Eng.*, 2009. ISSN: 01480731. DOI: 10.1115/1.3127260.
26. S. Geethanath, J. Kabil, and J. Thomas Vaughan Jr., In ISMRM 2 workshop on Machine Learning, Washington, D.C., 2018. ISMRM.
27. S. Ding, H. Zhao, Y. Zhang, X. Xu, and R. Nie, *Artif. Intell. Rev.*, 2015. ISSN: 15737462. DOI: 10.1007/s10462-013-9405-z.
28. T. H. Jochimsen and M. Von Mengershausen, *J. Magn. Reson.*, 2004. ISSN: 10907807. DOI: 10.1016/j.jmr.2004.05.021.
29. J.-F. Nielsen and D. C. Noll, *Magn. Reson. Med.*, 2018, **79**, 3128. ISSN: 07403194. DOI: 10.1002/mrm.26990.
30. K. Sravan Ravi, S. Potdar, P. Poojar, A. Kumar Reddy, S. Kroboth, J. Fredrik Nielsen, M. Zaitsev, R. Venkatesan, and S. Geethanath, *Magn. Reson. Imaging*, 2018. ISSN: 18735894. DOI: 10.1016/j.mri.2018.03.008.
31. T. Stöcker, K. Vahedipour, D. Pflugfelder, and N. Jon Shah, *Magn. Reson. Med.*, 2010. ISSN: 15222594. DOI: 10.1002/mrm.22406.
32. M. Weigel, *J. Magn. Reson. Imaging*, 2015, **41**, 266.
33. H. Benoit-Cattin, G. Collewet, B. Belaroussi, H. Saint-Jalmes, and C. Odet, *J. Magn. Reson.*, 2005. ISSN 10907807. DOI: 10.1016/j.jmr.2004.09.027.
34. F. Liu, J. V. Velikina, W. F. Block, R. Kijowski, and A. A. Samsonov, *IEEE T. Med. Imaging*, 2017. ISSN 1558254X. DOI: 10.1109/TMI.2016.2620961.
35. S. J. Inati, J. D. Naegele, N. R. Zwart, V. Roopchansingh, M. J. Lizak, D. C. Hansen, C. Y. Liu, D. Atkinson, P. Kellman, S. Kozerke, H. Xue, A. E. Campbell-Washburn, T. S. Sørensen, and M. S. Hansen, *Magn. Reson. Med.*, 2017. ISSN: 15222594. DOI: 10.1002/mrm.26089.
36. L. Winter, Open source imaging, 2018. http://www.opensourceimaging.org/.
37. J. F. Magland, C. Li, M. C. Langham, and F. W. Wehrli, *Magn. Reson. Med.*, 2016. ISSN: 15222594. DOI: 10.1002/mrm.25640.

FURTHER READING

J. T. Vaughan and J. R. Griffiths (eds), 'RF coils for MRI', John Wiley & Sons, 2012.

I. Graesslin, H. Homann, S. Biederer, P. Börnert, K. Nehrke, P. Vernickel, G. Mens, P. Harvey, and U. Katscher, *Magn. Reson. Med.*, 2012, **68**, 1664.

G. Eichfelder and M. Gebhardt, *Magn. Reson. Med.*, 2011, **66**, 1468.

T. H. Jochimsen, A. Schäfer, R. Bammer, and M. E. Moseley, *J. Magn. Reson.*, 2006, **180**, 29.

K. J. Layton, S. Kroboth, F. Jia, S. Littin, H. Yu, J. Leupold, J.F. Nielsen, T. Stöcker, M. Zaitsev, *Magn. Reson. Med.*, 2017, **77**, 1544.

K. S. Ravi, S. Potdar, P. Poojar, A. K. Reddy, S. Kroboth, J. F. Nielsen, M. Zaitsev, R. Venkatesan, S. Geethanath, *Magn. Reson. Imaging*, 2018, **52**, 9.

Chapter 15

RF Heating Due to a 3T Birdcage Whole-body Transmit Coil in Anesthetized Sheep

Samat Turdumamatov[1], Çağdaş Oto[2], Oktay Algın[3], Hamza Ergüder[4], and Tahir Malas[5]

[1]*University of Central Asia, Bishkek, Kyrgyzstan*
[2]*Ankara University, Ankara, Turkey*
[3]*Atatürk Training and Research Hospital, Ankara, Turkey*
[4]*Yildiz Technical University, Istanbul, Turkey*
[5]*Lorentz Solution, Santa Clara, CA, USA*

15.1 INTRODUCTION

Nonuniform radiofrequency (RF) power is deposited to the body during magnetic resonance imaging (MRI). This nonuniformly deposited RF power induces nonuniform in vivo heating with the possibility of 'harmful' local hot spots or hot regions. Thus, to better characterize the induced heating and to develop ways to mitigate thermogenic hazards associated with such heating, several investigators have measured the induced heating in healthy humans and/or human-relevant animals in high (i.e., 1.5 and 3 T) and ultrahigh fields (i.e., >3 T).[1–12] For example, Kido *et al.* measured the average temperature rise of 0.2 ± 0.1 °C and 0.5 ± 0.1 °C in the axilla due to the scanner-reported whole-body average specific absorption rate (SAR) of ~0.2 and ~0.8 W kg^{-1}, respectively. The RF power was deposited for 17 min and measured in 14 volunteers during lumbar scans in 1.5 T.[1] Van Den Brink[2] reported the core temperature rise of ~1.0 °C, measured due to the whole-body average SAR of 4.0 W kg^{-1} deposited for 15 min in 1.5 T. Shuman *et al.*[3] measured the average temperature change ranging from 2.6 to 5.1 °C in anesthetized dogs due to the whole-body average SAR of ~2.5 W kg^{-1} deposited for 25.6 min in 1.5 T. Barber *et al.*[4] measured the rectal temperature change of 2.3 °C in anesthetized sheep due to the whole-body average SAR of ~4.0 W kg^{-1} deposited for 82 min in 1.5 T. Shrivastava *et al.* measured the temperature change of ~2.5 °C in the brain and ~1.5 °C in the rectum in anesthetized swine due to the whole-body average SAR of ~2.7 W kg^{-1} deposited for 60 min in 3 T,

Safety and Biological Effects in MRI.
Edited by Devashish Shrivastava and J. Thomas Vaughan
 ISBN: 978-1-118-82130-5
Also published in eMagRes (online edition)
DOI: 10.1002/9780470034590.emrstm1640

when the swine head was placed in the isocenter. When the swine trunk was placed in isocenter instead, they measured the temperature change of ~1.8 °C in the brain and ~1.6 °C in the rectum due to the whole-body average SAR of ~2.8 W kg^{-1} deposited for 60 min. Nadobny *et al.*[6] measured the temperature changes exceeding 1 °C in anesthetized swine due to the whole-body average SAR deposition of 2.5–5.2 W kg^{-1} deposited for 30 or 60 min in 3 T (exact temperature change is not clear due to the way data are presented).

The current study augments the existing set of limited RF heating data in human-relevant animal models[3–12] by making measurements in seven anesthetized fleeced sheep placed in a 3 T horizontal bore, whole-body clinical magnetic resonance (MR) scanner. The new data together with the existing set of data may allow us to better understand the induced heating due to power deposition from 3 T, whole-body transmit body coils.

15.2 METHODS

15.2.1 Animals

Anesthetized, fleeced sheep ($N = 7$, mass = 44–69 kg) were used to make the measurements. The first sheep was used to better evaluate the role of anesthesia on the sheep body temperature. Sheep 2–6 were exposed to the RF power deposition to study the induced heating. Sheep were chosen because mass, surface area, normal core body temperature, and thermoregulatory mechanisms of sheep are comparable to those of humans.[4,13,14]

15.2.2 Experiment Design

The animal experiment protocol was approved by the Institutional Animal Care and Usage Committee (IACUC) of the university.

The sheep were fasted for 24 h before the experiment. Water was provided ad libitum. The sheep were immobilized by injecting, first with 0.02 mg kg^{-1} of subcutaneous atropine (0.2%) and ~20 min later with 0.5 mg kg^{-1} of intramuscular xylazine HCl (Alfazyne 2%). Next, 2.5 mg kg^{-1} of intramuscular ketamine HCl (Ketasol 10%) was injected to induce general anesthesia. Intubation was performed with a 7.5 cuff endotracheal tube. A 24 G cannula was inserted into the ear vein (vena auris) to keep animals anesthetized and hydrated during the experiment. The animals were kept anesthetized during the experiment (~4–5 h) via total intravenous anesthesia (TIVA). For this purpose, 16 mg kg^{-1} of propofol (Profol 1%) was mixed with 230 mL of physiological saline solution and injected into sheep at the average rate of ~16 mg kg^{-1} min^{-1}. After the experiment, sheep were euthanized using high dose of pentobarbital, per the approved protocol.

MR-compatible safe fluoroptic temperature probes (Neoptix) were inserted into the subcutaneous tissue, muscle, rectum, and, in a few experiments, into the brain. In some of the experiments, the temperature was also measured in the blood and/or inner organs, such as the bladder. Subcutaneous and inner-muscle probes were secured with sutures. Catheters were used for the blood or inner-organ measurements.

The heating is measured in a commercial, clinical, whole-body MR scanner with horizontal cylindrical bore. The study protocol consisted of ~30 min of thermal equilibration in the MR scanner, 1 h of RF exposure using a high-SAR TRUFI (true fast imaging with steady-state free precession) sequence, and ~30 min of post-RF observation in the MR scanner. The scanner-reported whole-body average SAR is recorded for each experiment. The true whole-body average SAR is unknown. The temperature of the scanner room was maintained between 20 and 22 °C.

15.3 RESULTS

15.3.1 Effect of Anesthesia on the Sheep Body Temperature

Figure 15.1 shows the effect of the anesthesia on the rectal temperature of a 42 kg sheep over the experimental duration of 3 h. The figure shows that the anesthesia may induce a linear temperature drop in the body. The temperature rise due to the RF power deposition may be estimated by subtracting such subject-specific anesthesia-induced temperature drop from the absolute temperature measurements.[5–12] The results presented herein do not correct for the anesthesia-induced cooling. Thus, the reported temperature changes are likely to underestimate the RF-induced temperature change.

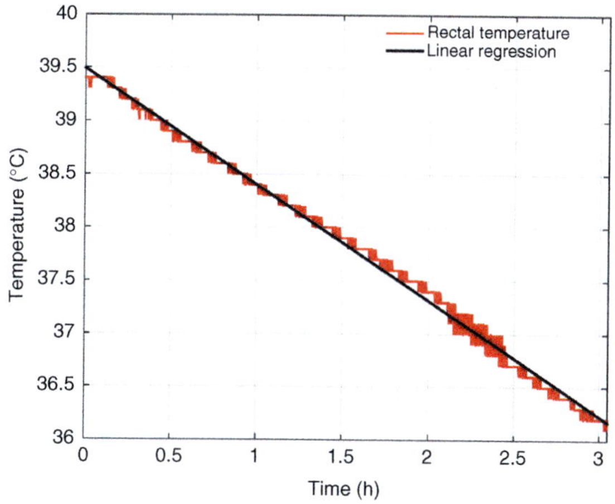

Figure 15.1. The effect of the anesthesia on the rectal temperature of a sheep. The temperature is shown to drop approximately to 1 °C h^{-1}

15.3.2 Effect of RF Heating

Figures 15.2–15.4 present the RF-induced heating in three sheep ($N = 3$) when the sheep head is placed in the isocenter. Likewise, Figures 15.5–15.7 present the RF-induced heating in three sheep ($N = 3$), when the sheep trunk is placed in the isocenter. The black vertical lines in the figures show the start and end of the RF power deposition.

Figure 15.2 presents the absolute temperatures and temperature changes for the first head-in-the-isocenter experiment. A linear increase in the temperatures is observed due to the RF exposure. The temperatures in the brain and rectum are shown to exceed 1.6 °C due to the MR scanner-reported whole-body average SAR deposition of 1.6 W kg^{-1} continuously for 60 min (mass of sheep = 69 kg).

Figure 15.3 presents the absolute temperatures and temperature changes for the second head-in-the-isocenter experiment. Additional probes were inserted into muscle and bladder to gather additional insight into the heating of body. The effect of the anesthesia on the RF-induced temperature rise is clearly depicted. The temperature rise of ~0.5 °C is measured due to the MR scanner-reported whole-body average SAR of 2.1 W kg^{-1} deposited continuously for 60 min. The result appears to show smaller temperature rise due to the RF power compared to the first experiment. However, noticing that the temperature drops at the rate of ~1 °C h^{-1} (~0.5 °C drop in pre-RF duration of 30 min), the RF-induced temperature rise is expected to be ~1.5 °C. Given the uncertainty regarding the true whole-body average SAR (the true and scanner-reported whole-body average SAR may be different from scan to scan and from one subject to another), the result appears comparable to the first experiment (mass of sheep = 50 kg).

Figure 15.4 presents the absolute temperatures and temperature changes for the third

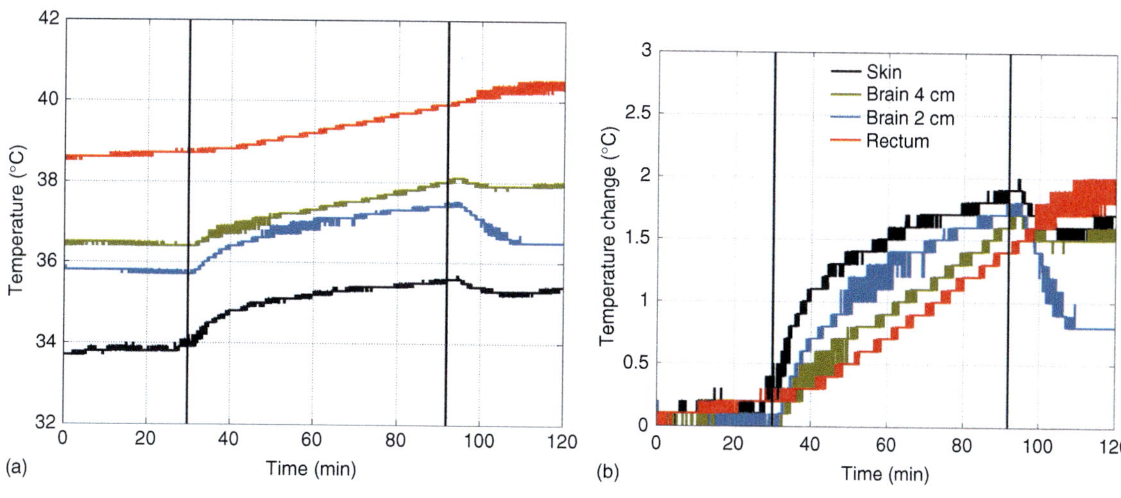

Figure 15.2. Absolute temperature (a) and temperature-change curves (b) for the first head-in-the-isocenter experiment. The MR-reported whole-body average SAR is 1.6 W kg^{-1}

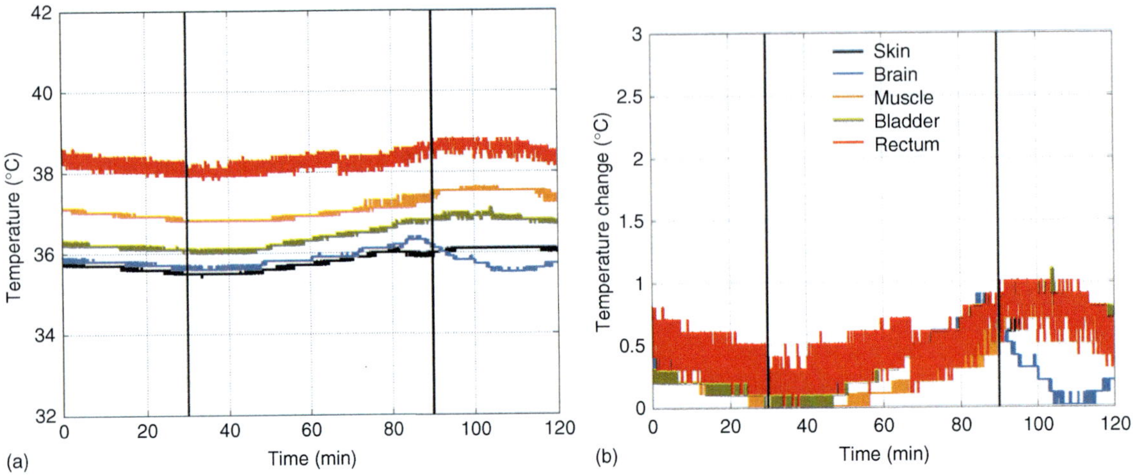

Figure 15.3. Absolute temperature (a) and temperature-change curves (b) for the second head-in-the-isocenter experiment. The MR-reported whole-body average SAR is 2.1 W kg^{-1}

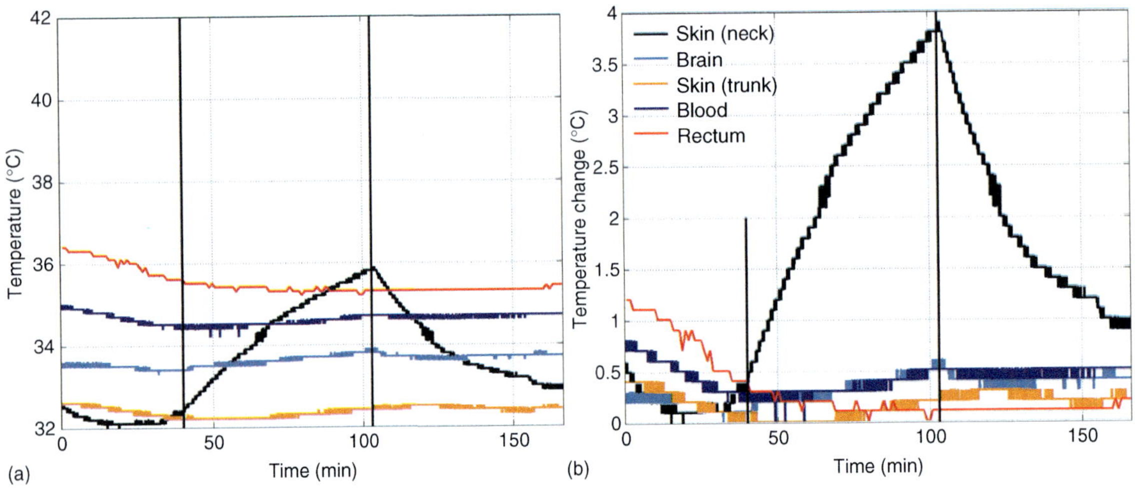

Figure 15.4. Absolute temperature (a) and temperature-change curves (b) for the third head-in-the-isocenter experiment. The MR-reported whole-body average SAR is 1.8 W kg^{-1}

head-in-the-isocenter experiment. The blood temperature was directly measured in the jugular vein. It is noted that while the rectal reading does not show a temperature increase due to the anesthesia-induced cooling, the temperature in the brain and blood is shown to rise. The RF-induced temperature rise in brain and blood is estimated to be ~1 °C due to the scanner-reported whole-body average SAR of ~1.8 W kg^{-1} deposited for 60 min (mass of sheep = 48 kg).

Figure 15.5 presents the absolute temperatures and temperature changes for the first trunk-in-the-isocenter experiment. All temperature changes exceeded 2 °C due to the scanner-reported whole-body average SAR of 3.6 W kg^{-1} deposited for 60 min (mass of sheep = 63 kg).

Figure 15.6 presents the absolute temperatures and temperature changes for the second trunk-in-the-isocenter experiment. All temperature changes exceeded ~2.8 °C due to the scanner-reported

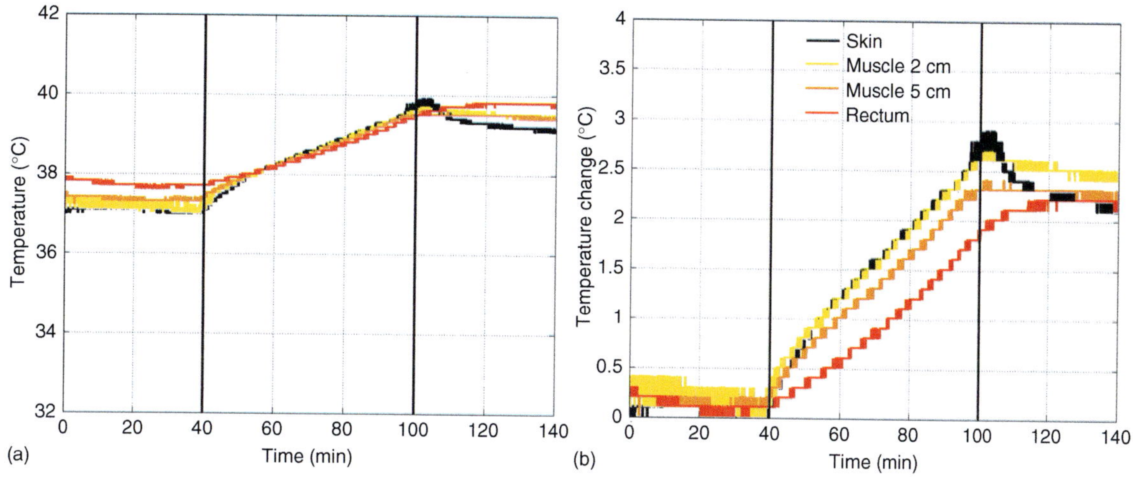

Figure 15.5. Absolute temperature (a) and temperature-change curves (b) for the first trunk-in-the-isocenter experiment. The MR-reported whole-body average SAR is 3.6 W kg^{-1}

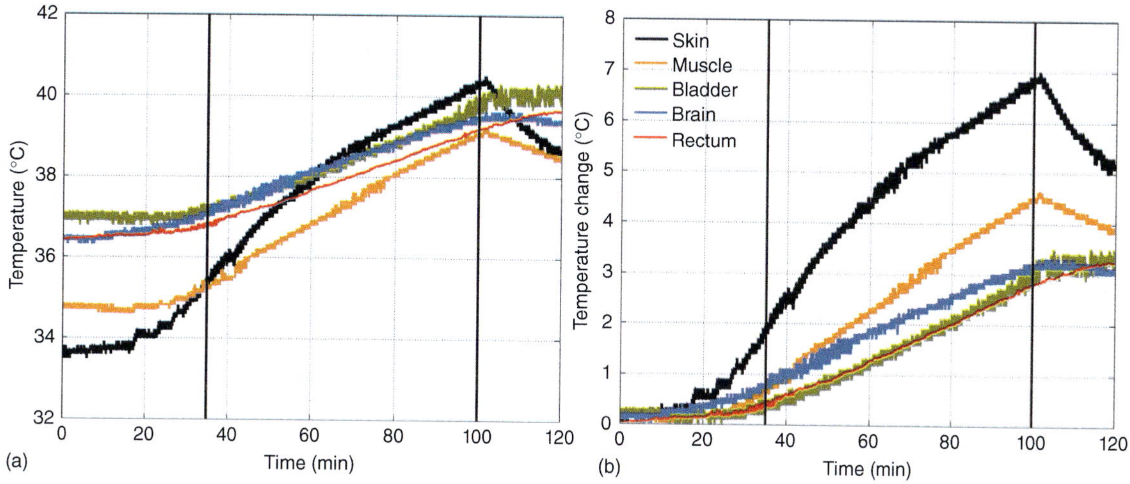

Figure 15.6. Absolute temperature (a) and temperature-change curves (b) for the second trunk-in-the-isocenter experiment. The MR-reported whole-body average SAR is 2.8 W kg^{-1}

whole-body average SAR of 2.8 W kg^{-1} deposited for 60 min (mass of sheep = 48 kg).

Figure 15.7 presents the absolute temperatures and temperature changes for the third trunk-in-the-isocenter experiment. All deep body temperature changes exceeded ~4.0 °C due to the scanner-reported whole-body average SAR of ~4.3 W kg^{-1} deposited for 60 min. The temperature change in the muscle exceeded 6.0 °C (mass of sheep = 42 kg).

15.4 DISCUSSION

Three main observations are made. First, allowable whole-body average SARs (i.e., ≤4.0 W kg^{-1}), when deposited for sufficient duration, may induce temperature changes that exceed the maximum allowable safe temperature change limit in the body (i.e., ≤1 °C in the deep tissue).[15,16] This observation is consistent with the measurements published before.[1–12] This observation suggests the need to monitor core

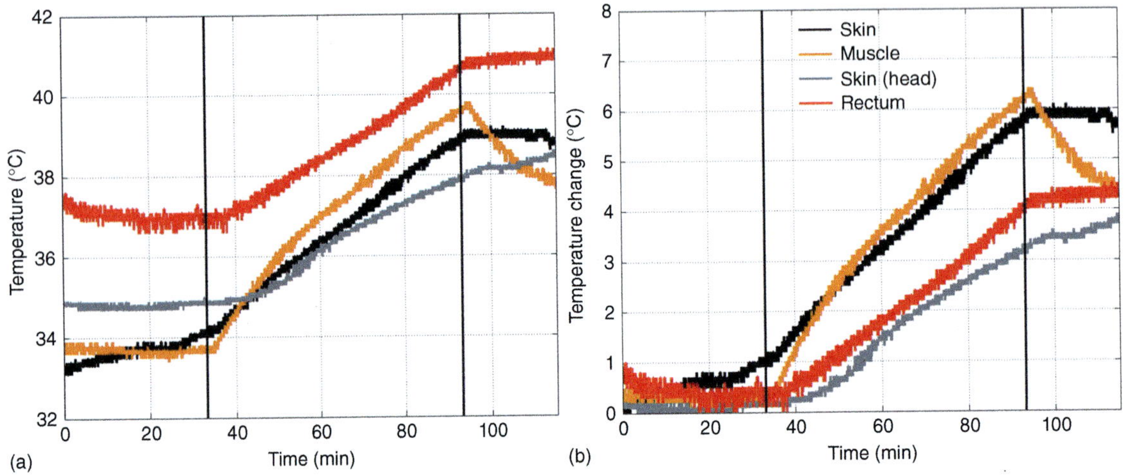

Figure 15.7. Absolute temperature (a) and temperature-change curves (b) for the third trunk-in-the-isocenter experiment. The MR-reported whole-body average SAR is 4.3 W kg^{-1}

body temperature of patients during 'long' scans to keep temperatures within allowable limits to avoid thermogenic hazards (e.g., in pregnant women since temperature is a known teratogen).

Second, temperature changes on the skin are variable and should not be used as a marker of the in vivo temperature change and/or safety. This observation suggests that new tools and/or methods are needed to reliably detect and control temperature changes everywhere in the body to improve safety.

Third, temperature in the blood and rectum may be different, and the difference is expected to be a function of space and time. Thus, the bioheat models that assume constant or quickly stabilizing body/blood temperature (such as the Pennes bioheat model) may not present reliable results.[5,17–19] More advanced models as the generic bioheat transfer model may present more reliable results due to their ability to model tissue and blood temperatures separately.[20]

Regarding the limitations of the study, the measurements are reported as a function of the scanner-reported whole-body average SAR. Scanner-reported whole-body average SAR may be different than the truly deposited whole-body average SAR. Further, the 'true' SAR may be different from one scan to the next and from one sheep to the next for the same 'reported' whole-body average SAR. Thus, our results need to be evaluated further to develop correlations between the whole-body average SAR and the RF-induced heating. The 'true' RF-induced temperature change need to be obtained from the measured temperatures by correcting for the anesthesia-induced cooling.

ACKNOWLEDGMENTS

The authors wish to thank the Scientific and Technological Research Council of Turkey (TUBITAK) for supporting the project under Grant No. 113E187.

RELATED ARTICLES IN EMAGRES

Radiofrequency Heating Models and Measurements

REFERENCES

1. D. K. Kido, T. W. Morris, J. L. Erickson, D. B. Plewes, and J. H. Simon, *Am. J. Neuroradiol.*, 1987, **8**, 263.
2. J. S. Van Den Brink, *Concepts Magn. Reson. B*, 2019, **2019**, 9618680.
3. W. P. Shuman, D. R. Haynor, A. W. Guy, G. E. Wesbey, D. J. Schaefer, and A. A. Moss, *Radiology*, 1988, **167**, 551.
4. B. J. Barber, D. J. Schaefer, C. J. Gordon, D. C. Zawieja, and J. Hecker, *AJR Am. J. Roentgenol.*, 1990, **155**, 1105.

5. D. Shrivastava, L. Utecht, J. Tian, J. Hughes, and J. T. Vaughan, *Magn. Reson. Med.*, 2014, **72**, 1141.
6. J. Nadobny, R. Klopfleisch, G. Brinker, and G. Stoltenburg-Didinger, *Int. J. Hyperther.*, 2015, **31**, 409.
7. D. Shrivastava, T. Hanson, J. Kulesa, J. Tian, A. Gregor, and J. T. Vaughan, *Magn. Reson. Med.*, 2011, **66**, 255 (PMC3339408).
8. D. Shrivastava, T. Hanson, R. Schlentz, W. Gallagher, C. Snyder, L. DelaBarre, S. Prakash, P. A. Iaizzo, and J. T. Vaughan, *Magn. Reson. Med.*, 2008, **59**, 73.
9. D. Shrivastava, T. Hanson, J. Kulesa, L. DelaBarre, G. Adriany, P. A. Iaizzo, and J. T. Vaughan, *Magn. Reson. Med.*, 2009, **62**, 888.
10. D. Shrivastava, J. Kulesa, J. Tian, G. Adriany, L. DelaBarre, and J. T. Vaughan, Radio-frequency heating in swine with a 12' ID, 8 channel 7 T (296 MHz) head coil, In *ISMRM Annual Meeting*, Montreal, Canada, 2011.
11. D. Shrivastava, J. Kulesa, T. Hanson, J. Tian, and J. T. Vaughan, Radio-frequency heating due to a 9' ID, 8 channel 7T (296 MHz) head coil, In *8th Biennial 2011 Minnesota Workshops*, Minneapolis, USA, 2011.
12. D. Shrivastava, L. Utecht, J. Tian, T. Hanson, and J. T. Vaughan, Radiofrequency heating in swine due to a 3T (123.2 MHz) and 7T (296 MHz) head coil, In *ISMRM Annual Meeting*, Melbourne, Australia, 2012.
13. D. R. Ames, J. E. Nellor, and T. Adams, *J. Anim. Sci.*, 1971, **32**, 784 DOI: 10.2134/jas1971.324784x.
14. K. Johnson, *Aust. J. Agric. Res.*, 1987, **38**, 587 DOI: 10.1071/AR9870587.
15. ICNIRP, *Health Phys.*, 1998, **74**, 494.
16. International Electrotechnical Commission, Medical Electrical Equipment—Part 2–33: Particular Requirements for the Basic Safety and Essential Performance of Magnetic Resonance Equipment for Medical Diagnosis [60601-2-33 Ed 3.2b], International Electrotechnical Commission: Geneva, 2015.
17. H. H. Pennes, *J. Appl. Physiol.*, 1998, **85**, 5.
18. E. H. Wissler, *J. Appl. Physiol.*, 1998, **85**, 35.
19. L. Zhu, in 'Standard Handbook of Biomedical Engineering and Design', ed. M. Kutz, McGraw-Hill: New York, 2003.
20. D. Shrivastava (ed), Theory and Applications of Heat Transfer in Humans, John Wiley & Sons, Inc: Hoboken, NJ, 2018.

Chapter 16

In Vivo Radiofrequency Heating due to 1.5, 3, and 7 T Whole-body Volume Coils

Shuo Song[1], Ji Chen[1], Rongxing Zhang[2], Qiang He[2], J. Thomas Vaughan[3], and Devashish Shrivastava[4]

[1] *University of Houston, Houston, TX, USA*
[2] *Shanghai United Imaging Healthcare Co., Ltd, Shanghai, China*
[3] *Columbia University in the City of New York, New York, NY, USA*
[4] *In Vivo Temperatures, LLC, Burnsville, MN, USA*

16.1 INTRODUCTION

In vivo heating due to radiofrequency (RF) power deposition from transmit coils is a safety concern during magnetic resonance imaging (MRI). MRI requires depositing RF power in the body to produce images. The deposited RF power is absorbed nonuniformly and together with the nonuniform blood flow that redistributes this energy, nonuniform tissue heating is induced, which may result in one or more local regions of clinically harmful temperature rise.

To mitigate the concern of undesirable thermal hazards, the International Electrotechnical Commission (IEC) recommends safe absolute temperature and temperature change thresholds that should not be exceeded during MRI (maximum core and local temperature ≤39 °C, maximum core temperature change of ≤0.5 °C in the normal mode; maximum core and local temperature ≤40 °C, maximum core temperature change of ≤1 °C in the first level mode).[1] However, since it is difficult to determine local temperature change deep inside the body noninvasively with sufficient accuracy and precision, and unpleasant/time-consuming to measure core temperature using temperature probes in every patient undergoing MRI, values of relatively easy to implement net, maximum, forward RF power (or RF power per unit mass or specific absorption rate or SAR) were determined instead, that could be deposited in the body to comply with the temperature guidelines. The values for the RF power (or SARs) were computed using simple thermal models (e.g., two-node model of Drs Adair and Berglund, Pennes bioheat transfer equation).[1–5] Unfortunately, the models employ such simplifying assumptions that make them invalid

Safety and Biological Effects in MRI.
Edited by Devashish Shrivastava and J. Thomas Vaughan

ISBN: 978-1-118-82130-5
Also published in eMagRes (online edition)
DOI: 10.1002/9780470034590.emrstm1570

and/or result in underestimated local and/or systemic tissue heating for a given SAR. For more on the applicability and limitations of these models, please refer to.[6,7]

The IEC recommends the maximum whole-body average SAR of $2\,W\,kg^{-1}$ in the normal mode and $4\,W\,kg^{-1}$ in the first level mode for transmit, volume body coils to comply with the temperature guidelines. Maximum SAR limit for the whole-head exposure is $3.2\,W\,kg^{-1}$ in the normal and first level modes. The maximum allowable RF energy deposition is recommended as $4\,W\,kg^{-1} \times 60\,min = 240\,W\,min\,kg^{-1}$. No limits are recommended for the local SAR values for volume coils.

In this chapter, we reevaluate the magnitude and distribution of the MRI induced heating using the new, state-of-the-art, validated, two-compartment generic bioheat transfer model (GBHTM) for various human body models (adult male, adult female, 9-month pregnant woman) placed inside a 1.5, 3, and 7 T whole body volume coil, in various landmark positions. The results of the GBHTM are compared to those of the conventional, 'simplified', empirical Pennes bioheat transfer equation (BHTE).[7,8] Since thermal hazards are a function of the temperature-time history – and not just the temperature – corresponding thermal dose (TD) values are computed, as well, per two frequently employed methods, the cumulative equivalent minutes at 43 °C (*CEM*43) and Arrhenius equation.

16.2 METHODS

16.2.1 Anatomical Models

Three whole-body human models are used – an adult male (Duke), and adult female (Ella), and a 9-month pregnant woman. These body models belong to virtual population (IT'IS Foundation, Switzerland). Duke is ~1.77 m tall and weighs ~70.2 kg. Ella is ~1.63 m tall and weighs ~57.3 kg. The pregnant woman is ~1.58 m tall and weighs ~68.5 kg. The pregnant woman model includes a detailed 9-month old fetus model and amniotic fluid.

16.2.2 Coils and Simulation Setup

Three whole-body coils are considered. The 1.5 T whole-body volume coil is modeled as a birdcage, resonates at 64 MHz, and has two excitation ports I and Q. The coil has 16 rungs and the diameter and length of 313.2 and 600 mm, respectively. The coil has two sets of capacitors of 50 pF to connect the gaps between the adjacent sections of the end rings and tune the coil to appropriate frequency. Two other capacitors of 75 pF each are used parallel to the two ports for impedance matching. The shielding of the coil has the diameter and length of 350 and 1200 mm, respectively.

The 3 T whole-body coil is modeled as a birdcage, resonates at 128.23 MHz, and has two excitation ports I and Q, as well. The coil has 16 rungs, and the diameter and length of 310 and 550 mm, respectively. The coil has two sets of capacitors of 13.5 pF each for tuning and matching. The shielding has the diameter of 334 mm and length of 1454 mm, respectively.

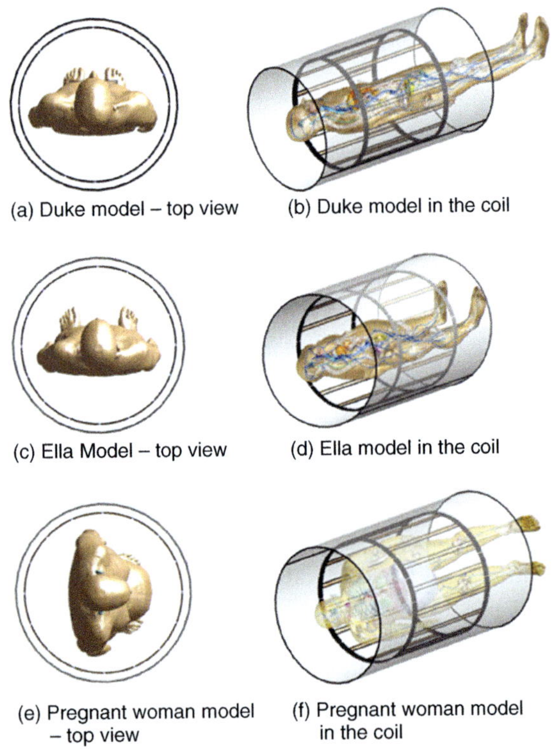

Figure 16.1. (a) Top view of Duke inside in the coil; (b) Duke orientation in coil, lying on the back; (c) Top view of Ella inside in the coil; (d) Ella orientation in coil, lying on the back; (e) Top view of pregnant woman inside in the coil; (f) pregnant woman orientation in coil, lying on the side

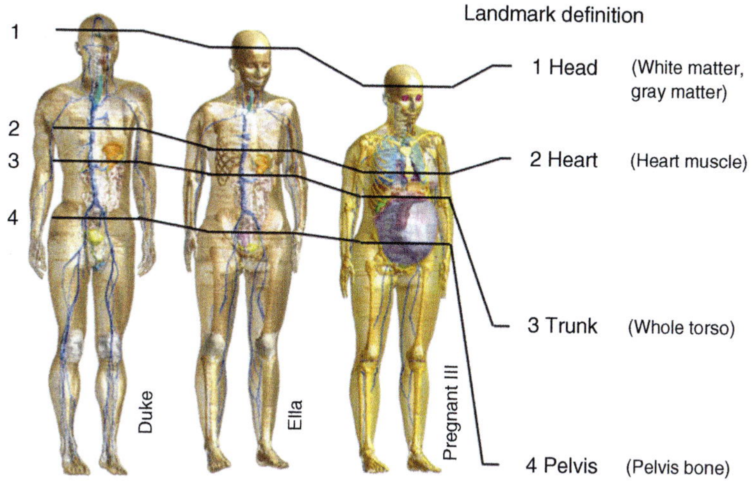

Figure 16.2. Landmark positions

The 7 T whole-body volume coil is modeled as a transverse electromagnetic (TEM) mode coil, resonates at ~300 MHz, and has 16 independent elements. The coils are modeled as a TEM coil because at ultra high frequencies (>3 T or 128.23 MHz), TEM structure provides better efficiency and field homogeneity compared to the birdcage structure, when loaded with the human body. The 16 independent elements of the coil are connected to the same grounded shielding. Each copper microstrip line propagates TEM mode and is excited by the source between one end of the microstrip line and the outer shielding. Two sets of shunt capacitors are connected between the microstrip lines and shielding to adjust the electrical length to tune each element to resonate at the appropriate 7 T Larmor frequency of ~300 MHz. The coil has the microstrip line resonant elements with the diameter of 313 mm and length of 450 mm. The shielding has the diameter of 317 mm and length of 950 mm.

The coil and human model alignments are shown in Figure 16.1. Notice that pregnant woman model is rotated 90° compared to Ella. This is because in practice, typically, normal patients lie on the back while full-term or near full-term pregnant women are more likely to lie on the side. It should be noted, however, that such position does not change the distribution of the RF energy with respect to a pregnant women lying on her back inside the coil since the coil is azimuthally symmetric around the body.

Four landmark positions are studied – head, heart, trunk, and pelvis. The head landmark is chosen such that the center of the human brain overlaps with the isocenter of the coil. For other landmark positions, the human models are moved along the coil. Landmark positions are presented in Figure 16.2.

The electromagnetic (EM) simulations are performed using commercial FDTD software Sim4Life (ZMT, Zurich, Switzerland) with the grid resolution of ~2.5 mm in the whole-body models. Broadband simulations are performed for I and Q channel separately to tune the 1.5 and 3 T birdcage coils. For the 7 T TEM coil, broadband simulations are performed with only one source on. All S11 values for the broadband simulations were below −20 dB. Single frequency harmonic simulations are then performed for circularly polarized (CP) mode to verify that uniform rotating magnetic field (B_1) field is generated.

16.2.3 SAR Modeling and Normalization

RF power deposition per unit volume or SAR is computed per equation (16.1). Necessary electric field (E) distribution is computed by solving Maxwell equations in the body models.

$$\mathrm{SAR} = \frac{1}{2}\frac{\sigma E^2}{\rho} \tag{16.1}$$

where E is the electrical field, σ is the electrical conductivity, and ρ is the density. Local SAR is computed in each voxel. 1 and 10 g average SAR are calculated by integrating local SAR in nearby 1 and 10 g mass, respectively, per equation (16.2).

$$\mathrm{SAR}_{\mathrm{mass}} = \frac{\int_{\mathrm{mass}} \left(\frac{1}{2}\,\sigma E^2\right) \mathrm{d}V}{\mathrm{mass}}, \ \mathrm{mass} = 1 \text{ or } 10\,\mathrm{g} \quad (16.2)$$

16.2.4 Thermal Simulation Setup

RF heating is simulated, by solving the two-compartment GBHTM and conventional, 'simplified' Pennes BHTE (In Vivo Temperatures, LLC, Burnsville, MN, USA).[7] The thermal models take RF power distribution (obtained by solving the Maxwell equations) as one of the inputs. The heating is simulated for the whole-body average SAR of $4\,\mathrm{W\,kg^{-1}}$ deposited continuously for 60 min (total energy $= 4\,\mathrm{W\,kg^{-1}} \times 60\,\mathrm{min} = 240\,\mathrm{W\,min}$). The GB-HTM is used since (i) the model is a first principle based, rigorously derived bioheat transfer model with minimum number of assumptions; (ii) the model has been validated using ~50–120 kg swine to predict tissue heating for MRI applications; and (iii) it has been shown to predict, relatively more accurate, in vivo tissue heating compared to the Pennes BHTE.[7–10] The conventional, 'simplified', empirical Pennes BHTE is used since the predictions of the 'simplified' BHTE has been used, traditionally, to develop SAR exposure thresholds to limit local in vivo heating. It should be noted, however, that the Pennes BHTE has never been validated for MRI application; violates conservation of energy; and underestimates tissue heating deep under the skin due to the overestimation the blood-tissue heat transfer rate. For simplicity, thermal simulations were performed by considering that the body models are made up of only the following materials: air, skin, fat, bone, lungs, and muscle. This thermal simulation approach is consistent with the one used for the validation of the GBHTM.[9,10] For more on the origin, assumptions, and applicability of different bioheat models, interested readers are encouraged to refer to the material presented in Ref. 7.

16.2.5 Thermal Dose Calculation

Thermal hazards and tissue effects are a function of the temperature-time history – and not just the temperature. Therefore, the simulated heating results are used to compute TD per two frequently employed methods, the *CEM*43 and Arrhenius equation. The *CEM*43 based TD is computed using equation (16.3), given below.

$$CEM43 = \int_0^{\tau} R^{43-T}\,\mathrm{d}t \quad (16.3)$$

where T is temperature (°C), t is time (minutes), τ is total time (minutes), and the weighting factor R is equal to 0.5 for $T \geq 43\,°\mathrm{C}$, and 0.25 for $T < 43\,°\mathrm{C}$. R is independent of the tissue type.[11]

Arrhenius equation based nondimensional TD (Ω) is computed using equation (16.4), given below.

$$\Omega = \int_0^{\tau} A e^{\frac{-E_a}{RT(t)}}\,\mathrm{d}t \quad (16.4)$$

where T is absolute temperature (K), t is time (s), τ is total time (s), A is the frequency factor ($\mathrm{s^{-1}}$), E_a is an activation energy barrier ($\mathrm{J\,mol^{-1}}$), and R is the universal gas constant ($8.3143\,\mathrm{J\,mol^{-1}\,K^{-1}}$). The value of the frequency factor A and activation energy barrier E_a is chosen as $3.1 \times 10^{98}\,\mathrm{s^{-1}}$ and $6.28 \times 10^5\,\mathrm{J\,mol^{-1}}$, respectively. These values were proposed originally in 1947 by Henriques and Moritz in their seminal papers investigating the effect temperature and time on the induced thermal damage.[12–14] Since then, several values of A and E_a have been published for various tissue types and with significant variation. To explain these variations, it has been shown that A and E_a are, in fact, dependent on each other and not independent.[7] TD is computed only for the duration of the heating and thus, presents the minimum total TD that might be accumulated due to the heating as well as cooling of tissue. The baseline temperature is assumed to be 37 °C. For more on the origin, assumptions, and applicability of different ways to compute TD, interested readers are encouraged to refer to the material presented in Ref. 7.

16.3 RESULTS

16.3.1 RF Heating and Thermal Dose in an Adult Male

Table 16.1 presents the peak 10 g and 1 g average SAR, maximum temperature change (dT) in the plane of peak 10 g and 1 g average SAR, and peak TD at the end of the heating in the plane of 10 g average SAR, for an adult male as a function of the field strength (i.e., 1.5, 3, and 7 T) and landmark positions (i.e., head, heart, trunk, and pelvis).

Table 16.1. SAR and thermal simulation results for the adult male whole-body model

Landmark position		Peak 10 g SAR ($W\,kg^{-1}$)	Peak 1 g SAR ($W\,kg^{-1}$)	d*T* in peak 10 g SAR plane (°C) GBHTM/ Pennes	d*T* in peak 1 g SAR plane (°C) GBHTM/ Pennes	*CEM*43 in peak 10 g SAR plane (min) GBHTM/ Pennes	*Ω* in peak 10 g SAR plane GBHTM/ Pennes
1.5 T	Head	116.2	138.5	16.6/12.1	16.2/11.7	>500.0/>500.0	12.42/1.33
	Heart	42.9	50.7	8.6/4.3	8.5/4.2	106.04/4.53	0.03/0.01
	Trunk	39.2	52.5	8.0/3.8	8.0/3.8	69.45/2.30	0.02/0.01
	Pelvis	44.1	86.3	12.7/8.5	14.4/10.1	>500.0/298.56	0.75/0.10
3 T	Head	67.7	85.9	11.1/6.9	11.1/6.9	>500.00/91.88	0.23/0.03
	Heart	41.2	76.8	9.1/4.9	9.3/5.1	159.07/10.33	0.05/0.01
	Trunk	56.8	103.6	10.6/6.2	11.4/7.0	437.36/57.01	0.15/0.02
	Pelvis	46.4	78.5	9.6/5.5	9.8/5.6	224.84/25.05	0.07/0.01
7 T	Head[a]	109.8	330.6	12.2/8.1	11.1/7.0	>500.00/222.15	0.52/0.07
	Heart	114.0	123.7	16.1/11.3	16.1/11.3	>500.00/>500.00	8.07/0.67
	Trunk	160.1	203.7	21.7/16.7	21.7/16.7	>500.00/>500.00	424.12/33.25
	Pelvis	167.9	209.9	22.3/17.1	22.4/17.2	>500.00/>500.00	>500.00/42.74

The heating is simulated for the whole-body average SAR of $4\,W\,kg^{-1}$ deposited continuously for 60 min (total energy = $4\,W\,kg^{-1} \times 60$ min = 240 W min).

[a]For 7 T simulations, the temperature data presented in the table are true for most of the tissue. Small regions of excessive heating (i.e., ≥50 °C) are found in regions with low cross sectional area for current flow. These high temperature numbers are not reported here. It is unclear if such high values of SAR (columns 3, 4) and associated temperature change (not reported) and thermal dose (last two columns) are induced due to the coil and/or numerical artifact in the body model. Such results should be verified in human-relevant animals (e.g., swine) and/or humans.

Figure 16.3(a) shows the 10 g average SAR distribution and associated temperature rise in a coronal plane near the center of the adult male model as a function of the field strength and landmark locations. Figure 16.3(b) shows the corresponding *CEM*43 and *Ω* values, at the end of heating.

16.3.2 RF Heating and Thermal Dose in an Adult Female

Table 16.2 presents the peak 10 g and 1 g average SAR, maximum temperature change (d*T*) in the plane of peak 10 g and 1 g average SAR, and peak TD at the end of the heating in the plane of 10 g average SAR, for an adult female as a function of the field strength (i.e., 1.5, 3, and 7 T) and landmark positions (i.e., head, heart, trunk, and pelvis).

Figure 16.4(a) shows the 10 g average SAR distribution and associated temperature rise in a coronal plane near the center of the adult female model as a function of the field strength and landmark locations. Figure 16.4(b) shows the corresponding *CEM*43 and *Ω* values, at the end of heating.

16.3.3 RF Heating and Thermal Dose in a Pregnant Female

Table 16.3 presents the peak 10 g and 1 g average SAR, maximum temperature change (d*T*) in the plane of peak 10 g and 1 g average SAR, and peak TD at the end of the heating in the plane of 10 g average SAR for a 9 month pregnant woman as a function of the field strength (i.e., 1.5, 3, and 7 T) and landmark positions (i.e., head, heart, trunk, and pelvis).

Figure 16.5(a) shows the 10 g average SAR distribution and associated temperature rise in a coronal plane near the center of the pregnant woman model as a function of the field strength and landmark locations. Figure 16.5(b) shows the corresponding *CEM*43 and *Ω* values, at the end of heating.

16.4 DISCUSSION

Several important observations are made regarding the in vivo tissue heating induced due to the RF power deposition during MRI. First, the induced heating is nonuniform (Figures 16.3a, 16.4a, 16.5a). This is so

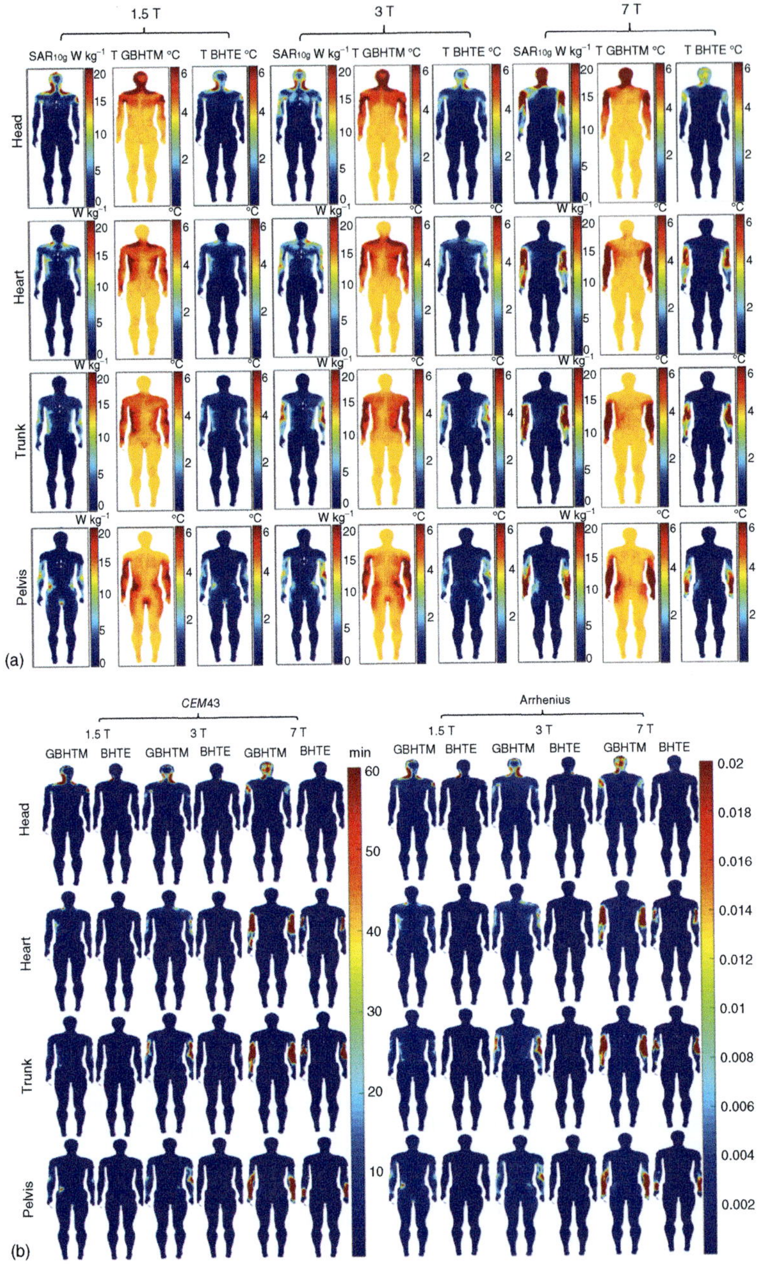

Figure 16.3. (a) 10 g average SAR and associated temperature change in a coronal plane near the center of the body of the adult male model in 1.5 T (columns 1–3), 3 T (columns 4–6), and 7 T (columns 7–9) as a function of landmark positions (head – row 1, heart – row 2, trunk – row 3, and pelvis – row 4). The temperature change is computed based on the GBHTM and 'simplified', traditional Pennes BHTE. (b) Thermal dose distribution in the same coronal plane as in Figure 16.3(a) in the adult male model. Thermal dose is computed at the end of the RF power deposition using the temperatures predicted by the GBHTM and 'simplified', traditional Pennes BHTE. Columns 1–6 present thermal dose calculated per *CEM*43 approach (1.5 T – columns 1–2, 3 T – columns 3–4, 7 T – columns 5–6). Columns 7–12 present thermal dose calculated per Arrhenius equation based approach (1.5 T – columns 7–8, 3 T – columns 9–10, 7 T – columns 11–12). Thermal dose is presented as a function of the landmark position (head – row 1, heart – row 2, trunk –row 3, and pelvis – row 4)

Table 16.2. SAR and thermal simulation results for the adult female whole-body model

Landmark position		Peak 10 g SAR ($W kg^{-1}$)	Peak 1 g SAR ($W kg^{-1}$)	dT in peak 10 g SAR plane (°C) GBHTM/ Pennes	dT in peak 1 g SAR plane (°C) GBHTM/ Pennes	*CEM*43 in peak 10 g SAR plane (min) GBHTM/ Pennes	Ω in peak 10 g SAR plane GBHTM/ Pennes
1.5 T	Head	101.0	156.2	15.5/10.7	15.5/10.7	>500.00/>500.00	5.18/0.45
	Heart	65.2	106.7	11.2/6.8	12.0/7.5	>500.00/84.08	0.24/0.03
	Trunk	59.5	95.2	10.8/6.4	11.4/6.9	>500.00/62.68	0.18/0.02
	Pelvis	46.1	73.0	10.7/6.4	11.6/7.4	479.56/70.56	0.17/0.02
3 T	Head	76.6	112.1	12.9/8.5	13.1/8.6	>500.00/273.03	0.84/0.09
	Heart	49.9	68.1	9.4/4.9	9.2/4.7	180.26/10.40	0.06/0.01
	Trunk	46.6	68.3	10.1/5.8	9.6/5.2	313.29/36.91	0.11/0.01
	Pelvis	40.1	64.8	9.1/4.9	17.1/13.0	156.16/10.18	0.05/0.01
7 T	Head	66.7	113.1	11.5/7.3	17.4/13.2	>500.00/130.48	0.30/0.04
	Heart[a]	106.7	351.5	13.5/8.8	13.4/8.7	>500.00/339.06	1.25/0.11
	Trunk[a]	155.1	518.0	16.7/11.8	16.5/11.6	>500.00/>500.00	12.25/1.00
	Pelvis[a]	201.5	627.8	27.3/22.0	21.4/16.2	>500.00/>500.00	>500.00/>500.00

The heating is simulated for the whole-body average SAR of 4 $W kg^{-1}$ deposited continuously for 60 min (total energy = 4 $W kg^{-1}$ × 60 min = 240 W min).

[a]For 7 T simulations, the temperature data presented in the table are true for most of the tissue. Small regions of excessive heating (i.e., ≥50 °C) are found in regions with low cross sectional area for current flow. These high temperature numbers are not reported here. It is unclear if such high values of SAR (columns 3, 4) and associated temperature change (not reported) and thermal dose (last two columns) are induced due to the coil and/or numerical artifact in the body model. Such results should be verified in human-relevant animals (e.g., swine) and/or humans.

because EM and thermal properties of the body are nonuniform resulting in nonuniform RF power deposition and heating. The observation suggests that the rectal or core temperature change measurement alone may have limited applicability in helping determine if an MRI study produced local temperatures that exceeded recommended safe temperature thresholds. Local heating must be determined with sufficient accuracy to ensure compliance with the IEC recommended safe temperature thresholds and improve patient safety.

Second, the new validated, mechanistic GBHTM predicts greater in vivo heating compared to the conventional, simplified Pennes BHTE (Figures 16.3a, 16.4a, and 16.5a). This is because the GBHTM allows for the blood temperature to vary per conservation of energy. However, the Pennes BHTE does not allow for the blood temperature to vary. Keeping the blood temperature artificially and nonphysiologically constant at the baseline core temperature and using blood perfusion values with nonequilibration constant of zero to compute blood–tissue heat transfer rate makes the Pennes BHTE violate conservation of energy, and overestimate the blood–tissue heat transfer rate consequently underestimating the tissue temperature rise compared to the predictions of the GBHTM.

Fifth, thermal hot regions may be produced deep inside the body away from the skin and its thermal receptors. Therefore, the absence of patient thermal sensation may not be interpreted as the absence of local in vivo heating exceeding the recommended safe temperature thresholds. Excessive, local in vivo heating away from the skin and its thermal receptors cannot be consciously ‘felt’ by a person, which could prevent a patient/technician/clinician from responding until it is too late to avoid redness, burning, etc. Computational tools, like the GBHTM, may help accurately determine in vivo RF heating to keep temperatures below desired thresholds during MRI. *CEM*43 value of ≥60 min and Arrhenius equation based nondimensional TD value of ≥0.02 are computed for various locations inside the body for maximum allowable whole-body average SAR (i.e., 4 $W kg^{-1}$) and energy (i.e., 240 $W min kg^{-1}$) (Figures 16.3b, 16.4b, and 16.5b). The *CEM*43 of ≥60 min (and equivalent Arrhenius equation based nondimensional TD value of ≥0.02) has been shown to reduce cell viability by 90% in in vitro experiments.[7,11]

Comparing the present study with previous studies, Shuman *et al.* measured an average deep tissue in vivo temperature change of 4.2 $°C h^{-1}$ in dogs exposed to

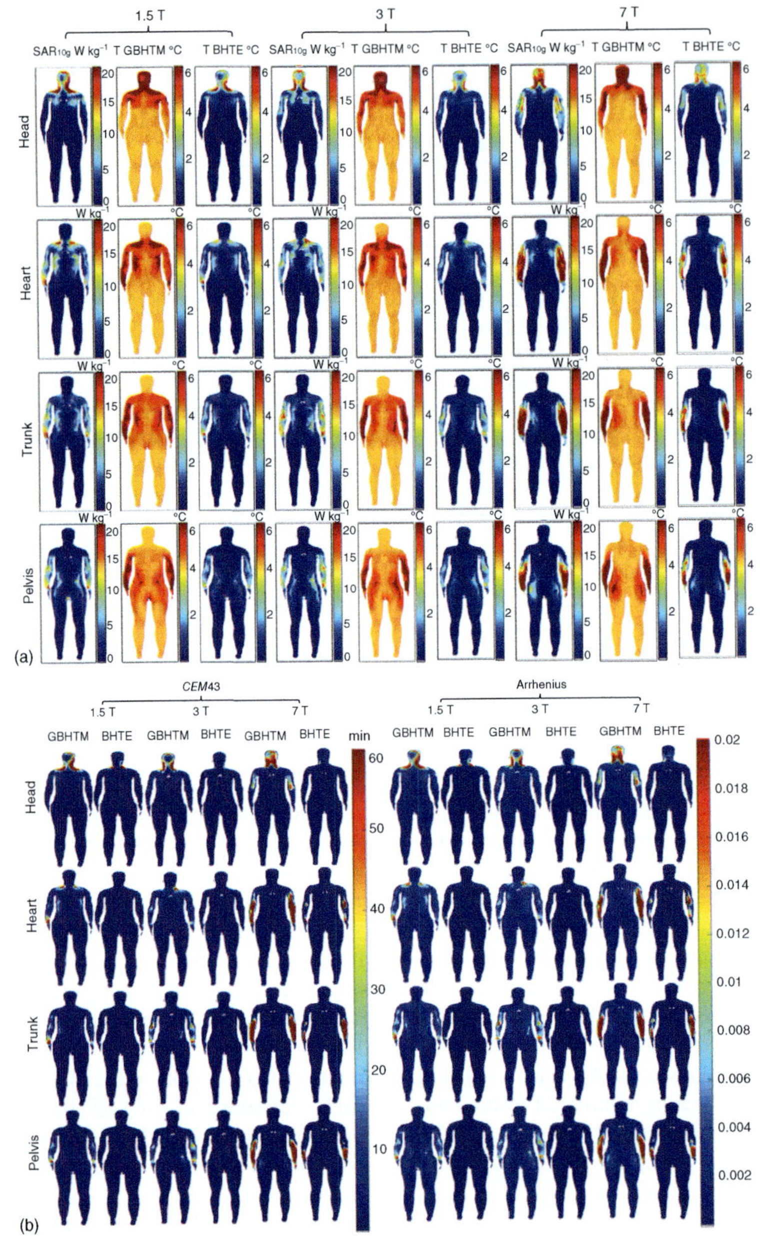

Figure 16.4. (a) 10 g average SAR and associated temperature change in a coronal plane near the center of the body of the adult female model in 1.5 T (columns 1–3), 3 T (columns 4–6), and 7 T (columns 7–9) as a function of landmark positions (head – row 1, heart – row 2, trunk – row 3, and pelvis – row 4). The temperature change is computed based on the GBHTM and 'simplified', traditional Pennes BHTE. (b) Thermal dose distribution in the same coronal plane as in Figure 16.4(a) in the adult female model. Thermal dose is computed at the end of the RF power deposition using the temperature changes predicted by the GBHTM and 'simplified', traditional Pennes BHTE. Columns 1–6 present thermal dose calculated per *CEM*43 approach (1.5 T – columns 1–2, 3 T – columns 3–4, 7 T – columns 5–6). Columns 7–12 present thermal dose calculated per Arrhenius equation based approach (1.5 T – columns 7–8, 3 T – columns 9–10, 7 T – columns 11–12). Thermal dose is presented as a function of the landmark position (head – row 1, heart – row 2, trunk – row 3, and pelvis – row 4)

Table 16.3. SAR and thermal simulation results for the pregnant woman whole-body model

Landmark position		Peak 10 g SAR ($W\,kg^{-1}$)	Peak 1 g SAR ($W\,kg^{-1}$)	dT in peak 10 g SAR plane (°C) GBHTM/Pennes	dT in peak 1 g SAR plane (°C) GBHTM/Pennes	*CEM*43 in peak 10 g SAR plane (min) GBHTM/Pennes	Ω in peak 10 g SAR plane GBHTM/Pennes
1.5 T	Head	113.8	165.1	17.4/12.8	22.6/18.5	>500.00/>500.00	21.41/2.05
	Heart	57.0	123.1	12.1/7.7	12.5/8.1	>500.00/169.76	0.46/0.05
	Trunk	45.2	89.7	9.2/4.9	10.9/6.6	167.83/10.90	0.06/0.01
	Pelvis	41.5	71.0	8.8/4.5	9.5/5.2	125.21/6.42	0.04/0.01
3 T	Head	92.7	124.9	14.4/9.8	15.1/10.6	>500.00/>500.00	2.48/0.24
	Heart	51.6	67.8	9.5/5.4	9.6/5.3	215.36/19.73	0.07/0.01
	Trunk	45.8	62.6	8.8/4.5	8.9/4.7	119.74/5.96	0.04/0.01
	Pelvis	47.9	103.4	14.5/10.4	13.9/9.8	>500.00/>500.00	2.76/0.39
7 T	Head	72.5	130.4	12.8/8.7	19.2/15.0	>500.00/341.34	0.83/0.11
	Heart[a]	129.9	360.6	13.1/8.5	12.3/7.8	>500.00/250.63	0.83/0.08
	Trunk[a]	157.3	413.1	12.6/8.0	13.3/9.2	>500.00/191.05	0.64/0.06
	Pelvis[a]	192.9	330.8	15.7/11.0	18.1/13.1	>500.00/>500.00	6.51/0.57

The heating is simulated for the whole-body average SAR of $4\,W\,kg^{-1}$ deposited continuously for 60 min (total energy = $4\,W\,kg^{-1} \times 60\,min = 240\,W\,min$).
[a]For 7 T simulations, the temperature data presented in the table are true for most of the tissue. Small regions of excessive heating (i.e., ≥50 °C) are found in regions with low cross sectional area for current flow. These high temperature numbers are not reported here. It is unclear if such high values of SAR (columns 3, 4) and associated temperature change (not reported) and thermal dose (last two columns) are induced due to the coil and/or numerical artifact in the body model. Such results should be verified in human-relevant animals (e.g., swine) and/or humans.

the whole-body average SAR of $4\,W\,kg^{-1}$ in 1.5 T. The temperature increase in deeper tissue was found to be greater than the temperature increase in superficial tissue.[15] Barber *et al.* measured the core temperature change of 1.26–1.80 °C h^{-1} and the subcutaneous skin temperature change of up to ~6.3 °C h^{-1} in sheep exposed to the whole-body average SAR of $4\,W\,kg^{-1}$ in 1.5 T.[16] Kido *et al.* measured a mean temperature change of 0.5 °C in the axilla due to the whole-body average SAR exposure of $0.8\,W\,kg^{-1}$ for 17 min in 1.5 T (i.e., mean temperature change rate of 8.82 °C h^{-1} at the whole-body average SAR of $4\,W\,kg^{-1}$).[17] Shellock *et al.* measured a scrotal skin temperature change of 0.2–3.2 °C due to the whole-body average SAR exposure of 0.56–0.84 $W\,kg^{-1}$ for 23 min in 1.5 T.[18] Shellock *et al.* measured an insignificant change in the rectal temperature and a change of up to 7.5 °C in the skin temperature due to the whole-body average SAR exposure of 2.7–4.0 $W\,kg^{-1}$ for 30 min in 1.5 T.[19] Shellock *et al.* measured a mean tympanic membrane temperature change of 0.4 °C and a mean skin temperature change of −0.5–3.6 °C due to the whole-body average SAR of $6\,W\,kg^{-1}$ for 16 min in 1.5 T.[20] Boss *et al.* measured skin temperature changes of 0.88 °C in human volunteers due to the whole-body average SAR exposure of $1.60\,W\,kg^{-1}$ for ~6.75 min and $2.85\,W\,kg^{-1}$ for an additional 4.25 min (i.e., total exposure of ~10 min).[21] Shrivastava *et al.* measured and simulated the core, brain, and hot region temperature of 1.5, 2.5, and 3.8 °C, respectively, in swine when the swine head was placed in the isocenter of a 3 T coil due to the whole-body average SAR of $2.7\,W\,kg^{-1}$ deposited for an hour. Further, they measured and simulated the core, brain, and hot region temperature of 1.6, 1.8, and 5.2 °C, respectively, in swine when the swine trunk was placed in the isocenter of a 3 T coil due to the whole-body average SAR of $2.8\,W\,kg^{-1}$ deposited for an hour.[9] All of these previously published values are comparable to the data presented here for the temperature change.

Regarding the limitations of this study, the heating depends on the human geometry, tissue composition and relative distribution, coil configuration, placement of human body inside the coil, EM and thermal properties of the body, skin surface conditions (e.g., clothing, sweating, etc.), and ambient conditions. Thus, the results presented herein are limited to the cases studied. Readers are encouraged to solve the GBHTM using additional body models, coils, placement of body models inside coils, and skin surface and ambient conditions

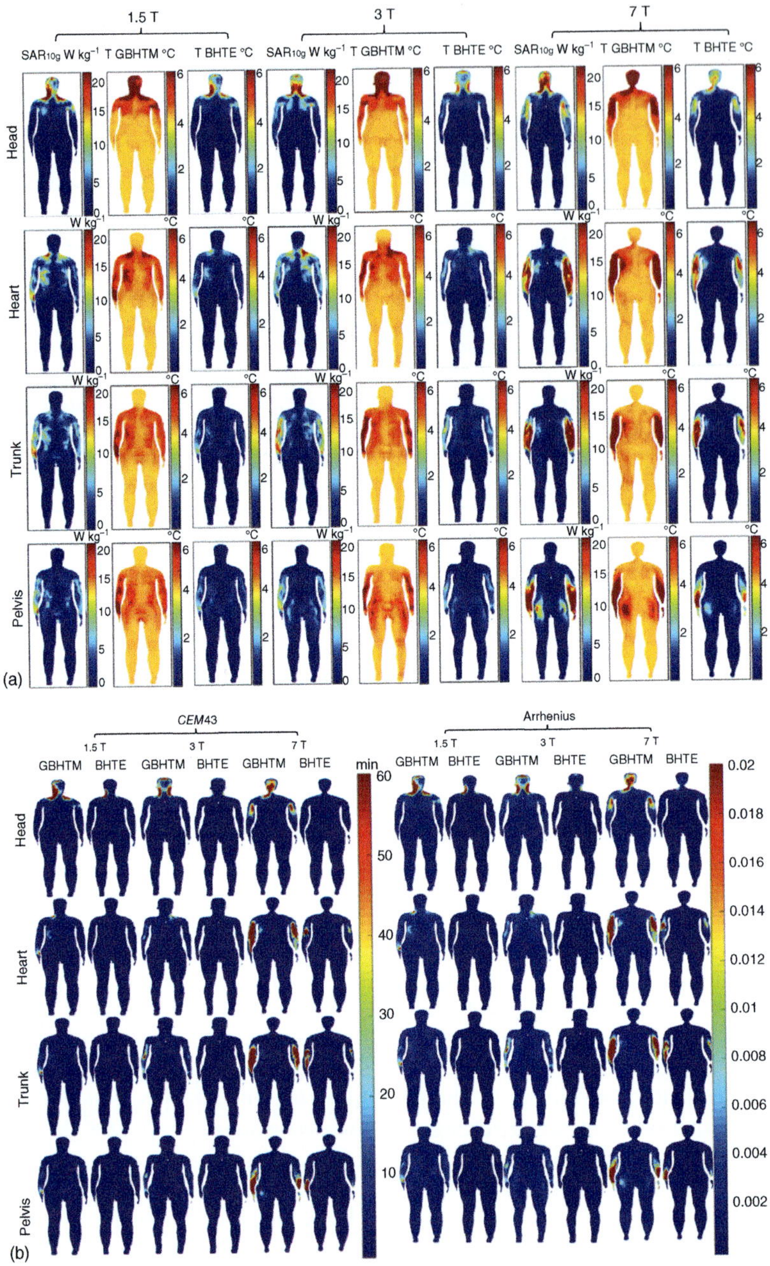

Figure 16.5. (a) 10 g average SAR and associated temperature change in a coronal plane near the center of the body of the pregnant woman model in 1.5 T (columns 1–3), 3 T (columns 4–6), and 7 T (columns 7–9) as a function of landmark positions (head – row 1, heart – row 2, trunk – row 3, and pelvis – row 4). The temperature change is computed based on the GBHTM and 'simplified', traditional Pennes BHTE. (b) Thermal dose distribution in the same coronal plane as in Figure 16.5(a) in the pregnant woman model. Thermal dose is computed at the end of the RF power deposition using the temperature changes predicted by the GBHTM and 'simplified', traditional Pennes BHTE. Columns 1–6 present thermal dose calculated per *CEM*43 approach (1.5 T – columns 1–2, 3 T – columns 3–4, 7 T – columns 5–6). Columns 7–12 present thermal dose calculated per Arrhenius equation based approach (1.5 T – columns 7–8, 3 T – columns 9–10, 7 T – columns 11–12). Thermal dose is presented as a function of the landmark position (head – row 1, heart – row 2, trunk – row 3, and pelvis – row 4)

to develop deeper understanding of the magnitude and distribution of the MRI induced tissue heating in humans to improve safety as well as performance.

16.5 SUMMARY

A computational study is performed to systematically analyze the RF power distribution, related temperature rise, and accumulated TD during heating, in an adult male, an adult female, and a pregnant woman whole-body model due to power deposition from a 1.5, 3, and 7 T whole-body volume coil placed in four landmark positions (i.e., head, heart, trunk, and pelvis). The RF heating is computed using the new, validated mechanistic GBHTM and empirical, simplified Pennes BHTE. Results show that the temperatures, exceeding recommended safe thermal thresholds of 1 °C, may be produced deep inside the body away from the skin and its thermal receptors with allowable whole-body average SAR values. Measuring rectal and skin temperature changes may not be sufficient for determining temperature changes in hot regions deep inside the body, and thus, in concluding a thermally safe MRI scan. Future studies employing the GBHTM to predict in vivo heating along with appropriate verification of the GBHTM results in humans may help significantly enhance our understanding of the RF safety in high and ultra-high field MRI and develop next generation of faster, safer, and more flexible SAR as well as temperature controlled MR systems.

Third, recommended safe in vivo temperature change thresholds are exceeded with allowable whole-body average SAR values, when heart, trunk, or pelvis (Figures 16.3a and 16.5a) is in the isocenter. This is expected because the maximum allowable whole-body average SAR exposure values were determined using the two-node model of Drs Adair and Berglund, which is unable to account for the nonhomogeneous distribution of RF power, and the conventional, simplified Pennes BHTE, which overestimates the thermal interaction between the blood and tissue.

Fourth, temperature in the brain and most of the core is not expected to exceed ~1.5 °C during a properly conducted head exam. However, local temperatures in limited regions may still exceed this value. This is so since RF power during a head exam is limited by the whole-head average SAR of 3.2 W kg^{-1} – instead of the whole-body average SAR. Since temperature change scales linearly with power, appropriate scaling for a realistic head exam will suggest that the brain and most of the core temperature is not likely to exceed 1.5 °C due to the whole-head average SAR deposition of 3.2 W kg^{-1} for an hour. It should be added, however, that in case an MR system assumes that the whole-body average SAR of 3.2 W kg^{-1} is equivalent to the whole-head average SAR of 3.2 W kg^{-1}, temperature changes are expected to exceed 1.5 °C, as can be seen from Figures 16.3(a), 16.4(a), and 16.5(a) by scaling the temperature change results by 80%.

DISCLAIMER

The subject matter, content, and views presented are mine and do not represent the views of the Department of Health and Human Services (HHS), US Food and Drug Administration (FDA), and/or the United States.

REFERENCES

1. IEC, Medical Electrical Equipment – Part 2-33: Particular Requirements for the Basic Safety and Essential Performance of Magnetic Resonance Equipment for Medical Diagnosis, 3rd edn, International Electrotechnical Commission, 2010; 60601-2-33 ed. 3.0B.
2. H. H. Pennes, *J. Appl. Physiol.*, 1998, **85**, 5.
3. E. R. Adair and L. G. Berglund, *Magn. Reson. Imag.*, 1986, **4**, 321.
4. E. R. Adair and L. G. Berglund, *Ann. NY Acad. Sci.*, 1992, **649**, 188.
5. ICNIRP, *Health Phys.*, 2004, **87**, 197.
6. D. Shrivastava and J. T. Vaughan, in 'RF Coils for MRI', eds J. T. Vaughan and J. Griffiths, Wiley: Chichester, 2012, p 425.
7. D. Shrivastava (ed), Theory and Applications of Heat Transfer in Humans, Wiley, 2018.
8. D. Shrivastava and J. T. Vaughan, *ASME – J. Biomech. Eng.*, 2009, **131**, 074506.
9. D. Shrivastava, L. Utecht, J. Tian, J. Hughes, and J. T. Vaughan, *Magn. Reson. Med.*, 2014, **72**, 1141.
10. D. Shrivastava, T. Hanson, J. Kulesa, J. Tian, A. Gregor, and J. T. Vaughan, *Magn. Reson. Med.*, 2011, **66**, 255.
11. S. A. Sapareto and W. C. Dewey, *Int. J. Radiat. Oncol. Biol. Phys.*, 1984, **10**, 787.

12. F. C. Henriques and A. R. Moritz, *Am. J. Pathol.*, 1947, **23**, 531.

13. A. R. Moritz and F. C. Henriques, *Am. J. Pathol.*, 1947, **23**, 695.

14. A. R. Moritz, *Am. J. Pathol.*, 1947, **23**, 915.

15. W. P. Shuman, D. R. Haynor, A. W. Guy, G. E. Wesbey, D. J. Schaefer, and A. A. Moss, *Radiology*, 1988, **167**, 551.

16. B. J. Barber, D. J. Schaefer, C. J. Gordon, D. C. Zawieja, and J. Hecker, *AJR Am. J. Roentgenol.*, 1990, **155**, 1105.

17. D. Kido, T. Morris, J. Erickson, D. Plewes, and J. Simon, *AJR Am J. Roentgenol.*, 1987, **148**, 1215.

18. F. Shellock, B. Rothman, and D. Sarti, *AJR Am. J. Roentgenol.*, 1990, **154**, 1229.

19. F. G. Shellock, D. J. Schaefer, and J. V. Crues, *Br. J. Radiol.*, 1989, **62**, 904.

20. F. G. Shellock, D. J. Schaefer, and E. Kanal, *Radiology*, 1994, **192**, 865.

21. A. Boss, H. Graf, A. Berger, U. A. Lauer, H. Wojtczyk, C. D. Claussen, and F. Schick, *J. Magn. Reson. Imag.*, 2007, **26**, 1334.

Chapter 17

Temperature Management and Radiofrequency Heating During Pediatric MRI Scans

Stanley Thomas Fricke[1,2], Marjean H. Cefaratti[2], and Andrew Matisoff[2]

[1]*Georgetown University Medical Center, Washington, DC, USA*
[2]*Children's National Medical Center, Washington, DC, USA*

Safety and Biological Effects in MRI.
Edited by Devashish Shrivastava and J. Thomas Vaughan

ISBN: 978-1-118-82130-5
Also published in eMagRes (online edition)
DOI: 10.1002/9780470034590.emrstm1576

17.1 INTRODUCTION

Children undergoing magnetic resonance imaging (MRI) scans are at risk for temperature derangements, including hypothermia and hyperthermia, both of which can have several harmful clinical consequences, leading to worse patient outcomes. Smaller, younger patients with more disease burden are at the highest risk of temperature alterations during MRI scans and developing complications from these changes in temperature. There are limited, costly methods to both monitor temperature as well as to maintain normothermia in patients during MRI scans. Good clinical practice is necessary to prevent untoward consequences of hypothermia and hyperthermia on pediatric patients undergoing MRI scans. Larger studies to evaluate the effect of various MRI protocols on radio frequency (RF) heating and on methods to maintain normothermia in pediatric patients are needed.

17.2 CLINICAL EFFECTS OF HYPOTHERMIA IN CHILDREN

Infants and neonates are at high risk of developing hypothermia due to a high surface area-to-volume ratio, which is highest in very low birth weight neonates.[1] Heat loss occurs via radiation, evaporation, conduction, and convection. With radiation, the loss of heat to the cooler environment is the most important contributor to hypothermia. While the use of incubators in the Neonatal Intensive Care Unit (NICU) provides a neutral thermal environment, which can prevent the majority of this heat loss, infants cared for in other environments are at risk for hypothermia.[2] Perioperative hypothermia (temperature below 36.0 °C) has been documented in up to 40% of patients from the NICU who require surgery.[3] Hypothermia invokes several harmful physiological responses which can increase morbidity in neonates. Cooling can induce non-shivering thermogenesis via release of norepinephrine in brown fat, increasing metabolic rate and oxygen consumption up to three times. This metabolic derangement can inhibit growth, and increase the risk of infection.[1–3] In a neonate with threatened oxygen delivery due to respiratory failure, congenital heart disease, and infection, increased oxygen consumption can result in tissue hypoxia and organ injury. Although not a direct cause of death, it is postulated that globally hypothermia 'contributes to a substantial proportion of neonatal mortality globally, mostly as a comorbidity of severe neonatal infections, preterm birth, and asphyxia.'[1] Avoidance of perioperative hypothermia is a standard of care and is currently a metric being used in the evaluation of neonatology programs and is linked to merit-based incentive programs in Medicaid reimbursement.[4]

17.3 HYPOTHERMIA DURING MRI SCANS IN CHILDREN

Pediatric patients, most notably younger, smaller patients who undergo MRI scans, are at the highest risk for developing hypothermia during scanning. Pediatric patients often require sedation due to the need for immobility during scans, procedural anxiety, and young age. Anesthesia is provided by various techniques, but often includes a combination of general anesthesia and deep sedation using various inhalational and intravenous anesthetic agents.[5,6] Patients under anesthesia experience hypothermia in a dose-dependent manner due to reduced activation of neural control mechanisms such as vasoconstriction of peripheral afferents, reduced heat production due to reduced metabolism and skeletal muscle inactivation, and heat loss to their surrounding environment via radiation, convection, evaporation, and conduction.[7,8] In infants and neonates, where normothermia is critical for survival, their large surface area-to-body volume ratio leads to a greater degree of heat loss and thus hypothermia under anesthesia. Children who require anesthesia for MRI scans typically are induced under anesthesia in a designated area outside of the scanning environment and then moved to the scanning environment. The scanning environment is typically kept cool 18 ± 3 °C with a low humidity 45 ± 15%. Heat loss to the surrounding cool environment after induction of anesthesia, during transport into the scanning environment and upon arrival to the scanning environment, can occur.[9,10] The smallest and the higher acuity patients, such as preterm neonates, are mostly at risk to develop hypothermia and complications related to hypothermia. Children who require MRI scans of the thorax or abdomen may have large areas of body surface exposed for heat loss during scanning. While application of warm blankets and other methods of insulation may reduce heat loss, there are no approved methods to actively warm patients during this period. MRI conditional chemical warmers such as the Transwarmer™ which use an exothermic reaction to generate heat for up to 2 h, have been tested in nonclinical situations for safety, but there are no data documenting their efficacy in reducing hypothermia during MRI scans.[11] In addition, they may cause image artifacts which might reduce image quality. MRI-compatible incubators are useful in selective patients, but due to increased cost (that can easily exceed $500 000) and their sometimes detrimental effect on image quality, cannot be generalized to most pediatric patients who require MRI scans.[12] Clinical studies documenting the incidence and clinical consequences of hypothermia in children undergoing MRI scans as well as the efficacy of various methods to warm pediatric patients undergoing MRI scans are greatly needed. Within the small group of existing studies, Lo *et al.* measured core temperatures in children before and after sedated MRI scans in 193 children and documented a 52% incidence of hypothermia after the scans with a mean post-scan temperature of 35.9 °C.[10] Paul *et al.* measured core temperatures continuously in 21 preterm neonates receiving brain MRI scans and found that 57% of these developed hypothermia during the MRI scan with a mean decrease in core temperature of 0.41 °C during the scan.[13] For details on how to quantitatively evaluate the effective ambient conditions, surface area, volume, reduced ability of vasoconstriction, and reduced metabolism on the core body temperature, readers are recommended to refer to Ref. 14.

17.4 RECOMMENDATIONS TO PREVENT HYPOTHERMIA DURING PEDIATRIC MRI SCANS

Given the high incidence and potentially negative clinical consequences of hypothermia during pediatric MRI scans, it is imperative for clinicians to follow measures to minimize its occurrence. The author recommends the following:[6,9]

1. All pediatric patients undergoing MRI scans should have continuous temperature monitoring, if possible. This is most important in anesthetized patients and preterm neonates. Axillary temperature probes are acceptable in most patients. Patients who are intubated should have esophageal temperature probes, which most accurately measures core temperature.
2. Methods to reduce heat loss should include minimizing exposure to the cold environment and insulation with warm blankets and/or other methods of insulation. MRI-compatible incubators are recommended for preterm neonates, when possible.
3. Patients who develop clinically significant hypothermia during scans may require termination or interruption of the scan to apply active warming measures in a more neutral thermal environment until normothermia is achieved.
4. In all patients, clinicians must weigh the benefit of diagnosis against the risk and harms of hypothermia during the procedure.

17.5 HYPERTHERMIA DURING MRI SCANS

Children undergoing MRI scans may also be at risk for systemic hyperthermia (temperature >38.5 °C) or burns due to magnetic resonance (MR) radiofrequency heating. Radiofrequency-induced currents lead to power dissipation within the body's tissues, causing increases in body temperature. Heat generation depends on coil design, and magnetic field strength. The specific absorption rate (SAR) is a measure of the RF-power absorbed per mass of tissue.[14] Relatively larger surface area-to-volume ration in small children may not be sufficient to mitigate the risk of systemic hyperthermia due to RF heating. Systemic hyperthermia has several harmful clinical consequences affecting multiple organ systems. Hyperthermia increases the permeability of the GI tract, increasing the rate of gut bacterial translocation. Hyperthermia increases heart rate and can cause malignant arrhythmias and cardiac dysfunction. Liver and renal dysfunction can occur at high temperatures.[15] Coagulopathy is common, with a reported incidence of 45% in classical heatstroke.[15] Most concerning is the neurological effects of hyperthermia. Neurological damage and cognitive dysfunction may occur within minutes after an episode of hyperthermia and may lead to chronic damage, with the cerebellum at greatest risk for injury.[16] The pathophysiological mechanisms are unclear, but may be due to disruption of the blood brain barrier (BBB), leading to increased bacterial translocation, direct cellular damage, and the release of cytokines and other inflammatory mediators.[17] Mortality has been shown to increase at temperatures above 37.9 °C in stroke patients and at temperatures of above 38 °C in traumatic brain injury patients.[18] Since many pediatric patients who require MRI scans have or are at risk for brain injury, even a slight increase in brain temperature may be harmful. Thankfully, the limited studies thus far have shown no clinically significant hyperthermia. Cawley studied 25 neonates (gestational age ranged from 37 + 6 to 42 + 0 weeks, and median birth weight was 3385 g) undergoing brain MRI scans and found no significant change in core temperature between the start and end of scanning and no infant with a core temperature that exceeded 37.5 °C during scanning.[19] Bryan measured pre- and post-MRI tympanic temperatures in 30 children undergoing sedated MRI scans. Temperature increased by 0.5 °C (0.3–0.7 95% CI) during scan, but no patients developed hyperthermia.[20] Fricke *et al.* measured temperature on 458 anesthetized pediatric patients. Four percent of the patients had a temperature increase of more than 1 °C and no patients developed hyperthermia.[21] As noted earlier, above, sedation is expected to decrease core body temperature in dose, ambient conditions, and patient-dependent manner. Thus, the effect of MRI-induced RF heating on increasing body temperature in these sedated patients with decreasing core temperature may or may not be apparent. Future studies will look at the effect of different MRI pulse sequences (protocols) on the induced non-uniform (local, organ level, and core) temperature changes during scanning to adequately prepare with specific attention given to temperature fluctuations in patients at risk of local, organ level, and/or systemic hyperthermia and burns related complications during certain scanning protocols.

17.6 RECOMMENDATIONS FOR PREVENTING RF HEATING DURING PEDIATRIC MRI SCANS

In addition to monitoring temperature during MRI scans, the following manufacturer's recommendations are given to minimize the risk of RF heating during MRI scans.[22]

1. As is the case for all MR imaging, follow good clinical practices: continuous patient observation and contact are required. *All patients should be monitored for increased temperature during the scan acquisition.*
2. Monitor temperature continuously during MRI scans in anesthetized patients. Extra attention should be given when scanning patients who are unconscious, sedated, or may have loss of feeling in any body part (temporary or permanent paralysis). They may not be able to alert the operator to RF heating.
3. If the patient reports discomfort due to excessive warming, stop the scan.
4. Give patient breaks to cool down, provide light clothing, limit room temperature to $18 \pm 3\,°C$ ($64.4 \pm 5.4\,°F$), and maximize air flow.

Furthermore, it is recommended that any temperature rise beyond 1 °C should alert to stop a scan in progress with a full stop order if the patient's body temperature reaches 40 °C. And again, at either indication, allow the patient to cool down before proceeding with the scanning session.

17.7 COST OF MONITORING TEMPERATURE DURING MRI

Given the risk of temperature derangements in children during MRI scans, and the significant clinical consequences of hypo/hyperthermia, it is recommended that temperature is monitored in all patients undergoing MRI scans. In fact, the mandate to monitor temperature during MRI scanning sessions was formally stated in a letter from General Electric Healthcare's JW Dennison (Vice President of Quality and Regulatory) and Hersh J. (Chief Medical Officer – Medical Solutions), Entitled Urgent Medical Device Correction: Potential Safety Issue with Head SAR and Recommendations for Scanning Patients with Medical Implants Using GE Healthcare 3.0 T MR Scanners.[22] Temperature monitoring during MRI is associated with increased cost arising from maintenance and consumable costs associated with the temperature probe (end effector) used for temperature monitoring, but does not incorporate depreciation of the capital equipment (physiological monitor) or maintenance of the same. In the Fricke study of 485 patients, it was determined that the approximate cost of performing a temperature monitoring during MRI was about $22.26 per patient (Table 17.1).[21]

Table 17.1. Cost analysis of temperature monitoring of patients

Month	Total patients	No change	Change	Increase >1 °C	% of patients with change	% patients >1 °C	Temperature probes replaced @ $1212 ea.	Disposable temperature probe sleeves @ $9/patient
November	122	87	35	6	28.70	4.90	1	122
December	151	109	42	4	27.80	2.60	3	151
January	94	76	18	6	19.10	6.40	0	94
February	91	71	20	3	22	3.30	1	91
Total patients	458	343	115	19	21.50	4.10	5	458
Costs							$6075.00	$4122.00
Total costs								$10 197.00
Total costs per patient								$22.26

Patients that were sedated were monitored with the InVivo (subsidiary of Philips Medical) temperature probe in the axillary position. As part of a process improvement to better understand equipment failure rate data was taken over a four month period to determine (i) the need for monitoring, (ii) the percent of patients that would benefit from monitoring, (iii) failure rate of monitoring equipment, (iv) the cost of temperature monitoring.

Part of the information that this study renders is that the temperature probe used in this study has a mean free time between failure (MTBF) of approximately 91 uses. Given that there were only five failures during the entire study period confidence in this number is low and actually ranges (per data period) from 50 uses to 122 uses before failure. More data are needed to pin down the actual failure rate. Using a failure rate of once per 50 uses, the cost of temperature monitoring patients could be as much as $33.24.

In addition to the increased cost of temperature measurement, there are questions about the appropriate method for measuring temperature during MRI scans. Given that it is impossible to measure every point on and in the human body, the problem of 'hot spots' is impossible to account for. Nonetheless, some groups have indicated that an esophageal measurement of core temperature would render accurate measurement.[23] However, an esophageal measurement is a relatively invasive method that is hard to imagine being widely accepted apart from patients scheduled to be intubated. While axillary temperature measurement is less invasive and easy to apply, there are concerns about its accuracy with one study showing a difference of ±0.45 °C compared to true core temperature.[24] Again here, the core temperature measurement still ignores the reality of hot spots occurring at different places on or in the body during an MRI scan. As a case study of an implanted object an expert implanted device testing firm [MR:COMP gmbh] showed that within 5 s an implanted electrode with a 48 in. lead wire could heat up by 25 °C or more. Hence, using the patient as an indicator of temperature would necessarily fail especially if one considers that reaction time of the patient to the heat added to the reaction time of the MRI scanning personnel (that would stop a scan in progress) could easily take more than 5 s thus resulting in tissue temperatures in excess of 60 °C and probable irreversible tissue damage would result.

To prevent damage from excess heating and burns, the American College of Radiology established the following safety guidelines during MRI scans:[25]

1. Remove metallic objects and all conductive materials including drug patches containing conductive metal particles contacting the patients skin.
2. Use insulation material of 1 cm or thicker to prevent skin-to-skin contact and the formation of closed-loops from touching body parts.
3. Allow only devices, equipment, accessories, and material that have been thoroughly tested and determined to be MRI safe.

17.8 CONCLUSION

Children undergoing MRI scans are at significant risk of clinically significant temperature derangements which might have harmful clinical consequences. The changes in temperature depend on several factors, including the patients size, clinical condition, the effects of anesthesia, the type of scanner used, as well as the RF sequences applied. Little data exists in pediatric patients to evaluate the true incidence and clinical consequences of these alterations in temperature, the effect of various MRI sequences on temperature changes, and the proper methods to maintain normothermia. Until then, good clinical practice should include monitoring patients for both hypothermia and hyperthermia with the ability to address both problems rapidly when present. The lack of thermoregulation and communication skills in the pediatric population indicates that constant and direct monitoring from beginning to end of each case is required.

DISCLAIMER

The subject matter, content, and views presented do not represent the views of the Department of Health and Human Services (HHS), US Food and Drug Administration (FDA), and/or the United States.

RELATED ARTICLE IN EMAGRES

Radiofrequency Heating Models and Measurements

REFERENCES

1. K. Lunze, D. E. Bloom, D. T. Jamison, and D. H. Hamer, *BMC Med.*, 2013, **11**, 24.
2. A. Russo, M. McCready, L. Torres, C. Theuriere, S. Venturini, M. Spaight, R. Jean Hemway, S. Handrinos, D. Perlmutter, T. Huynh, A. Grunebaum, and J. Perlman, *Pediatrics*, 2014, **133**, e1055.
3. D. Morehouse, L. Williams, C. Lloyd, D. S. McCoy, E. Miller Walters, C. E. Guzzetta, S. Baumgart, A. Sill, D. Mueller-Burke, and B. L. Short, *Adv. Neonatal Care*, 2014, **14**, 154.
4. J. Oberlander and M. J. Laugesen, *N Engl. J. Med.*, 2015, **373**, 1185.

5. O. J. Arthurs and M. Sury, *Curr. Opin. Anaesthesiol.*, 2013, **26**, 489.
6. L. Borghi, *Anesthesiology*, 2015, **122**, 495.
7. D. I. Sessler, *Anesthesiology*, 2001, **95**, 531.
8. L. Feinstein and M. Miskiewicz, *Int. J. Anesthesiol.*, 2009, **27**.
9. B. M. Engorn, S. L. Kahntroff, K. M. Frank, S. Singh, H. A. Harvey, C. T. Barkulis, A. M. Barnett, O. O. Olambiwonnu, E. S. Heitmiller, and R. S. Greenberg, *Paediatr. Anaesth.*, 2017, **27**, 196.
10. C. Lo, G. Ormond, R. McDougall, S. J. Sheppard, and A. J. Davidson, *Anaesth. Intensive Care*, 2014, **42**, 333.
11. S. Chawla, A. Amaram, S. P. Gopal, and G. Natarajan, *J. Perinatol.*, 2011, **31**, 780.
12. K. O'Regan, P. Filan, N. Pandit, M. Maher, and N. Fanning, *Br. J. Radiol.*, 2012, **85**, 363.
13. J. M. Don Paul, E. J. Perkins, P. M. Pereira-Fantini, A. Suka, O. Farrell, J. K. Gunn, A. E. Rajapaksa, and D. G. Tingay, *J. Paediatr. Child Health*, 2018, **54**, 426.
14. D. Shrivastava, in *Theory and Applications of Heat Transfer in Humans*, John Wiley & Sons: Chichester, 2018.
15. L. R. Leon and A. Bouchama, *Compr. Physiol.*, 2015, **5**, 611.
16. H. S. Sharma and P. J. Hoopes, *Int. J. Hyperth.*, 2003, **19**, 325.
17. P. Sminia, J. van der Zee, J. Wondergem, and J. Haveman, *Int. J. Hyperth.*, 1994, **10**, 1.
18. R. H. Sacho, A. Vail, T. Rainey, A. T. King, and C. Childs, *J. Neurotrauma*, 2010, **27**, 2157.
19. P. Cawley, K. Few, R. Greenwood, P. Malcolm, G. Johnson, P. Lally, S. Thayyil, and P. Clarke, *J. Pediatr.*, 2016, **175**, 228.
20. Y. F. Bryan, T. W. Templeton, T. G. Nick, M. Szafran, and A. Tung, *Anesth. Analg.*, 2006, **102**, 1674.
21. S. Fricke, In *ISMRM Workshop Series, 28 September-01 October 2017, ISMRM Workshop on Ensuring RF Safety in MRI: Current Practices & Future Directions*, Hilton McLean Tysons Corner, McLean, VA, 2017. https://www.ismrm.org/workshops/Safety17/program.htm
22. J. Dennison and J. Hersh, Urgent Medical Device Correction: Potential Safety Issue with Medical Implants Using GE 3.0T MR Scanners, GE Healthcare: Wauwatosa, WI, 2015.
23. V. G. Nasr, R. Schumann, I. Bonney, L. Diaz, and I. Ahmed, *Anesth. Analg.*, 2012, **114**, 1230.
24. J.-Y. Lefrant, L. Muller, J. E. de La Coussaye, M. Benbabaali, C. Lebris, N. Zeitoun, C. Mari, G. Saïssi, J. Ripart, and J. J. Eledjam, *Intensive Care Med.*, 2003, **29**, 414.
25. Expert Panel on MR Safety, E. Kanal, A. J. Barkovich, C. Bell, J. P. Borgstede, W. G. Bradley Jr, J. W. Froelich, J. R. Gimbel, J. W. Gosbee, E. Kuhni-Kaminski, P. A. Larson, J. W. Lester Jr, J. Nyenhuis, D. J. Schaefer, E. A. Sebek, J. Weinreb, B. L. Wilkoff, T. O. Woods, L. Lucey, and D. Hernandez, *J. Magn. Reson. Imaging (JMRI)*, 2013, **37**, 501.

Chapter 18

Failure to Monitor and Maintain Thermal Comfort During an MRI Scan: A Perspective from a Thermal Physiologist Turned Patient

Christopher J. Gordon

Retired, U.S. Environmental Protection Agency, Research Triangle Park, NC, USA

18.1 SUMMARY

Safety and the wellbeing of the patient subjected to an MRI scan are of utmost importance. The author of this communication has had decades of training in thermal physiology and has participated in discussions on the thermal issues of MRI safety at national meetings for many years. One issue of patient safety widely discussed is the potential for hyperthermia and/or the elicitation of localized heating (i.e., hot spots) in susceptible tissues and organs. The overall thermal comfort of the patient during a scan is also important, but it is not clear how this parameter is evaluated or considered by staff performing a scan. This author was under the impression that overt thermal discomfort of the patient was likely not a problem for most scans. However, a recent hospitalization involving a 1 h spinal column scan has changed the author's opinion on this issue. The thermal discomfort experienced during the procedure and apparent lack of awareness of this stress from the medical staff performing the scan has compelled the author to prepare this communication. A first had description of an MRI scan from the perspective of a trained thermal physiologist is given with the goal to describe the significant issues of thermal discomfort that was encountered during this scan. A list of relatively simply guidelines and recommendations for new research are provided with the intention of improving protocols and to encourage the collection of more data to assess how MRI scans lead to perception of thermal stress. It is this author's hope that these recommendations will lead to improvements to minimize stress of MRI scans by focusing on the all important issue of thermal discomfort.

Safety and Biological Effects in MRI.
Edited by Devashish Shrivastava and J. Thomas Vaughan

ISBN: 978-1-118-82130-5
Also published in eMagRes (online edition)
DOI: 10.1002/9780470034590.emrstm1631

18.2 AUTHOR'S ACADEMIC AND RESEARCH BACKGROUND

The author of this communication is a thermal physiologist with over four decades of research experience. He has published extensively on the thermoregulatory effects of radiofrequency (RF) radiation in experimental animals and humans when he worked with the U.S. Environmental Protection Agency's program in the 1980s to study the health effects of RF radiation. He was later involved in studies on the thermal responses of human subjects when subjected to clinical MRI scans.[1] In addition, he has been an invited expert in several meetings sponsored by the International Society of Magnetic Resonance in Medicine (ISMRM) that have focused on the thermal safety of MRI and gave presentations on the thermoregulatory effects of RF radiation, MRI, and the general effects of heat stress on the human body (e.g., in ISMRM Workshop on Ensuring RF Safety in MRI: Current Practices & Future Directions, Arlington, VA, USA, 2017).

18.3 MEDICAL CONDITIONS LEADING TO THE MRI SCAN

I was hospitalized in February 2018 (Duke University Medical Center, Durham, NC, USA) for eight days while being treated for several significant health issues associated with multiple myeloma, including renal dysfunction, high serum calcium, skeletal and muscle weakness. While in the hospital, my physician ordered an MRI of the entire spinal column to assess for possible bone lesions of the vertebrae. At the time of the scan, I was in poor health. I was being given IV fluids to improve kidney function and to rehydrate. Around this same time, I was also being treated for a supraventricular tachycardia (SVT) and had to undergo two cardiac ablations (~7 days after the MRI). Patient physical characteristics: 65 years old male; 86.4 kg (weight); 1.82 m (height); BMI of 25.

18.4 A BRIEF SUMMARY OF MY SCAN

18.4.1 Physical Environment and Preparation for the Scan

There was essentially no warning for me that my physician had ordered a scan. I suspect that this is probably not unusual for a patient hospitalized. It is mentioned here to note that there was little or no time to prepare for the scan (e.g., drink additional fluids).

I wore the typical hospital gown and slip-proof socks when I was transported into the MRI facility. It felt relatively cold in the room to me (no data on room temperature). I was very weak with rib pains and needed considerable help to be placed on the scan table in a supine position. My head was placed in a plastic head fixation frame to limit the movement of my head and spine. There was a relatively small opening in the frame allowing bare skin of my face to be exposed directly to the ambient environment. The frame itself is solid acrylic and may impede airflow around the head and thus heat loss from the head to the ambient.

The technicians asked if I would like a blanket after I was placed on the table. At the time, I felt very cold and two blankets were wrapped securely around my legs and feet. With the hospital gown, blankets, and helmet on my head, there was very little bare skin exposed to the ambient air and I was thermally comfortable.

I had the typical air bulb in my hand to squeeze if I needed assistance during scan along with a microphone and speaker system. No devices were used to monitor basic life functions and no temperature data of my core or skin were taken before or after the scan. The only questions regarding my thermal comfort during the entire scan was, whether or not I was comfortable at the start of the scan.

The scan lasted approximately 1 h. Approximately 40 min into the scan, a contrast agent was administered IV. Whole-body average specific absorption rate (SAR) of the MRI procedures is unknown to me.

18.4.2 Heat Stress During the Scan

The combined insulation from the gown, blankets, and socks I wore in the relatively cool room was adequate to provide an overall state of thermal comfort at the start of the scan. On the other hand, the combined stresses mentioned earlier, in addition to the heat load, was a physiological and psychological challenge for me. The very close quarters of being in the bore with my head in the helmet, the loud noise of the scan, and tight quarters of the bore were very stressful to me. I would suspect that my state of thermal stress might be due to the combination of whole-body average SAR, duration of exposure and my medical condition. I should note that I have had a head scan and an abdominal scan MRI scans in the past, both lasting

~30 min. During those scans, I was in good health and I did not feel the stress as I did with the scan of my spinal column.

Within ~15 min of scanning, I started to feel warm. As the scan continued, my thermal sensation was shifting from a feeling of warmth to feeling uncomfortably hot. I believe that the sensations of warmth were worsened by the limited movement due to the head restricting device and the blankets wrapped around my legs. It is also my opinion that being subjected to other stressors of the scan mentioned above, combined with the heat load of the MRI, were all significant factors contributing to a state of duress that grew rapidly in intensity as the scan progressed.

As I recall I finally squeezed the ball after ~30 min to alert the technicians of my state of duress. They pulled me out of the bore and I asked them to remove the blankets. There was another 20 or 30 min of scan remaining at that point, including the administration of the contrast agent. When I was pulled out of the bore, I was very upset, so much so that I later apologized to the technicians for my outburst. This is a simple reflection of how I felt after just 30 min of the scan. It was difficult for me to go back into the bore and complete the scan. At the termination of the scan, I was placed back in the wheelchair and eventually moved back to my room. There was very little communication between the technicians and myself. One of the first things I did was ask for some water when I was removed from the MRI.

18.4.3 Communication with Medical Staff During the Scan

I was offered but declined to use earphones to listen to music during the scan. I declined because, with my previous experience, it is very difficult to hear music with the scan. Reflecting later on how warm I felt during the scan, I suspect that the plastic earphones would have added to my thermal discomfort and would have further limited the surface area of my head that could dissipate excess heat from the scan. I would expect perspiration to build up under the headphones during a scan of this nature. Hence, I was communicating through the microphone in the bore of device but it was relatively difficult to hear the technicians speaking to me. In fact, when I asked how much longer was remaining in the scan, I thought I heard 2 min but he claimed he said it was 20 min. This clearly added to the duress of the scan. In such an isolated environment and with no indication of time (i.e., not knowing elapsed time or time remaining for the scan is another issue that contributes to the stress). It becomes a challenge to deal with estimating a duration of time unless one is given frequent updates from the technicians.

Days afterward as I was recovering from my hospitalization, I often asked myself why I did not squeeze the ball earlier in the scan to let medical staff know that I was very uncomfortable. My attitude, and I suspect this would be typical of most patients, is that I wanted to be cooperative and complete the scan as soon as possible and not interfere with the technician's task of completing their job. I believe this attitude of the patient affects his/her decision processes to not interrupt the scan and inform the technician that there may be a problem.

18.5 TWO CRITICAL THERMOREGULATORY FACTORS TO CONSIDER

1. *Thermal perception.* Considering all of the undesirable aspects of my MRI scan, I conclude that my perception of feeling hot, especially during the early stages when the blankets were wrapped around my legs, was the most stressful part of the scan. My thermal sensations were not evaluated or assessed by the medical staff. I was never asked if I felt warm or hot at any time. I found this to be the most significant oversight considering the focus on the patient's thermoregulatory system in the MRI safety conferences that I have attended.
2. *Convective heat loss.* The room housing the scanner felt very cold and there was excellent circulation of air within the room to encourage forced convective heat loss. Natural and forced convection from the body to the ambient environment are important avenues of heat loss. Forced convection, resulting from air movement over the clothing and skin would be crucial avenue of heat loss during the scan. However, when a full-size adult is placed entirely in the bore, the area for air circulation through the bore is clearly going to be limited. With the blankets and helmet around the bare skin of my head, I would predict that forced convective heat loss was very limited during the scan. I do not have exact values but I would estimate

that the cross-sectional area of the bore is reduced by well over 50% with a full-sized adult placed completely in the bore. It is this author's opinion that air movement is restricted significantly, limiting forced convective heat loss. In addition, heat loss from the head with the head restriction device would also be limited. I predict that this would contribute to an increased sense of thermal stress as my body warmed during the scan.

18.6 RECOMMENDATIONS: NEW GUIDELINES AND RESEARCH TO IMPROVE QUALITY OF PATIENT HEALTH

I have several recommendations to improve the safety and wellbeing of patients subjected to MRI scans that involve high SARs' of relatively long duration. When attending the MRI conferences, I found that thermoregulation, especially the potential for the generation of hot spots that could lead to irreversible tissue damage represent a significant part of the agenda. There are many talks that deal with predicting hot spots. There are also a few experimental studies that typically involve exposing healthy, young adults under controlled conditions. These areas of study are important but I conclude that fundamental thermoregulatory responses to the MRI scan may not be receiving adequate attention.

Being in the unique position as a thermal physiologist and patient, I would thus like to propose the following to be considered in the future development of safety guidelines for MRI scans. These guidelines should be applied to scans involving relatively high SAR's that are capable of leading to significant heating of the core or trunk of the body. These SAR × time relationships are well known and it is simply a matter of developing guidelines for scans that will or will not lead to significant heating. Clearly, better protocols are needed to minimize thermal stress of the patient:

1. *One of the most important questions that needs to be asked at frequent intervals throughout a scan is, "Do you feel warm or hot"?* A standard protocol needs to be established for high SAR scans of the trunk that assures that patient thermal comfort is maintained. This would call for education of the medical staff performing the scans and physicians ordering the scans. The physicians need to consider any obvious health issues that might be associated with a thermoregulatory process, such as prescription drug medications (see the following discussion).

   For the medical staff, the critical parameters to consider is whether or not the patient's thermal comfort could be compromised. Considering the patients' age, weight, gender, and overall health would likely have a significant impact on his/her thermal comfort during a scan. The ambient temperature of the facility is also crucial but the guidelines for this parameter are well established and the room is typically maintained relatively cold. But as pointed out earlier, the ambient temperature of the facility will not necessarily match the predicted heat loss and thermal comfort of the patient once he/she is in the bore and wrapped with insulating blankets. I would predict that these parameters would be the most important that would affect thermal comfort during a scan and warrant further research.

   Even without additional research, the MRI technicians must be cognizant of how the thermoregulatory system is going to respond as an internal heat load is applied to a patient that is wrapped in insulating blankets; their thermal comfort is likely to change rapidly during the scan. Considering the experience from my scan, I would strongly urge that the scan be initiated with the blankets wrapped around the patient's legs as I described earlier. However, after ~15 min (more or less depending on body mass), the blankets need to be replaced with a less insulating fabric such as linen or equivalent material. Simply removing all the blankets with no insulation could result in a situation here the patient becomes uncomfortably cold due to perspiration on the legs as heating progresses. A thin blanket of insulation as heating progresses would likely be an ideal replacement for the thick blankets. In addition, removing the socks to facilitate heat loss from the feet might also be useful to achieve thermal comfort.
2. *Measure oral temperature of patients before and after a scan.* For hospitalized patients, I would recommend that a pre-scan and post-scan body temperature being taken soon after the scan as well as approximately 1 h after the scan and possibly again at a later time after completion of the scan. In terms of my scan, basic clinical functions (blood pressure, oral temperature) were measured several

times per day when hospitalized. My core temperature was in fact elevated but not in the febrile range on the day of the scan. I was not asked any questions regarding my health before the scan (e.g., any shivering, feeling cold or hot, sweating, or a fever). A post-scan temperature measurement taken 1 h after the scan may provide some additional assurances on the health and wellbeing of hospitalized patients.

3. *Assess medical history of patient relevant to potential thermoregulatory response to MRI scan.* This is an important topic and is frequently discussed at the national MRI meetings. However, the medical history of a patient in terms of treatment with prescription drugs or drugs of abuse that can interfere with thermal perception as well as the activation of thermoregulatory effectors that can increase core temperature.[2]

18.7 ADDITIONAL RESEARCH AND FUTURE DIRECTIONS

During a scan, a patient may be subjected to many forms of stress, including physiological as occurs from thermal discomfort as well as psychological stress that many patients may encounter from the unique environment of the MRI device. In fact, a stress such as thermal discomfort may well exacerbate the perceived psychological stress of the scan. All would agree that minimizing patient stress but without compromising the quality of the scan, should be an ultimate goal. I recommend the development of prospective studies to better evaluate the potential thermal stress patients may encounter during a scan. It would be important to consider the factors such as body weight and overall health and to assess basic thermoregulatory changes before and after a scan.

1. *Quantify thermal sensation during scans.* Behavioral thermal sensation and responses to heat and cold stimuli are one of the most well-studied areas of human temperature regulation.[3] For example, simply asking the patient the state of their thermal comfort during the scan is an approach that is relatively simple and easy to perform. Thermal physiologists often study thermal sensory function of humans subjects by using a simple numerical scale of subjective measure of thermal comfort.[4] For example, using a five point scale, a subject feeling uncomfortably cold would give a score of 1; mildly cold, a score of 2; ideal thermal comfort would be a score of 3, and on up to uncomfortably hot with a score of 5. Comfort scales ranging can range from 5 to 15.[4] Such a simple behavioral approach would be an ideal starting point in clinical MRI studies to begin to understand how the patient's body size, age, gender, health status, and other factors may impact on his/her thermal comfort. I strongly urge such an approach to be taken in future work to understand the fundamental behavioral thermoregulatory responses to the MRI scan.
2. *Better understand how heat stress from scan affects psychological response to other stressors.* With apparently very little or no research in this area, it would be pure speculation at this time to predict how the stress of the MRI scan (e.g., tight space, noise, limited movement) could exacerbate the perceived thermal stress of the scan. There is considerable database on the interactions between thermal stress and performance of mental tasks and overall psychological stress. However, I know of no research on this as it pertains to RF heating during an MRI scan.

If these recommendations can be implemented, it will be important to consider the impact of the patient's health status and anthropomorphic characteristics. In terms of the experience with my scan, I considered myself to be in reasonably good physical condition to endure this scan despite my health issues. Obesity, heart disease, and type 2 diabetes, to name a few, are likely to have an undesirable impact on the thermal comfort of a patient during a scan.

REFERENCES

1. C. J. Gordon, in 'Theory and Applications of Heat Transfer in Humans', ed D. Shrivastava, John Wiley and Sons, 2018, p 501.
2. M. E. Musselman and S. Saely, *Am. J. Health Syst. Pharm.*, 2013, **70**, 34.
3. Z. J. Schlader, S. R. Stannard, and T. Mündel, *Physiol. Behav.*, 2010, **M99**, 269.
4. H. Hensel, Thermoreception and Temperature Regulation, Monographs of the Physiological Society No. 38, Academic Press, 1981.

Chapter 19

MR Thermometry to Assess Heating Induced by RF Coils Used in MRI

Henrik Odéen, John Rock Hadley, Dylan Palomino, Katelynn Stroth, and Dennis L. Parker

University of Utah, Salt Lake City, UT, USA

19.1 INTRODUCTION

Despite all the values of magnetic resonance imaging (MRI) in providing information for improved health care that can be obtained in no other way, there are risks associated. One of the primary risks is the unpredictable, nonuniform temperature increase due to the deposition of nonuniform radio frequency (RF) power in tissues by RF coils used in MRI.[1–4] Although the body maintains tissue temperatures at or near 37 °C, most tissues can be heated a small amount for short period of times without incurring any damage. To establish the effects of heating within the human body caused by MRI, it is necessary to be able to accurately monitor the temperature increase that occurs in vivo. Because accurate in vivo temperature maps have not been made within the human body during heating caused by the MRI scanner, there is very little knowledge of the effects of this heating in vivo. Because of the lack of knowledge of the effects of temperature on the different body tissues, safety committees around the world, such as the International Commission on Non-Ionizing Radiation Protection (ICNIRP)[5] and the International Electrotechnical Commission (IEC),[6] and US regulatory agencies such as the US Food and Drug Administration (US FDA)[7] have set guidelines for MRI operations that are intended to maintain temperature increases below levels that are believed to be safe.

Currently, there is no method established to measure the distribution of the temperature increase associated with the RF fields used in MRI. Ideas of the temperature increase have been obtained by placing temperature sensors at specific locations within anthropomorphic phantoms and human-sized animals.[1,2] However, these only provide temperature estimates at a finite set of points, and phantoms do not always accurately mimic the in vivo situation in terms of tissue inhomogeneities and physiological effects, such as perfusion (especially if they are temperature sensitive). Estimates of RF-power distributions have been made using full wave numerical simulations of

Safety and Biological Effects in MRI.
Edited by Devashish Shrivastava and J. Thomas Vaughan
 ISBN: 978-1-118-82130-5
Also published in eMagRes (online edition)
DOI: 10.1002/9780470034590.emrstm1580

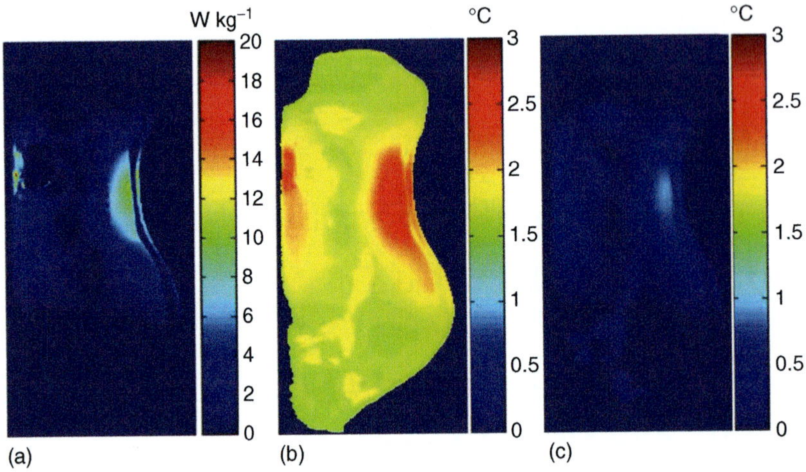

Figure 19.1. Simulated local SAR distribution in a swine (a). The associated temperature changes simulated using a 'mechanistic generic bioheat transfer model (GBHTM)' that takes into account heating of the blood (b) compared to the simulated temperature changes simulated using the standard Pennes BHTE (c). The images are in the sagittal plane 5 mm lateral to the central plane at the end of the heating when the swine trunk was placed in the isocenter of a 3 T birdcage body coil. (Reproduced with permission from Ref. 2. © John Wiley & Sons, 2014)

the RF fields associated with the MRI transmit coils in conjunction with detailed numerical human tissue models.[8–11] Resultant tissue heating has been estimated using validated as well as unvalidated bioheat models (Figure 19.1).[2] The point measurements in phantoms and animals do not provide temperature distributions, and the simulated temperature distributions in numerical models are not necessarily accurate, and both methods have limited applicability in providing estimates of any hot spots that may occur during human scans.

In addition to causing heating, it has been shown since 1980 that MRI can be used to make images of temperature change.[12–15] However, the ability of MRI to monitor temperature change accurately over large tissue volumes, over long periods of time, and to within 1 °C has not been established. In this chapter, we review MRI techniques that can be used to measure temperature with special consideration to temperature measurements needed for heating that can occur due to the RF fields used in MRI. We give special consideration to the problems of detecting small changes over large image volumes in the presence of respiratory, peristalsis, and other motions, and field drift. We also consider measuring the temperature changes with high spatial and temporal gradients that can occur near implants.

For the purposes of this chapter, heating is caused by the electric currents that flow in the tissue or phantom in response to both the conservative and nonconservative electric fields induced by the MRI transmit RF coils. The conservative fields are due to charge buildup on coil components and decrease with distance from the coil components. The nonconservative fields are due to the changing magnetic field, which is generally more uniform across the body than the conservative fields. Because the currents also depend on the tissue conductivity and geometry, the magnitude and position of temperature increases observed will likely vary between subjects. Areas of major concern include regions where there is very little cooling from perfusion.

19.1.1 Different Pulse Sequences' Effect on Heating

In general, RF coils and pulse sequences for MRI are designed to result in very low heating. For example, some pulse sequences, such as basic gradient echo sequences (gradient echo – GRE; spoil gradient echo – SPGR; fast low angle shot – FLASH; segmented echo planar imaging – EPI; and single shot EPI) use low flip angle RF pulses and thus have very low specific absorption rates (SAR). To cause heating, sequences with high SAR are required. These sequences include those with many short duration, high-amplitude RF pulses, such as turbo spin echo (TSE) or fast spin echo (FSE) sequences, and sequences with large amplitude magnetization transfer (MT) or preparation pulses (such as inversion or saturation pulses). Even for high SAR sequences, it is expected that maximum heating due only to the applied RF fields from the imaging coils will be slow and on the order of just a few degrees centigrade. Further, hot spots could occur anywhere, but are more likely at the edges of large body cross sections, where the body is close to the coil components, near places with high electrical conductivity, in locations where perfusion is low, or in regions with high current density.

19.1.2 Bioheat Transfer Equation

The relationship between temperature change and SAR is often described to first order by the 'simplified' Pennes' bioheat transfer equation (BHTE)[16]:

$$\rho C_t \frac{\partial T}{\partial t} = k\nabla^2 T - WC_b(T - T_b) + Q \qquad (19.1)$$

where ρ is the tissue density (kg m^{-3}); C_t and C_b are the specific heats (at constant pressure) of tissue and blood (J kg^{-1} °C^{-1}); T and T_b are the tissue and blood temperature (°C); k is the thermal conductivity (W m^{-1} °C^{-1}); W is the Pennes' perfusion-related parameter (kg m^{-3} s^{-1}); and Q/ρ is the SAR (W kg^{-1}). It has been shown that the Pennes' BHTE does not properly account for blood temperature, which heats during long duration studies (Figure 19.2).[2] For more information on the derivation and validity of the simplified Pennes BHTE, readers are encouraged to refer to the text 'Theory and Applications of Heat Transfer in Humans' edited by Dr. Shrivastava.[17]

19.1.3 SAR from MRI RF coils

Tissue heating occurs due to currents that arise from voltages induced in the tissue or phantom by the oscillating RF magnetic field:

$$\text{emf} = -\frac{\mathrm{d}}{\mathrm{d}t}\int B_1(t) \cdot \hat{n}\mathrm{d}a \qquad (19.2)$$

where $B_1(t)$ is the applied RF field, and $\hat{n}$ is the unit vector normal to the surface of the integral. Because this induced voltage increases with tissue or phantom cross-section area, da, and the resistance increases with the circumference, the heating from a changing magnetic field tends to be greater at the edge of a subject than near the center (Figures 19.3 and 19.4).[11,18–21]

For time scales such that the thermal effects of perfusion and diffusion may be neglected (< ~30 s), and where heating is mostly uniform ($\nabla^2 T \sim 0$) so that thermal conductivity has less of an effect, SAR can be directly estimated from the rate of temperature increase[22]:

$$\text{SAR} \approx C_t \frac{\partial T}{\partial t} \qquad (19.3)$$

Measurements can also be made in vivo, to the extent that safety limits are not exceeded.

19.1.4 Temperature Determination with MRTI

Because MRI methods have been used to monitor temperature change in a variety of thermal treatments such as focused ultrasound, laser interstitial thermal therapy, microwave, and radiofrequency, for both ablative and hyperthermia applications, it is logical to question whether sequences for magnetic resonance (MR) temperature imaging could be used to monitor the heating that occurs with MRI. For magnetic-resonance temperature imaging (MRTI) to be useful in measuring temperature change, at least three requirements must be met. The MRTI sequence must be able to: (i) heat the tissue sufficiently for the temperature increase to be measured; (ii) monitor and correct for any phase shift (from, e.g., B_0-drift) not associated with temperature; and (iii) measure the temperature change with sufficient precision and accuracy.

In general, MRI pulse sequences are not designed to measure temperature increases. Further, the temperature may increase outside of the desired imaging volume. Therefore, it is unlikely that MRI can be used to self-monitor during actual scanning. Instead, it would make sense to use a separate, large volume MRTI method designed to measure temperature over the entire volume of the RF coil to determine distribution of the rate at which temperature increases as a function of the power output of the RF coil. To first approximation this could be determined from the SAR distribution of equation (19.3). If the heat capacity is not known, the distribution of SAR to heat capacity could be determined from equation (19.3) and would be sufficient to predict patient-specific heating for each

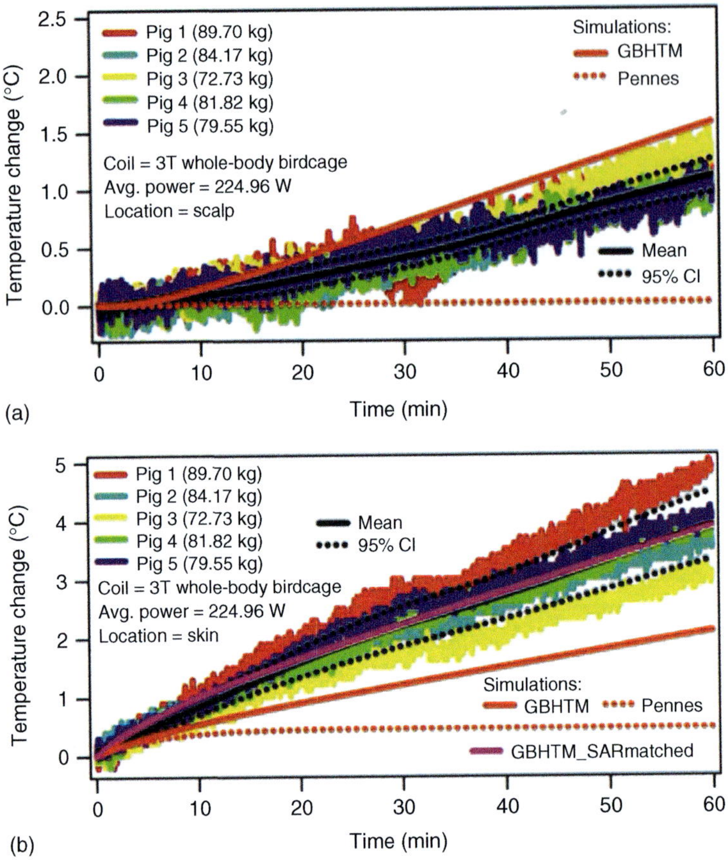

Figure 19.2. RF-power-induced temperature changes in the subcutaneous layer of the scalp (a) and in the subcutaneous layer of the skin in the plane of the isocenter (b) when the swine trunk was placed in the isocenter of a 3 T birdcage body coil. While the Pennes' model shows very little heating, the GBHTM model is likely more accurate because it accounts for the heating of the blood over time. (Reproduced with permission from Ref. 2. © John Wiley & Sons, 2014)

pulse sequence. Note that the SAR distribution will be different for different subjects and should be determined on a patient-specific basis.

In the following section we discuss the basics principles, strengths, and limitations of several methods that can be used for MRTI. Each of these could be modified to deposit energy while at the same time measuring the energy that is being deposited. Because the temperature increase is expected to be small, on the order of 1 or 2 °C, it is essential that the MRTI measurement accuracy is better than 1 °C, which is a formidable requirement, but possible because the temperature change is generally slow and extensive averaging is possible.

19.2 MR TEMPERATURE IMAGING (MRTI) METHODS

There are several MRI parameters, including the relaxation rates T_1 and T_2, the water diffusion coefficient, and the resonance frequency of protons on water molecules that are sensitive to temperature and change as temperature changes. Techniques to use these parameters in MRTI are discussed in a number of excellent reviews.[14,15,23–25] Although T_1 was the first parameter used for MRTI,[12] it is generally less accurate than the proton resonance frequency shift (PRFS) method. The temperature dependence of proton resonance frequency (PRF) is nearly the same for all aqueous-based tissue types,[26] and thus is less sensitive

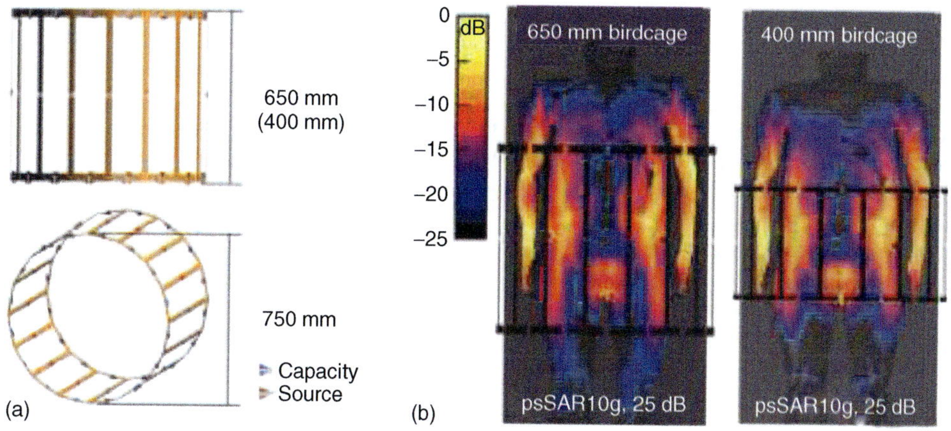

Figure 19.3. (a) Models of 16-Rung birdcage coils of 750 mm diameter and 650 and 400 mm length used in general for the simulation of heating in a numerical human phantom. (b) Illustrative SAR distribution for the numerical phantom in the pelvis imaging position within the two birdcages. The simulations demonstrate the greater power (SAR) deposition in the periphery than in the center

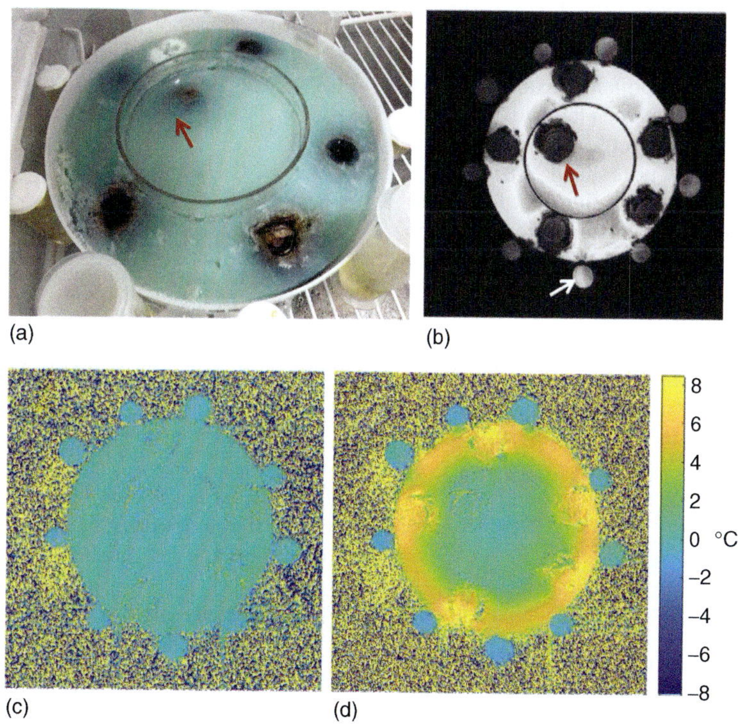

Figure 19.4. (a) Agar phantom doped with copper sulfate to shorten the MRI relaxation times and with NaCl added to approximately match tissue conductivity. Six cow eyeballs are placed in the agar as indicated by the red arrows, and nine vials of oil are placed around the outside to control magnetic field drift. (b) A magnitude image from a PRFS sequence that also applied a large tip angle RF pulse for heating. (c) A temperature image obtained at the start of the sequence before temperature increase was observed. (d) A temperature image obtained about 20 min after start showing about 8 °C temperature increase at the edge of the phantom

to thermally induced changes in tissue than the other MRI parameters. However, lipids and nonaqueous tissues do not exhibit a temperature-dependent PRFS, and for these tissues, other methods such as T_1, T_2, or the diffusion coefficient may be needed. In general, T_1, T_2, and the diffusion coefficient depend on other tissue properties and may be less useful if heating causes changes such as local edema.

In the following section, we discuss the several most likely methods in terms of capabilities to measure temperatures over extended periods of time with high accuracy. We review the physical basis of each technique, the intrinsic sensitivity, sources of potential errors, and ideas for correction.

19.2.1 Longitudinal Relaxation Time (T_1) Measurement Methods

19.2.1.1 Physical Mechanism and Temperature Dependence

In biological tissues the longitudinal relaxation time is due to both intramolecular (between the two hydrogen protons in the same water molecule) and intermolecular (between protons in water and surrounding macromolecules) dipolar interactions, where the former has the largest effect. Magnetic field interactions between the two hydrogen protons in the water molecule are created due to random thermal motion of water molecules. These intramolecular interactions can be described by the frequency spectral density $J(\omega)$, Figure 19.5. The frequency spectral density describes the number of interactions occurring at different frequencies. If a spin system has a large spectral density at or close to the Larmor frequency (where the Larmor frequency is the precession frequency of a proton magnetic moment around the B_0-field), it will have many opportunities to transfer energy and relax from its excited state. This will result in a short T_1 value. As examples, free water molecules experience fast motion and have a spectral density that is too wide, and frozen tissues experience slow motion and have a spectral density that is too narrow, for efficient energy transfers. This reduced spectral density at the Larmor frequency results in longer T_1 relaxation times.[27] For increased B_0-field strengths, the Larmor frequency is also higher, and T_1 is longer since the spectral densities decrease with higher ω.

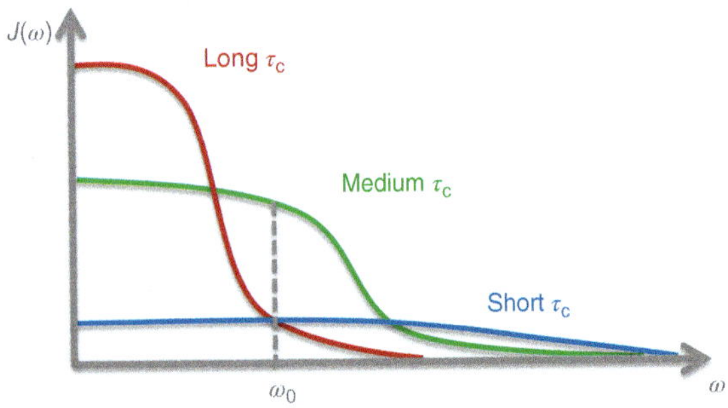

Figure 19.5. Schematics of frequency spectral density, $J(\omega)$, as a function of resonance frequency, ω, for different correlation times, τ_c. The longitudinal relaxation time, T_1, is proportional to the number of protons that are tumbling at the Larmor frequency, ω_0. Pure water and water molecules bound to large slow-moving macromolecules have a wide flat spectrum and a narrow spectrum, respectively. In both the cases there is relatively little energy around the Larmor frequency. The largest contribution to T_1 comes from water bound to intermediate-sized molecules

The rate of motion of water molecules can be described by the so-called correlation time, τ_c, which is related to the time a water molecule spends in a specific position. T_1 and τ_c are related by:

$$\frac{1}{T_1} = \frac{2\gamma^2 B_{\mathrm{loc}}^2}{3} \frac{\tau_c}{1+\omega_0^2\tau_c^2} \tag{19.4}$$

where B_{loc} is the local field experienced by the nucleus and consists of the external B_0-field plus fields due to local magnetic moments. For field strengths and temperatures experienced in most MRI studies $\omega_0\tau_c \ll 1$, and equation (19.4) can hence be approximated as:

$$\frac{1}{T_1} \propto \tau_c \tag{19.5}$$

It can be further shown that τ_c is inversely proportional to the temperature, Figure 19.6. Thus, to this approximation, T_1 is directly proportional to temperature.

Since the body mainly consists of nearly free water, the spectral density at the Larmor frequency is low. However, as temperature decreases, the kinetic motion reduces, and the spectral density at the Larmor frequency increases, resulting in shortening of T_1. Thus, for tissues composed mainly of free water, T_1 will increase as temperature increases. Values have been found to be around 2% per °C.[12,28] The temperature dependence varies with tissue type, hydration, and other molecular environmental factors (an excellent review is available in Ref. 29). Within a small temperature

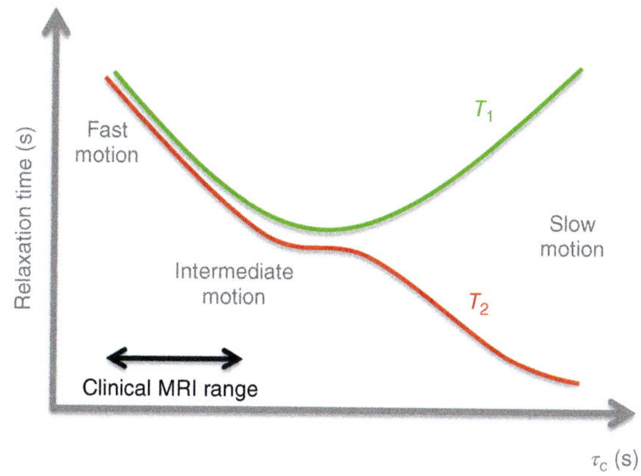

Figure 19.6. T_1 and T_2 relaxation times as a function of correlation time, τ_c. Modern MRI scanners operate at rather low τ_c as indicated by the black arrow. In this range, both T_1 and T_2 increase as a function of decreased correlation time, resulting in both T_1 and T_2 increase as a function of increased temperature

range, T_1 varies linearly with temperature and can be described by[15]:

$$T_1(T) = T_1(T_{ref}) + m(T - T_{ref}) \quad (19.6)$$

where m is the change in T_1 (in ms per °C) with temperature.

19.2.1.2 *Measurement Methods*

The ability to use T_1 to monitor temperature change will depend on the accuracy with which T_1 can be measured. Probably the most accurate methods are inversion recovery (IR)- or saturation recovery (SR)-based methods, but both are time-consuming, requiring measurements at multiple recovery times. Although IR methods can be slow, one very rapid method was developed to monitor T_1 and T_1 change in blood.[30] Because the blood equilibrates with the core body temperature, this method might be a very rapid method to track the effect of MRI RF on core body temperature. The T_1 by multiple readout pulses (TOMROP) can acquire multiple slices in about 4 min and may be adequate for assessing heating due to RF.[31] Another relatively fast method is the multiple-flip angle method, where T_1 is calculated based on the signal intensities from multiple images acquired with different flip angles.[32,33] It has been shown that using flip angles on either side of the Ernst angle, so that each angle produces a signal that is 0.71 times the signal produced at the Ernst angle, high precision T_1 measurements can be achieved with only two images.[33,34]

19.2.1.3 *Limitations*

Limitations include the different dependencies for different tissues (a different m for each tissue type in equation (19.6) the small percentage change in T_1 value with temperature, and the fact that T_1 will change with the various other tissue properties in addition to temperature). *Tissue dependence*: The temperature dependence (m) is different for different tissues, and m for each tissue must be calibrated separately. *Temperature dependence*: Further, m is very small, corresponding to about 2% per °C. So for monitoring very small temperature changes, e.g., which might occur with heating due to the MRI transmit RF coils, the standard deviation in the T_1 measurements needs to be on the order of 1% of the T_1 value. This can be attained with averaging over large region of interest and/or for longer time periods. *Other factors*: Unfortunately, T_1 as well as its temperature dependence will also change with the hydration and macromolecular state of the tissue.[35] If the tissue state changes with the procedure, the ability of T_1 to follow small temperature changes may be lost.

19.2.2 Transverse Relaxation Time (T_2) Measurement Methods

19.2.2.1 *Physical Mechanism and Temperature Dependence*

The transverse component of the magnetization signal relaxes both due to static field variation within a voxel and field fluctuations at very low frequencies and fluctuations at the Larmor frequency. The effect of static field variation in space is eliminated using spin echo-type pulse sequences. The remaining magnetic field experienced by a spin depends both on the partner hydrogen-proton in the water molecule as well as spins in neighboring molecules and varies in time due to random motion of the molecules. Since $\omega = \gamma B$, the time varying B will result in time-dependent variations in the precession rate ω, and hence result in a dephasing and loss of the spin coherence. Since this loss of spin coherence is due to random motions, it cannot be reversed. The relaxation due to these random fluctuations, which is described by the transverse relaxation coefficient T_2, is also a function of temperature. The resulting dependence of the transverse relaxation on the correlation time is given by the relation:

$$\frac{1}{T_2} = \gamma^2 B_{\text{loc}}^2 \left(\tau_c + \frac{\tau_c}{1 + \omega_0^2 \tau_c^2} \right) \quad (19.7)$$

Thus, because $\omega_0 \tau_c \ll 1$, T_2 will be inversely proportional to τ_c. Just as for T_1, it can further be shown that τ_c is inversely proportional to the temperature, Figure 19.6, and to this approximation, changes in T_2 are hence directly proportional to temperature changes.

In aqueous tissue, T_2 seems to depend on many factors, including temperature. However, in fat, the temperature dependence is more stable.[36,37] Kuroda showed that the temperature dependence of T_2 is different for the CH_2 protons (4–5% per °C) and CH_3 protons (3–6% per °C).[38] Multiple studies have shown that T_2 increases linearly and reversibly with temperature.[36–39]

19.2.2.2 Measurement Methods

T_2 is generally measured using multiple spin echoes. If gradient recalled echoes were used, the signal decay would include the effects of the static field component, for which the temperature dependence is not well understood. To avoid the effects of the RF variation across the slice, the phase of the refocusing pulses is shifted 90° from the excitation pulse.

19.2.2.3 Limitations

Limitations include the restriction of validity to measurement in fat mentioned before and the relatively inefficient acquisition, which is limited to multiple 2D slice acquisition rather than 3D. Because of the refocusing pulses, it is necessary to add a delay between repeat excitations of the same slice to allow the signal to regrow. Thus, interleaving multiple slices can be done to improve measurement efficiency.

19.2.3 Proton Density and Signal Intensity

19.2.3.1 Physical Mechanism and Temperature Dependence

In addition to the signal dependence on relaxation times as discussed before, the MRI signal in each voxel is directly proportional to the density of the magnetization within a voxel. For the two-state proton system in a magnetic field, the relative populations in the two states are given by the Boltzmann distribution, which is temperature dependent. The magnetization density, M_o, is related to this difference and reduces to

$$M_o \approx n \frac{\gamma^2 \hbar^2 |B|}{4kT} \quad (19.8)$$

where n is the density of protons (number per unit volume), $\hbar$ is Planck's constant, and k is the Boltzmann constant. The temperature dependence of the equilibrium magnetization can be detected in the proton density (PD), which is directly proportional to the equilibrium magnetization, $\text{PD} \propto M_o$. The fractional change in magnetization with temperature can be written as:

$$\Delta M_o \approx -n \frac{\gamma^2 \hbar^2 |B|}{4kT^2} \Delta T \quad (19.9)$$

so that

$$\frac{\Delta M_o}{M_o} \approx -\frac{\Delta T}{T} \quad (19.10)$$

At room temperatures near 300 K, a one-degree change in temperature corresponds to approximately a 0.3% fractional change in the magnetization (and hence also in the PD).

19.2.3.2 Measurement Methods

Since many factors contribute to the MRI signal intensity, and it also depends on the pulse sequence used, it can be challenging to account for all other temperature dependencies and measure a pure change in PD with temperature. Chen *et al.*, in one of the few studies to date, measured the temperature dependence of the apparent proton density (APD) in porcine muscle and abdominal fat.[40] For adipose (i.e., fatty) tissue, a linear and reversible change in APD of approximately 0.29% per °C in the range of 30–75 °C was observed, in good agreement with theory. For muscle samples, on the other hand, the change in APD was linear but not reversible. A larger APD was observed during heating (approximately 0.40% per °C) than during cooling (approximately 0.28% per °C).

19.2.3.3 Limitations

In addition to the difficulty in developing a pulse sequence that is sensitive only to the PD and not to T_1 and T_2, the biggest challenge is the high signal accuracy required for 1 °C measurement precision – the signal change must be measured to within 0.3% to detect a 1 °C temperature change. This may be feasible when imaging at low spatial and temporal resolution or averaging over large regions in the image volume.

19.2.4 Diffusion

19.2.4.1 *Physical Mechanism and Temperature Dependence*

In general, the water molecules with their protons experience the random thermal motions known as diffusion. Once the magnetization has been tipped from the equilibrium direction, and becomes transverse to the main B_0 field, the effect of diffusion is evident and can be measured using gradients in the main field to cause signal loss due to the diffusion motion. The diffusion itself is energy activated, and the diffusion coefficient, D, is proportional to:

$$D \propto e^{E_a(D)/kT} \tag{19.11}$$

where E_a is the activation energy specific to diffusion.[14,15,41] By measuring a change in D and knowing E_a for a specific tissue type, the corresponding change in temperature can be calculated.

19.2.4.2 *Measurement Methods*

Diffusion consists of random Brownian motion that results in a three-dimensional Gaussian distribution of displacements, which increases in width as a function of time. The diffusion constant is measured by applying large diffusion encoding gradients (in addition to the gradient fields necessary to spatially encode the MRI signal), which cause a dispersion of the signal phase. The random Brownian motion coupled with this phase dispersion results in signal loss that is related to the displacement distribution. The signal loss can be described as an exponential according to e^{-bD}, where b is a function of the magnitude and duration of the applied gradients. Applying stronger and longer duration gradients results in more signal loss and higher diffusion weighting.

The temperature dependence of D can be derived by taking the derivative of equation (19.11) with respect to temperature, and normalizing, resulting in:

$$\frac{\mathrm{d}D}{D\mathrm{d}T} = \frac{E_a(D)}{kT^2} \tag{19.12}$$

which can be rearranged according to:

$$\Delta T = T - T_{ref} = \frac{kT_{ref}^2}{E_a(D)}\left(\frac{D - D_{ref}}{D_{ref}}\right) \tag{19.13}$$

where D_{ref} is the diffusion coefficient at a known reference temperature, and D is the dynamically acquired diffusion coefficients, which are assumed to vary with temperature. The temperature sensitivity of the diffusion coefficient is approximately 2% per °C.[42,43]

As outlined below, there are a number of difficulties and challenges associated with measuring the diffusion coefficient. Despite these challenges, diffusion has recently been used to measure the absolute temperature of the cerebrospinal fluid (CSF).[44–46] This absolute temperature measurement works because of the similarity of CSF macromolecular content between subjects and the resulting relative subject independence of the activation energy in CSF.

19.2.4.3 *Limitations*

Despite the relatively high temperature sensitivity of the diffusion coefficient, it has not been routinely used to track temperature changes due to several practical difficulties. The encoded diffusion distances are on the order of 10 μm and hence naturally very sensitive to both physiological motion and bulk motion of the patient.[14] Since the diffusion depends on the tissue structure, it can also change significantly and become nonlinear when tissue properties change. Irreversible tissue coagulation and reversible ischemia are two examples where the tissue structure changes, and both lead to significant changes in the diffusion. This can also result in competing effects where, e.g., the diffusion increases with temperature, but at the same time decreases due to ischemia.[47] Another challenge is the anisotropic nature of biological tissues. For many tissues, such as muscle and white matter in the brain, the mobility of water molecules is directionally dependent (anisotropic). Because of tissue structure, the diffusion coefficient is described by a full nine-element tensor (with six independent elements). The full tensor can be measured with diffusion gradients applied in at least six directions. Rotationally invariant measures of D, such as the trace of the tensor or fractional anisotropy, can also be measured.[48,49]

Since the diffusion in fat-based tissues is very low, diffusion is not well suited for temperature measurements in fat. For diffusion measurements in water-based tissues, the fat signal should be saturated to not underestimate the measured diffusion constant in the water.

Diffusion pulse sequences can be relatively slow and are not ideal to monitor rapid temperature changes that might occur around metal implants. However, some fast pulse sequences have been suggested.[50,51]

19.2.5 Proton Resonance Frequency Shift (PRFS)

19.2.5.1 Physical Mechanism and Temperature Dependence

At this time, the most widely used method for monitoring temperature changes with MRI is based on the shift in the water proton resonant frequency with temperature. The temperature dependence of the PRF was first described by Hindman in 1966.[52] The PRFS method has become the current standard for MR-based temperature measurements since it provides relatively high sensitivity and is, to a large extent, tissue-type independent.

From the resonance equation ($\omega = \gamma B_{\text{loc}}$), it is known that a proton's resonance frequency depends on the local magnetic field (B_{loc}) it experiences. According to Maxwell's equations, the magnetic field in matter can be approximated as:

$$B_{\text{loc}} \cong B_0 \left(1 - \frac{2\chi_0(T)}{3} - \sigma(T)\right) \tag{19.14}$$

where the magnetic susceptibility, χ_0, becomes a source term that distorts the main magnetic field, while the electronic screening constant, σ, describes the reduction of the field at the nucleus due to the electron cloud surrounding the nucleus. Both coefficients are functions of temperature. For aqueous (i.e., water-based) tissues, the electronic screening constant is at least an order of magnitude larger than the magnetic susceptibility, and the local magnetic field can therefore be approximated as:

$$B_{\text{loc}} \cong B_0(1 - \sigma(T)) \tag{19.15}$$

On water molecules, the oxygen atom attracts much of the protons electron cloud, reducing the electronic screening of the field at the hydrogen nucleus (i.e., the proton). The cloud is further reduced by hydrogen bonding of the proton with the oxygen atoms on neighboring water molecules, Figure 19.7. As temperature increases, this hydrogen bonding reduces, returning some of the proton's electron cloud and thereby increasing the screening and reducing the local field

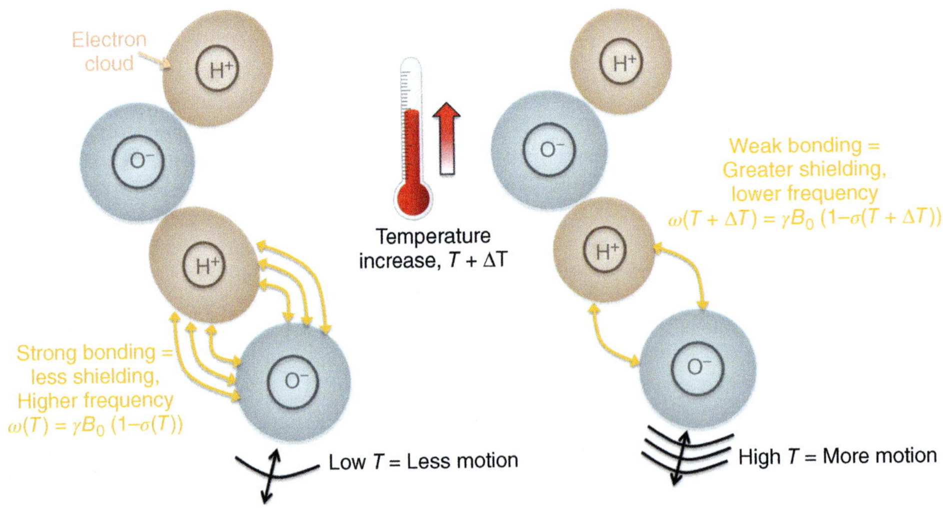

Figure 19.7. Schematic diagram depicting the PRF effect. At lower temperatures, strong hydrogen bondings exist between water molecules, resulting in weak shielding of the hydrogen proton. As temperature increases, the molecular movements increase and the hydrogen bonds start to break. This results in greater shielding from the electron cloud and a lower resonance frequency

B_{loc} experienced by the nucleus. This increased screening is nearly linear with temperature over a wide range of temperature:

$$\sigma(T) = \alpha T \tag{19.16}$$

where α is the PRFS temperature coefficient. Hindman found $\alpha = -0.0103$ ppm per °C in the range of −15 to 100 °C for pure water, and in more recent validation studies, values for various tissue types have been reported.[26] Not only is α nearly independent of tissue type, it does not seem to depend strongly on the hydration state of tissue or the various effects of thermal therapy, unlike the relaxation and diffusion coefficients.[53]

Because adipose tissues do not have the same hydrogen bondings as aqueous tissues, the electron screening coefficient in fatty tissue is not temperature dependent. In adipose tissue, the resonance frequency shift with temperature is dominated by the change in magnetic susceptibility, which has a substantially lower temperature sensitivity, and the PRFS method is therefore only applicable in aqueous tissues.

19.2.5.2 Measurement Methods

The PRF in MRI is directly proportional to the local field, B_{loc}, at the nucleus, and the image phase is directly proportional to this frequency and the time, TE, between the excitation of the magnetization and time of the data sampling: $\phi = \omega\text{TE}$. Combining all of these factors, the change in temperature can be related to the change in phase between a reference image and one during heating:

$$\Delta\phi = \phi(T) - \phi(T_{ref}) = \gamma\alpha B_0 \text{TE} \Delta T \tag{19.17}$$

or, rearranging, the change in temperature becomes:

$$\Delta T = \frac{\Delta\phi}{\gamma\alpha B_0 \text{TE}} \tag{19.18}$$

By calculating the temperature based on the difference in phase between a reference image and the current image, most static non-temperature-dependent contributions to the phase, from, e.g., RF coil sensitivities and inhomogeneities in the B_0 field, are eliminated.

Note that the PRFS method determines changes in temperature, rather than absolute values of the temperature. If the reference temperature (i.e., the temperature at the start of the experiment) is known, the absolute temperature is then:

$$T(t) = T_{ref} + \Delta T(t) \tag{19.19}$$

19.2.5.3 Limitations and Challenges

Despite many advantages of the PRFS method, there are a number of challenges that must be addressed, especially to accurately measure very small temperature changes over long time periods. The measurement precision and accuracy are affected by a number of factors.

Measurement Noise

The intrinsic precision (standard deviation) of the temperature change measurement is a function of TE since both the phase and the standard deviation of the phase depend on TE. The phase increases linearly with TE, while the standard deviation in the phase, $\sigma(\phi)$, is equal to the standard deviation of the signal divided by the signal magnitude, M, which decreases exponentially with TE[15] $M_{TE} = M_0 e^{-\text{TE}/T_2^*}$:

$$\sigma(\Delta T) = \frac{\sigma(\Delta\phi)}{\gamma\alpha B_0 \text{TE}} = \frac{\sigma(M)}{M_0}\frac{e^{+\text{TE}/T_2^*}}{\gamma\alpha B_0 \text{TE}} \propto \frac{1}{\text{SNR}_0}\frac{e^{+\text{TE}/T_2^*}}{\text{TE}} \tag{19.20}$$

This is minimized when $\text{TE} = T_2^*$, where T_2^* is the transverse relaxation time due to both random field fluctuations (which itself is described by T_2) and B_0-field inhomogeneities. Usually, T_2^* is longer than the chosen TE, such that using a longer TE would result in a more accurate phase measurement, but at the same time require a longer total scan time.

Field Drift

Over long time periods the main magnetic field of the MRI scanner (B_0) is found to drift. The drift is due to the slow loss in current in the superconducting windings as well as the change due to the heating and subsequent susceptibility change of the iron pieces that are used to passively shim the B_0 field. The iron shims are typically placed in trays that are installed between the primary and shield windings of the gradients. The heating of the shim iron is caused by the large currents used to create the gradient fields. If undetected or uncorrected, this field drift results in a corresponding error in the measured temperature due to the phase differencing with the baseline phase in equation (19.17).

Phase Variations Due to Motions

PRFS temperature measurements are affected by motion occurring both inside and outside the imaging field of view (FOV). These motions can occur both during a single scan (intrascan motion) and between scans (interscan motion). If motion occurs inside the imaged FOV and the acquisition time is too long to effectively 'freeze' the motion, the acquired images will be blurred. In these cases, the subtraction between the baseline and the dynamic images will not be clean and results in errors in the temperature map. This will also happen if bulk patient motion occurs throughout a heating experiment. Respiration and cardiac motions occurring outside the imaged FOV result in changes in the susceptibility distribution inside the imaged FOV, yielding field variations throughout the imaging volume. The variation in the field results in non-temperature-induced phase variations, which add to the temperature-induced phase variations. In all types of motion, the observed effect depends on the type of pulse sequence used. Fast pulse sequences such as single shot and segmented (i.e., multishot) EPI can be used to reduce the acquisition time and 'freeze' the motion. However, the sampling bandwidth in the phase encoding direction is generally fairly low in these sequences, making them more sensitive to off-resonance effects. Non-Cartesian methods using, e.g., radial and spiral sampling, are inherently less sensitive to motion as the center of *k*-space is sampled more frequently.

Temperature-dependent Changes in Electrical Properties

Peters *et al.* showed that RF fields undergo both amplitude attenuation and phase retardations in conductive materials such as the body.[54] In MRI, this results in spatially nonuniform flip angles and also nonuniform phase of the transverse magnetization. The phase retardation increases with temperature, resulting in temperature errors when applying the baseline subtraction. The effect was also shown to be worse for larger heating volumes such as regional hyperthermia, and can therefore be a problem for the regional heating that might occur with MRI RF coils.

Presence of Fat

Many tissue types are composed of a mixture of fat- and water-based tissues. In an imaging voxel containing both fat- and water-based tissues, the resonance frequency of the water-based tissue will change with temperature, whereas the resonance frequency of the fat-based tissue will not, resulting in an underestimation of the total frequency shift. This in turn will lead to an underestimation of the temperature changes.

Susceptibility Change Due to Heating in Fat

Although fat does not have a PRF dependence on temperature, the temperature dependence of the susceptibility coefficient of fat is much higher than that of aqueous tissue.[55,56] Changes in susceptibility due to temperature increase in fat or other tissues can cause distortions in the magnetic field and errors in temperature measurements in adjacent tissues.[57–61] Similar temperature measurement errors can occur when moving an ultrasound transducer or other metallic heat applicator.[62] Peters *et al.* also showed that PRF errors caused by temperature-induced changes in the tissue volumetric magnetic susceptibility can be dependent on the orientation and geometry of the heat applicator and its associated heating pattern.[63]

19.2.5.4 Addressing Limitations and Challenges

Measurement Noise

There is an inherent trade-off among the spatial resolution, temporal resolution, temperature precision, and the FOV that can be imaged. Assuming a standard MRTI pulse sequence for a PRFS measurement, when all other factors are held constant, the image signal-to-noise ratio (SNR) is proportional to the product of voxel volume ($\Delta x\Delta y\Delta z$) and the square root of the number of measurements acquired in *k*-space ($N_xN_yN_z$):

$$\mathrm{SNR} = \frac{\mathrm{SI}}{\sigma(\mathrm{SI})} = M_o e^{-\mathrm{TE}/T_2^*} \frac{1 - e^{-\mathrm{TR}/T1}}{1 - e^{-\mathrm{TR}/T1}\cos\theta} \sin\theta \cdot \Delta x \Delta y \Delta z \sqrt{N_x N_y N_z \Delta t} \tag{19.21}$$

where θ is the flip angle. The standard deviation in the phase measurement is just the inverse of the measurement SNR, so:

$$\frac{\Delta\phi}{\sigma(\Delta\phi)} = \alpha\gamma B_o \mathrm{TE} \cdot \Delta T \cdot M_o e^{-\mathrm{TE}/T_2^*} \frac{1 - e^{-\mathrm{TR}/T1}}{1 - e^{-\mathrm{TR}/T1}\cos\theta} \sin\theta \cdot \Delta x \Delta y \Delta z \sqrt{N_x N_y N_z \Delta t} \tag{19.22}$$

From equations (19.21) and (19.22) it can be seen that increased spatial (i.e., making Δx, Δy, and Δz smaller) and temporal resolution (i.e., shorter Δt) comes at the cost of a decrease in SNR. This will increase the phase standard deviation, resulting in lower precision in the PRF measurements.

For the low-level heating expected with the RF coils in MRI, the spatial distribution of temperature change will likely be very broad. However, when measuring the temperature near implants, it is possible that the SAR distribution may be very local, causing a rapid temporal and spatial variation in the temperature. In the case of a very focal SAR distribution, the accuracy of MRTI will depend on both the spatial resolution and the position of the voxel grid in the MR images.[64,65] The voxel size necessary for accurate temperature measurements depends on the dimensions of the SAR distribution used and should typically be on the order of the dimensions of the energy deposition source.[65] For implants, the accuracy of the temperature maps will likely also depend on the temporal resolution. No detailed studies have been performed evaluating temperature errors as a function of temporal resolution, and the temporal resolution needed depends on how fast the tissue is being heated.

Field Drifts

Field drifts can be corrected by placing reference phantoms that remain at constant temperature or do not change with temperature around the body.[66–69] The phase change observed in the phantoms will then be purely due to the drift in the B_0 field, and can be used to correct the effect of the field drift inside the body. Since fat-based tissues do not have hydrogen bonds and therefore do not experience a temperature-dependent change in resonance frequency, the phase of these tissues can also be used to correct for field drifts and other disturbances such as motion.[30,46,68,70–76] This method requires that both aqueous and lipid-based tissues are present in the FOV, and has recently been evaluated in vivo for breast and prostate applications of MR-guided focused ultrasound.[75] When fat and aqueous tissues are in the same image voxel, spectroscopic methods can be used to calculate absolute temperature based on the separation between the fat and aqueous peaks.[15,77]

A method using the apparent diffusion coefficient (ADC) in conjunction with PRF thermometry has also been described for achieving field drift correction.[78]

Motion

To alleviate the problem of intrascan motion, faster imaging can be applied to 'freeze' the motion. This has successfully been done with both single- and multishot EPI approaches. To alleviate problems from physiological motion such as cardiac and respiratory motion, the MR scans can be gated to the cardiac and/or respiratory cycle so that the data is only sampled during (quasi)-calm parts on the motion cycle.[79,80] However, gating the acquisition will significantly slow down the acquisition speed and leads to lower temporal resolution. Attempting to acquire MR images faster also often results in lower SNR and lower accuracy of the temperature measurements.

Interscan motion occurring from one image to the next can be especially challenging for PRFS imaging since the temperature maps are calculated based on the phase difference between a baseline reference image and the current heating image. One of the largest sources of interscan motion is respiration. Respiratory motion results both in motion of the organs, especially in the upper abdominal region, and can also result in large temperature errors due to susceptibility changes. To alleviate the respiratory motion, many types of MR imaging are performed during breath holds. Breath-hold acquisition is in general not possible when the acquisition time is on the order of minutes. Since the respiratory motion is cyclic, one approach to achieve artifact-free temperature maps is to build up a library of reference images before the start of the treatment, where each image in the library is acquired at a different position in the respiratory cycle.[15,81–84] During the heating, each dynamic image is then compared to all the images in the library, and the one that is the closest match in the respiratory cycle is used as the baseline image (Figure 19.8).

For highly localized heating, such as due to implants, a method called referenceless thermometry can be used to remove the need for baseline images all together.[85,86] Here the reference baseline phase is estimated from each image itself by fitting a polynomial surface to the background phase of unheated regions of the image. The fitted phase is extrapolated onto the heated region and used as reference that is subtracted from the measured phase. The referenceless technique has been validated in many studies, and multiple variations and improvements to the method have been published in recent years.[15,82–84,87–92]

Temperature-dependent Changes in Electrical Properties

Peters *et al.* presented a dual-echo method to correct for the induced error, and this method has since been validated in other studies.[67,93,94]

Presence of Fat

To alleviate problems caused by its presence, the fat signal can either be saturated before the signal readout, or the fat and water signals can be separated using,

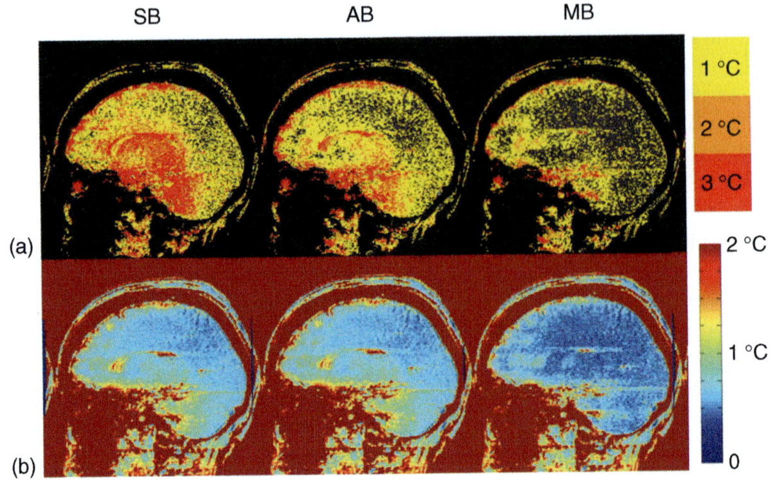

Figure 19.8. Demonstration of multibaseline MRTI. (a) Maximum absolute error of three different temperature reconstruction methods over five images in a volunteer without heating. SB, single baseline subtraction; AB, average of baseline images; and MB, multibaseline reconstruction. (b) Temporal temperature uncertainty over 50 treatment images in the same dataset. SB subtraction results in substantial errors across the brain. Averaging the baseline images (AB) achieves only minor improvements. MB reduces the errors considerably. (Reproduced with permission from Ref. 59. © John Wiley & Sons, 2013)

e.g., multiecho readouts and Dixon fat–water separation techniques. Selective fat saturation will eliminate both the effects of the fat shift relative to water and also any errors due to the non-temperature-dependent phase of fat combined with the temperature-dependent phase of water. It is also possible to sample the data with high enough bandwidth that the fat-water shift becomes negligible; however, using high bandwidth will reduce the imaging SNR and hence also the MRTI precision.

Susceptibility Change Due to Heating in Fat

For the most part, temperature changes in fat due to heating by the imaging RF coils in the MRI scanner should be small because of the low electrical conductivity of fat. If heating does occur, then correction could be performed by establishing the 3D geometry of the fat, measuring the temperature distribution in the fat, and using standard susceptibility equations to predict the resulting distribution of the induced field.[57]

19.3 LOGISTICS OF MRTI MEASUREMENT

In this section, we specifically consider the logistics of using MRTI to measure the heating due to the transmit RF used in MRI. We consider the RF coils to be used in heating, the pulse sequences to be used to create heating, and review some specific experiments that have been performed using MRTI to measure heating due to different RF coil configurations.

In designing MRTI methods, consideration must be given to the rate and distribution of heating as there is a general trade-off among spatial, temporal, and temperature resolution and coverage. When motion is not a consideration, MRTI can be applied using a 3D acquisition with large FOV. For most RF-induced heating from MRI coils, the temperature variation is spatially slowly varying, and low spatial resolution (i.e., large imaging voxels) can be used to enable large FOV and volumetric acquisitions. If needed, the acquisition can be sped up with k-space undersampling in conjunction with, e.g., parallel image- or constrained-reconstruction methods.[95]

19.3.1 Whole Body Transmit Coils vs Local Transmit Coils and Coil Arrays

Both large volume whole-body transmit coils and small volume local transmit coils and coil arrays are used in MRI and should be evaluated for SAR distributions.

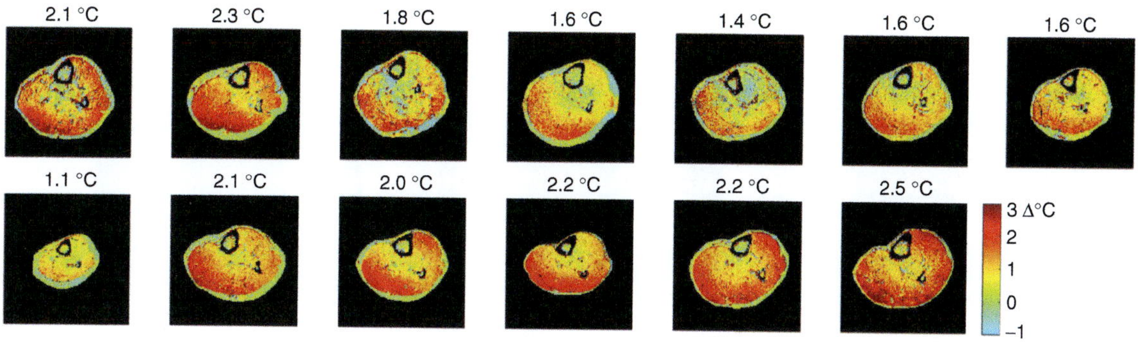

Figure 19.9. Temperature images obtained from 13 volunteers after 16 min of RF heating, where temperature measurements were obtained with a 2D PRFS sequence, and heating was performed by interleaving a large tip angle RF pulse during temperature measurements. The values above the maps portray the 90th percentile (only 10% of the values are higher) of the temperature distribution. (Reproduced with permission from Ref. 98. © John Wiley & Sons, 2016)

Large volume transmit RF coils expose a much larger volume to the RF field and require a corresponding large imaging volume for SAR distribution determination. In fact, it is possible that the volume exposed to the RF field may be larger than the homogeneous B_0 imaging volume of the MRI scanner, in which case it is not technically possible to use MRI to measure the full volume experiencing the temperature increase. The trade-offs among spatial and temporal resolution, FOV, and temperature measurement precision as well as motions make it difficult to perform MRTI and calculate SAR over the entire volume. Instead, it is likely that measurements will be made in subsets of the full volume, with a need to repeat to obtain SAR over the full volume.

Local transmit coils and coil arrays generally have very limited regions of heating, making it easier to obtain direct MRTI measurements of SAR over the entire heated volume. Several studies have been performed to use MRTI to measure SAR in local transmit coils.[18,95–99]

19.3.2 Pulse Sequence to Use – MRTI Before and After Heating vs During Heating

MRTI sequences are typically GRE-based sequences that do not cause significant heating due to the low flip-angles used. For that reason, several of the studies using MRTI to investigate SAR induced by MRI imaging coils have been performed using TSE or similar sequences to cause measurable heating, and then GRE-based MRTI is applied before and after the heating sequence.[18,95–97] More recently, Simonis *et al.* added a high SAR off-resonance pulse to an MRTI sequence, demonstrating the ability to heat the tissue and measure the heating simultaneously with the same sequence[98,99] (Figure 19.9).

19.3.3 Other MRTI Methods Used for SAR Determination

There are a number of other interesting techniques that have been used for SAR measurements, including the use of the temperature dependence of the water diffusion coefficient to monitor temperature increases for RF-induced hyperthermia[100] and recently for measuring SAR induced from the body transmit coil in body equivalent phantoms.[101] More recently, there have been studies using sodium or other agents with increased temperature sensitivity.[102–106] Although these have increased temperature sensitivity, the concentration appears to remain low, resulting in a low net measurement precision. Further, these methods would not be possible in humans, in vivo. Examples of studies include the phantom studies at 1.5, 3, and 7 T, using a FSE sequence with increased RF amplitude to heat for 300 s, performed by Cline *et al.*[4] The PRF method was then used to measure the phase distribution after the heating, and temperature was determined by comparing the phase change from a measurement made before the FSE sequence. For the spherical phantoms studied, the measured temperature profiles matched qualitatively well with their theoretical predictions. In a proof of concept, Oh *et al.* demonstrated heating in a phantom and a human

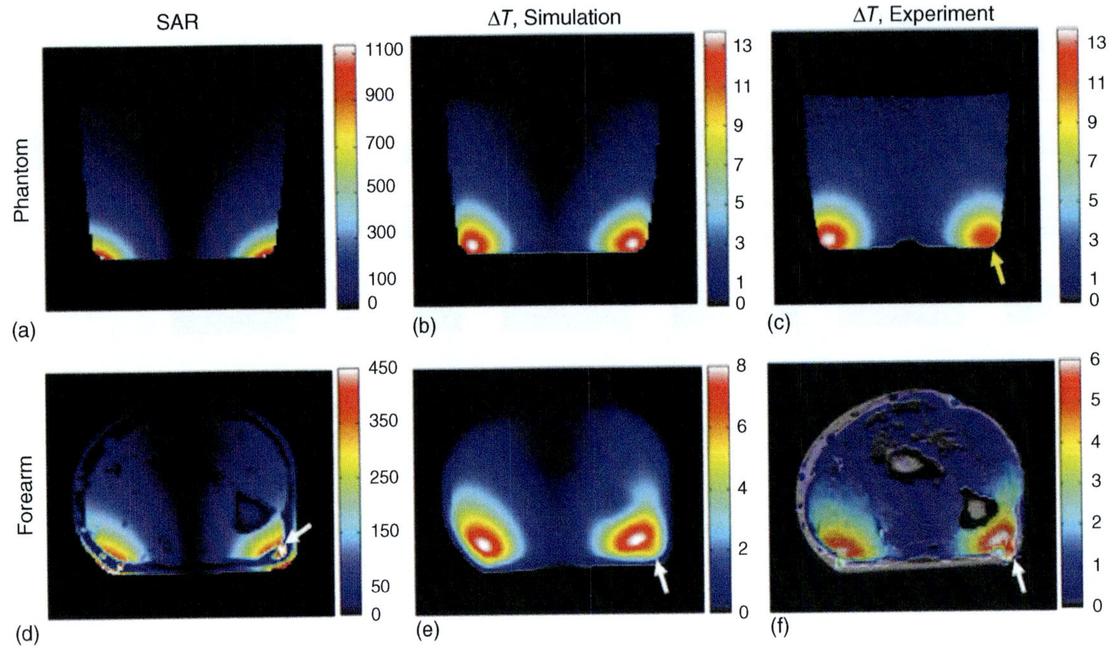

Figure 19.10. Simulated unaveraged SAR ($W\,kg^{-1}$) map (a, d), simulated temperature increase (°C) (b, e), and experimentally measured PRF temperature increase (°C) (c, f) for an agar-gel phantom (a–c) and an in vivo forearm (d–f). Yellow arrow indicates region of highest disagreement between experiment and simulation in phantom. White arrow indicates blood vessel having high SAR but only moderate temperature increase in forearm. The plane shown passes through the center of the coil and is transverse to the long axis of the phantom or forearm. (Reproduced with permission from Ref. 96. © John Wiley & Sons, 2014)

forearm using an adjacent (nonimaging) circular loop coil and simulating the heating and comparing with a basic PRF MRTI measurement.[96] Good agreement was observed between the simulated and measured heating in both the cases (Figure 19.10).

19.3.4 Monitoring RF-induced Heating Around Metal Implants

We briefly discuss issues involved in using MRI to monitor the heating that occurs in tissues that are close to metal implants and conductive wires (such as from pacemakers, electrodes, or catheters). Issues that must be dealt with are the effects of magnetic susceptibility and the relatively rapid heating that may occur because of the increased SAR around the implant.

Because metals tend to have magnetic susceptibilities that differ from water, large phase variations due to large magnetic field variations are observed, causing substantial signal loss next to the implant. Further, the metal itself can locally focus the transmit RF field, causing substantial increase in local SAR, resulting in faster heating that is more comparable to local heat deposition methods such as lasers and focused ultrasound. Thus, MRTI must deal with both the faster heating where there is extensive experience as well as the signal loss that occurs near the implant.

In regions where adequate signal can be observed, the temperature measurement can be made with corrections for field fluctuations and field drift. Detti *et al.* measured the temperature increase around metal wires using the signal intensity from T_1w images from a True FISP sequence.[107] The heating was induced by the imaging RF pulses, and increasing the flip angle increased the observed heating. Gensler *et al.* used an IR snapshot FLASH sequence where the added off-resonant inversion pulses were used to cause heating around metal wires.[108] With image acceleration and sliding-window reconstruction, temperature maps could be reconstructed every 7.6 s. Weber *et al.* described a two-dimensional inversion-recovery – prepared multispectral imaging pulse sequence for artifact reduced T_1 mapping near metal.[109,110] Finally, Zhang *et al.* demonstrated a dual-echo GRE sequence for PRF MRTI near metal implants. The first echo was either under- or over-refocused in the slice encoding dimension to recover signal and temperature precision near the metal.[111] The second echo was fully refocused to obtain image signal everywhere else in the slice, and a penalized maximum likelihood algorithm was used to combine the information from the two echoes into a single temperature map. Although these experiments provide encouraging results, more work is needed to develop methods that can assess heating near implants.

19.4 CONCLUSION

This chapter considers the problem of using MRTI to assess the heating caused by the transmit RF field in MRI scanners and has reviewed the theoretical and practical considerations for the most commonly used approaches of performing MRTI. Currently, the PRFS technique is the most commonly used MRTI method and is also likely the most suitable method to monitor heating induced from MRI coils. The specific pulse sequence and type of postprocessing needed will depend on the size of the coil (body vs local) and the anatomy being imaged. The inherent tradeoffs in spatial and temporal resolution, FOV, and measurement accuracy will further impose constraints on the selected methods.

On the basis of the MRTI studies from fields such as hyperthermia, in which applicators are used to induce slowly varying (temporally and spatially) temperature increases over potentially large FOVs, and on the other preliminary studies discussed here, it is likely that MRTI can achieve accurate assessment of the power deposition and resulting temperature increase caused by the RF coils used in MRI. Such measurements will require imaging over large volumes to capture all heating induced within the RF coil's sensitivity volume and compensation for long-term field drift and body motions. With proper attention to these details, volumetric temperature measurements of heating due to MRI coils are likely to be more accurate than temperature estimates obtained with simulations and will provide substantially more information than can be achieved with invasive probe measurements.

DISCLAIMER

The subject matter, content, and views presented do not represent the views of the Department of Health and Human Services (HHS), US Food and Drug Administration (FDA), and/or the United States.

RELATED ARTICLES IN EMAGRES

Jolesz, Ferenc A.: The Development of Interventional MRI

Bioeffects and Safety of Radiofrequency Electromagnetic Fields

Hydrogen Bonding

Thermometry

Therapy Monitoring by MRI

Thermal Therapies in the Body Monitored by MRI

Safety Considerations in MRI

Temperature Monitoring Using Chemical Shift

Radiofrequency Fields: Interactions, Biological Effects, and Safety Issues

Radiofrequency Gradient Pulses

Radiofrequency Pulses: Response of Nuclear Spins

Radiofrequency Systems and Coils for MRI and MRS

Temperature Measurement In Vivo Using NMR

Safety Regulation in MR

RF Device Safety and Compatibility

Radiofrequency Fields and SAR for Transverse Electromagnetic (TEM) Surface Coils

Radiofrequency Fields and SAR for Bird Cage Coils

Radiofrequency Heating Models and Measurements

Safety and Sensory Aspects of Main and Gradient Fields in MRI

MRI for Noninvasive Thermometry

REFERENCES

1. D. Shrivastava, T. Hanson, J. Kulesa, L. DelaBarre, P. Iaizzo, and J. T. Vaughan, *Magn. Reson. Med.*, 2009, **62**, 888 PMCID: PMC2782895.
2. D. Shrivastava, L. Utecht, J. Tian, J. Hughes, and J. T. Vaughan, *Magn. Reson. Med.*, 2014, **72**, 1141 PMCID: PMC4041852.
3. E. Balidemaj, C. A. van den Berg, A. L. van Lier, A. J. Nederveen, L. J. Stalpers, H. Crezee, and R. F. Remis, *Med. Biol. Eng. Comput.*, 2017, **55**, 225 PMCID: PMC5272903.
4. H. Cline, R. Mallozzi, Z. Li, G. McKinnon, and W. Barber, *Magn. Reson. Med.*, 2004, **51**, 1129.
5. International Commission on Non-Ionizing Radiation Protection, *Health Phys.*, 1998, **74**, 494.
6. IEC, *Medical Electrical Equipment: Part 2–33. Particular Requirements for the Safety of Magnetic Resonance Equipment for Medical Diagnosis*, 2008.
7. Administration (FDA), *Usfad. Staff Criteria for Significant Risk Investigations of Magnetic Rresonance Diagnostic Devices*, 2003.
8. O. Kraff, A. K. Bitz, P. Dammann, S. C. Ladd, M. E. Ladd, and H. H. Quick, *Med. Phys.*, 2010, **37**, 6368.
9. M. Murbach, E. Neufeld, E. Cabot, E. Zastrow, J. Corcoles, W. Kainz, and N. Kuster, *Magn. Reson. Med.*, 2016, **76**, 986.
10. M. Murbach, E. Neufeld, M. Capstick, W. Kainz, D. O. Brunner, T. Samaras, K. P. Pruessmann, and N. Kuster, *Magn. Reson. Med.*, 2014, **71**, 421.
11. M. Murbach, E. Neufeld, W. Kainz, K. P. Pruessmann, and N. Kuster, *Magn. Reson. Med.*, 2014, **71**, 839.
12. D. L. Parker, V. Smith, P. Sheldon, L. E. Crooks, and L. Fussell, *Med. Phys.*, 1983, **10**, 321.
13. Y. Ishihara, A. Calderon, H. Watanabe, K. Okamoto, Y. Suzuki, K. Kuroda, and Y. Suzuki, *Magn. Reson. Med.*, 1995, **34**, 814.
14. B. Quesson, J. A. de Zwart, and C. T. Moonen, *J. Magn. Reson. Imaging*, 2000, **12**, 525.
15. V. Rieke and P. K. Butts, *J. Magn. Reson. Imaging*, 2008, **27**, 376.
16. H. Pennes, *Appl. Physiol.*, 1948, **1**, 93.
17. D. Shrivastava, Theory and Applications of Heat Transfer in Humans, Wiley: Hoboken, NJ, 2018.
18. L. Alon, C. M. Deniz, G. Carluccio, R. Brown, D. K. Sodickson, and C. M. Collins, *Concepts Magn. Reson. B Magn. Reson. Eng.*, 2016, **46**, 8 PMCID: PMC4847547.
19. P. L. Davis, C. Shang, L. Talagala, and A. W. Pasculle, *IEEE Trans. Biomed. Eng.*, 1993, **40**, 1324.
20. J. W. Hand, Y. Li, and J. V. Hajnal, *Phys. Med. Biol.*, 2010, **55**, 913.
21. D. Simunic, P. Wach, W. Renhart, and R. Stollberger, *IEEE Trans. Biomed. Eng.*, 1996, **43**, 88.
22. R. B. Roemer, A. M. Fletcher, and T. C. Cetas, *Int. J. Radiat. Oncol. Biol. Phys.*, 1985, **11**, 1539.
23. B. Denis de Senneville, B. Quesson, and C. T. Moonen, *Int. J. Hyperthermia*, 2005, **21**, 515.
24. I. Rivens, A. Shaw, J. Civale, and H. Morris, *Int. J. Hyperthermia*, 2007, **23**, 121.
25. K. Kuroda, *J. Magn. Reson. Imaging*, 2017, **47**, 316.
26. N. McDannold, *Int. J. Hyperthermia*, 2005, **21**, 533.
27. A. B. Wolbarst, P. Capasso, and A. R. Wyant, Medical Imaging: Essentials for Physicians, John Wiley & Sons: Hoboken, NJ, 2013.
28. D. L. Parker, *IEEE Trans. Biomed. Eng.*, 1984, **31**, 161.
29. P. A. Bottomley, T. H. Foster, R. E. Argersinger, and L. M. Pfeifer, *Med. Phys.*, 1984, **11**, 425.
30. J. Guo, S. E. Kim, E. K. Jeong, D. L. Parker, L. Zhang, and R. Roemer, In *Proc ISMRM, Kyoto, Japan*, 2004, 2587.
31. M. Peller, H. M. Reinl, A. Weigel, M. Meininger, R. D. Issels, and M. Reiser, *Magn. Reson. Med.*, 2002, **47**, 1194.
32. S. C. Deoni, B. K. Rutt, and T. M. Peters, *Magn. Reson. Med.*, 2003, **49**, 515.
33. S. C. Deoni, T. M. Peters, and B. K. Rutt, *Magn. Reson. Med.*, 2004, **51**, 194.
34. M. C. Schabel and G. R. Morrell, *Phys. Med. Biol.*, 2009, **54**, N1.
35. I. R. Young, J. W. Hand, A. Oatridge, and M. V. Prior, *Magn. Reson. Med.*, 1994, **32**, 358.
36. P. Baron, R. Deckers, F. M. Knuttel, and L. W. Bartels, *NMR Biomed.*, 2015, **28**, 1463.
37. P. Baron, M. Ries, R. Deckers, M. de Greef, J. Tanttu, M. Kohler, M. A. Viergever, C. T. Moonen, and L. W. Bartels, *Magn. Reson. Med.*, 2014, **72**, 1057.

38. K. Kuroda, T. Iwabuchi, M. Obara, M. Honda, K. Saito, and Y. Imai, *Magn. Reson. Med.*, 2011, **10**, 177.

39. E. Ozhinsky, M. P. Kohi, P. Ghanouni, and V. Rieke, *J. Ther. Ultrasound*, 2015, **3**, 15 PMCID: PMC4567827.

40. J. Chen, B. L. Daniel, and K. B. Pauly, *J. Magn. Reson. Imaging*, 2006, **23**, 430.

41. D. Le Bihan, J. Delannoy, and R. L. Levin, *Radiology*, 1989, **171**, 853.

42. J. Delannoy, C. N. Chen, R. Turner, R. L. Levin, and D. Le Bihan, *Magn. Reson. Med.*, 1991, **19**, 333.

43. K. A. Il'yasov and J. Hennig, *J. Magn. Reson. Imag. JMRI*, 1998, **8**, 1296.

44. L. R. Kozak, M. Bango, M. Szabo, G. Rudas, Z. Vidnyanszky, and Z. Nagy, *Acta Paediatr.*, 2010, **99**, 237 PMCID: 2816360.

45. K. Sakai, K. Yamada, S. Mori, N. Sugimoto, and T. Nishimura, *NMR Biomed.*, 2011, **24**, 1063.

46. K. Sumida, N. Sato, M. Ota, K. Sakai, Y. Nippashi, D. Sone, K. Yokoyama, K. Ito, N. Maikusa, E. Imabayashi, H. Matsuda, K. Yamada, M. Murata, A. Kunimatsu, and K. Ohtomo, *Brain Behav.*, 2015, **5**, e00340 PMCID: PMC4467774.

47. M. E. Moseley, Y. Cohen, J. Mintorovitch, L. Chileuitt, H. Shimizu, J. Kucharczyk, M. F. Wendland, and P. R. Weinstein, *Magn. Reson. Med.*, 1990, **14**, 330.

48. P. J. Basser, J. Mattiello, and D. LeBihan, *Biophys. J.*, 1994, **66**, 259 PMCID: PMC1275686.

49. P. van Gelderen, M. H. de Vleeschouwer, D. DesPres, J. Pekar, P. C. van Zijl, and C. T. Moonen, *Magn. Reson. Med.*, 1994, **31**, 154.

50. A. R. Bleier, F. A. Jolesz, M. S. Cohen, R. M. Weisskoff, J. J. Dalcanton, N. Higuchi, D. A. Feinberg, B. R. Rosen, R. C. McKinstry, and S. G. Hushek, *Magn. Reson. Med.*, 1991, **21**, 132.

51. D. Morvan, A. Leroy-Willig, A. Malgouyres, C. A. Cuenod, P. Jehenson, and A. Syrota, *Magn. Reson. Med.*, 1993, **29**, 371.

52. J. C. Hindman, *J. Chem. Phys.*, 1966, **44**, 4582.

53. R. D. Peters, R. S. Hinks, and R. M. Henkelman, *Magn. Reson. Med.*, 1998, **40**, 454.

54. R. D. Peters and R. M. Henkelman, *Magn. Reson. Med.*, 2000, **43**, 62.

55. J. De Poorter, *Magn. Reson. Med.*, 1995, **34**, 359.

56. I. R. Young, J. V. Hajnal, I. G. Roberts, J. X. Ling, R. J. Hill-Cottingham, A. Oatridge, and J. A. Wilson, *Magn. Reson. Med.*, 1996, **36**, 366.

57. P. Baron, R. Deckers, M. de Greef, L. G. Merckel, C. J. Bakker, J. G. Bouwman, R. L. Bleys, M. A. van den Bosch, and L. W. Bartels, *Magn. Reson. Med.*, 2014, **72**, 1580.

58. A. Boss, H. Graf, B. Muller-Bierl, S. Clasen, D. Schmidt, P. L. Pereira, and F. Schick, *J. Magn. Reson. Imag. JMRI*, 2005, **22**, 813.

59. V. Rieke, R. Instrella, J. Rosenberg, W. Grissom, B. Werner, E. Martin, and K. B. Pauly, *J. Magn. Reson. Imag. JMRI*, 2013, **38**, 1462 PMCID: PMC3775924.

60. S. M. Sprinkhuizen, M. K. Konings, M. J. van der Bom, M. A. Viergever, C. J. Bakker, and L. W. Bartels, *Magn. Reson. Med.*, 2010, **64**, 1360.

61. M. N. Streicher, A. Schafer, E. Reimer, B. Dhital, R. Trampel, D. Ivanov, and R. Turner, *MAGMA*, 2012, **25**, 41.

62. A. G. Webb, T. Neuberger, E. J. Park, and N. Smith, *IEEE Trans. Ultrason. Ferroelectr. Freq. Control*, 2009, **56**, 1145.

63. R. D. Peters, R. S. Hinks, and R. M. Henkelman, *Magn. Reson. Med.*, 1999, **41**, 909.

64. L. J. Pisani, A. B. Ross, C. J. Diederich, W. H. Nau, F. G. Sommer, G. H. Glover, and K. Butts, *J. Magn. Reson. Imaging*, 2005, **22**, 109.

65. N. Todd, U. Vyas, J. de Bever, A. Payne, and D. L. Parker, *Magn. Reson. Med.*, 2011, **65**, 515 PMCID: 3015010.

66. D. L. Carter, J. R. MacFall, S. T. Clegg, X. Wan, D. M. Prescott, H. C. Charles, and T. V. Samulski, *Int. J. Radiat. Oncol. Biol. Phys.*, 1998, **40**, 815.

67. T. Dadakova, J. Gellermann, O. Voigt, J. G. Korvink, J. M. Pavlina, J. Hennig, and M. Bock, *MAGMA*, 2015, **28**, 305.

68. W. Wlodarczyk, R. Boroschewski, M. Hentschel, P. Wust, G. Monich, and R. Felix, *J. Magn. Reson. Imaging*, 1998, **8**, 165.

69. C. Wyatt, B. Soher, P. Maccarini, H. C. Charles, P. Stauffer, and J. Macfall, *Int. J. Hyperthermia*, 2009, **25**, 422 PMCID: PMC2946346.

70. J. Gellermann, W. Wlodarczyk, B. Hildebrandt, H. Ganter, A. Nicolau, B. Rau, W. Tilly, H. Fahling, J. Nadobny, R. Felix, and P. Wust, *Cancer Res.*, 2005, **65**, 5872.

71. A. V. Shmatukha, P. R. Harvey, and C. J. Bakker, *J. Magn. Reson. Imag. JMRI*, 2007, **25**, 579.

72. J. Gellermann, M. Weihrauch, C. H. Cho, W. Wlodarczyk, H. Fahling, R. Felix, V. Budach, M. Weiser, J. Nadobny, and P. Wust, *Med. Phys.*, 2006, **33**, 3912.

73. J. Gellermann, B. Hildebrandt, R. Issels, H. Ganter, W. Wlodarczyk, V. Budach, R. Felix, P. U. Tunn, P. Reichardt, and P. Wust, *Cancer*, 2006, **107**, 1373.

74. L. W. Hofstetter, D. T. B. Yeo, W. T. Dixon, L. Marinelli, and T. K. Foo, *Magn. Reson. Imaging*, 2018, **49**, 86.

75. L. W. Hofstetter, D. T. Yeo, W. T. Dixon, J. G. Kempf, C. E. Davis, and T. K. Foo, *J. Magn. Reson. Imaging*, 2012, **36**, 722.

76. P. Baron, R. Deckers, J. G. Bouwman, C. J. Bakker, M. de Greef, M. A. Viergever, C. T. Moonen, and L. W. Bartels, *Magn. Reson. Med.*, 2016, **75**, 1187.

77. K. Kuroda, *Int. J. Hyperthermia*, 2005, **21**, 547.

78. S. K. Das, J. Macfall, R. McCauley, O. Craciunescu, M. W. Dewhirst, and T. V. Samulski, *Int. J. Hyperthermia*, 2005, **21**, 657.

79. B. D. de Senneville, S. Roujol, P. Jais, C. T. Moonen, G. Herigault, and B. Quesson, *NMR Biomed.*, 2012, **25**, 556.

80. V. Auboiroux, L. Petrusca, M. Viallon, A. Muller, S. Terraz, R. Breguet, X. Montet, C. D. Becker, and R. Salomir, *Biomed. Res. Int.*, 2014, **2014**, 421726 PMCID: PMC3925565.

81. S. Hey, G. Maclair, B. D. de Senneville, M. Lepetit-Coiffe, Y. Berber, M. O. Kohler, B. Quesson, C. T. Moonen, and M. Ries, *Magn. Reson. Med.*, 2009, **61**, 1494.

82. W. A. Grissom, V. Rieke, A. B. Holbrook, Y. Medan, M. Lustig, J. Santos, M. V. McConnell, and K. B. Pauly, *Med. Phys.*, 2010, **37**, 5014 PMCID: PMC2945742.

83. B. D. de Senneville, S. Roujol, C. Moonen, and M. Ries, *Magn. Reson. Med.*, 2010, **64**, 1373.

84. S. Roujol, M. Ries, B. Quesson, and C. Moonen, *Magn. Reson. Med.*, 2010, **63**, 1080.

85. V. Rieke, K. K. Vigen, G. Sommer, B. L. Daniel, J. M. Pauly, and K. Butts, *Magn. Reson. Med.*, 2004, **51**, 1223.

86. K. Kuroda, D. Kokuryo, E. Kumamoto, K. Suzuki, Y. Matsuoka, and B. Keserci, *Magn. Reson. Med.*, 2006, **56**, 835.

87. V. Rieke, A. M. Kinsey, A. B. Ross, W. H. Nau, C. J. Diederich, G. Sommer, and K. B. Pauly, *IEEE Trans. Med. Imaging*, 2007, **26**, 813 PMCID: PMC2780365.

88. W. A. Grissom, M. Lustig, A. B. Holbrook, V. Rieke, J. M. Pauly, and K. Butts-Pauly, *Magn. Reson. Med.*, 2010, **64**, 1068 PMCID: PMC3155729.

89. A. B. Holbrook, J. M. Santos, E. Kaye, V. Rieke, and K. B. Pauly, *Magn. Reson. Med.*, 2010, **63**, 365 PMCID: PMC3212435.

90. N. McDannold, C. Tempany, F. Jolesz, and K. Hynynen, *J. Magn. Reson. Imaging*, 2008, **28**, 1026 PMCID: PMC2574694.

91. R. Salomir, M. Viallon, A. Kickhefel, J. Roland, D. R. Morel, L. Petrusca, V. Auboiroux, T. Goget, S. Terraz, C. D. Becker, and P. Gross, *IEEE Trans. Med. Imaging*, 2012, **31**, 287.

92. C. Zou, H. Shen, M. He, C. Tie, Y. C. Chung, and X. Liu, *Phys. Med. Biol.*, 2013, **58**, 5735.

93. J. Gellermann, W. Wlodarczyk, A. Feussner, H. Fahling, J. Nadobny, B. Hildebrandt, R. Felix, and P. Wust, *Int. J. Hyperthermia*, 2005, **21**, 497.

94. R. D. Peters, E. Chan, J. Trachtenberg, S. Jothy, L. Kapusta, W. Kucharczyk, and R. M. Henkelman, *Magn. Reson. Med.*, 2000, **44**, 873.

95. Z. Cao, S. Oh, R. Otazo, C. T. Sica, M. A. Griswold, and C. M. Collins, *Magn. Reson. Med.*, 2015, **73**, 1420 PMCID: PMC4205230.

96. S. Oh, Y. C. Ryu, G. Carluccio, C. T. Sica, and C. M. Collins, *Magn. Reson. Med.*, 2014, **71**, 1923 PMCID: PMC3842374.

97. S. Oh, A. G. Webb, T. Neuberger, B. Park, and C. M. Collins, *Magn. Reson. Med.*, 2010, **63**, 218 PMCID: PMC2836721.

98. F. F. Simonis, E. T. Petersen, J. J. Lagendijk, and C. A. van den Berg, *Magn. Reson. Med.*, 2016, **75**, 1743.

99. F. F. Simonis, A. J. Raaijmakers, J. J. Lagendijk, and C. A. van den Berg, *Magn. Reson. Med.*, 2017, **77**, 1691.

100. J. Delannoy, D. LeBihan, D. I. Hoult, and R. L. Levin, *Med. Phys.*, 1990, **17**, 855.

101. Y. Seo and Z. J. Wang, *J. Appl. Clin. Med. Phys.*, 2017, **18**, 224.

102. S. Dharmadhikari, J. R. James, J. Nyenhuis, and N. Bansal, *Magn. Reson. Med.*, 2016, **75**, 2121.

103. N. N. Graedel, J. R. Polimeni, B. Guerin, B. Gagoski, and L. L. Wald, *Magn. Reson. Med.*, 2015, **73**, 442 PMCID: PMC4136997.

104. E. M. Shapiro, A. Borthakur, N. Bansal, J. S. Leigh, and R. Reddy, *J. Magn. Reson.*, 2000, **143**, 213.

105. E. M. Shapiro, A. Borthakur, and R. Reddy, *MAGMA*, 2000, **10**, 114.

106. E. M. Shapiro, A. Borthakur, M. J. Shapiro, R. Reddy, and J. S. Leigh, *Magn. Reson. Med.*, 2002, **47**, 492 PMCID: PMC2855824.

107. V. Detti, D. Grenier, E. Perrin, and O. Beuf, *Magn. Reson. Med.*, 2011, **66**, 448.

108. D. Gensler, F. Fidler, P. Ehses, M. Warmuth, T. Reiter, M. During, O. Ritter, M. E. Ladd, H. H. Quick, P. M. Jakob, W. R. Bauer, and P. Nordbeck, *Magn. Reson. Med.*, 2012, **68**, 1593.

109. H. Weber, P. Ghanouni, A. Pascal-Tenorio, K. B. Pauly, and B. A. Hargreaves, *Magn. Reson. Med.*, 2018, **80**, 259 PMCID: PMC5876098.

110. H. Weber, V. Taviani, D. Yoon, P. Ghanouni, K. B. Pauly, and B. A. Hargreaves, *Magn. Reson. Med.*, 2017, **77**, 1162 PMCID: PMC5532173.

111. Y. Zhang, M. E. Poorman, and W. A. Grissom, *Magn. Reson. Med.*, 2017, **78**, 2299 PMCID: PMC5552453.

Chapter 20
Heating of RF Coil

Joseph Murphy-Boesch
National Institutes of Health, NINDS, Bethesda, MD, USA

Safety and Biological Effects in MRI.
Edited by Devashish Shrivastava and J. Thomas Vaughan

ISBN: 978-1-118-82130-5
Also published in eMagRes (online edition)
DOI 10.1002/9781119441649.emrstm1585

20.1 SUMMARY

- Radio frequency (RF) transmit fields can cause heating of coil parts, affecting safety of coils and coil reliability.
- Careful design of RF blocking circuits can prevent the induction of excessive currents from transmit B_1 fields and can reduce the heating of parts near patient surfaces.
- High-impedance cable baluns installed on connecting cables provide protection from the effects of strong electric fields of the body transmit coil.
- Supply currents from DC control lines and power connections can contribute to over-all heating of the coil former, reducing the marginal allowable temperature rise from other sources of heating.

20.2 INTRODUCTION

High-field (1.5 and 3 T) MRI systems are generally constructed with a body transmit coil separate from the receive coil or receive coil array positioned near the patient. The RF fields of the transmit body coil are of primary concern for local heating and core heating of tissues. But, these same fields also induce currents and heating of the electronic parts of receive arrays, which can be destructive and can create excessive heating of coil surfaces. In this presentation, the heating of coil parts from the transmit magnetic (B_1) and the

This chapter contains material presented at the 'ISMRM Workshop on Ensuring RF Safety in MRI: Current Practices & Future Directions,' held on 28 Sept.–1 Oct. 2017 in McLean, VA, USA.

transmit electric fields of standard body coils are examined as it affects patient safety and coil reliability. The goal of the discussion is to protect the coil and to operate within the limits of the regulatory standards for surface heating for medical equipment as prescribed by the IEC[1,2] and the Food and Drug Administration (FDA). In industry, coil safety tests associated with parts heating are among a group of tests normally performed on clinical coils to verify safety and reliability as they are being developed. Preliminary to testing, a stress analysis of a coil circuit can reveal the magnitude of voltage stress from the body coil and the blocking impedances that would be required to protect a coil element from large induced currents. Verification tests that reveal elevated temperatures and component heating are described, and methods for reducing coil heating are reviewed. Separate from the transmit fields, DC power is required to power preamplifiers and PIN diode control lines. PIN diodes are found in the RF blocking circuits of receive arrays, and blocking circuits are the primary means of preventing high currents in the receive loops. For large arrays, the number of resistive DC connections multiply, contributing to an overall temperature rise of a coil housing. Current sharing and use of lower power transistors and preamplifiers can help reduce this dissipation. Techniques for reducing coil heating continue to evolve and benefit from new technology as it becomes available, and some promising new approaches are reviewed in a later section. While many of the aspects of heating in transmit arrays are similar, a review of the specific problems associated with transmit arrays is not covered here and is reviewed elsewhere.

20.3 TRANSMIT BODY COILS

As described above, most heating of receive coils is derived from the RF magnetic and electric fields generated by a high-field body coil. A snap-shot of the typical field patterns for a birdcage-type body coil is shown in Figure 20.1. When the coil is driven in circularly polarized (CP) mode, this snap-shot pattern of the impressed field is roughly maintained as it rotates about the axis of the body coil. Within the tissue, however, this impressed field can be strongly modified by the dielectric and conductive properties of the tissue. Both the RF electric and magnetic fields of the body coil induce heating. Electric fields of the body coil couple to coil conductors and connecting cables and induce RF currents. RF magnetic or B_1 fields couple to the loops of an array and induce large RF voltages or 'emfs' (for electromotive force). The emfs in receive loops can be quite large and require blocking circuits with high impedances to prevent large currents from circulating in them. The secondary B_1 flux from these currents can concentrate in tissues near the coil, causing excessive tissue heating.

The body coils for 1.5 and 3 T systems are located inside the gradients and are enclosed within an RF shield

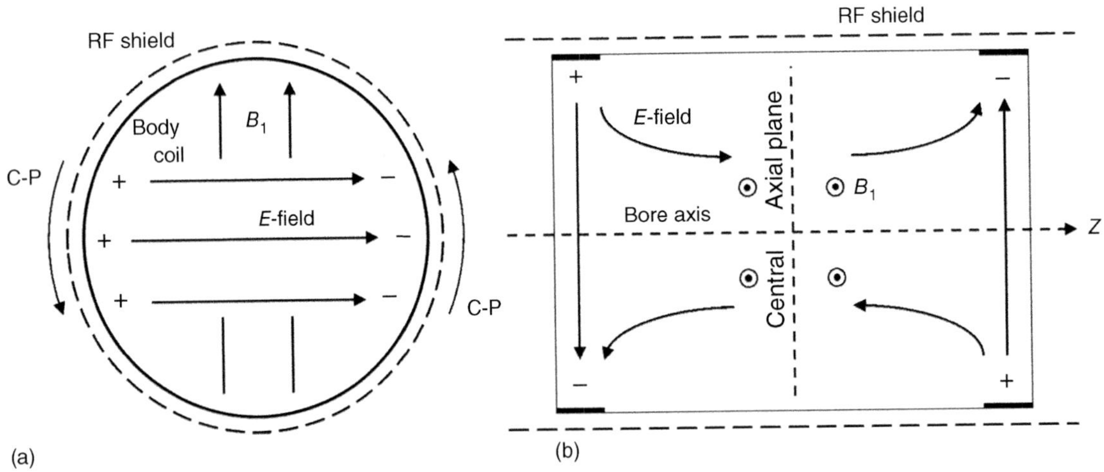

Figure 20.1. In (a), the electric field of the body coil is illustrated in the axial plane of the forward end ring. The B_1 field in the interior of the coil is transverse to this electric field. In (b), the ***E***-fields of the body coil are illustrated in a Coronal cross-section. A virtual ground is developed along the axis of the bore and in the central axial plane of the coil

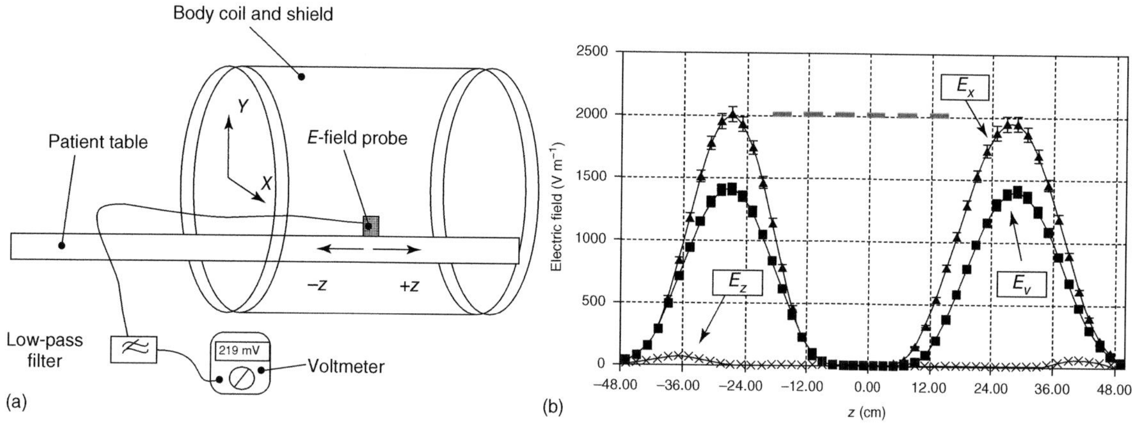

Figure 20.2. In (a), electric field measurements were plotted in the z-direction for one linear mode of a 1.5 T high-pass body coil. In (b), maximum $\boldsymbol{E}$-fields occur at the level of the coil end rings. At maximum B_1 strength, fields in transverse directions (x, y) reach maxima of approximately 20 V cm^{-1}. (Guclu.[3] Reproduced with permission of John Wiley & Sons)

to provide electrical isolation from the gradient. The RF shield has the effect of terminating most of the externally directed electric fields (***E***-fields) from the body coil conductors. Still, substantial ***E***-fields are set up in the interior of the body coil, which induce RF currents in the conductors and components of the receive coil. In Figure 20.2, the electric fields of a 1.5 T high-pass birdcage were measured along the axis of the bore at the level of the patient table.[3] At maximum power, strong electric fields in the x- and y-directions could be measured in the planes of each end ring of the coil, reaching a maximum of about 20 V cm^{-1}. Because the length of the transmit coil is approximately equal to its diameter and because the potentials on the end rings are the same, z-directed ***E***-fields of similar magnitude can found running parallel to the struts of the birdcage.

To verify and quantify the ***E***-field distributions in a high-field (1.5 T) body coil, measurements of ***E***-field intensity and temperature were performed by Nordbeck *et al.*[4] on the ASTM F2182-02a standard head/torso phantom.[5] ***E***-fields were measured by a dipole-type ***E***-field probe that was inserted and moved within the phantom solution. Figure 20.3(a) shows the result for the x-directed ***E***-field of a 1.5 T body coil, which shows the strong fields in the end-ring planes of the body coil. Figure 20.3(b) is a plot of the magnitude of the total ***E***-field of the coil, and it shows that the fields parallel to the struts of the birdcage are oppositely directed, resulting in the virtual ground along the z-axis of the coil. The strength of these electric fields is roughly proportional to the inductance of the struts of the birdcage, and they are generally constructed with wide conductors to lower their inductance. This inductance becomes even more important at 3 T because for the same conductor layout, the reactance of the struts is doubled, and the voltage across them is doubled. To reduce strut inductance, newer designs, such as the one shown in Figure 20.4 by Weyers *et al.*[6] double the number of struts from 16 to 32. ***E***-fields are further reduced by increasing the diameter of the two end rings and placing them closer to the RF shield. As can be seen in plot for B_1, increasing the number of struts provides about a 20% increase in B_1 for an average size patient (75 kg).

In summary, the electric fields of a circularly polarized body coil of birdcage design are strongest near the conductors of the coil. Voltage potentials are highest on the end rings of the coil, and they set up strong ***E***-fields in the planes of the end rings and along the struts of the coil that connect to the end rings. Because the potentials of the birdcage are quadrupolar in nature, a virtual ground is established along the z-axis of the coil. A virtual ground is also established in the central axial plane of the body coil, although z-directed ***E***-fields are quite large along walls of the bore. As a consequence, if a subject is positioned close to the axis of the bore, the body will assume an average potential close to earth ground. Because of the high conductivity and high dielectric constants of tissue, ***E***-fields from the large potentials of the body coil will tend to terminate on the body. Coils placed close to a patient also tend to assume the potential of the body and provide

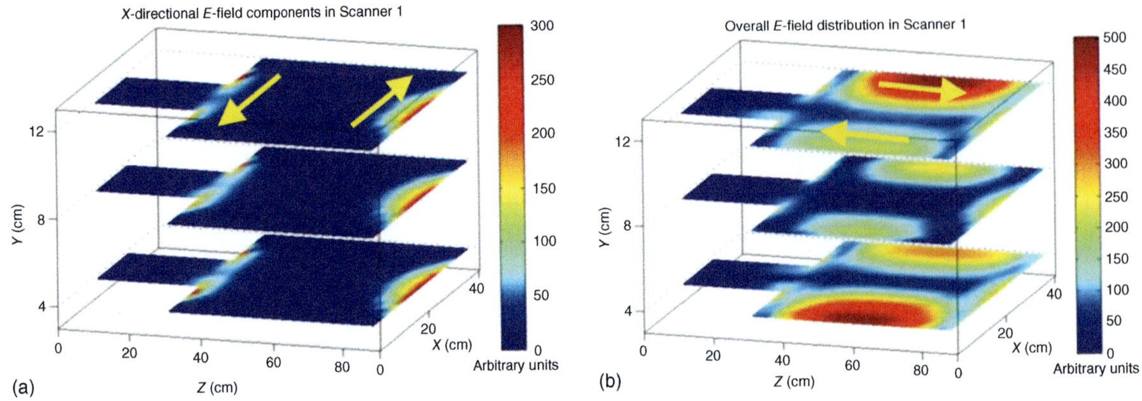

Figure 20.3. ***E*****-fields measured at the 1.5 T frequency using the standard head/torso phantom (ASTM F2182-02a phantom). In (a), the *x*-component of the *E*-field only is shown; in (b) the total *E*-field is shown. (Reference Nordbeck *et al.*[4] with permission)**

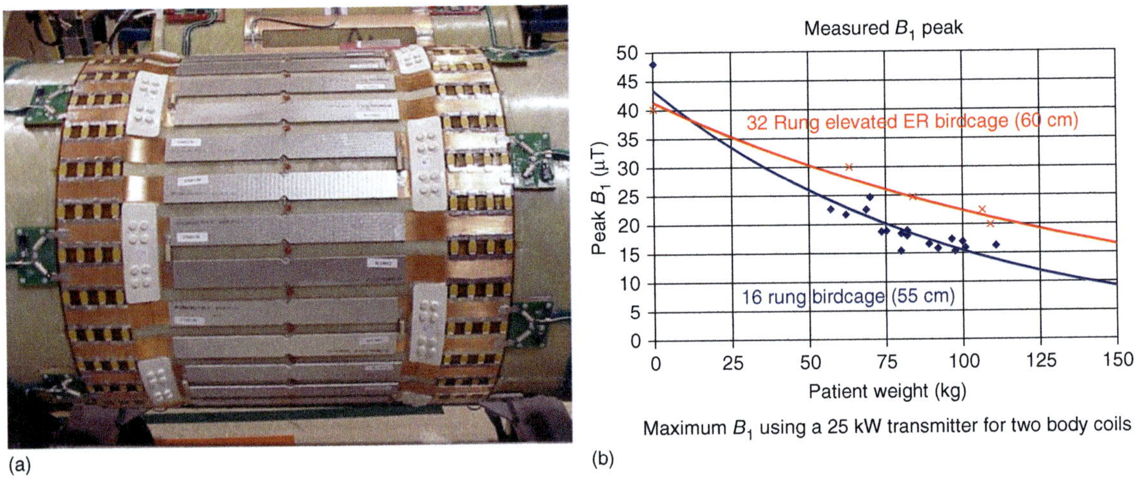

Figure 20.4. In (a), the strut inductance of the high-pass birdcage is reduced by increasing their number to 32. In (b), the resulting B_1 field for a 75 kg patient increases from 20 μT to more than 25 μT for 25 kW of transmit power. (Weyers *et al.*[6] by permission)

new pathways for ***E***-fields coupling. ***E***-fields also couple strongly to the wires and cables internal to the coil and produce currents that cause heating of its parts.

In tandem with the ***E***-fields of the body coil, Faraday induction from the radio frequency B_1 fields of the body coil can induce large voltages (emfs) and currents in the loops of the receive elements. The tuned nature of the elements has the effect of transferring dangerous levels of energy from the body coil to a small region of tissue defined by the size of the receive element. Carefully constructed blocking circuits are, therefore, required to limit this energy transfer, and receive elements are rendered largely transparent to the B_1 field of the body coil. Parts heating in receive elements from large induced currents and the means for protecting against them are reviewed in the next sections.

20.4 COIL SAFETY TESTS

Coils are designed to meet the clinical requirements for diagnostic imaging. Once a coil design has been

	DESIGN VERIFICATION ANALYSIS & TEST GUIDELINES				
		Test / Report Description	**Test Standard(s)**	**Company Req.**	**CE Mark**
Feasibility and Analysis	1	B1 Uniformity and Coverage		X	
Feasibility and Analysis	2	Hazard Analysis	ISO 1497-1	X	X
Feasibility and Analysis	3	Failure Mode and Effect Analysis	ISO 1497-2	X	X
Feasibility and Analysis	4	Component Stress Analysis		X	X
Feasibility and Analysis	5	Flammability Rating	UL 94	X	X
Feasibility and Analysis	6	Mechanical Feasibility / Safety Analysis	UL 2601-1 d, IEC 601-1	X	
Coil Testing	7	Component Stress Test		X	X
Coil Testing	8	Surface Temperature Test	IEC 601-1, 42.3.3	X	
Coil Testing	9	Dielectric Strength Leakage Current	IEC 601-2, 19.4-5, 20.3	X	X
Coil Testing	10	Spillage Test	IEC 601-3, 44.3	X	X
Coil Testing	11	Mechanical Durability: Patient Weight Test	IEC 21.3	X	
Coil Testing	12	Cable Strain Relief Test	UL 544 7.2, 3.4-5	X	X
Coil Testing	13	Cable Bend Test		X	
Coil Testing	14	Connector Life Test			X
Coil Testing	15	Impact Test	UL 2601, US Deviation 55	X	X
Coil Testing	16	Rigidity of Enclosure/Mechanical Strength	IEC 601-1: 21.1.a	X	X
Coil Testing	17	Drop Test	IEC 601-1, 21.5, 21.6	X	X
Coil Testing	18	Proton Signal From Housing			
Coil Testing	19	Electrostatic Discharge Immunity	IS / EN 6100-4.2, 8.3.1.	X	X
Coil Testing	20	B0 Distortion Test (Parts Magnetism)			
Coil Testing	21	B1 Distortion Test			
Coil Testing	22	Component Temperature Test			
Coil Testing	23	Temperature Exposure Test	IEC 601-1: 10.6.8.3(d), 6.1(v)		X
Coil Testing	24	Durability of Markings	IEC 601-1: 6.1.z		X
Coil Testing	25	Creepage and Air Clearances	IEC 601-1: 57.10		X
Coil Testing	26	Insulation - Dielectric Strength Test	IEC 601-1: 59.2		X

CE

Figure 20.5. A representative design verification checklist (circa 2001) for the development of a product coil for clinical MRI and meeting the listed IEC 60601[1] and Underwriter Laboratories™ (UL) requirements

settled upon, it moves to the realm of engineering for construction and integration into an MRI system. In industry, the analysis and testing of a coil to meet its engineering and safety requirements is referred to as design verification. An example list of the tests and the requirements they are intended to meet is shown in Figure 20.5. A few of these tests are meant to meet requirements of a particular country, such as for Japan, but most are designed to meet the international requirements of the IEC and its IEC 60601 document for medical equipment.[1,2] Devices that meet all of the IEC clinical and safety requirements can then be marked with the CE label.

Tests in the list related to heating of the parts of a coil, including the coil surfaces, are tests 4, 7, 8, and 22. Test 4 is not a test per se, but an engineering analysis to determine if individual components of the coil will remain within their specifications for temperature, voltage, and current. Evaluated here are the induce stresses on array elements from the B_1 field of the body coil. The maximum stated B_1 field for the body coil for 1.5 and 3 T systems is typically 25–30 μT, and the maximum duty cycles for excitation are typically 5–6%. These values are generally listed by a manufacturer in their Coil Test Specification for the MR system.

Test 7 is the Component Stress Test. For it, a coil is tested in the MRI system under maximum RF conditions (B_1 and duty cycle) for a period of time comparable to the examination time for a patient. Both before and after the stress is applied, images are acquired and the coil SNR evaluated to determine if there is any degradation in SNR or image quality. Test 8 is the surface temperature test. For it, the coil is placed in the MRI system itself and a test sequence is run that produces the conditions described above. The test is critical enough that during development, coils are often placed in a simulator containing a body coil that replicates the fields of an actual MRI system. The test is designed to reveal any elevated temperatures on patient surfaces originating from heating of the internal components of the coil. The choice of these surfaces is generally related to the location of RF blocking and other circuits that produce heat from the transmit field. Test 22 is the component stress test to determine if the temperatures of internal components remain within their specifications. As for the surface temperature test, this test is generally performed in the MRI system, but the simulator is often used during coil development.

20.5 REDUCTION OF RF CURRENTS FROM TRANSMIT ELECTRIC FIELDS

The strong electric fields of the body coil can couple to connecting cables of a coil, as illustrated in Figure 20.6. The voltages developed on the cables can be passed to the coil and are strong enough to cause arcing, overheating of coil parts, and tissue heating if tissue is inadequately insulated from the coil. Body coils are located behind the shroud or cover of the magnet but inside the gradient coil. To prevent the body coil from coupling to the conductors of the gradient coil, an RF shield is inserted between them and is gapped in such a way that the magnetic field of the gradient can pass through it without causing large eddy currents. There is also enough capacitance in the gaps of the shield to pass the RF currents of the body coil and prevent it from coupling to the windings of the gradient coil. A large fraction of electric fields of the body coil near its end rings is terminated by the RF shield. But, as described above, a typical 1.5 T body coil still produces ***E***-fields in the neighborhood of $20\ \mathrm{V\,cm^{-1}}$ in its interior.[3,4] An object, including the patient, centered in the bore of the magnet will experience capacitive couplings to the body coil that are roughly balanced in the x–y directions, and, to a lesser extent, in the z-direction depending upon positioning. The average potential of the body of a patient, therefore, remains close to earth ground. Balanced ***E***-fields do, however, enter and exit the body from the body coil and can cause an increase in SAR. Without the protection of cable baluns, voltages developed on the cables are strong enough to cause arcing and overheating of coil internal parts. Cables passing near a patient can produce tissue heating and require some protection.

20.6 ISOLATION OF CONNECTING CABLES USING CABLE BALUNS

The most common device for blocking RF currents induced by body coil ***E***-fields is the RF 'balun,' a term that was coined for a device that converts balanced signals to unbalanced signals. Some possible pathways for currents induced on the shield of a cable are shown in Figure 20.7. The circuit is completed with return currents that are set up on the shield or possibly on other nearby cables or conductors. As indicated in Figure 20.7(a), an RF balun is constructed by enclosing the cable shield with another conductor that develops some external inductance with the shield. Capacitors are then added across the inductance to tune the balun to the NMR frequency. Blocking impedances in series with shield conductor obtained for this type of balun range from 500 to 4000 Ohms (Ω). An example of a high-impedance balun for a single coaxial cable

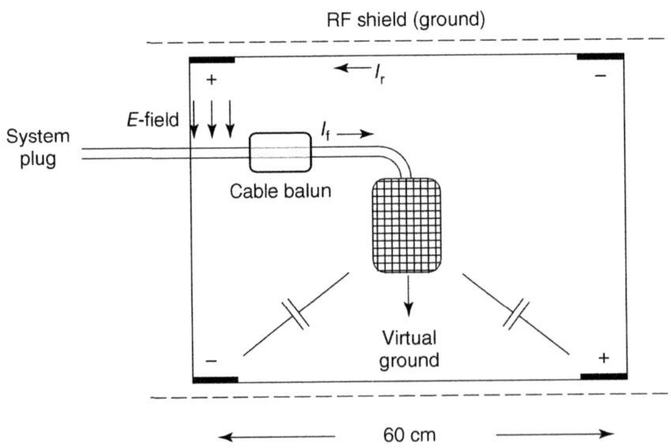

Figure 20.6. A coil or other device centered in the body coil (hatched area) assumes a potential close to that of ground. ***E***-fields of the body can then induce currents on the outer shield of the cable unless they are blocked by the high impedance of a cable balun

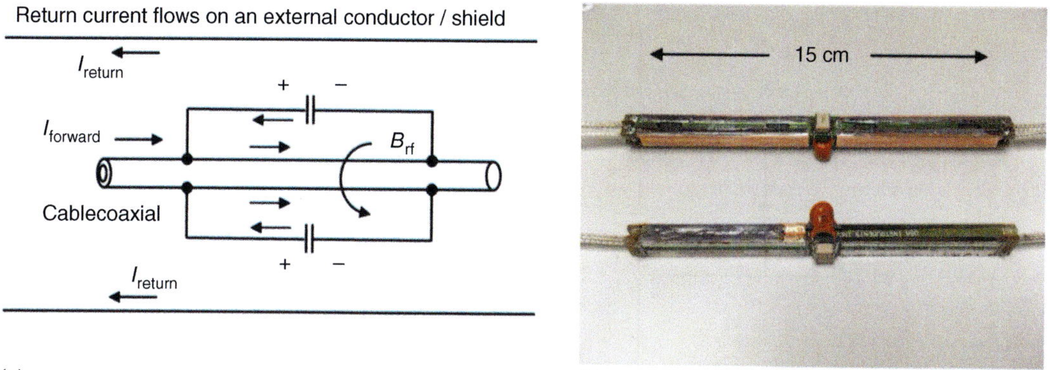

(a) (b)

Figure 20.7. In (a) the parallel resonance of a cable balun presents a large blocking impedance to currents on the shield of a cable. An example of a high-voltage balun is shown in (b) which for an applied ***E***-field of 20 V cm^{-1}, blocks a minimum of 300 V (by Pei Chan, USA Instruments, OH)

is shown in Figure 20.7(b). Baluns are also effective when they enclose bundles of cables surrounded by a single shield. Several cable baluns are often placed in series on system cables to block the distributed effects of body coil ***E***-fields. Tuning of RF baluns can be difficult owing to the difficulty of compensating for the effect of stray capacitance. The effectiveness of a balun can be tested in the MRI system by subjecting it to a high level of RF excitation and measuring components of the coil for increases in temperature. For thoroughness, a coil should be tested for a range of likely positions in the magnet to identify worst-case heating.

20.7 REDUCTION OF RF CURRENTS FROM TRANSMIT B_1 FIELDS: RF BLOCKING CIRCUITS

Radio frequency B_1 fields from the body coil can induce strong currents in resonant surface coils. Coil currents can cause heating of the components of the coil, and concentrated flux in the coil can cause heating of tissues beneath it. The induction of a voltage or 'electromotive force' (emf) in a loop is described in Figure 20.8. As indicated on the right-hand side of the coil, high impedance blocking circuits are placed in series with the coil to limit coil current.[7,8] Detuning of a surface coil is not enough because a detuned element can still concentrate flux from the transmit coil.[9] If the transmit B_1 field is uniform, the magnitude of the emf is given by,

$$|\text{emf(V)}| = \omega_o \cdot \text{Area}(\text{m}^2) \cdot B_1(\text{T})$$

where, $\omega_o = 2\pi \cdot f_o$, is the NMR frequency (in radians s^{-1}). The maximum B_1 provided by the body coil is specified by the original equipment manufacturer (OEM) for the MRI system. For a 1.5 T system with a 60 cm diameter bore, it is typically 25–30 μT. For example, the emf generated within a 10 × 10 cm coil element tuned for 3 T (127.7 MHz) would be 200 V

$$\text{emf (V)} = -\frac{d\Phi}{dt}$$

where

$$\Phi(t) = \int \vec{B_1}(t) \cdot \vec{n}\, da$$

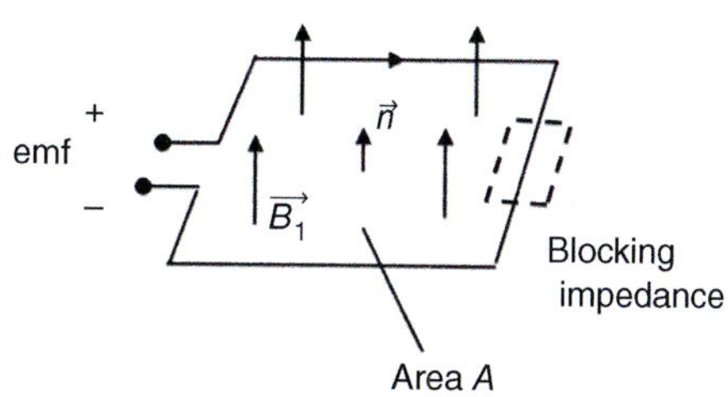

Figure 20.8. The transmit B_1 field of the body coil produces a voltage or emf in a coil by induction. Placement of a blocking impedance in series with the coil prevents large currents from flowing

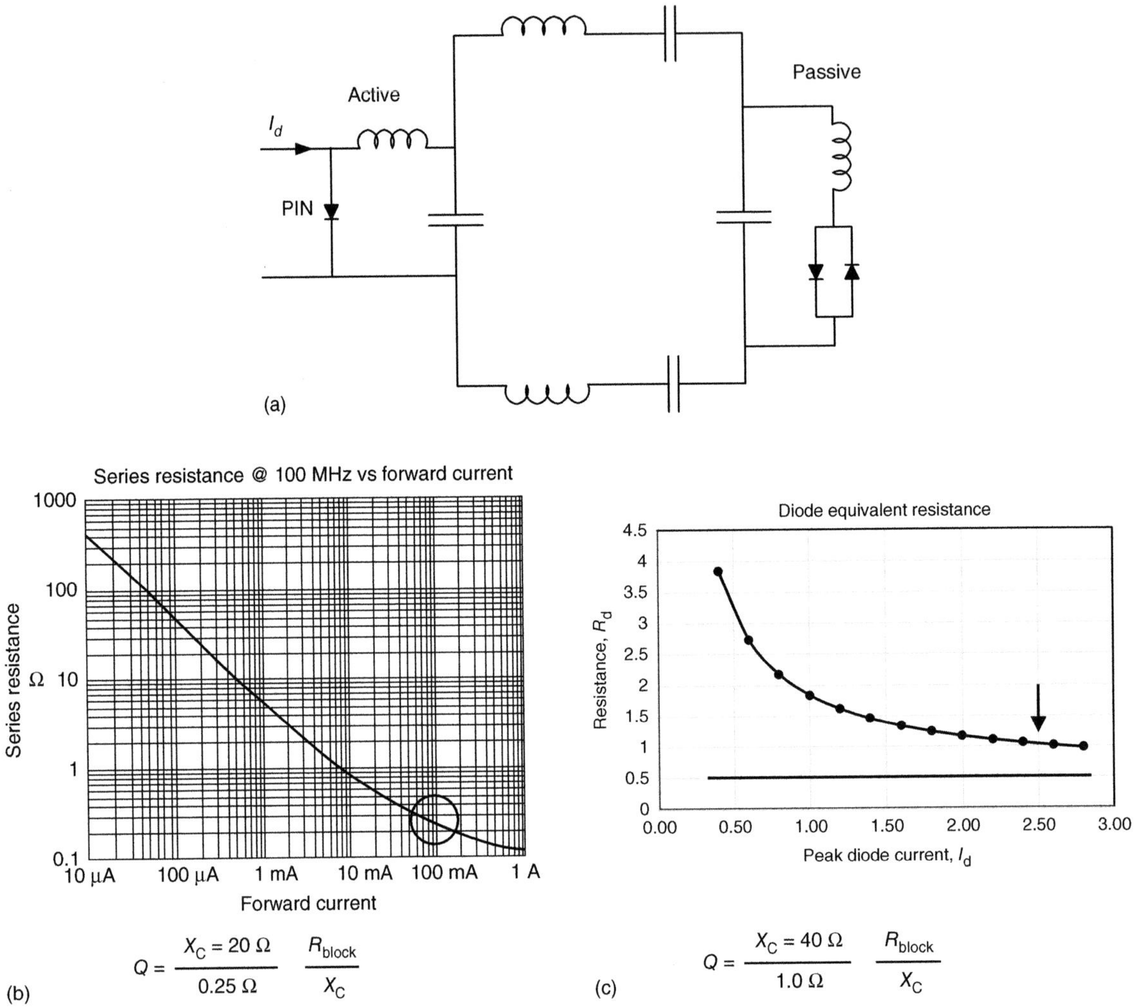

Figure 20.9. In (a), two types of RF blocking circuits are illustrated, an active blocking circuit on the left using a PIN diode, and a passive blocking circuit on the right using two crossed diodes. In (b), a PIN diode (example type MA4P1250) activated with a control current from the system of 50–100 mA develops a dynamic resistance of 0.25–0.5 Ω. In (c), a crossed pair of RF diodes develops an on-resistance that decreases with increasing RF current in the blocking circuit. The dashed line indicates the minimum diode resistance from contact resistance (0.5 Ω)

when excited with a transmit field of 25 μT. A blocking impedance of 1000 Ω would limit the current to 0.2 A and limit the average power dissipated to 1 W (5% Duty Cycle).

Blocking circuits are parallel resonant circuits, and two types of these circuits are illustrated in Figure 20.9. The first uses a PIN diode to short the matching inductor of the input circuit, a common configuration used in phased arrays. When the PIN diode is biased on, the matching inductor resonates with the adjacent capacitor to develop a (resistive) blocking impedance across the input. PIN diodes are typically activated with DC currents of 50–100 mA supplied by the system controller of the MRI system. At these current levels, on-resistances for the diode range from 0.25 to 0.5 Ω, as indicated in the chart of Figure 20.9(b). The expressions for the Q shown in the figure can be used to compute the blocking resistance of a circuit. The impedance of the matching inductor is likely about 20 Ω (the square root of 50 Ω times the series resistance of the coil). Using 0.25 Ω for the dynamic resistance of the PIN diode, we obtain a blocking resistance of 1600 Ω.

A second type of blocking circuit that uses a pair of crossed diodes is shown on the right-hand side of the coil. This 'passive' blocking circuit is activated by strong currents in the coil induced by the transmit B_1 field. Computation of the blocking impedance for the passive circuit is more complicated, but an estimate can be obtained by using a simple model for the equivalent series resistance, R_s, of a crossed pair of diodes. The model is based on the assumption that the forward voltage drop across each diode is constant at high current levels. The sinusoidal variation of the current in the blocking circuit assures that very little time will be spent during a cycle at low voltage and current. Assuming then that each diode experiences a forward voltage drop of V_d, the average power dissipated in the diode pair, P_d, can be obtained by multiplying V_d by the current averaged over one cycle of the RF. If I_d is the amplitude of the sinusoidal current in the blocking circuit and R_s is the equivalent series resistance for the diode pair, then,

$$
\begin{aligned}
P_d &= \frac{1}{2} {I_d}^2 R_s \\
&= \frac{2}{T} \times V_d \int_0^{T/2} I_d \sin(2\pi f_o t)\, dt = 2\, V_d I_d/\pi
\end{aligned}
$$

which yields the equivalent resistance,

$$R_s \approx 4V_d/\pi I_d$$

For a diode voltage drop of 1.0 V, R_s is approximately $4/(\pi\, I_d)$. As a refinement, we add to this a fixed contact resistance of 0.5 Ω, taken from the diode specification for a 1N4148 diode, and this sum is used in the plot of Figure 20.9(c). For a circulating current of 2.5 A, the equivalent resistance for the diodes would be about 1 Ω. The reciprocal relationship with current means that the diodes become more conductive at higher transmit power, and blocking impedance rises monotonically with the transmit B_1 field. If the passive blocking circuit in this example is located across a distributed capacitor in a coil, the reactance of the capacitor will be higher than for the matching circuit. Using a value of 40 Ω for the capacitive reactance and 1 Ω for the equivalent diode resistance, we again obtain a blocking impedance 1600 Ω for the circuit.

One misconception that this discussion dispels is that very little current flows in a well-tuned blocking circuit. While current circulating in the coil element is certainly reduced, large currents still circulate in the reactive elements of the blocking circuit. If large currents flow in the inductor of the blocking circuit, its local field can modify the transmit B_1 field and produce an image distortion. Large circulating currents in a blocking circuit create heat in its components, and the heat can make its way through the coil former to a surface in contact with the patient. An example of a coil where problems of this type are encountered is the 1.5 T spine coil, shown in Figure 20.10. This coil was constructed of loop-saddle pairs that provide quadrature reception in the region of the spine. The loop element of one section of the array is quite large at 14 × 14 cm, and the peak emf generated in the loop from a 30 μT pulse (test B_1 for General Electric coils) would be 236 V. The loop has two passive and one active blocking circuits and has a total blocking impedance estimated to be 3200 Ω. One passive circuit of the loop has a blocking impedance of approximately 1100 Ω, so its voltage drop is 81 V or about one-third of the emf. The reactance of this blocking circuit is 33 Ω, so during transmit, the amplitude of the diode current is about 2.5 A. RF diodes used in passive circuits have characteristics similar to the 1N4148 diode used in NMR spectrometers, which can sustain relatively high currents. Poor quality or 'leaky' diodes can appear resistive in their off-state, so for these reasons manufacturers often specify proprietary diodes with improved electrical and thermal characteristics. If diodes cannot sustain a high peak current, then more blocking circuits are needed, and which might reduce coil sensitivity. IEC rules stipulate that a medical device (the coil) should be able to sustain one component failure and remain safe for the patient.[1] For that reason, coil elements typically incorporate at least two blocking circuits. Because PIN diode blocking circuits are generally provide higher blocking impedances, at least one PIN diode circuit is generally incorporated into an element that absorbs most of the voltage stress. If only one blocking circuit is required, a pair of crossed diodes can serve as a backup by placing them in parallel with the PIN diode. The crossed diodes are normally off, but if the PIN diode fails (opens) or if the PIN control line becomes disconnected (the coil becomes unplugged), the passive diodes will activate and provide protection.

Heating of coil elements is computed as part of the stress analysis, Test 4. In the example above, the loop of the spine coil develops a peak emf of 236 V. If the total blocking impedance is 3200 Ω, the peak power dissipated in the loop is 8.7 W, and the average

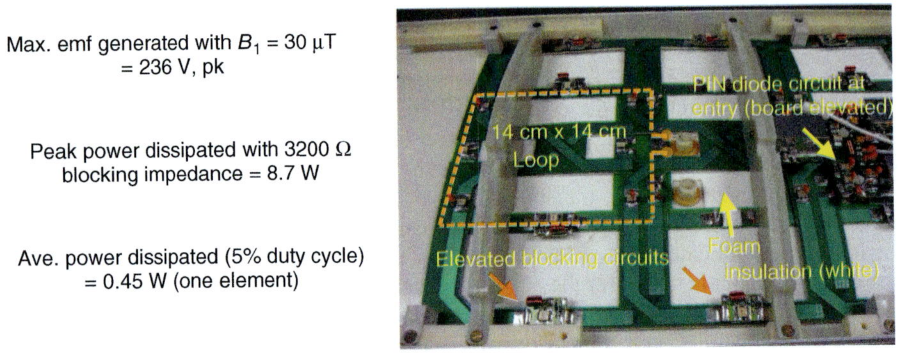

Figure 20.10. A six station USAI 1.5 T spine coil (circa 2001) illustrating construction and methods for limiting surface heating. A 14 × 14 cm loop is illustrated with the feed board removed

dissipation in the element with 5% duty cycle is 0.44 W. The blocking circuits of the element absorb most of this heating. The copper conductors connected to the blocking circuits will move much of this heat away, but for the spine coil, even this was not enough. So, as indicated in Figure 20.10, the blocking circuits were elevated, and the entire coil was insulated with foam to keep heat away from the coil former.

When a large current is induced in a surface coil, an image current is induced in the tissue beneath the coil conductors, which can cause tissue heating. As a secondary effect, the RF B_1 field created by this current can nutate spins near the element, causing an image distortion. Because the two are related by B_1, image distortion is often used to identify coil elements that have inadequate blocking impedance. B_1 distortions can be created by a mistuned blocking circuit, but they can also be created by lack of adequate blocking impedance in the element. How much blocking impedance is required? Because the emf induced in an element is proportional to its area, a design criterion for minimum blocking impedance can be specified in ohms per square centimeter, which in effect places a limit on the amount of current that is allowed to flow. This question was investigated using a 1.5 T clinical system, and the blocking impedances of coil elements with areas 100, 300, and 500 cm^2 were evaluated using a large phantom.[10] The study determined that a minimum factor of 2.8–3.0 $\Omega\,\text{cm}^{-2}$ is required at the 1.5 T field strength to maintain image distortion to less than 1%. This factor, however, was obtained by averaging the image intensity over the entire field of view (FOV). In another study, investigators used an analytical approach to set a limit on B_1 distortion from a surface coil, as described in Figure 20.11.[11] In their approach, a limit of 5% is set on the change in B_1 at a location 1 cm below the conductor of a surface coil. The results they obtained are also shown in the figure. Using an NMR frequency of 64 MHz, their approach yields a much more conservative factor of 16 $\Omega\,\text{cm}^{-2}$ for the minimum blocking impedance for 1.5 T. To be sure, the ability of both of these approaches to predict the temperature increase of tissue or the heating of the coil parts is qualitative in nature. Observation of image distortion does not mean that the coil is unsafe or that it will experience undue heating. Calculation of the heat deposited in individual coil parts using an engineering analysis remains a better approach for quantifying heating, and this is performed during the stress analysis of Test 4. These analyses are then verified with stress testing in Test 22, where the temperatures of parts are measured under load. To evaluate tissue heating, electromagnetic simulations or at minimum, temperature measurements on phantoms are generally required.

20.8 PROGRESS IN BLOCKING CIRCUIT DESIGN

PIN diode-controlled circuits have the disadvantage that active control lines from the MR system need to be connected to the individual coil elements. A typical control line can source up to 10 V and deliver 100 mA of forward current, which amounts to as much as 1 W of power if supplied continuously. As an alternative, a circuit referred to as an 'auto-bias circuit' by its inventors derives a bias current for the PIN diode directly from the RF field of the body coil.[12] The auto-bias circuit, shown in Figure 20.12, functions by rectifying a portion of the current circulating in the

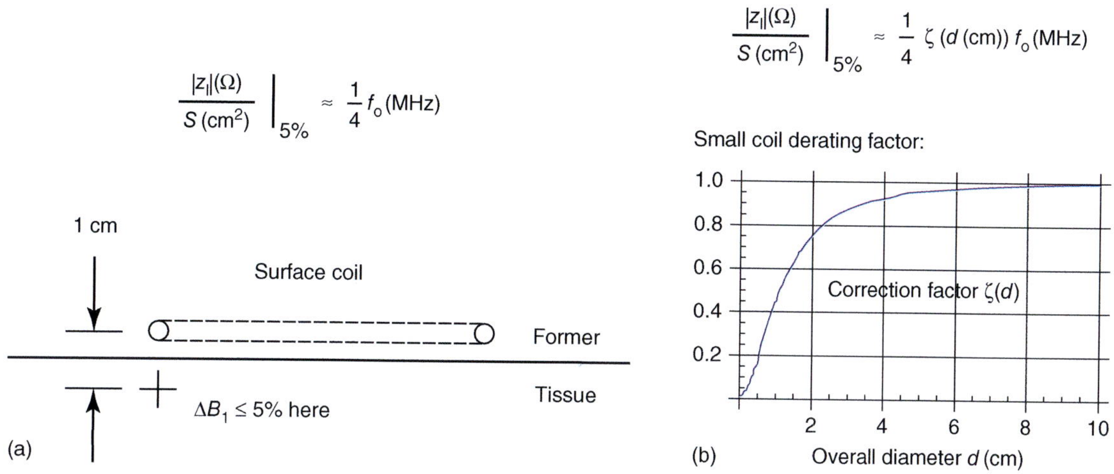

Figure 20.11. In (a) this analytical approach[11] evaluates the blocking impedance for a circular loop by setting a limit of 5% on the deviation of the B_1 field at 1 cm from the coil conductor. In (b), a derating factor is included for coil diameters less than 5 cm

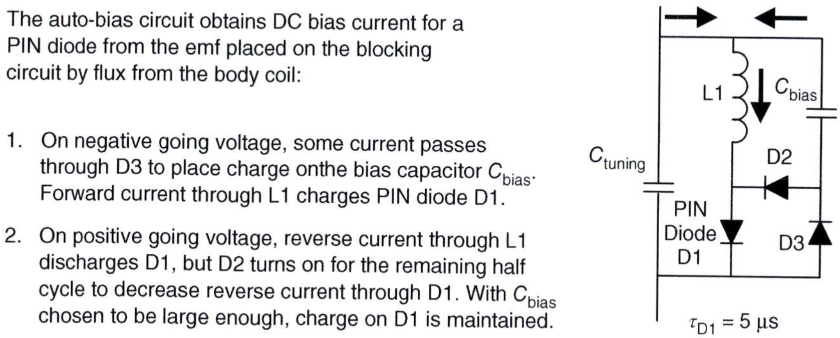

Figure 20.12. A blocking circuit using the auto-bias circuit[12] placed across one distributed capacitor of the coil

blocking circuit and using it to replace charge in the PIN diode normally lost to recombination. The efficiency of the auto-bias circuit approaches that of the active PIN diode circuit and is likely higher than that of the crossed-diode circuit under conditions of high transmit power.

In another type of blocking circuit, an active transistor replaces the PIN diode as a switch.[13] Transistors have long been used to switch audio frequency signals, such as for sample-and-hold circuits in multiplexers. With the advent of GaAs and GaN materials, FET transistors have become both high-power and fast. In a recent study, several of these transistors were investigated, and the blocking impedances obtained with them were found to be comparable to those of good quality PIN diodes.[13] Because switching of the transistor was controlled via its gate terminal, control currents were very low, much less than the 50–100 mA typically used for a PIN diode. Dissipation from the device was thereby minimized.

Microelectromechanical (MEMS): In the example above, the transistors of a blocking circuit were employed as 'switches', but what if one could fabricate an actual switch? Two examples of how switches might be used are shown in Figure 20.13(a) and (b). Switches of this type have been a primary focus of MEMS devices development, and their use as a coil switch was the subject of an early patent claim.[14] More recently, some MEMS switching devices have been developed that are both compatible with use in MRI magnets (mainly for their packaging) and exhibit resistances

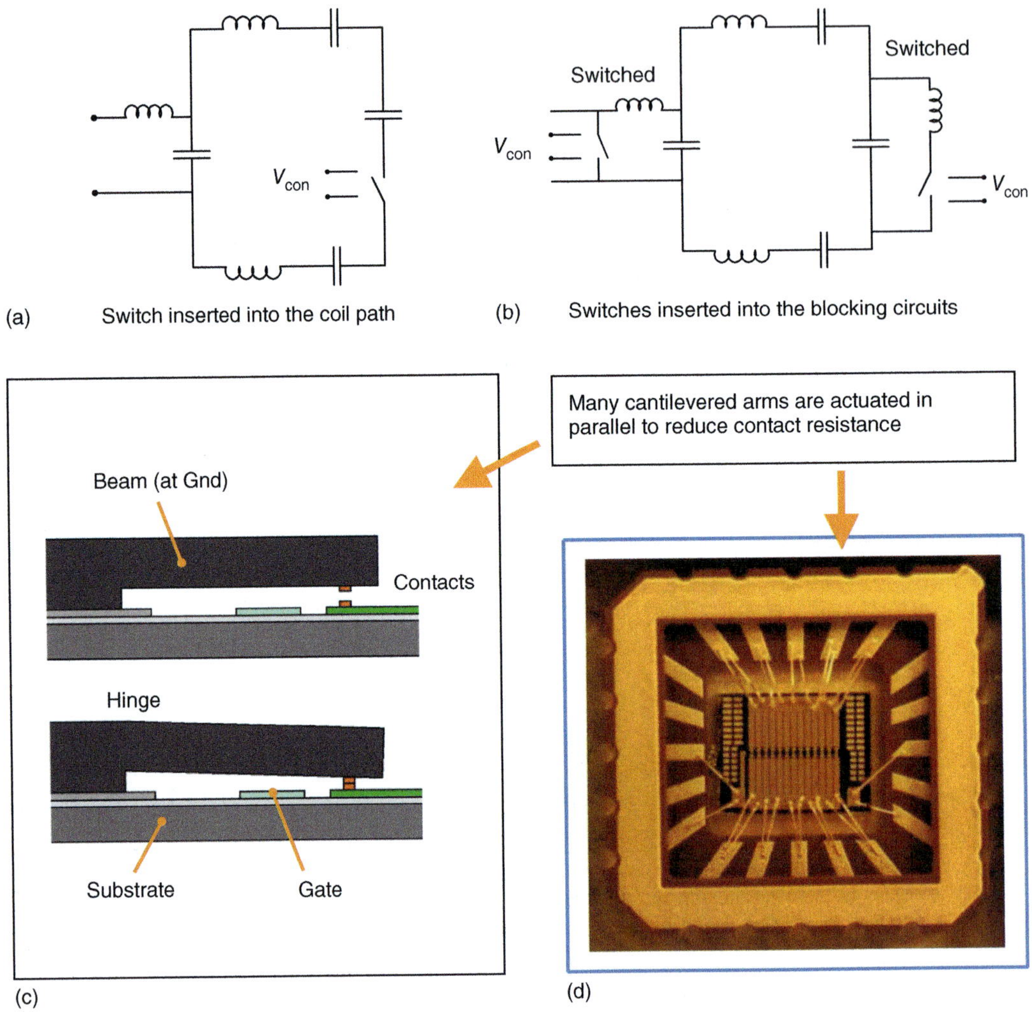

Figure 20.13. Fabrication and use of MEMS switch in blocking circuits for array coils. In (a) the switch is placed in series with the coil, the simplest implementation. In (b) they take the place of diode in the blocking circuits. In (c) a Gate voltage of ~50 V closes the many actuators of the device using electrostatic attraction.[16] In (d), a photo of an MRI compatible MEMS switch placed in series with array elements to acquire an image of the spine.[17]

low enough to replace diodes.[15–17] These devices use multiple cantilevered arms suspended over electrical contacts, as shown in Figure 20.13(c). The contacts are closed when an electrostatic potential is applied and a force is created that pulls the arms down and onto their individual contacts. As indicated in the photo of Figure 20.13(d), dozens of these arms are paralleled within a single device to achieve a low on-resistance. Devices have been fabricated that can switch currents of 5 A or more while sustaining 100 V or more across the contacts in the off-state.[15] Switching times as low as 10 microseconds have been achieved, which is fast enough for MRI applications.[17] The contact resistances are low enough that they can be placed in series with the coil conductors, permitting rapid reconfiguration of the array.[18]

A special advantage of a MEMS switch is the logic of their switching when placed in series with the coil. In the absence of a control signal, the actuators default to the open state. A receive coil can, therefore, function only if it is connected to the MRI system providing the control. The disadvantage is that a high-voltage drive circuit is required to close the contacts. MEMS devices are currently rather expensive and remain a work-in-progress, while reliability and manufacturing issues are worked out.

20.9 MINIMIZING HEAT FROM PIN CONTROL LINES AND PREAMPLIFIERS

DC control lines and power supply lines are also exposed to the transmit fields of the body coil. In the cable that connects them to the system, they are generally bundled together with coaxial cables for the receiver. Since electric fields from the body coil induce common mode currents in the cable conductors, cable baluns placed around the cable bundle are effective in blocking them. Within the coil assembly, body coil ***E***-fields can be quite high, and liberal use of RF inductors and shunt capacitors is needed to protect control lines and power connections for the preamplifiers. Heating of coil parts can be a volume effect as well as a local effect. If the temperature of the entire coil increases, the marginal allowable temperature increases from blocking circuits and other components will be reduced in order to maintain surface temperatures below the 41 °C limit. In order to obtain an idea of how various parts of the contribution to the total heating of a coil, heat dissipation in the coil from three source groups were compiled in Table 20.1. The assumptions that were used in the computations are included as separate entries within each sub-table, and heating from blocking circuits was compiled for some typical arrays at the 1.5, 3, and 7 T field strengths. The results suggest that for blocking circuits, the heating per coil element is about the same, owing to a decrease is size for elements implemented at the higher field strengths. Total dissipation increases, however, because of the increase in the number of elements. The assumptions here are somewhat arbitrary, of course, but they illustrate trends.

Heat dissipation from PIN diode control lines is also compiled. Field strength for this compilation is not a significant factor, so it was not included. Instead, heating was compiled for different numbers of channels and a difference in duty cycle. The results suggest that the heat generated by control lines is of less concern.

Finally, the heat generated by the preamplifiers of an array was compiled for two different types of preamplifiers. The first ones are of an older design that requires a 10 V power supply and substantial current for gain and stability. Newer ones use a 3.3 V

Table 20.1. Estimates of parts dissipations, including preamplifiers

Bo	fo (MHz)	Area (cm^2)	Maximum B_1	emf	R_{block}	Duty cycle	Average power	Number of elements	Total power
Examples for 1.5 T. 3 T and 7 T arrays									
Dissipation from coil blocking circuits									
1.5 T array	64	196	30	236.4	3136	0.05	0.45	4	1.78
3 T array	128	100	30	241.3	3200	0.05	0.45	8	3.64
7 T head coil	298	32	30	179.7	2384	0.05	0.34	32	10.84

	PIN diode (V)	DC current	Series R	Pk power (W)	Duty cycle	Average power	Number of elements	Total power
Dissipation from PIN diode control lines								
8 Channels	0.8	0.100	9.00	0.17	0.05	0.0085	8	0.068
8 Channels, disabled	0.8	0.100	9.00	0.17	1.00	0.17	8	1.36
32 Channels	0.8	0.100	12	0.20	0.10	0.02	32	0.64

	V supply	DC current	Duty cycle	Single power	Number of elements	Total power
Dissipation from 10 V and 3.3 V preamplifiers						
32 Preamplifiers	10	0.035	1.00	0.35	32	11.20
32 Preamplifiers	3.3	0.070	1.00	0.231	32	7.39

power supply and separate current connections for the two stages of the amplifier, approximately doubling the current. The actual supply current for the 3.3 V designs may be somewhat less than this, so it is likely that the 3.3 V amplifiers provide a net power reduction of a factor of two. Even with this improvement, however, the total power dissipation from preamplifiers is significant and is a problem for the construction of large arrays.

20.10 MEASUREMENT TOOLS

Measurement of blocking impedance is generally performed with a network analyzer. While the shorting of a diode or diode pair is a useful method for tuning these circuits, shorting of diodes does not allow one to measure a true blocking impedance under dynamic conditions. A better approach is to develop a fixture in which bias-Ts can provide bias currents for PIN or crossed-diodes so that a better measure of the Q of the blocking circuit can be obtained. A two-port fixture provides for measurement of transfer impedance (S21), and measurement of transfer impedance provides a more accurate measurement of the blocking impedance than reflection coefficient from a single port. Most industry-grade network analyzers are programmed with the math for this type of measurement. Once calibrated, the measurement parameters for a fixture can be stored, and future measurements expedited.

The maximum allowed temperature of a patient's surface is 41 °C (see Appendix A). Given that the temperature of the body is already close to 37 °C, even a modest rise in temperature at the coil surface might cause a coil to fail the surface temperature test. The accuracy of the probe used for temperature measurement should be included in the measurement, so accurate probes contribute to the quality of the measurement. One method is to use an optical probe, such as the Opsens Model OTP-M probe connected to an AccuSens signal conditioner (Opsens Solutions, Inc., Quebec, Canada). The AccuSens instrument has up to eight inputs, and the OTP-M sensors have an absolute accuracy of ±0.3 °C in the physiological temperature range.

Another method is to use an infrared camera to obtain temperature via a temperature-sensitive photograph of the coil surface. One such device is the FLIR E6 infrared camera (https://www.flir.com/products/e6/) that has an absolute accuracy of ±2.0 °C degrees over its extended temperature range and an accuracy of ±0.75 °C in the physiological temperature range. While this accuracy is marginal, the camera also has an accuracy of < 0.1 °C for differential readings. So, while the absolute accuracy of the camera is marginal, temperature increases can be monitored accurately when comparing two nearby surfaces. Obviously, one can combine the two approaches to thermally image with the absolute accuracy of an optical sensor.

20.11 SUMMARY

For 1.5 and 3 T MRI systems, most sources of heating in RF coils originate from currents induced by the strong radiofrequency fields of the body coil. Strong electric fields that couple to the coil cables and conductors can induce strong currents and heating in the interior parts of a coil. Judicious use of cable baluns, inductors, and other components will reduce RF currents induced by electric fields of the body coil. Strong B_1 fields from a transmit coil can induce large RF voltages in the loops of receive elements. High-impedance blocking circuits placed in series with receive elements will reduce RF currents and minimize heating. Blocking circuits are effective in reducing RF currents in a coil and are important for protecting both the coil circuit and the tissue located beneath the coil. Reduction of RF currents is required to maintain the temperatures of coil components within their operating limits. Reduction of RF currents is also required to meet regulatory limits on the temperature of coil surfaces in contact with a human subject.

ACKNOWLEDGMENTS

This research was supported (in part) by the Intramural Research Program of the NIH, NINDS.

APPENDIX A. SURFACE TEMPERATURE LIMITS (IEC)*

11.1.2.2 APPLIED PARTS Not Intended to Supply Heat to a PATIENT*

The limits of Table 24 shall apply in both NORMAL CONDITION and SINGLE FAULT CONDITION. If the surface temperature of an APPLIED PART exceeds 41 °C:

- the maximum temperature shall be disclosed in the instructions for use;
- the conditions for safe contact, e.g., duration or condition of the PATIENT, shall be disclosed; and
- the clinical effects with respect to characteristics such as body surface, maturity of PATIENTS, medications being taken, or surface pressure shall be determined and documented in the RISK MANAGEMENT FILE.

where 41 °C is not exceeded, no justification is required.

If analyses documented in the RISK MANAGEMENT FILE demonstrate that APPLIED PART temperatures cannot be affected by operation of the ME EQUIPMENT including in SINGLE FAULT CONDITIONS, measurement of APPLIED PART temperature according to 11.1.3 is not required.

*IEC 60601-1 as amended in 2012, reference [2].

RELATED ARTICLES IN EMAGRES

Radiofrequency Fields and SAR for Bird Cage Coils

Radiofrequency Heating Models and Measurements

Safety Considerations in MRI

Impedance Matching and Baluns

REFERENCES

1. International Electrotechnical Commission, IEC 60601-2-33, Particular Requirements for Magnetic Resonance Equipment, 2nd Edition for 2002-2005, and 3rd Edition for 2010, Geneva, Switzerland.
2. International Electrotechnical Commission, IEC 60601-1:2005+AMD1:2012 CSV, Consolidated version. Medical electrical equipment – Part 1: General requirements for basic safety and essential performance, Section 11.1.2.2.
3. C. C. Guclu, *J. Magn Reson. Imaging*, 2001, **14**, 484.
4. P. Nordbeck, F. Fidler, I. Weiss, M. Warmuth, M. T. Friedrich, P. Ehses, W. Geistert, O. Ritter, P. M. Jakob, M. E. Ladd, H. H. Quick, and W. R. Bauer, *Magn. Reson. Med.*, 2008, **60**, 312.
5. American Society for Testing and Materials (ASTM), Standard test method for measurement of radio frequency induced heating near passive implants during magnetic resonance imaging (F2182–02a), ASTM International: West Conshohocken, PA, 2002.
6. D. Weyers, D. Keren, E. Boskamp, G. McKinnon, and K. Kinsey, *Proc. Intl. Soc. Mag. Reson. Med.*, 2004, **12**, 1548.
7. P. B. Roemer, W. A. Edelstein, C. E. Hayes, S. P. Souza, and O. M. Mueller, *Magn. Reson. Med.*, 1990, **16**, 192.
8. W. A. Edelstein, C. J. Hardy, and O. M. Mueller, *J. Magn. Reson.*, 1986, **67**, 156.
9. H. Merkle, J. Murphy-Boesch, P. van Gelderen, S. Wang, T.-Q. Li, A. Koretsky, and J. H. Duyn, *Magn. Reson. Med.*, 2011, **66**, 901.
10. A. Kocharian, P. J. Rossman, T. C. Hulshizer, J. P. Felmlee, and S. J. Riederer, *Magn. Reson. Mater. Phys. Biol. Med.*, 2000, **10**, 80.
11. V. Taracila, P. Chan, and F. Robb, *Proc. Int. Soc. Magn. Reson. Med.*, 2010, **18**, 3928.
12. M. Burl and M. X. Zou, Transmit Mode Coil Detuning for MRI Systems, U.S. Pat. 6850067 (Feb. 2005).
13. J. Y. Lu, T. Grafendorfer, T. Zhang, S. Vasanawala, F. Robb, J. M. Pauly, and G. C. Scott, *IEEE Trans. Med. Imaging*, 2016, **35**, 2558.
14. A. Reykowski and J. Wang, Magnetic Resonance Tomography Apparatus and Method for Operating Same Employing an Electrostatic Relay, U.S. Pat. 6710597 (March 2004).
15. M. Fuentes, E. Weber, S. Wilson, B. Li, and S. Crozier, *Proc. Int. Soc. Magn. Reson. Med.*, 2010, **18**, 422.
16. C. Keimel, G. Claydon, B. Li, J. N. Park, and M. E. Valdes, *IEEE Trans. Industry Appl.*, 2012, **48**, 1163.
17. D. Spence and M. Aimi, *Proc. Int. Soc. Magn. Reson. Med.*, 2015, **23**, 0704.
18. S. B. Bulumulla, K. J. Park, E. Fiveland, J. Iannotti, and F. Robb, *Rev. Sci. Intrum.*, 2017, **88**, 025003.

Chapter 21

RF-Induced Heating in Bare and Covered Stainless Steel Rods: Effect of Length, Covering, and Diameter

Sunder Rajan, Peter Serano, Joshua Guag, Tayeb Zaidi, Kyoko Fujimoto, Maria Ida Iacono, and Leonardo M. Angelone

Division of Biomedical Physics, Office of Science and Engineering Laboratories, CDRH/FDA, Silver Spring, MD, USA

21.1 INTRODUCTION

A major concern when performing MRI examinations in patients with electrically conductive medical implants (e.g. stents) is the increase in induced currents due to the 'antenna effect' along conductive components, leading to heating of the tissue near the tips.[1] A number of reports characterizing this behavior have been published for various constructs in the context of active implants with long leads and for interventional procedures.[2–4] It has been demonstrated that the exposed conductive tip of an insulated lead can lead to higher heating in the conductive medium. A systematic study looking into the effect of insulation on the induced heating, however, has not been yet presented.

Computational electromagnetic modeling is increasingly being used to complement experimental testing, as it allows for extensive, cost-effective, and systematic analysis of several variables that can influence the induced heating. Thus, in this chapter, we present computational analysis of specific absorption rate (SAR) in cylindrical rod-like constructs to better understand the dependence of device length and diameter on the induced heating. A parametric analysis is performed to establish the RF-induced heating characteristics by calculating peak 1 g-averaged SAR within 1 cm from the implant. In addition, RF heating measurements are made in a subset of structures to confirm the trends observed in the results of EM simulations.

21.2 METHODS

Numerical simulations: numerical simulations were carried out using the commercial finite element method (FEM) solver ANSYS Electronics Desktop

Safety and Biological Effects in MRI.
Edited by Devashish Shrivastava and J. Thomas Vaughan
 ISBN: 978-1-118-82130-5
Also published in eMagRes (online edition)
DOI: 10.1002/9780470034590.emrstm1630

v18 (ANSYS, Canonsburg, PA). Simulations were performed at three discrete Larmor frequencies for 1.5 T (64 MHz), 3.0 T (128 MHz), and 7.0 T (300 MHz) RF exposure. Rods were exposed to a homogenous incident electric field over the entire volume and oriented along the length of the device (Ex = 0, Ey = 0, Ez = 100 V m^{-1}). Homogeneity of the Ez field was 0.5%, 2.5%, and 12% over the distance of 400 mm for the 64, 128, and 300 MHz exposures, respectively. The 1 g-averaged SAR was calculated for each design variation as prescribed by IEEE Standard 1528. The peak SAR located in the region within 1 cm of the stent was used as the convergence criterion with acceptable convergence occurring when the value of this parameter changed less than 2% between successive runs of increasing mesh density. All SAR results are reported as a ratio to the peak SAR value found across all models and design variations. In other words, in Figure 21.1 a value of 1 W kg^{-1} represents the maximum value across all constructs. Rod lengths were varied from 5 to 400 mm in 5 mm increments. Copper was selected as the material for the rods and Teflon was selected as the material for the rod covers due to ease of fabrication in related experimental studies.

Experimental Measurements: Hollow stainless-steel rods of various lengths and 3 mm diameter were used for the measurements. In addition, one set of rods was covered on the outside with Teflon heat-shrink tubing (henceforth called 'covered rods'). Flurooptic temperature probes were placed inside precision holes drilled at the edge of the rod. The heating tests were performed as per the ASTM 2182-11a Standard. Two MITS body MR coils resonating at 64 and 128 MHz (Zurich Med Tech, Zurich, Switzerland) and operating in the circular polarized mode, using a 240 s RF exposure were used.[5] The rods were placed on a holder 2 cm away from the wall of the phantom in the X-direction, and at $y = 0$, inside a gelled saline phantom as prescribed by the ASTM 2182-11a Standard. A 10 cm hollow rod was also placed as a control on the contralateral side to ensure scaling for run to run variations. Care was taken to ensure that the hollow regions were filled with gel. The point SAR at the tip of the rod was estimated (based on linear line fitting) from the slope of the first 5 s of temperature changes during the RF exposure. The mean of three measurements was reported. From repeated measurements by repositioning the rod, the standard deviation of the measurements was found to be <25%.

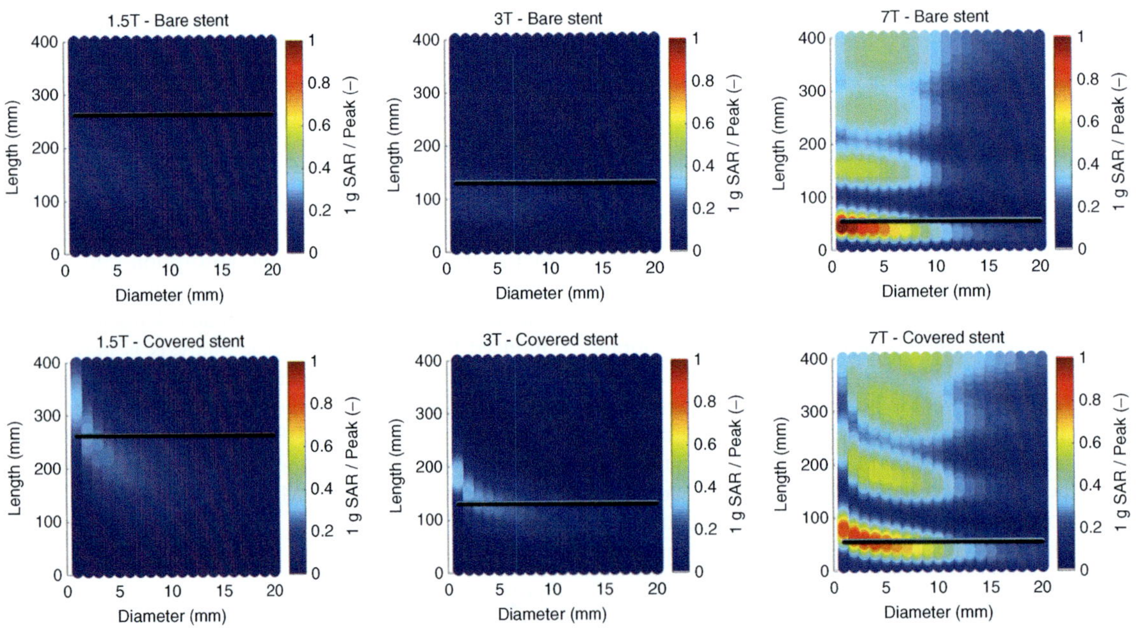

Figure 21.1. Results of HFSS simulation showing the maximum relative 1 g average SAR around the tip of hollow rod devices, as a function of length and internal diameter. The black horizontal line denotes the resonant length for the covered rods

Table 21.1. Relative SAR derived from EM simulations at the tip of 3 mm diameter hollow rods

Field	Length (mm)	Relative SAR bare rods ($W\,kg^{-1}$)	Relative SAR covered rods ($W\,kg^{-1}$)
1.5 T	150	0.122	0.109
	250	0.072	0.262
3.0 T	110	0.149	0.203
	150	0.064	0.279
7 T	45	0.854	0.512
	60	0.47	0.801

21.3 RESULTS

Figure 21.1 shows the results of the HFSS simulation across the range of parameters (diameter of hollow rod: *X*-axis, length: *Y*-axis, and color: relative 1 g average SAR). The top row depicts the results for bare rods and bottom row for the covered rods. The relative SAR values extracted from the chart for resonant heating lengths are shown in Table 21.1. It has been well established that the maximum SAR occurs near the tips of the rods. In addition, the behavior of rod diameter is more striking for the covered rods, with non-linear drop in the 1 g SAR with increase in diameter.

Figure 21.2 shows the measured relative SAR at the tip of the rods from the slope of the heating curve for different lengths ($°C\,s^{-1}$). At 64 MHz, the bare rods show maximum heating at a length of 150 mm as expected ($0.38\,°C\,s^{-1}$), whereas the covered rods show most heating ($2\,°C\,s^{-1}$ which is >5 times that of bare) at the longest length tested (250 mm). At 128 MHz, the bare rods show maximum heating at a length of 110 mm ($0.8\,°C\,s^{-1}$) and the covered rods show most heating ($9.3\,°C\,s^{-1}$) at the longest length tested (200 mm).

21.4 DISCUSSION

Computational results demonstrate that the heating effects of bare metal constructs are consistent with what has been reported previously.[6] A maximum in 1 gm SAR is observed for characteristic resonant lengths (20, 10, and 5 cm for 64, 128, and 300 MHz). The term 'resonant length' is used to denote the rod length that shows maximum peak heating. Interestingly, the maximum value increases with frequency (from 0.1 at 64 MHz to 1 at 300 MHz), for a given incident electric field ($Ez = 100\,V\,m^{-1}$). As has been previously reported there is a slight decrease in heating with diameter, more pronounced at lower frequencies. A significant increase is seen in the resonant heating lengths and the local 1 g average SAR upon covering the bare rod on the outside. It has been hypothesized that the higher heating is caused by the build-up of electric fields due to the insulation and the focused dissipative pathways for the insulated constructs. The increase in resonant length due to insulation is less intuitive and has been described by Bottomley *et al.*[3]

Experimental results of heating rates (at 64 and 128 MHz), at the tips of the rods, confirm the trends observed in computational modeling for the behavior of induced heating versus length. Significantly higher heating is observed using the covered rods, compared to the bare rods. In addition, the resonant lengths for the covered rods have been markedly altered due to the presence of covering and appear to be not included within the range of lengths tested.

Regarding the limitations of the study, the comparisons of 1 g average SAR (in simulations) to point SAR measurements (ASTM) show some disparities, possibly due to differences in simulations and measurements and/or averaging effects. For example, in simulations, the 150 mm bare rod at 64 MHz shows higher values compared to the covered rod, whereas measurement showed higher values of SAR for the covered rod. Also, the SAR for the measured values of 200 mm covered rod at 128 MHz, is higher than that of 150 mm as derived from modeling. The modeling uses a plane wave exposure versus the experiments which were performed in a body coil and hence subject to E-field variations. The modeling was performed with copper, whereas the experiments were carried out with stainless-steel rods. The modeling studies 1 gm average SAR, whereas the experiments yield an estimate of point SAR in the holes that are drilled at the tip of the rod.

21.5 SUMMARY

Computational modeling, as well as ASTM measurements, shows that the magnitude of the induced heating and the length where the induced heating is maximum (i.e. resonant length) may be significantly altered due to the material (such as insulation) present around a bare metallic construct. Careful characterization of such effects is needed to evaluate safety of patients wearing conductive devices and undergoing MRI.

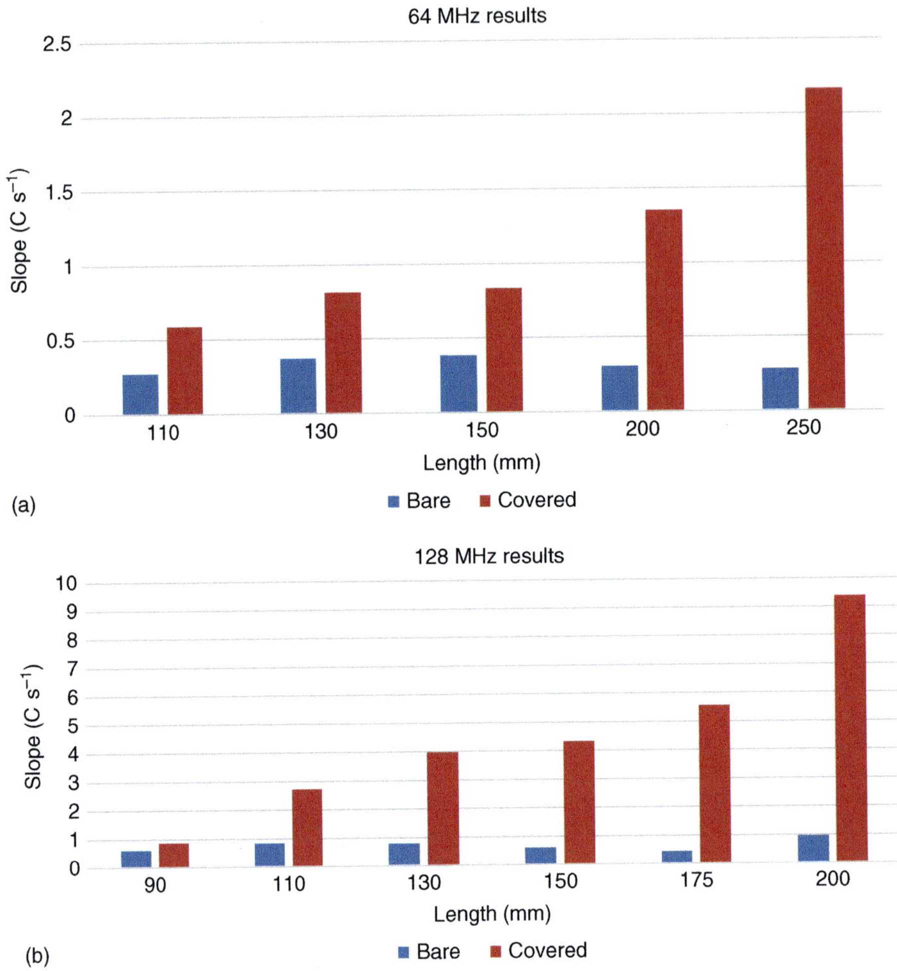

Figure 21.2. Values of the slope of temperature change at the tip of the hollow stainless steel rod, measured using the first 5 s of RF exposure as a function of the length, for bare and covered constructs, at 64 MHz (a) and 128 MHz (b)

DISCLAIMER

The mention of commercial products, their sources, or their use in connection with material reported herein is not to be construed as either an actual or suggested endorsement of such products by the Department of Health and Human Services.

RELATED ARTICLES IN EMAGRES

High-Field Whole Body Systems

Conradi, Mark S.: Evolution of NMR Hardware

TEM Fields and SAR

A Standard Procedure for Analyzing Radio Frequency MRI Coils

Radiofrequency Fields and SAR for Bird Cage Coils

Radiofrequency Heating Models and Measurements

Safety Considerations in MRI

Imaging around Orthopedic Hardware: Clinical Applications

REFERENCES

1. H. Bassen, W. Kainz, G. Mendoza, and T. Kellom, *Minim. Invasive Ther. Allied Technol.*, 2006, **15**, 76. DOI: 10.1080/13645700600640931.
2. C. Armenean, E. Perrin, M. Armenean, O. Beuf, F. Pilleul, and H. Saint-Jalmes, *Magn. Reson. Med.*, 2004, **52**, 1200. DOI: 10.1002/mrm.20246.
3. P. A. Bottomley, A. Kumar, W. A. Edelstein, J. M. Allen, and P. V. Karmarkar, *Med. Phys.*, 2010, **37**, 3828. DOI: 10.1118/1.3439590.
4. D. Santoro, L. Winter, A. Müller, J. Vogt, W. Renz, C. Özerdem, A. Grässl, V. Tkachenko, J. Schulz-Menger, and T. Niendorf, *PLoS One*, 2012, **7**, e49963.
5. ASTM-F2182–11. Standard test method for measurement of radio frequency induced heating on or near passive implants during magnetic resonance imaging, http://www.astm.org/Standards/F2182.htm (2011).
6. T. Song, Z. Xu, M. I. Iacono, L. M. Angelone, and S. Rajan, *Magn. Reson. Med.*, 2018, **80**, 2726.

Chapter 22

On the Development of a Novel Leg Phantom for RF Safety Assessment for Circular Ring External Fixation Devices in 1.5 T

Xing Huang[1] and Ji Chen[2]

[1]*Abbott Laboratories, Chicago, IL, USA*
[2]*University of Houston, Houston, TX, USA*

22.1 INTRODUCTION

Circular external fixation devices are special forms of an external fixator module used in bone construction. Compared to modular external fixation, these circular devices help improve the stability and configurability and cause minimal invasive damage to soft tissue. For these reasons, within decades, people have come to prefer circular external fixators. However, on the flip side, circular external fixation devices tend to produce relatively more tissue heating due to the radio frequency (RF) power deposition during magnetic resonance imaging (MRI). This chapter discusses the assessment of tissue heating near circular external fixation devices induced due to the RF power deposition from whole-body coils in MRI. To help evaluate the RF-induced heating, a novel testing leg phantom is proposed and examined. Later, numerical studies are performed for the worst-case RF heating determination.

To analyze the RF-induced heating effects of circular external fixation devices, the ASTM standard to assess the RF-induced heating F2182 is not applicable.[1] The fact that the circular external fixation devices are not implantable prevents the applicability of the standard. The large metallic conductive loop induces extra current and impacts RF heating.[2] Additionally, the geometry of the fixation devices precludes using the standard ASTM phantom for such devices. This is so because the existing ASTM phantom is a rectangular container, which is not physically robust enough to enforce every pin around the ring frame of circular external fixation device to be inserted into the phantom from any direction.

Under certain circumstances, it is possible to use virtual family human models to help evaluate the RF-induced heating effects (e.g., Refs 3,4). However, those human models have limitations as well. First and foremost, virtual family models are computational models that are developed from a series of MR scan pictures with finite spatial resolution and limited contrast. Although widely used, appropriate in vivo validation of the suitability of the tissue segmentation,

Safety and Biological Effects in MRI.
Edited by Devashish Shrivastava and J. Thomas Vaughan
 ISBN: 978-1-118-82130-5
Also published in eMagRes (online edition)
DOI: 10.1002/9780470034590.emrstm1573

tissue properties, etc. of these models in predicting electromagnetic fields, induced power deposition, etc. in humans or human-relevant animals for MR applications is still eluding. Thus, simulation results alone may not be sufficient to 'truly' evaluate the RF Safety of devices. Second, the virtual family human models contain about 80 different tissues. The large heterogeneity and fine mesh used to distinguish organs requires long simulation time and large GPU memory. For instance, a single DUKE simulation with the presence of a circular external fixation device using 2 mm grid resolution takes about 10 h and 6G GPU memory to arrive at converged results. For GPUs with smaller memory capacity, the simulation will be much more time-consuming. Last but not least, the effects of different variables can be confounded with each other when using the human models. Unlike the ASTM phantom, which has a regular shape and uniform properties, the human models do not have uniform geometry and properties. Even if we are able to get the simulation results after a long simulation time, a robust conclusion cannot be easily drawn because multiple parameters are changing at the same time. Thus, in order to assess the MRI RF coil-induced heating effects for circular external fixation devices efficiently, there is a need for developing a novel testing phantom which is regular in shape, as simple as possible to reduce simulation complexity, and representative for human models.

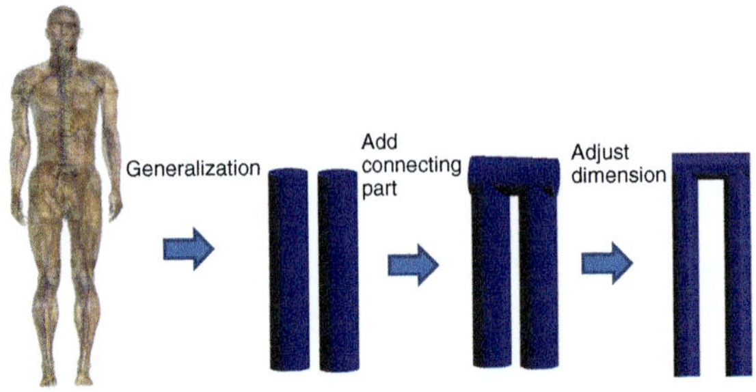

Figure 22.1. Procedures to design the leg phantom

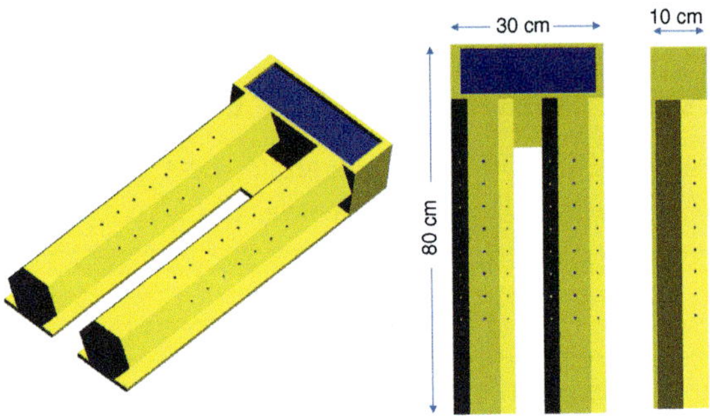

Figure 22.2. Basic dimensions of the leg phantom

22.2 METHODOLOGY

The basic idea of developing such a phantom is shown in Figure 22.1. Since we focus on the lower part of the human body, two cylinders are used to represent two legs. The connecting part is added to retain the connectivity of two legs as in human models. The shape and dimension of the testing leg phantom is then adjusted to get an optimal design.

When manufacturing the leg phantom for experiment test, the physical robustness of the liquid holder that can contain the leg phantom gel should also be considered. In accordance with the existing standard, the leg phantom gel should simulate the overall human body electromagnetic and thermal properties, where the holder needs to be electrically insulated. For ease of inserting the leg phantom inside MRI RF coil and keeping it stable, a hexagon-shaped leg instead of cylinder is used. As shown in Figure 22.2, the struts also improve the stability of leg phantom holder. On the upper surface of the holder, several holes with a diameter of $^1/_4$ in. are drilled for pin insertion. When the leg phantom is used for the experimental test, all the holes including the ones that are inserted with screws will be filled with engineering clay. The clay is an electrically insulating material so that the electric property of the liquid holder will not change. To approximate the size of human models, the leg phantom is designed to have a dimension of 80 cm length, 30 cm width, and 10 cm height, as indicated in Figure 22.2. Figure 22.3 shows the morphology comparison between the DUKE model and the leg phantom.

Before we use the leg phantom for numerical investigation of circular external fixation devices, it is critical to examine the validity of the novel testing phantom. The process of determining whether a leg phantom gets an optimal design is to inspect the electric field and/or specific absorption rate (SAR) distribution inside or around the leg phantom and to compare with the field distribution for human models. In the following section, two sets of simulations are conducted to develop the leg phantom: unloaded leg phantom/human model in MRI RF coil comparison and loaded leg phantom/human model in MRI RF coil comparison.

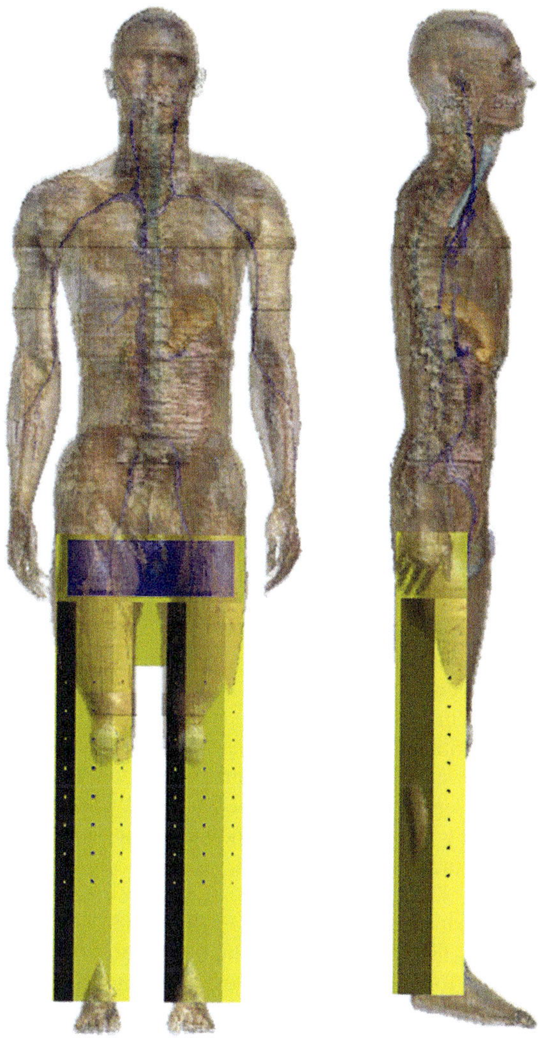

Figure 22.3. Morphology comparison between the DUKE model and the leg phantom

The first group of simulations is set up for an unloaded leg phantom and human model placed in a whole-body 1.5 T (resonant frequency = 64 MHz) MRI RF coil. No medical devices are present in this simulation study. Both the leg phantom and human model are placed in a similar position where most of the leg component is in the center of the RF coil as shown in Figure 22.4. The electromagnetic properties of human tissues are retrieved from the ITIS database.[3,4] Due to the absence of circular external fixation devices, there is no significant energy deposition inside the leg phantom or human body. In other words, SAR values are relatively small and thus are ignored. In these cases, only the electric field distribution is taken into consideration. Different loading positions are studied to evaluate the similarities and differences between the leg phantom and human model. Loading position is defined as the distance between the transverse (i.e., axial) center plane of the RF coil to the center axial plane of the leg phantom/human legs. The loading position is defined to be zero at the position shown in Figure 22.4, where positive loading position means that the leg phantom or human leg is moving upward in the longitudinal direction.

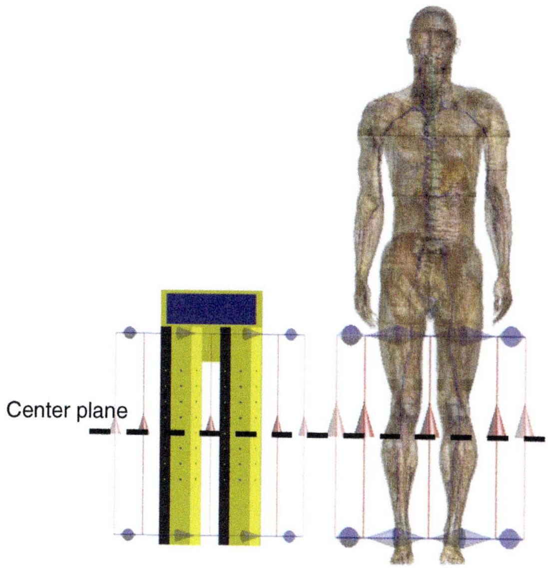

Figure 22.4. Illustration of center plane and 0 mm loading position for the leg phantom and the human model

Figure 22.5 shows a comparison of the electric field distribution between the leg phantom and human model in the center plane. The field patterns appear comparable. Electric fields in both the leg phantom and human simulations reach minimum near the inner side of the legs. Progressing outward, larger electric fields are observed. The electric field outside the leg phantom or human leg is even larger and reaches its maximum in the space between the legs.

In addition to the general distribution, a comparison of the amplitude of the electric field is essential to show that the leg phantom may be an effective tool to simulate relevant human environment and evaluate the effect of device parameters (such as geometry and dimensions) and positioning on the induced RF heating. The amplitude of the electric field is proportional to the square root of input power, which is referred to as the normalization factor in most simulation studies. Three normalization methods are commonly used and studied here: (i) Normal whole-body SAR (wbSAR) (i.e., $2\,W\,kg^{-1}$) method, (ii) partial body SAR (*pbSAR*) method, and (iii) B_1-field method.[5,6] For each method, the electric field in the center line that goes across the leg phantom or human knee position (denoted as the green line in Figure 22.5) is plotted.

The wbSAR method is commonly used for most situations. The input power is adjusted so that the whole-body SAR is normalized to the $2\,W\,kg^{-1}$ of absorbed power as specified in international standard ASTM F2182. The entire human body and the leg phantom weights were obtained by the integration of each small segment in the simulation domain. By following the wbSAR method, the electric field plot can be seen as in Figure 22.6. The two legs are positioned between the coordinates −0.15 to −0.05 m and 0.05 to 0.15 m. Although the electric field inside the phantom is of similar magnitude compared with human body simulation, the field between the two legs is about $700\,V\,m^{-1}$, which is smaller than the $\boldsymbol{E}$ field for human body (about $950\,V\,m^{-1}$).

Figure 22.6 shows that using wbSAR normalization method may give underestimated results. The reason can be explained by the power deposition difference between the leg phantom and the human body. For the leg phantom, most of the phantom portion is within the accessible region of the RF coil. For the human body, while the energy is still concentrated near the accessible region, the whole-body mass becomes large since the complete human body is included. Given the same input power, the whole-body SAR for the human body

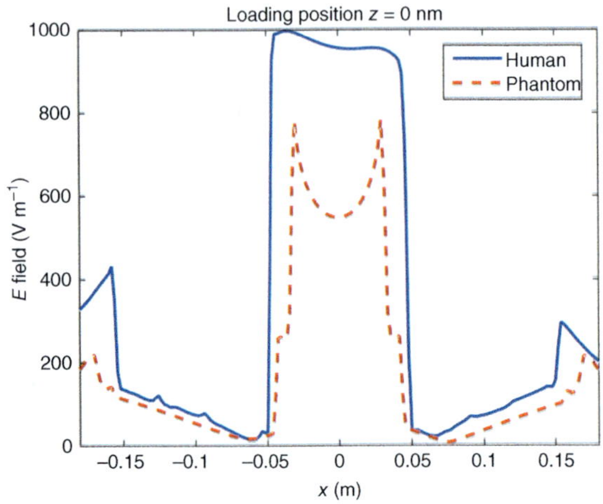

Figure 22.6. E_{RMS} field distribution along the center line for the leg phantom and the human model when the normal whole-body SAR is used for normalization

is less than that of the leg phantom since the weight of the leg phantom is less than that from the entire human body model. As a result, more input power is required for human models. Under this situation, the electric field in human model becomes relatively higher because most of the energy consumption is concentrated near the leg part of the human body. Thus, the leg phantom using wbSAR normalization may underestimate RF coil-induced heating.

The *pbSAR* is also used in some simulation studies. As described in standard IEC-60601-2-33, it is used for cases in which most of the human body part is outside the RF coil. The partial body SAR is defined as the SAR averaged over the mass of the body that is exposed by the RF coil. The mass used to determine

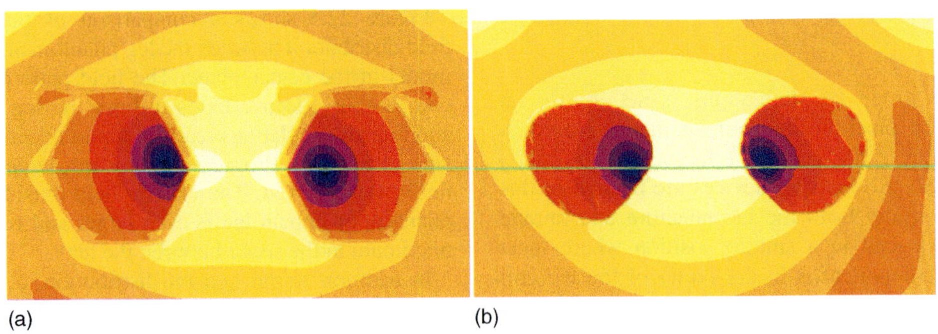

Figure 22.5. E_{RMS} field distribution pattern on the center plane for the leg phantom (a) and the human model (b). The green line denotes the center line

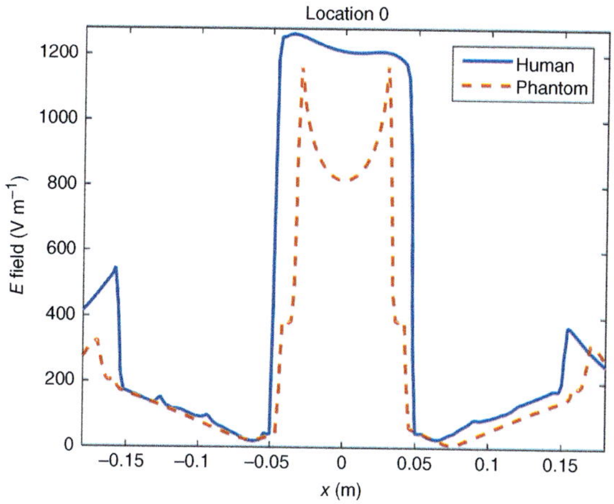

Figure 22.7. E_{RMS} electric field distribution along the center line for the leg phantom and the human model when partial body SAR normalization is used

the *pbSAR* is called the exposed mass. It is given by the mass within the effective volume of the RF coil. The effective volume of the RF transmit coil is the volume in which no more than 95% of the total absorbed RF power is deposited inside a homogeneous material which fills the volume normally accessible by the patient. For the partial body SAR, the SAR limit scales dynamically with the ratio of the exposed mass to the total mass. For a normal operating mode, the pbSAR limit is

$$\text{pbSAR} = 10 - 8\frac{m_{\text{exposed}}}{m_{\text{total}}}$$

where pbSAR is in unit of W kg^{-1}, m_{exposed} is the exposed mass, and m_{total} is the total mass.

The electric field plot along the center line using the pbSAR normalization is shown in Figure 22.7. Compared with the wbSAR plot in Figure 22.6, the ***E*** field difference between the leg phantom and the human model becomes less significant. The leg phantom using the pbSAR normalization may still, however, underestimate the RF heating because the electric field between the legs is still relatively less in the leg phantom compared to the human body model.

Both wbSAR and pbSAR normalizations are significantly affected by the mass that is present in the MRI system. Regardless of the mass, the B1+ normalization method is proposed based on the fact that the image quality of MRI is closely related to the amplitude of the MRI RF pulse. During MRI, the B1+ field remains unchanged to achieve good signal-to-noise ratio (SNR)

Table 22.1. B_1 field at the isocenter for different loading positions using 2 W kg^{-1} wbSAR normalization

Loading position	B_1 field in leg phantom (μT)	B_1 field in human model (μT)
−400	6.87	4.58
−300	5.80	4.67
−200	5.03	5.14
−100	4.46	5.68
0	4.16	6.78
100	3.92	7.67
200	3.85	8.31
300	3.94	8.90
400	4.24	9.87

for imaging. In the MR system, the B1+ and B1− fields are defined as the rotational components of the B_1 field (typically used for RF field analysis) with the formulae:

$$B_1+(r) = \frac{1}{2}(\text{B}(r)\cdot\hat{x} + j\text{B}(r)\cdot\hat{y})$$
$$B_1-(r) = \frac{1}{2}(\text{B}(r)\cdot\hat{x} - j\text{B}(r)\cdot\hat{y})^*$$

The B1+ and B1− fields are calculated at the isocenter, which is located at the geometric center of the RF coil. During the normalization process, the B_1 field, which is chosen from the B1+ or B1− field with larger amplitude, is normalized to a constant value. The scaled input power is then calculated by the square of B_1-field scaling. Table 22.1 lists the B_1 field at the isocenter for different loading positions when using 2 W kg^{-1} wbSAR normalization. As the loading position moves from −400 to 400 mm, the B_1 field in leg phantom first decreases and then increases, while the B_1 field in the human model grows continuously. At the loading position of −200 mm, the B_1 value in leg phantom is close to the B_1 value in the human body. By taking the average of these similar B_1-field values, the normalized B_1 field for all loading positions is chosen to be 5.08 μT.

Based on B_1 normalization, the *x*, *y*, and *z* components of electric field along the center line are presented in Figures 22.8, 22.9, and 22.10, respectively. By examining the real and imaginary parts of each component, the unloaded leg phantom is proved to be

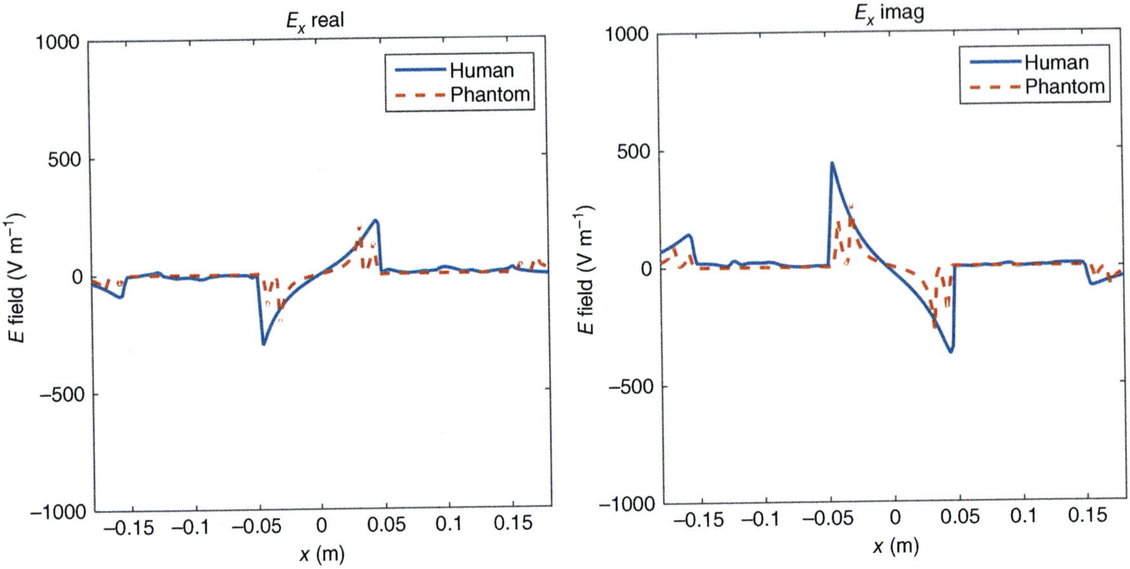

Figure 22.8. x component of the electric field along the center line using B_1-field normalization

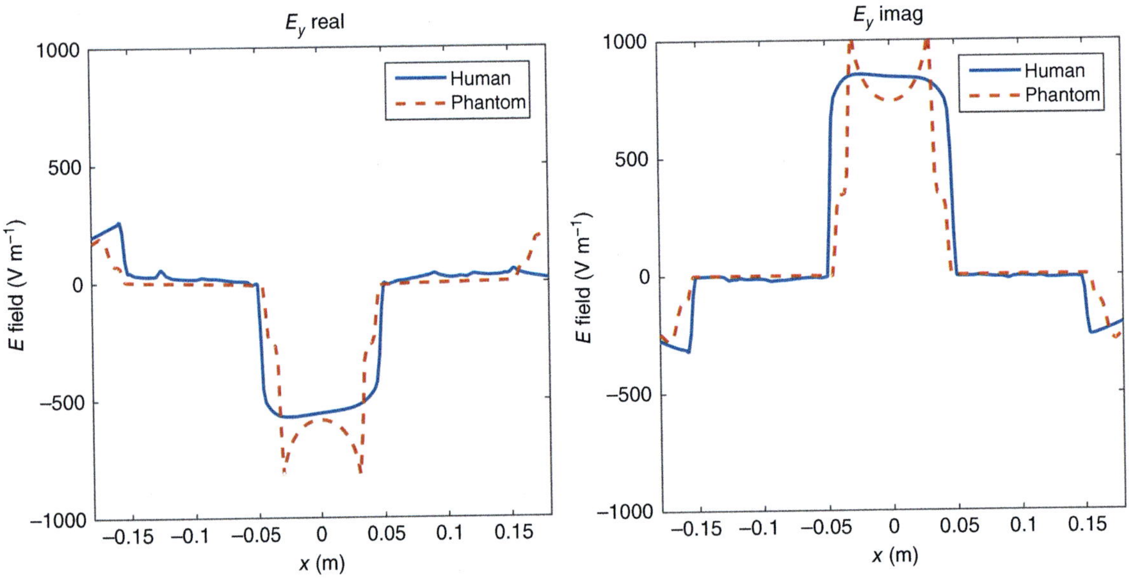

Figure 22.9. y component of the electric field along the center line using B_1-field normalization

consistent with the human model in terms of electric field distribution.

The RMS value of the total electric field along the center line is plotted in Figure 22.11. The two curves in Figure 22.11 are overlapping with each other, indicating that the overall impacts are similar.

Beyond case $z=0$, the B_1 normalization method is also valid for other loading positions.

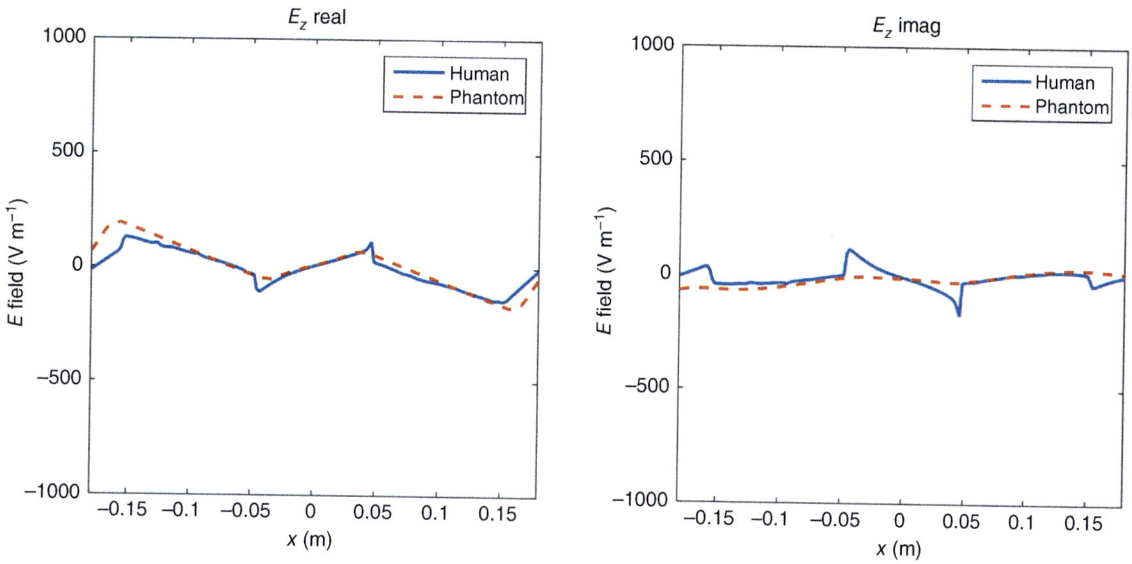

Figure 22.10. z component of the electric field along the center line using B_1-field normalization

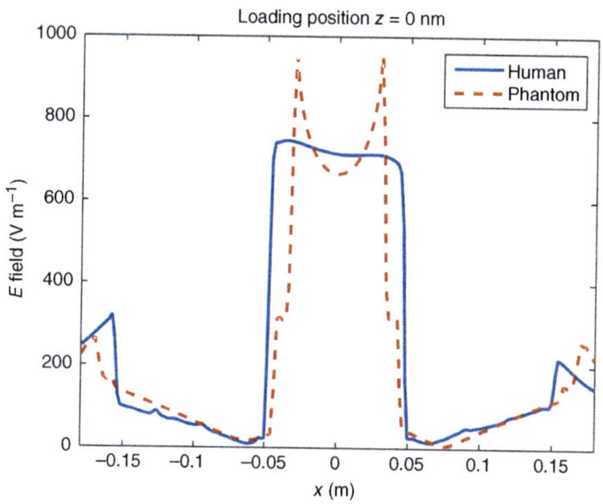

Figure 22.11. E_{RMS} field along the center line at 0 mm loading position using B_1-field normalization

Figures 22.12–22.15 show the electric field comparison between the leg phantom and the human model at different positions along the center line.

From the above plots, it is clear that the leg phantom can be used to represent human model simulations using the B_1 normalization method. The normalized field has a similar distribution to that of the human model for different loading positions ranging from −400 to 400 mm. The material below presents a comparison of the effect of the loading of a circular fixation device for the leg phantom and whole-body human model.

The simulation setup is depicted in Figure 22.16. The leg phantom and human model are placed at a loading position $z=0$. A typical circular external fixation device is placed near the knee position of the human body. The center of circular external fixation device coincides with the center of the RF coil in the longitudinal direction. The absolute position of the circular external fixation device is kept the same for the left and right configurations in Figure 22.16.

Due to the presence of the conductive device, the electric field distribution in both the leg phantom and human body is altered by the surface current induced by the device. The overall effect of the altered electric field is the accumulation of power dissipation near the tip of the screws that impinge into the leg phantom or human body. SAR is calculated to quantify the power dissipation. Figure 22.17 shows the SAR distribution for the circular external fixation device loaded into the leg phantom near the top ring frame. Energy is concentrated near the tip of the impinging screw and decays dramatically in the leg phantom gel.

The same SAR behavior is observed for circular external fixation devices loading into the human model. In Figure 22.18, the maximum SAR occurs at the tip of the screw. Although the field distribution shows some singularity due to the inhomogeneity of human body

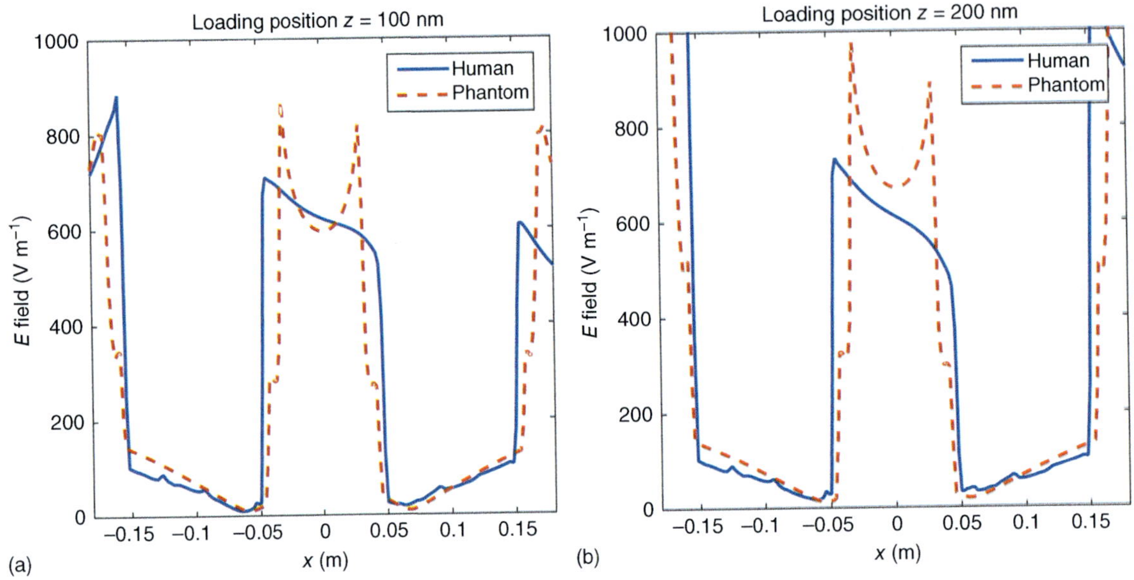

Figure 22.12. E_{RMS} field along the center line at 100 mm (a) and 200 mm (b) loading position using B_1-field normalization

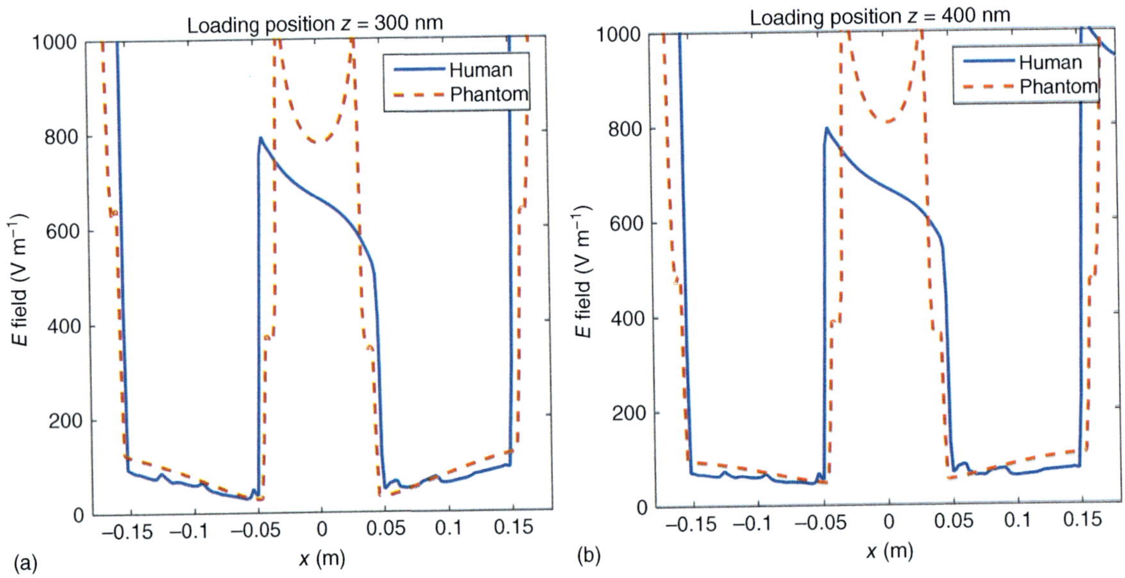

Figure 22.13. E_{RMS} field along the center line at 300 mm (a) and 400 mm (b) loading position using B_1-field normalization

tissue, the general pattern is still consistent with that of the leg phantom.

In addition to the SAR distribution pattern, the use of a normalization factor is also investigated. Due to the presence of large metallic medical devices, the conventional B_1 normalization method does not function well. Strong surface current on devices will induce a large scattered field, which has a notable impact on B1+ or B1− field computation. The B_1-field calculation at the isocenter will become more difficult

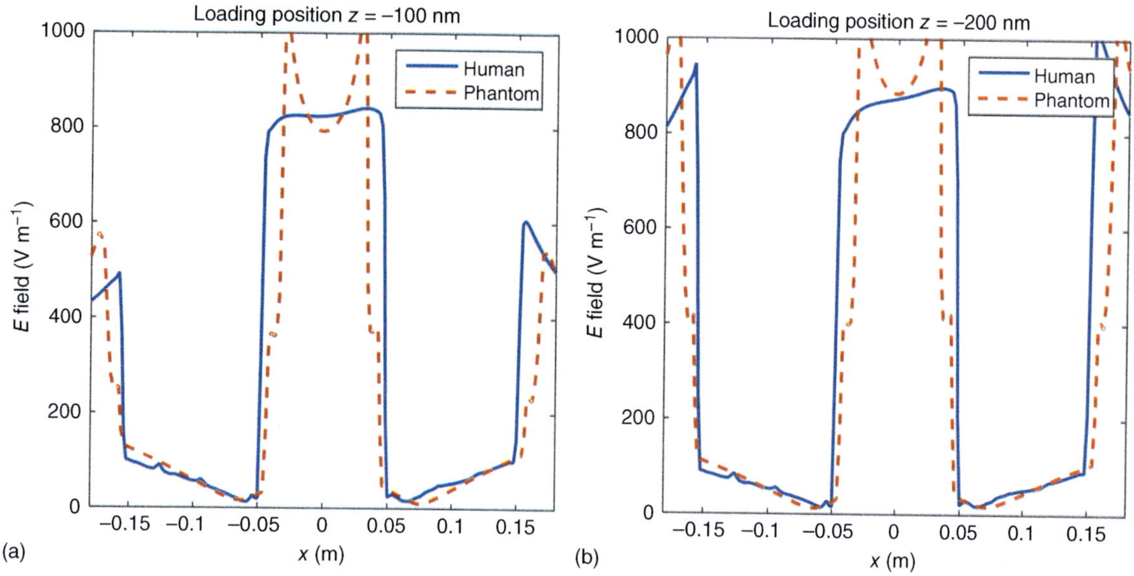

Figure 22.14. E_{RMS} field along the center line at −100 mm (a) and −200 mm (b) loading position using B_1-field normalization

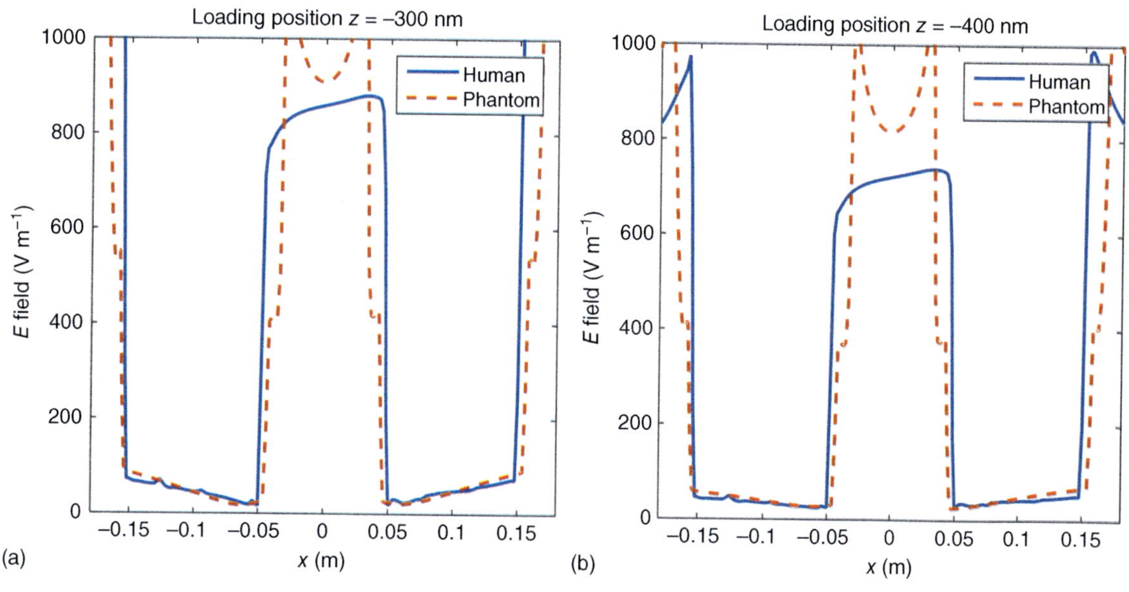

Figure 22.15. E_{RMS} field along the center line at −300 mm (a) and −400 mm (b) loading position using B_1-field normalization

for circular external fixation devices in this case because the location of the circular external fixation devices is very close to the RF coil isocenter. The incident B_1 field is used as normalization criteria instead of B_1 field. The incident field refers to the electric fields associated with the unloaded leg phantom or human body in MRI RF coil, which has been studied in the previous section. To distinguish from the incident field, the electric fields from induced current on circular external fixation devices are referred to

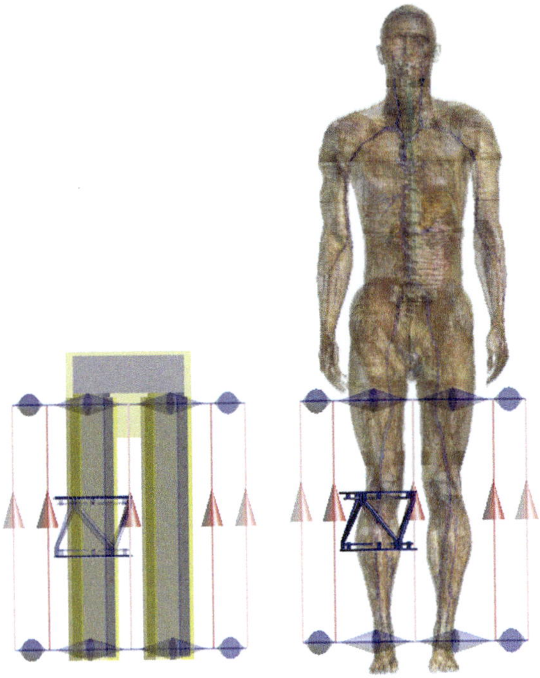

Figure 22.16. Simulation setup for the leg phantom and the human model with the presence of circular external fixation device

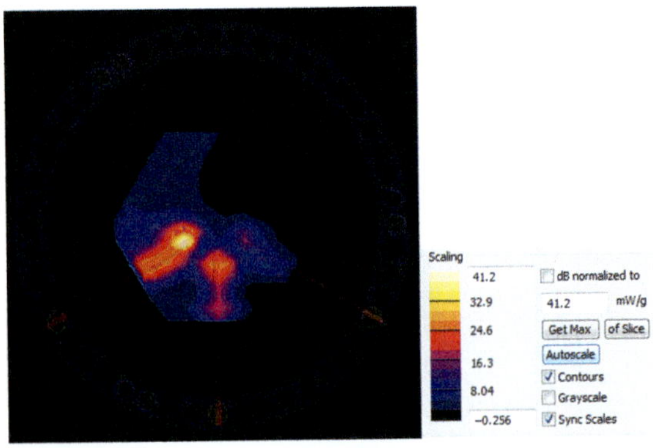

Figure 22.17. SAR distribution for circular external fixation device loaded into the leg phantom

as the induced field. The incident field is calculated without the presence of the circular external fixation device. No matter what the circular external fixation device is, the incident B_1 field is constant. The total electromagnetic field is the superposition of incident field and induced field.

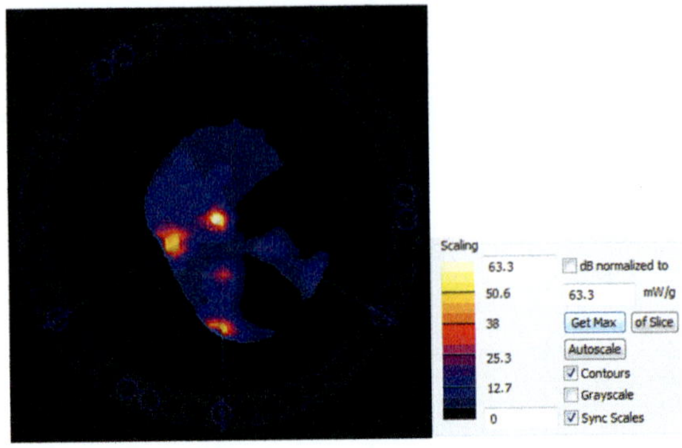

Figure 22.18. SAR distribution for circular external fixation device loaded inside the human model

The processes to obtain the same incident B_1 field are described as follows: (i) Use the conventional source settings to run an unloaded leg phantom/human simulation. Record the input power without any normalization. The power that excites the incident field is defined as the 'prenormalized incident power', which means the total input power when using the predefined source settings. (ii) Adjust the normalization factor so that the B_1 field at the isocenter is equal to 5.08 μT, which is derived in the previous section. The total input power is called the 'B_1-normalized incident power'. (iii) Apply the same source settings and run a simulation with the presence of the circular external fixation device. Input power is then obtained without normalization. The power is referred to as the 'prenormalized total power'. (iv) 'Incident B_1-normalized total power' is calculated by

$$P^{\text{tot}}_{B_{1_{\text{inc}}}} = \frac{P^{\text{tot}}}{P^{\text{inc}}} P^{\text{inc}}_{B_1}$$

where P^{inc} is prenormalized incident power, P^{tot} is prenormalized total power, $P^{\text{inc}}_{B_1}$ is B_1-normalized incident power, and $P^{\text{tot}}_{B_{1_{\text{inc}}}}$ is incident B_1-normalized total power. Using the incident B_1 normalization, the RF coil-induced heating effect can be quantified.

Figure 22.19 shows the induced surface current distribution for a typical circular external fixation device exposed in MRI RF environment. It is observed that currents are induced from ring and struts structure of circular external fixation as well as the pin. Different parameters of the external fixation device are studied including (i) insertion depth, (ii) ring frame size, (iii) strut height, and (iv) loading position. These parameters are chosen because the largest induced current appears at the ring frame structure, the struts, and the pins that enter the human body, as indicated

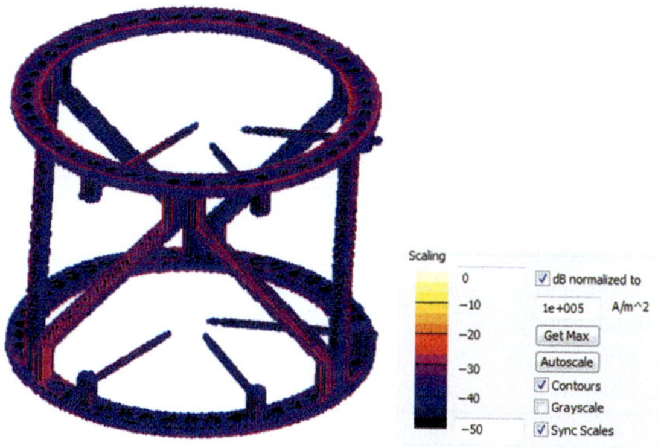

Figure 22.19. Induced surface current distribution for a typical circular external fixation device in an RF environment

in Figure 22.19. In addition, the effect of loading position needs to be assessed because patients with medical devices are frequently loaded in or out of the MR machine during the MR scanning procedure. By showing the maximum 1 g-averaged SAR tendency affected by each parameter, the leg phantom is proved to be representative for human model.

22.2.1 Insertion Depth

The insertion depth is the length that a screw is immersed inside the phantom gel or the human body as shown in Figure 22.20. It plays an important part in the RF coil-induced heating because the insertion depth determines the path that energy takes during dissipation in the leg phantom or the human model. Insertion depths are chosen as 25, 35, and 45 mm to show the validity of the leg phantom. For each insertion depth, the circular external fixation device is placed near the human model as well as leg phantom.

Table 22.2 shows the incident B_1-normalized total power for each simulation and maximum 1 g-averaged SAR. The relationship between maximum 1 g-averaged SAR and insertion depth is plotted in Figure 22.21. As the insertion depth increases, the RF heating effects tend to decrease. Because the leg phantom gel is electrically lossy like the human tissues, when the insertion depth gets larger, the induced energy that travels along the pin to the tip will lead to more power dissipation along the path. Less energy will be dissipated at the pin tip. On the other hand, if the insertion depth becomes very short, the dissipated power is concentrated on the tip of the pin.

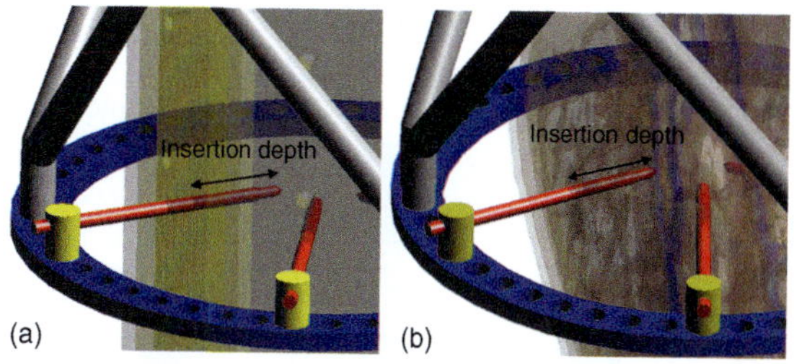

Figure 22.20. Illustration of insertion depth for circular external fixation device in the leg phantom (a) and the human model (b)

Table 22.2. Maximum 1 g-averaged SAR for different insertion depths

Model	Insertion depth (mm)	Incident B_1-normalized total power (W)	Maximum 1 g-averaged SAR (W kg^{-1})
Leg phantom	25	199.38	79.6
Leg phantom	35	199.38	60.6
Leg phantom	45	199.38	47.8
Human model	25	147.53	62.9
Human model	35	147.53	48.5
Human model	45	147.53	39.8

The pin will reserve the most power and generate the worst-case heating.

22.2.2 Ring Frame Size

Ring frame size can also affect the RF coil-induced heating. For the leg phantom validation process, the radius of the ring size is selected to be 89, 99, and 109 mm as shown in Figure 22.22.

When loading the leg phantom or the human model with the circular external fixation device with varying ring radii, the maximum 1 g-averaged SAR is calculated as shown in Table 22.3. Figure 22.23 shows the trend of the maximum 1 g-averaged SAR varying with the ring size. As the radius of the ring frame grows, the maximum SAR near the tip of the pins in the human body increases. The same tendency is observed for both leg phantom and human simulations. This observation suggests that a large conductive loop will easily receive RF signals and strongly impact the current distribution in tissue. The larger the ring size is, the higher the RF heating will be.

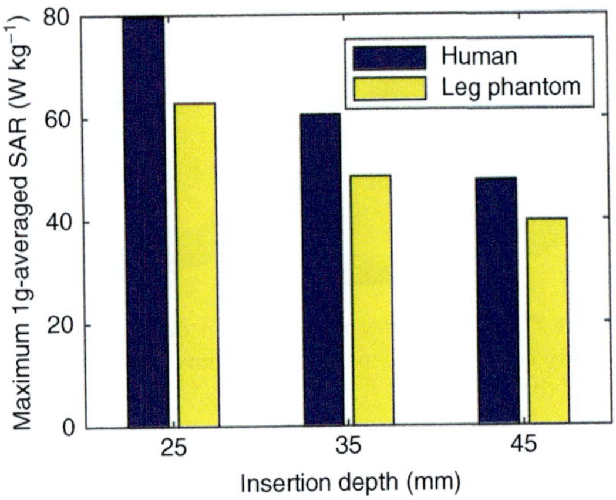

Figure 22.21. Maximum 1 g-averaged SAR versus insertion depth for the leg phantom and the human model

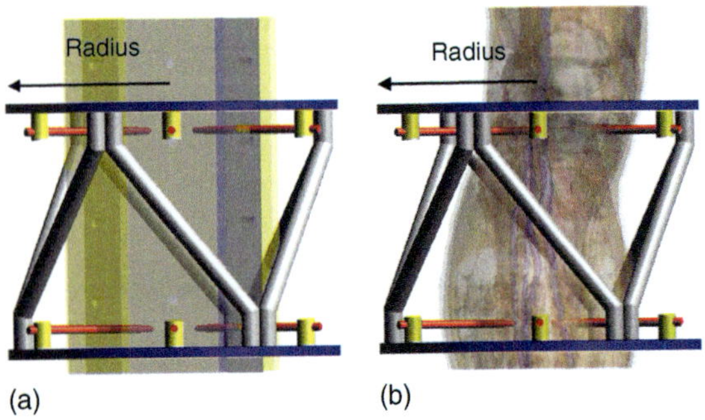

Figure 22.22. Illustration of ring frame radius for circular external fixation device in the leg phantom (a) and the human model (b)

Table 22.3. Maximum 1 g-averaged SAR for different ring frame radii

Model	Ring frame radius (mm)	Incident B_1-normalized total power (W)	Maximum 1 g-averaged SAR (W kg^{-1})
Leg phantom	89	199.38	57.3
Leg phantom	99	199.38	60.6
Leg phantom	109	199.38	66
Human model	89	147.53	41.7
Human model	99	147.53	48.5
Human model	109	147.53	53.5

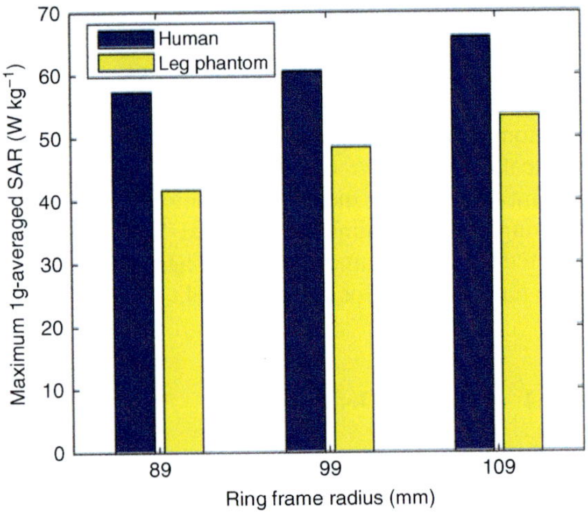

Figure 22.23. Maximum 1 g-averaged SAR versus ring frame radius for the leg phantom and the human model

22.2.3 Strut Height

Strut height is the vertical distance between the upper ring frame and the lower ring frame as described in Figure 22.24. To investigate the effect of strut height, the circular external fixation devices with different heights ranging from 140 to 170 mm are placed in leg phantom and the human model. The maximum 1 g-averaged SARs under MR environment are calculated after the incident B_1 normalization.

Table 22.4 shows how maximum 1 g-averaged SAR changes with strut height. To give a better illustration, the trend is also plotted in Figure 22.25. Because of the heterogeneity of human tissues and the irregular shape of human body, the fluctuation of maximum 1 g-averaged SAR versus strut height curve is expected. Although there is little deviation within the two curves, the basic trend is the same. The green dashed line in Figure 22.25 is a fitted line using linear regression. Generally speaking, the device with the shorter strut height will lead to the lower RF heating effect. The shorter the distance between the ring frames is, the weaker will be the coupling.

In addition to simulation results, an experiment was performed to estimate the MRI RF-induced heating inside an MRI shielding room. A testing 10 cm titanium rod is placed inside the leg phantom. The distance from the rod to the left inner edge of the phantom container is about 3 cm. The rod is located at the center plane of the left leg as shown in Figure 22.26.

In the experiment, the rod was fixed on a plastic frame and slides into the leg phantom as shown in Figure 22.27. The holes on the side wall are covered with engineering clay. The fishing line was used to

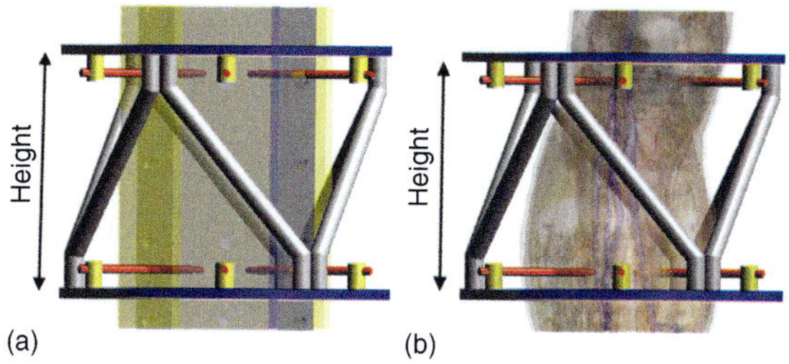

Figure 22.24. Illustration of strut height for circular external fixation device in the leg phantom (a) and the human model (b)

Table 22.4. Maximum 1 g-averaged SAR for different strut heights

Model	Strut height	Incident B_1-normalized total power	Maximum 1 g-averaged SAR
Human model	150	201.87	63.8
Human model	155	202.59	60.6
Human model	160	201.19	64.1
Leg phantom	150	162.25	47.4
Leg phantom	155	162.38	48.5
Leg phantom	160	161.83	50.6

push in or pull out the frame together with the rod. The employment of the fishing line and the plastic frame ensures that the rod is placed at the center of the leg phantom in the longitudinal direction.

The leg phantom loaded with the 10 cm rod is then placed at the center of the MRI bore (Figure 22.28). Before the thermal experiment was conducted, the H field at the isocenter of the RF coil was measured using H probe as shown in Figure 22.29.

The H field at the isocenter is 3.3 A m^{-1} when the MRI RF coil is turned on. The H field is used to normalize the input power in EM simulation. A temperature probe is attached at the tip of the rod and records the temperature during the 15 min MR exposure.

A verification simulation was run for comparison. When using H field normalization, the input power of the EM simulation is 102.6 W. The electric field, together with the normalization power factor, is used in thermal simulation. The thermal properties of the leg phantom gel, leg phantom shell, and the 10 cm rod are shown in Table 22.5. The EM source in the thermal simulation is turned on for 15 min and then turned off, so the rod will have 3 min cooling time. Figure 22.30 plots the temperature increase near the tip of the rod

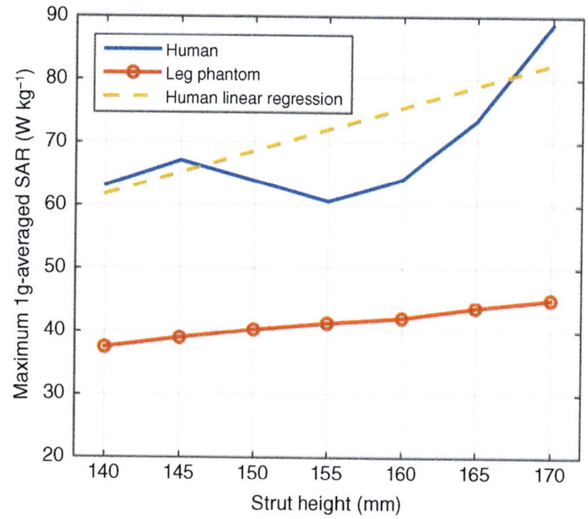

Figure 22.25. Maximum 1 g-averaged SAR versus strut height for the leg phantom and the human model. Dashed line denotes the linear regression of human data model

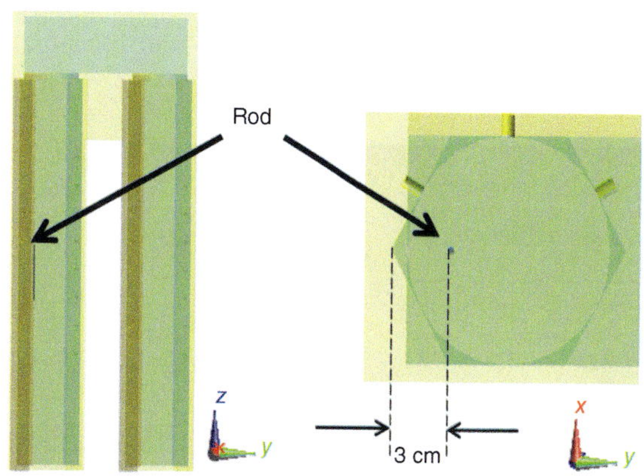

Figure 22.26. Illustration of experimental setup for leg phantom validation

in the experiment and the simulation and shows good agreement.[7]

22.3 CONCLUSION

The novel leg phantom has been shown to be a reasonable approximation to the complex human model to assess the RF heating effects of the circular external fixation devices in 1.5 T. For the generic circular external fixation devices used in this study, the maximum heating locations are close to the tips of the screws that

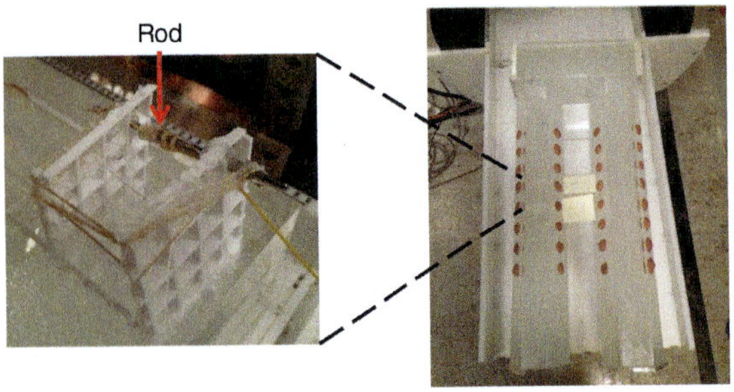

Figure 22.27. Experiment setup for rod with fixture and the placement in the leg phantom

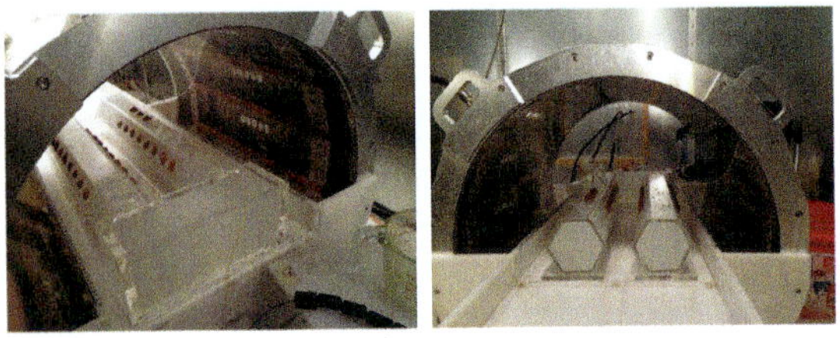

Figure 22.28. Side view of leg phantom with 10 cm rod loading inside the MRI bore

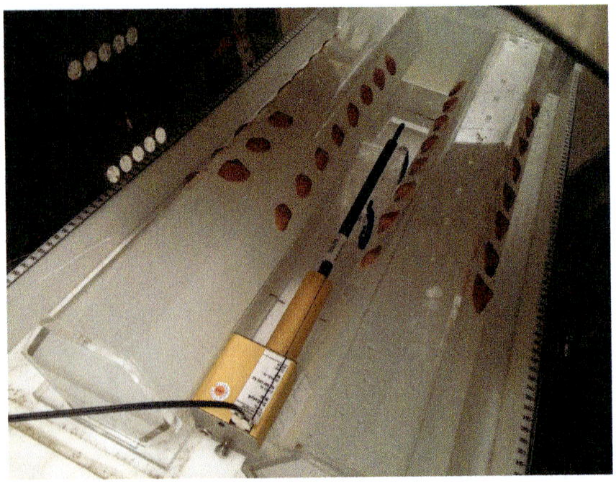

Figure 22.29. H probe measurement at isocenter

are inserted into the human body. Due to the presence of conductive loops, the circular external fixation can receive a large amount of RF power, and the induced energy is dissipated inside the human body or the phantom gel. Most of the energy is concentrated at the tips or edges of the impinging screws and thus causes significant RF heating effects near screw tips. The maximum 1 g-averaged SAR is shown to be a reasonable indicator of the induced temperature rise.

Table 22.5. Thermal properties of the materials

Model	Specific heat capacity ($J\,kg^{-1}\,K^{-1}$)	Thermal Conductivity ($W\,m^{-1}\,K^{-1}$)	Density ($kg\,m^{-3}$)
Leg phantom gel	4160	0.42	1000
Leg phantom shell	1000	0.2	1000
PEC	400	7	8000

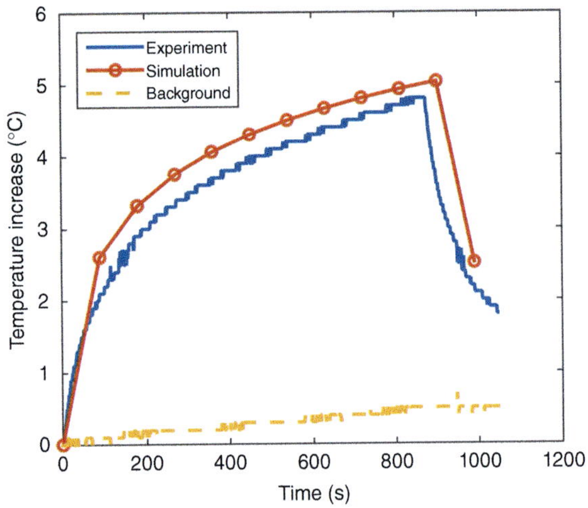

Figure 22.30. Temperature increase at the tip of 10 cm rod versus time

RELATED ARTICLES IN EMAGRES

Birdcage Resonators: Highly Homogeneous Radiofrequency Coils for Magnetic Resonance

Coils for Insertion into the Human Body

Design and Use of Internal Receiver Coils for Magnetic Resonance Imaging

Multifrequency Coils for Whole Body Studies

Radiofrequency Systems and Coils for MRI and MRS

Refrigerated and Superconducting Receiver Coils in Whole Body Magnetic Resonance

Spatial Encoding Using Multiple rf Coils: SMASH Imaging and Parallel MRI

Surface Coil NMR: Detection with Inhomogeneous Radiofrequency Field Antennas

Surface and Other Local Coils for In Vivo Studies

Whole Body Machines: NMR Phased Array Coil Systems

TEM Transceiver Head Array Coils for Ultra High Magnetic Fields

TEM Arrays, Design and Implementation

Quadrature Surface Coils

Double-Tuned Surface Coils

Quadrature Transverse Electromagnetic (TEM) Surface Coils

Radiofrequency Fields and SAR for Transverse Electromagnetic (TEM) Surface Coils

Double-Tuned Birdcage Coils: Construction and Tuning

Radiofrequency Fields and SAR for Bird Cage Coils

TEM Body Coils

Transverse Electromagnetic (TEM) Surface Coils for Extremities

Receiver Loop Arrays

Coil Array Design for Parallel Imaging: Theory and Applications

Millipede Coils

Microcoils

Catheter Coils

Radiofrequency Heating Models and Measurements

Characterization of Multichannel Coil Arrays on the Benchtop

A Standard Procedure for Analyzing Radio Frequency MRI Coils

Litz Coils for High Resolution and Animal Probes, Especially for Double Resonance

RF Field Modeling for Double-Tuned Volume Coils

An Historical Introduction to Surface Coils: The Early Days

Transceiver Loop Arrays

Radiofrequency Coils for NMR: A Peripatetic History of Their Twists and Turns

Nested Surface Coils for Multinuclear NMR

Birdcage Volume Coil Design

Bioeffects and Safety of Radiofrequency Electromagnetic Fields

Radiofrequency Fields: Interactions, Biological Effects, and Safety Issues

RF Device Safety and Compatibility

Safety Considerations in MRI

REFERENCES

1. ASTM F2182-19e2, Standard test method for measurement of radio frequency induced heating on or near passive implants during magnetic resonance imaging, ASTM International, West Conshohocken, PA, 2019.
2. J. D. Jackson, Classical Electrodynamics, 3rd edn, John Wiley & Sons: Chichester, UK, 1999.
3. A. Christ, W. Kainz, E. G. Hahn, K. Honegger, M. Zefferer, E. Neufeld, W. Rascher, R. Janka, W. Bautz, J. Chen, B. Kiefer, P. Schmitt, H.-P. Hollenbach, J. Shen, M. Oberle, D. Szczerba, A. Kam, J. W. Guag, and N. Kuster, *Phys. Med. Biol.*, 2010, **55**, N23.
4. M.-C. Gosselin, E. Neufeld, H. Moser, E. Huber, S. Farcito, L. Gerber, M. Jedensjö, I. Hilber, F. Di Gennaro, B. Lloyd, E. Cherubini, D. Szczerba, W. Kainz, and N. Kuster, *Phys. Med. Biol.*, 2014, **59**, 5287.
5. IEC, Medical electrical equipment – Part 2-33: particular requirements for the basic safety and essential performance of magnetic resonance equipment for medical diagnosis. International Electrotechnical Commission; 60601-2-33 ed. 3.0B (3rd Ed.3.0b), 2010.
6. ISO/TS 10974:2018, Assessment of the safety of magnetic resonance imaging for patients with an active implantable medical device, 2018.
7. D. Shrivastava (ed), Theory and Applications of Heat Transfer in Humans, John Wiley & Sons: Chichester, UK, 2018.

Chapter 23

RF Safety of Active Implantable Medical Devices

Berk Silemek[1], Volkan Açıkel[2], and Ergin Atalar[1]

[1]*Bilkent University, Ankara, Turkey*
[2]*ASELSAN, Ankara, Turkey*

23.1 INTRODUCTION

The maximum level of radiofrequency (RF) power used during magnetic resonance imaging (MRI) scanning is regulated.[1] These regulations are developed for patients without any metallic implants in their body. Because of this reason, MRI of the patients with active implantable medical devices (AIMDs) such as deep brain stimulators (DBS), pacemakers, implantable cardioverter defibrillator (ICDs), and spinal cord stimulators (SCS) are, typically, not recommended owing to the possibility of the excessive RF-induced heating and related thermal tissue damage. Fifty to seventy-five percent of the patients with AIMDs, however, need MRI scanning in their lifetime.[2]

Fundamentally, AIMDs have three main components. The first component is called the implantable pulse generator or IPG which is a metal case that encapsulates complex electronic circuits and a battery. The second component, the lead, is a long insulated electrical wire which is connected to the case. In some implants, more than one lead may exist. Finally, the electrode(s), which is located near the tip of the lead(s), delivers the electrical pulses to the target tissue.

MRI scanning of the patients with AIMDs may result in other unwanted effects as well. In the literature, there are some reports of device reset[3] and unwanted pacing[4,5] during the scanning. In modern pacemakers, these problems are resolved with relatively small modifications to the IPG electronics such as removal of the reed relays and other magnetic cores. Currently, the remaining main problem is the RF-induced heating. It is feared that the unintended and uncontrolled induced currents may damage the tissue next to the electrodes irreversibly. Different from the problems related with the electromagnetic incompatibility of the IPG electronics mentioned before, the modifications to the electronic circuits may not be enough

Safety and Biological Effects in MRI.
Edited by Devashish Shrivastava and J. Thomas Vaughan
 ISBN: 978-1-118-82130-5
Also published in eMagRes (online edition)
DOI: 10.1002/9780470034590.emrstm1587

to solve the RF safety problem since the source of the problem is the induced currents on the long metallic structures such as the leads of AIMDs. The amount of induced current and the tissue heating do not only depend on the device properties but also related to the complex electromagnetics and biophysical properties of the human body. Indeed, these complex interactions may cause fatal injuries.[6] Therefore, a deep understanding and control are needed about the RF safety of AIMDs.

In this chapter, we analyze and present solutions for the problem of unintended, induced tissue heating near AIMDs due to the RF power deposition during MRI. In Section 23.2, a variety of models and simulation methods are presented to capture the problem's essence. The Section 23.3 is devoted to the technology of the AIMDs relevant to study their RF safety during MRI. In Section 23.4, a different approach, implant-friendly MR imaging, is discussed. The Section 23.5 is related to in vivo validations. In Section 23.6, we briefly present the clinical experiences and reports on the MRI of patient populations implanted with AIMDs.

23.2 MODELING OF INDUCED RF HEATING NEAR AN IMPLANT

The complex problem of the RF-induced heating near AIMDs and associated damage can be analyzed in three simple steps (Figure 23.1). First step is the determination of the specific absorption rate (SAR) in the tissue due to the presence of the implants. Second step is the determination of the temperature rise due to the localized power around the electrode and/or the lead tip. Third and last step is the determination of the tissue damage due to the temperature rise.

In determining each of the steps of the RF heating problem, it is easy to see that the electrical and thermal properties of the body (tissue conductivity, permittivity, heat capacity, heat conductivity, perfusion), and electrical properties and position of the implant in the body play important role.

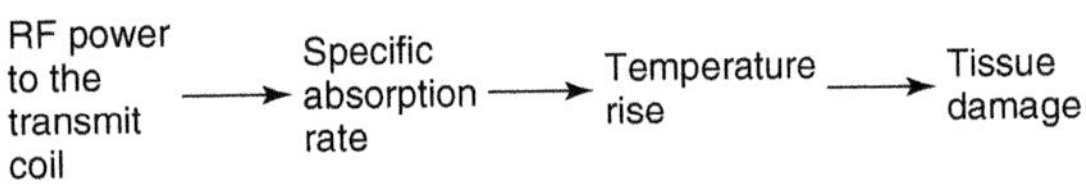

Figure 23.1. The analysis of RF-induced tissue damage

23.2.1 Specific Absorption Rate

SAR is a critical parameter in the RF safety problem and can be written in terms of the peak electric field (E), conductivity (σ), tissue mass density (ρ_t) as:

$$\text{SAR} = \frac{\sigma E^2}{2\rho_t} \tag{23.1}$$

Finding the SAR value inside the human body during an MRI examination is not trivial. The electric field is not only a function of the RF power transmit coil parameters but also the body conductivity and permittivity. To simplify the problem, some investigators use simple homogeneous cylindrical phantoms, some others, however, use complex electrical models of human body. The safety regulations recommend spatial averaging when using these values. IEC, for example, recommends 10-g averaging.[1] The importance of SAR averaging will be discussed later.

In the presence of AIMDs inside the body, the problem becomes significantly more complex because their position inside the body plays a very significant role in the SAR calculations. The RF-induced tissue heating is a result of the electromagnetic coupling of the implants to the transmitted RF field from the RF coils of the MRI scanner. The coupling between AIMDs and RF transmit coils will result in change in the E-field distribution inside the tissue as sketched in Figure 23.2.

Since there are many variables related to RF heating problem, the experiments conducted on phantoms became the basis of understanding. If one puts a bare wire inside a phantom and measures the RF electric field, SAR or temperature rise around the tip of the wire as a function of wire length, the maximum values are observed at a critical length. This length is called resonance length, which is approximately equal to the half of the wavelength inside the phantom material.[8] For a 1.5 T scanner, in a homogeneous phantom with dielectric constant of 77 and conductivity of 0.5 S m^{-1}, this length is about 18 cm. In Figure 23.3, the SAR gain (the ratio of the SAR with and without the wire) is plotted for various wire lengths. A very significant increase in SAR can be observed at the tips of the 18 cm wire.

Even a thin insulation on the wire has a significant effect on the resonance length. In addition, it has been showed that the SAR gain is inversely proportional with the wire diameter.[8,9]

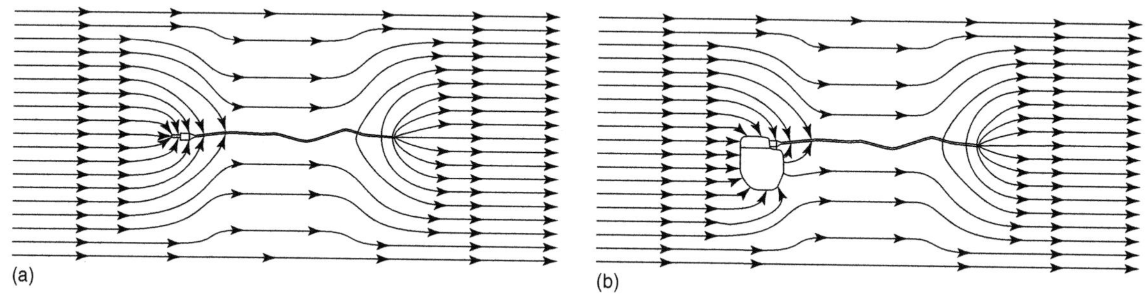

Figure 23.2. Sketches of the current pattern around (a) an isolated lead and (b) a lead connected to an IPG, respectively. (Reproduced with permission from Ref. 7. © John Wiley & Sons, 2015)

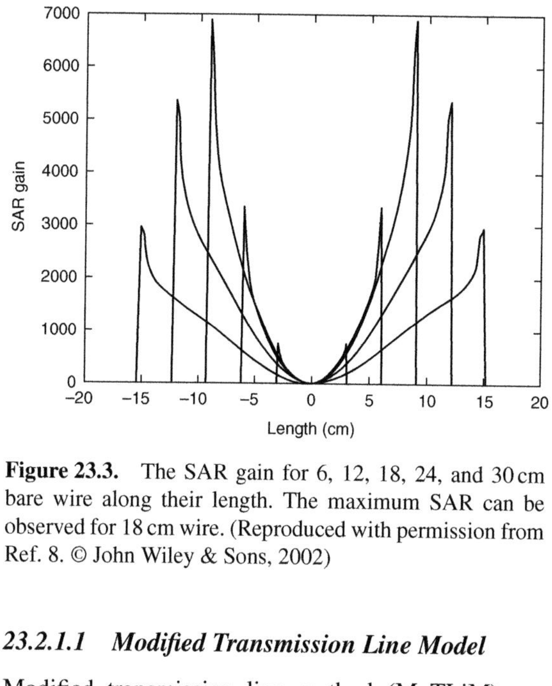

Figure 23.3. The SAR gain for 6, 12, 18, 24, and 30 cm bare wire along their length. The maximum SAR can be observed for 18 cm wire. (Reproduced with permission from Ref. 8. © John Wiley & Sons, 2002)

23.2.1.1 Modified Transmission Line Model

Modified transmission line method (MoTLiM) approach to model RF-induced currents on implant leads was proposed previously.[10] The model was derived from the theory of the lumped element model of transmission line used for analysis of dipoles inside the seawater.[11] In MoTLiM, the original method was modified by adding a series voltage source per unit length to model the effect of the tangential component of the incident *E*-field. Here, the induced current was represented, similar to the current on a transmission line, as superposition of two traveling waves and a DC term as:

$$I(s) = Ae^{-jk_t s} + Be^{jk_t s} + \frac{E_i}{Z} \tag{23.2}$$

The corresponding differential equation can be written as:

$$I(s) + \frac{1}{k_t^2}\frac{d^2 I(s)}{ds^2} = \frac{E_i(s)}{Z} \tag{23.3}$$

where k_t is the wavenumber along the lead, Z is the distributed impedance, s is the position along the lead, $I(s)$ is the current on the lead, and $E_i(s)$ is the tangential component of the incident *E*-field.

In MoTLiM, the case and electrodes of the implant are also modeled with lumped element circuit models using a voltage source and impedance[7] as shown in Figure 23.4.

If the tangential component of the *E*-field is known along the implant lead, the induced currents can be found analytically. In this method, the parameters A and B are the unknowns that are determined by the boundary conditions, which are the equivalent circuits of the electrode and the IPG case. Once these values are known, the temperature rise at the tip of a lead with a length of l_m, under uniform *E*-field (E_0) can be approximated as:

$$\Delta T \approx C\left|\frac{E_0}{k_t}\tan\left(\frac{k_t l_m}{2}\right)\right| \tag{23.4}$$

In equation (23.4), C is the constant that includes the thermal properties of the tissue. The calculated temperature rise at the lead tip when the lead is connected to the case, using the case model with MoTLiM is given in Figure 23.5. The current distribution has been solved using MoTLiM and verified with MoM (method of moments) simulations under uniform *E*-field incidence.[7]

The interaction between the lead, case, and electrode was investigated. It is shown that the connecting lead to a case changes its effective electrical length and causes a shift in the resonance length of the lead. Furthermore,

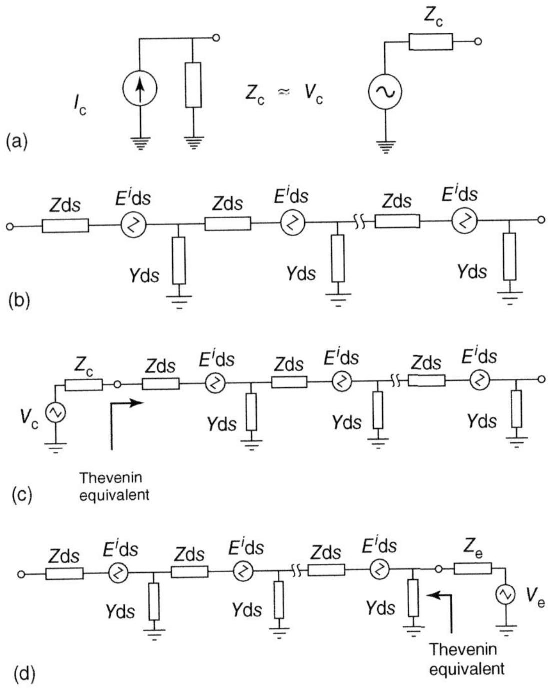

Figure 23.4. The IPG case and electrode models. (a) The Norton and Thevenin models of electrode and IPG case, (b) the modified transmission line model of the lead, (c) the model of the IPG case connected to the lead, and (d) the model of the electrode connected to the lead. (Reproduced with permission from Ref. 7. © John Wiley & Sons, 2015)

placing lumped impedance between the lead and the electrode is also shown to demonstrate the effect.[7]

A method to measure the lead parameters, k_t (or Y) and Z was described in detail.[12] In this method, a lead is connected to a coaxial line as shown in Figure 23.6 and immersed into a gel phantom with the coaxial line. For various lead lengths, the impedance is measured. The calculated impedance values are fitted to the measured results to find the two parameters.

The advantage of MoTLiM is that under changing lead length, electrode, and case and incident E-field; the temperature rise at the tip of the electrodes can be predicted precisely. This ability may help in the management of the scanning patients with AIMDs.

23.2.1.2 *Transfer Function*

The electric field transfer function is another modeling technique that describes the relationship between the incident electric field and the scattered electric field in the vicinity of the electrode. Park *et al.* transforms the vectoral relationship to a scalar relationship by assuming that the magnitude of the scattered electric field, $E_s(P)$ at location P around the implant is significantly higher than the incident field.[13] In this case, the lead a transfer function $S(l, P)$ can be found such that:

$$E_s(P) = \int_0^L S(l, P) E_{\tan}(l) \mathrm{d}l \tag{23.5}$$

The transfer function at the electrode can be calculated by applying sequential tangential fields along the lead and measuring related scattered electric fields around the electrode. Therefore, for any known tangential electric field around the lead, the magnitude of the scattered electric field can be calculated.

The transfer function method was improved.[14] In this method, the field inside a volume that contain the implant was calculated without implant then the scattered electric field is calculated using the implant with computer simulations in the small volume that contain the implant.

In another study, the transfer function is determined experimentally. In this technique, the induced current profile on the lead is calculated using reconstructed MR images. Using these current profiles, the corresponding transfer function is calculated.[15]

All above-mentioned techniques enable finding the current and/or electric field around the wire. Using this information, the SAR around the implant can be calculated in various conditions. Finding the temperature rise due to the SAR increase require additional work.

23.2.2 RF-induced Temperature Rise

The temperature in the body is highly regulated. Blood perfusion redistributes the heat generated in the tissue including the induced heating near AIMDs. Pennes modeled this effect with the bioheat equation.[16] Simplified Pennes bioheat equation is given below.

$$\frac{1}{\propto}\frac{\mathrm{d}T(r,t)}{\mathrm{d}t} = \nabla^2 T(r,t) - \frac{\rho_t \rho_b c_b m}{k}(T(r,t) - T_b) + \frac{\rho_t}{k}\mathrm{SAR}(r,t) + Q \tag{23.6}$$

where $\propto$ is thermal diffusivity; ρ_t, ρ_b are mass densities of the tissue and the perfusing blood respectively; c_b is the heat capacity of the blood and m is the volumetric flow rate of the blood per unit mass of the tissue; T_b is the temperature of the perfusing blood; k is the thermal conductivity; and Q is the metabolic heat. Equation (23.6) is a simplified version of the Pennes

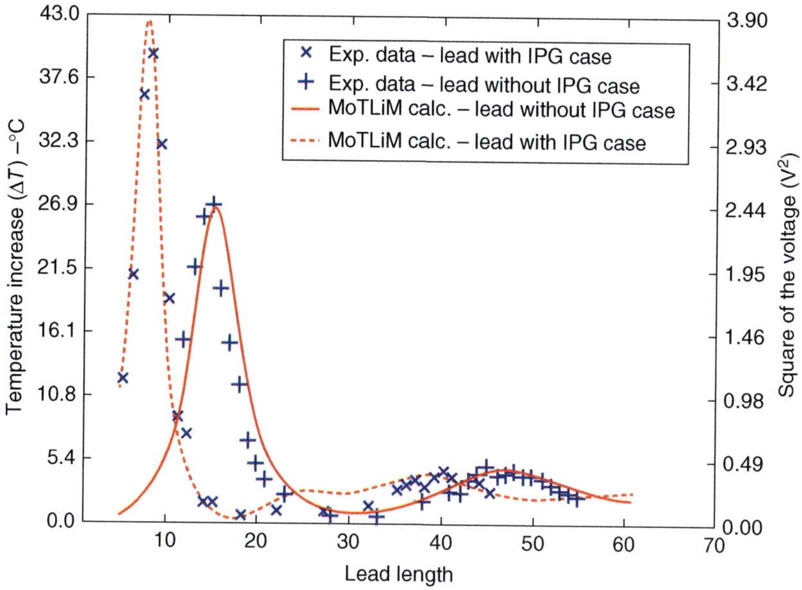

Figure 23.5. The MoTLiM prediction and experimental results for a lead with and without IPG case. (Reproduced with permission from Ref. 7. © John Wiley & Sons, 2015)

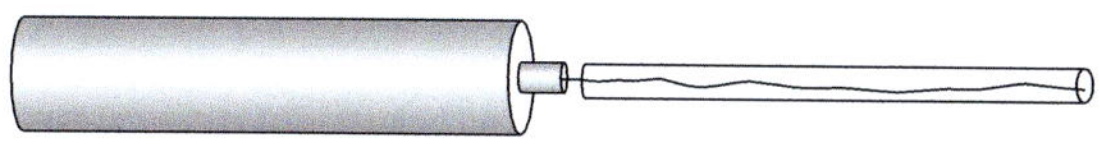

Figure 23.6. A lead is connected to inner conductor of a coaxial cable to form a loopless antenna. (Reproduced with permission from Ref. 12. © Bilkent University, 2014)

original equation that assumes 100% efficiency of energy exchange between the blood and surrounding tissue without any change in blood temperature. The assumption makes the simplified model overestimate the blood-tissue heat transfer rate and thus, underestimate related tissue heating in deep tissues alongside of violating conservation of energy. For more on the limited applicability of the simplified Pennes model, please refer to the additional material presented elsewhere in this book regarding modeling RF power-induced heating in MRI and Ref. 17.

A general analytical solution to the simplified Pennes' equation does not exist. Under linearity and time invariance, homogenous infinite medium assumptions, Green's function solution to the problem can be found.[18,19] For MRI heating application, Yeung and Atalar found the steady-state Green's function solution or spatial averaging kernel as:

$$G(R) = \frac{\rho_t}{4\pi k R}\exp(-\nu R) \qquad (23.7)$$

where ν is the perfusion constant and can be calculated as $\nu^2 = \rho_t \rho_b c_b m/k$.[20] Note that the above expression can be thought as a SAR to temperature conversion function and valid under the assumption that the temperature regulation does not exist, the thermal parameters are uniform within the local region of interest and the thermal parameters are not function of temperature including metabolic heat. Yeung and Atalar proposed this function as an alternative to 1 or 10 g averaging which have been proposed before.[20] They also showed in the same article that both 1 and 10 g averaging causes significant errors in predicting the effect of highly localized heating. As can be seen from the expression, $1/\nu$, the reciprocal of the perfusion constant, can be thought as the radius of averaging volume. For the body parts where the perfusion is high, a smaller averaging volume is needed. Therefore, if there is a localized heating in a highly perfused region, temperature rise will occur in only very close vicinity of the hot spot. It should be noted that high perfusion also decreases the maximum temperature rise.

Although this intuitive understanding of SAR-temperature relationship is critical, calculation of the temperature directly without making uniformity assumption is preferred.

Today, most commercial electromagnetic simulators come with the bioheat solver that employ simplified Pennes bioheat model. It should be noted that the accuracy of the solutions may be limited because of the limitations of the Pennes model and the human body models used. The electrical and thermal properties of the human body changes from person to person. In most simulators, the body thermal regulation, such as sweating, dilation of blood vessels in response to increased temperature has been ignored. However, these solvers are extremely useful in understanding the nature of the problem. For more accurate calculations, interested readers are encouraged to refer to material and software presented in Ref. 17.

In any case, for understanding RF safety of AIMDs, the temperature rise in the presence of these implants should be analyzed rather than SAR. Yeung *et al.* analyzed RF safety of the straight electrical wires that were placed completely inside a uniform object of average electrical and thermal properties of the human body.[8] They calculated the temperature rise at the tip of the wire for a uniform incident electric field and reported temperature rise per applied SAR as a safety index in Figure 23.7; the theoretical prediction of the temperature rise was given as a function of the wire length. As can be seen in the figure, there is a critical length, called the resonance length where the

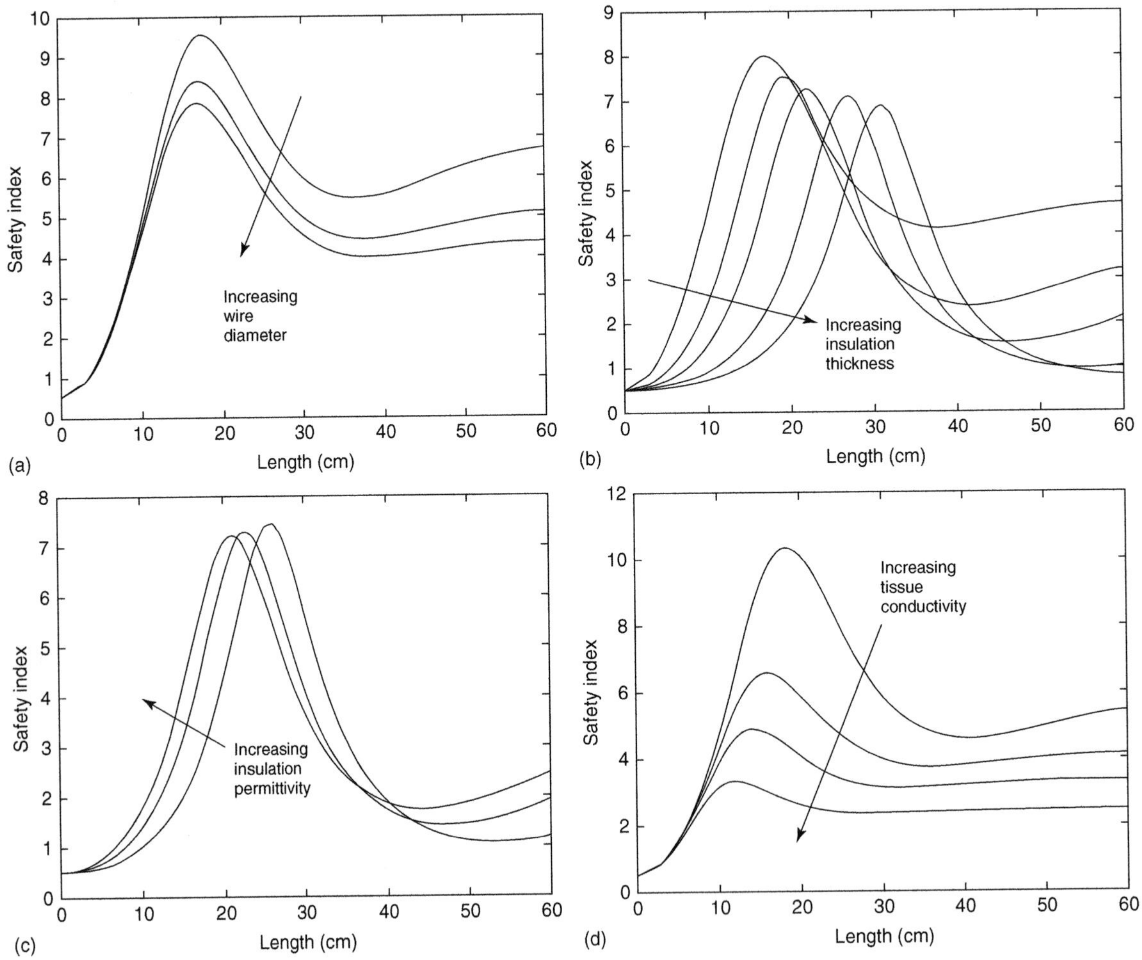

Figure 23.7. Theoretically predicted safety index when each of the following parameters varied: (a) wire diameter, (b) insulation thickness, (c) relative permittivity of the insulator, and (d) electrical conductivity of the tissue. (Reproduced with permission from Ref. 8. © John Wiley & Sons, 2002)

temperature rise is maximum. The resonance length and the maximum temperature rise depends on many parameters. For example, as given in Figure 23.7(a), increasing wire diameter reduces the maximum temperature which is experimentally verified.[9] Insulation thickness is an important parameter (the resonance length increases with the increase in the insulation thickness). The dielectric constant of the insulator and electrical properties of the medium also play role in the resonance length. Increasing dielectric constant of the medium decreases the resonance length. The electrical conductivity of the medium has a strong effect on the maximum temperature rise. As one can imagine, the whole analysis becomes very complex in an inhomogeneous medium such as human body. Nevertheless, average electrical properties may produce ballpark estimates shedding useful insight into what may happen in the body.

If the incident electric field is perpendicular to the wire of interest, there will be no induced current on the wire. Only the tangential component of the electric field is important. While the *z*-component (i.e., along the longitudinal axial direction of the RF coil) of the electric field is dominant in the body when it is exposed to a RF field from a birdcage body coil, the exact direction of the field varies highly because of the complex structure of the body and its inhomogeneity. Therefore, even when the wire is placed inside the body purely in the *z*-direction, some component of the electric field will not induce current. Therefore, the safety index may be considered as the worst-case scenario where incident electric field is parallel to the wire.[8] The transmit coil and wire can be considered independently while optimizing the properties of these structures using safety index. Therefore, the applied power or the worst-case peak SAR can be limited using safety index depending on the knowledge about the wire and RF coil structure.

Although the above argument is correct for the exposure from a conventional birdcage coil, one other parameter that may affect the maximum temperature rise is the phase of the incident field noting that in the conventional birdcage coils, the phase of the electric field is rather uniform. Because of this most simulations are conducted with constant phase incident electric field, however, this is not the worst condition for long wires. In fact, when the incident tangential electric field has a uniform magnitude and worst possible phase, there is no resonance length, longer the wire, higher the temperature rise.[21] For this case, the worst-case analysis has to be reconsidered.

The positions of AIMDs also affect the heating as shown by the investigators.[22] The authors have measured that when the implant lead is at the edge of the phantom and the RF coil, the induced temperature rise was higher compared to the center of the coil. This is expected since the electric field of a birdcage body coil is low at the center and high at its edges. The DBS devices were placed in the phantom and the lead path was configured as close as possible to a patient implanted with DBS; the results again showed the effect of the lead path on the heating.[23]

Another important parameter to consider in the implant heating problem is the static field strength. The static field strength dictates the operating frequency of the MRI scanners and the electric field pattern inside the body. The resonance length of the wires is a strong function of the frequency of the transmitted RF power. In one study, for example, experiments in gel phantoms were conducted in such a way that all other experimental parameters (i.e., sequence parameters and landmark positioning) were the same for a 3 and 1.5 T MRI scanners (thus changing the transmitted frequency of the RF power).[24] In this particular study, the resulting temperature rise at the electrode of the DBS lead was greater at 3 T than 1.5 T system. It should be noted, however, that this fact may change for different length and construction of the DBS leads.

In MRI, various pulse sequences are used. Fortunately, the temperature elevation is related to the time-averaged SAR distribution. Thus, analyzing a particular pulse sequence is not necessary in order to determine an AIMD's safety profile. It is, however, interesting to note that the appropriate duration for the spatial averaging depends on many parameters. The time-dependent Green's function analysis given in Ref. 20 shows that if the heated region is small, short-time averaging is necessary to find the peak temperature rise, which is dictated by the thermal diffusivity of the medium. For typical diffusivity values in the body, if the heated region is larger than 1 mm^3, 10-s averaging is enough. This is longer than most, if not all MR sequence repetition times (TR). Therefore, it is a common practice to average over one TR to figure out the average SAR value. In the case of more diffuse heating, the averaging must be carried out using the perfusion time constant. This time was estimated to vary between 15 s (for kidney) and 70 min (bone) depending on the tissue of interest.[20]

Although by definition, the AIMDs are completely immersed inside the body and, therefore; for the safety study of AIMDs, understanding partially immersed conductive wires is not critical. For the sake of completeness, however, it should be pointed that the amount of induced currents of the wires highly depend on the immersed length of the wires. This is especially important for guidewires, catheters,[25,26] and other similar wire-like structures such as stereo-electroencephalography electrodes[27] that are partially inserted inside the body during MRI. For more details regarding the safety analyses of the partially implanted conductive structures, please refer to the material presented elsewhere in the book.

23.2.3 Thermal Tissue Damage

To ensure RF safety near implanted conductive devices, the ultimate goal is to avoid possible thermal damage to the tissue around implants. Thermal damage is a function of the temperature-time history. Going into this relationship between the temperature-time history and tissue damage is beyond the scope of this chapter and the interested readers are encouraged to refer to material presented in Ref. 17 for more information. Briefly, if any part of the body is at or below 39 °C due to RF power, it is considered to be safe.[1] Going beyond this limit does not mean immediate tissue damage; however, it, also, does not mean perfectly healthy tissue. The temperature above 50 °C is very likely to produce adverse thermal effects. A study conducted for MRI application suggests that a thermal dose formulation (an integral of temperature over time), cumulative equivalent minutes at 43 °C or CEM43, may prove itself to be useful under limited conditions.[28]

Tissue damage due to MR scanning of patients with implants has been shown. In a case report, a patient with DBS implant showed transient dystonia following MRI.[29] In another case report, a patient with DBS was scanned using a 1.0 T MRI although the DBS used in the patient was marked as MRI incompatible and caused permanent right hemiparesis.[6] Another MRI scan was performed on the same patient to image the extent of the problem as shown in Figure 23.8.

As a summary of this section, the main safety problem of MRI scanning patients with AIMDs is the RF-induced heating. The source of the problem is well known. To understand the extent of the problem,

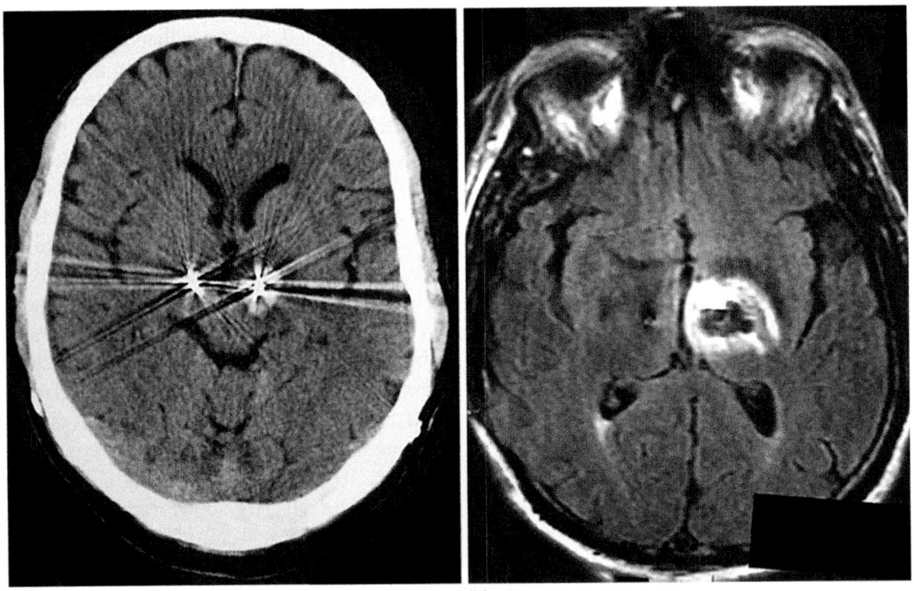

(a) (b)

Figure 23.8. (a) Computed tomographic scan performed immediately after the lumbar spine MRI scan of a patient with DBS revealed evidence of a hemorrhage surrounding the left DBS electrode. (b) T2-weighted MRI scan of the brain showing edema around the left DBS electrode. (Reproduced with permission from Ref. 6. © Oxford University Press, 2005) researchers have investigated some of the parameters affecting the safety profile of the implants. In vivo studies showing thermal damage is limited but there are at least two case reports showing the problem.

23.3 MRI CONDITIONAL AIMDS

The understanding of the RF-induced tissue heating using models and experiments led to possible solutions to the problem. Since tissue heating occurs due to coupling between MR coils and long conductive leads, there may be solutions by modifying the problematic leads of the implants. The most intuitive approach to this problem can be the replacement of the electrical wires to nonelectrical wires. Greatbatch *et al.* proposed to modify a pacemaker lead by implementing fiber-optic connection between the case and electrode.[30] They have claimed that pacing function of the pacemaker was preserved and reported less than 1 °C temperature rise for their RF heating experiments. Another major modification method has been shown using current traps to the lead which presented more than 50% reduction in heating.[25] Resistive leads are also presented,[31] and it is reported that $R \geq 3\,k\Omega$ required to keep temperature rise below 2 °C for ~75 cm leads with the whole body average SAR of $4\,W\,kg^{-1}$ for a 5 min scan at 1.5 T. The Billabong design requires a special winding of the electrical wires inside the implant lead.[32] A temperature rise of below 2 and 0.5 °C, relative to the reference temperature was measured for 1.5 and 3 T, respectively. In the above designs, the mechanical properties of the leads and the effect of the design modifications on the normal operation of the AIMDs were not analyzed. The full analysis was left to the development teams of the implant manufacturers.

There were similar set of studies on MRI conditional guidewires and catheters. Active decoupling method was proposed for loopless catheter antenna design[33] and later applied to guidewires[34] reaching sizes that could be used in coronary interventions.[35]

Since 2005, ASTM International recommends identifying the MR compatibility of the AIMDS in three categories: MRI safe, MRI conditional, or MRI unsafe.[36] Of course, MR conditional means, the patients with these devices can be scanned using MRI under a specific set of conditions. Although design details have not been published, successful test results of the first commercial MR conditional AIMD designs were shown.[37–39] Immediately following the commercial success of an MRI conditional pacemaker design, other designs were developed.[40] No AIMD can be considered to be MRI safe at this time. The patients with MR conditional AIMDs can be scanned under specified conditions. Widespread use of these devices will be required to fully understand the implications of using MRI conditional AIMDs. For example, in one study investigators have questioned the possibility of cardiac perforation and lead dislodgement.[41]

Of course, even after these technical developments, still a significant body of the patients should not be scanned using MRI because they have MRI unsafe AIMDs in their body. The replacement of the millions[42] of MRI unsafe implants with the MRI conditional ones is unreasonable. In that point, modifying MRI scanners could be another approach to the problem.

23.4 IMPLANT FRIENDLY IMAGING

Today, most of the MRI scanners are equipped with a birdcage body coil. The *E*-fields generated by these coils are well known, and therefore their interactions with AIMDs can be analyzed as discussed earlier. Although the phase distribution of the *E*-field of a birdcage coil is almost uniform (as the field strength and therefore the Larmor frequency increases this assumption starts to fail), its influence on the AIMD heating problem has been analyzed.[21] The results from the study indicate that the safety of the implant can be altered (can be made worse or better) using different phase distributions. Using the variation of the phase, the 'implant-friendly' electromagnetic transmitter concept was hypothetically introduced.[21]

The transmitter in a 1.5 and 3 T MR system, typically, is a birdcage body coil, which creates homogeneous forward polarized magnetic field. The standard implementation for creating forward polarized magnetic field depends on the rungs that are used. A phase shift between currents is given to each neighboring channels by a factor of $2\pi/N$ where N is the number of rungs in the birdcage coil.[43] In quadrature mode, there are two feeding points with a phase difference of $\pi/2$ between them. If the phase difference is different than the proposed values, the birdcage coil generates linearly polarized magnetic field. The theoretical derivation and experimental validation in gel phantoms of implant-friendly coil was introduced by Eryaman *et al.* using birdcage coils.[44] First, the *E*-field distribution of the forward polarized, quadrature, birdcage coil can be modeled. The approximation in equation (23.8) was derived for an infinitely long homogeneous model by not taking the end-ring currents into account.[44]

$$E_z = \frac{-H_f \omega \mu_0 \theta}{2} e^{-j\phi}, \quad E_\phi = 0, E_r = 0 \qquad (23.8)$$

In equation (23.8), the E-field components E_z, E_ϕ, and E_r are longitudinal, angular, and radial components respectively. ω, μ_0 are the Larmor frequency and permeability, respectively. The imaginary number j is represented as $\sqrt{-1}$ and H_f is the transmit sensitivity of the coil. The linearly polarized birdcage coil's E-field is expressed in equation (23.9).

$$E_z = -H_f j \omega \mu_0 \theta \sin \phi, \quad E_\phi = 0, E_r = 0 \qquad (23.9)$$

These E-field equations for the quadrature and linear birdcage coils illustrate the difference between two E-field distributions. The transmit sensitivities of the coils are similar. The detailed derivation can be found in Ref. 44. In equation (23.9), it is important to note that E-field component of the plane $\phi = 0$ is zero over entire plane which can be steered to any angular direction, $\phi = \phi_0$. This is critical because the source of the RF-induced heating of implants is the E-field as it is described in the models. If a zero E-field plane is steered to the plane where implant conductors lies, no induced currents on these conductors will be present.

It is interesting to note that the method described here holds true even when the implant conductor does not lie in a plane. In another work by the same investigators, the investigators show that significant reduction in the induced heating can be achieved for very complex implant geometries by simply controlling the currents' amplitudes and phases of the two ports of a conventional birdcage coil.[45]

In dual drive birdcage coils, the ports of the birdcage channels can be weighted by $\cos \theta$ and $\sin \theta$ provided that θ is a variable between $[0, \pi]$. The implant tip current relationship between θ and the lead located in $\phi = \phi_0$ plane can be denoted as $I[\theta, \phi]$. When the off-set flip angle due to RF coil excitation is small, the flip angle near the tip is linearly dependent on the induced current. If the product of transmit sensitivity and nominal flip angle are denoted as α, then, $\alpha = A \cdot I[\theta, \phi]$, where A is a constant that depends on geometric parameters. Finally, using the trigonometric approximations ($\sin \alpha \approx \alpha$ and $\cos \alpha \approx 1$), when the flip angle α due to the RF-induced current is small, the signal intensity from the implant artifact can be approximated as follows:

$$\mathrm{SI} = C \cdot A \cdot I[\theta, \phi] \qquad (23.10)$$

When dual drive mode is used, the current on the implant can be formulated as

$$S = |S_1 \cos \theta + S_2 \sin \theta e^{-j\beta}| \qquad (23.11)$$

where S_1 and S_2 are the currents at a specific position on the wire when a fixed amplitude and phase voltage is applied to each of the two ports of the birdcage coil. In equation (23.11), S is the total current induced on the wire, when the amplitude of the current is changed by $\cos \theta$ for the first port, $\sin \theta$ for the second port, and the phase for the second port is changed by β. Note that for arbitrary values of S_1 and S_2, one can always find a pair of θ and β values such that the S becomes zero. Therefore, the induced current on the wire can be nulled by simply adjusting these two parameters.[45]

In the same article, measuring the current on the implant, the flip-angle artifact due to the scattered magnetic field around the implant lead was used. The flip-angle artifact is detectable even in low field excitations. Thus, this approach can provide a noninvasive RF-induced safety assessment of the implants when the complex properties of the tissue are considered and also it can be used to nullify the induced currents on the implants.[45]

The technique was tested in phantoms using various wire trajectories and different wire types: helical wire, copper wire, and DBS lead. The artifact intensity measurements were done using gradient echo pulse sequence with 2° flip angle. The artifact intensity can be seen in Figure 23.9(a) with a gradient echo pulse sequence, at flip angle of 25°. The signal artifact intensities are plotted after flip angle was reduced to 2° and the theta values are swept between 0 and 180. The calculated and measured values are in agreement (Figure 23.9b–d). In all cases, the peak artifact signal intensity is observed where the heating is maximum; and the base artifact signal intensity is observed where the heating is minimum. For the ex vivo animal experiment (Figure 23.9d), the behavior is similar, confirming that the technique can be used for complex tissue properties.

Several cautions must be considered while using this technique. The flip angle value must be low for measuring the RF-induced current artifacts because higher flip angles may create measurement errors and unwanted heating during measurements. In addition, the signal measurements must be made as close as possible to the tip location for precise heating assessment.

As an alternative to the above-mentioned E-field steering methods, Golestanirad *et al.* proposed to use a rotating linearly polarized birdcage coil.[46]

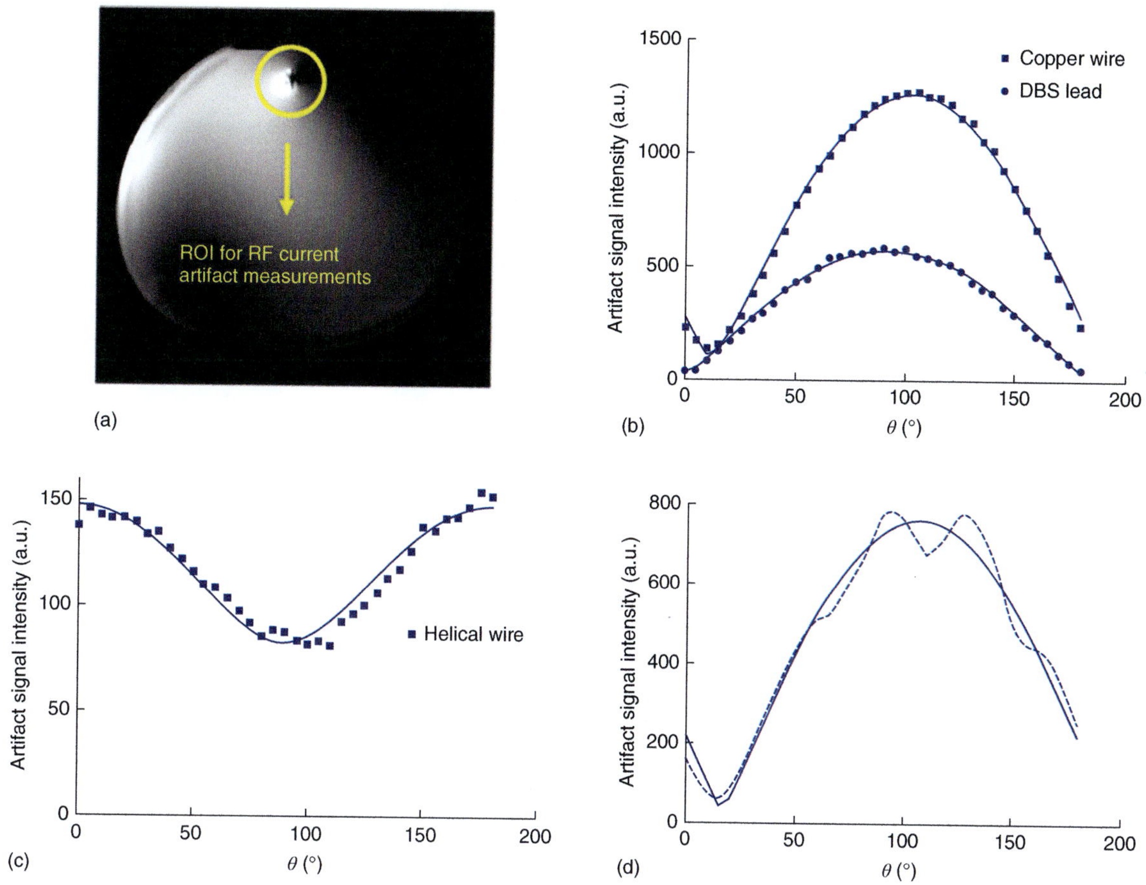

Figure 23.9. Panel a shows the induced current artifact near the lead in a phantom. The region of interest that is used to measure the maximum level of the image artifact (bright region) is also presented. The image in Panel a is obtained with a flip angle of 25° to clearly show the position of the artifact in the phantom. Panel b and c shows estimated and measured signal intensity curves of copper wire, helical wire and the DBS lead. The signal intensity curve for animal experiment can be seen in Panel d. All quantitative artifact signal intensity measurements were made with a 2° flip angle excitation. (Reproduced with permission from Ref. 45. © John Wiley & Sons, 2013)

The simulated coil sensitivities for the quadrature (Figure 23.10a) and linear polarized coils (Figure 23.10d) indicate relatively higher SAR for linear excitation.[47] The *E*-fields in a trans-axial plane are shown in Figure 23.10(b) and (e), and in a $\phi=0$ half-plane are shown in Figure 23.10(c) and (f) for the quadrature and linear polarized coils, respectively. The linear polarized coil has zero *E*-field planes at the cost of increased SAR.

Generating zero *E*-field planes on the implant may solve the RF-induced heating; however, safe imaging of other locations without losing tissue information is desirable. To achieve this, transmit field optimization is needed to increase signal level at desired locations without creating *E*-field on the implant. The transmit field optimization for implant heating problem was examined in Eryaman's paper using simulations which introduce implant friendly coils.[44] The coil sensitivity (Figure 23.11a) on the nonoptimized transmit field is worse at the edges of the phantom but optimized transmit field (Figure 23.11d) has better homogeneity in the sample, again at the cost of increased SAR (Figure 23.11c and f). The different sets of zero *E*-fields on the implant lead can be seen in Figure 23.11(b) and (e).

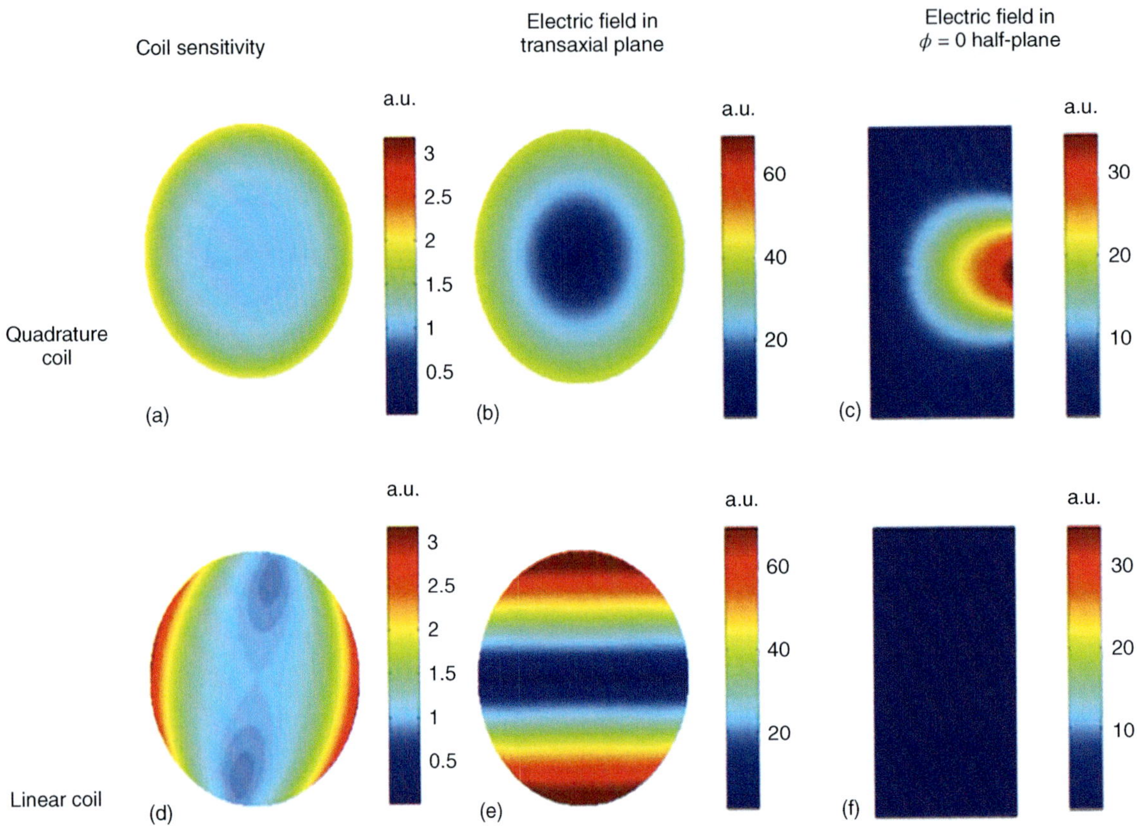

Figure 23.10. Transmit sensitivity (a and d), electric field in the trans-axial plane (b and e), and electric field in the $\phi = 0$ half-plane (c and f) generated by quadrature and linear coils. Note that all field solutions are in arbitrary units. (Reproduced with permission from Ref. 44. © John Wiley & Sons, 2011)

Implant friendly coils with homogenous transmit magnetic field may require more degree of freedom. Conventional two-channel birdcage coil can reduce *E*-field with an increased whole-body SAR. Multi-channel transmit arrays coils may be better suited for implant-friendly MR scanning. The numerical simulations showing the effect of number of channels have been carried out.[48] RF shimming method is used to design safe excitation fields. As can be seen in Figure 23.12(a), a normal quadrature coil has much more *E*-field distribution around the lead (red bright line). For the same setup, *E*-field is reduced for the 2, 4, and 8 channel configurations (Figure 23.12b–d). The magnetic field homogeneity improves with an increase in the number of channels, as can be seen in Figure 23.13. The signal variation of birdcage coil is much less than a two-channel parallel transmit but homogeneity improves as the number of channel increases.[48]

As can been in the above-mentioned body of work, implant friendly MR imaging is possible. One important challenge in converting these techniques into clinical practice is to determine the location of the implant in a short time without causing safety hazard.

23.5 EXPERIMENTAL METHODS TO DETERMINE AIMD SAFETY AND IN VIVO VALIDATION

23.5.1 Noninvasive Implant Safety Assessment Methods

Computing reliable RF-induced heating near AIMDs depends on the realistic input of electromagnetic and

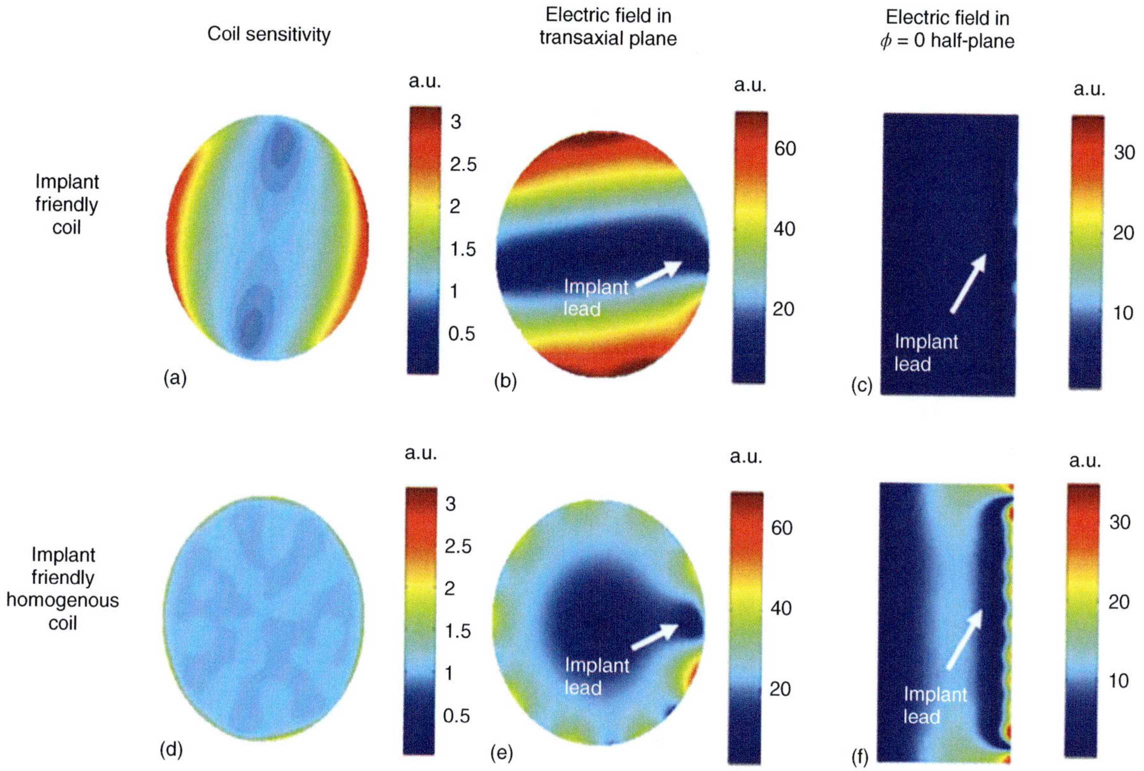

Figure 23.11. Transmit sensitivity (a and d), electric field in the trans-axial plane (b and e), and electric field in the $\phi = 0$ half-plane (c and f) generated by implant-friendly coils and implant-friendly homogeneous coils. Locations of the implant lead are denoted by arrows in the figures. Note that all field solutions are in arbitrary units. (Reproduced with permission from Ref. 44. © John Wiley & Sons, 2011)

biophysical properties. The electromagnetic property distribution in humans is complex and time varying. Thus, for simplicity, most of the RF heating studies are conducted in uniform phantoms. Only a handful of simulation studies have cared to consider the complex nature of the body[49] and complex lead geometries.[46,50] Nonuniform, sometimes unknown, and time-varying electromagnetic and biophysical properties make the assessment of the RF heating near AIMDs in uniform phantoms insufficient. In vivo, measurements are expected to provide better understanding and improve safety. In this section, we will briefly discuss in vivo measurement techniques for implant safety.

One method for safety assessment is to measure the induced currents on the leads because the induced currents can be related to heating. For this, some of the studies have used pickup coils or embedded optocouplers.[51,52] The feasibility of the *E*-field adjustments using measured currents was demonstrated on pTx.[53] It is, however, may be impractical to place these bulk devices on the implants for measuring currents on the wires in vivo.

The presence of a metallic conductor inside MRI produces image artifacts. This is because the induced currents on the wire change the polarization of the RF field around the wire. Figure 23.14 shows the magnitude and phase images of a phantom with a wire. The observed bright spots are the signal enhancements due to the RF-induced currents on the wire.[54]

The apparent RF-induced image artifact near a lead is characterized using the contribution of B_{1+} from the coil and the lead. The total B_{1+} field is the vector sum up of the incident B_{1+} field from the coil and the scattered field from wire. The local signal increase is related to the induced current on the wire which can be quantified on the image.[55]

Another interesting approach is to find the wire location in vivo and use the, so-called, reverse polarization

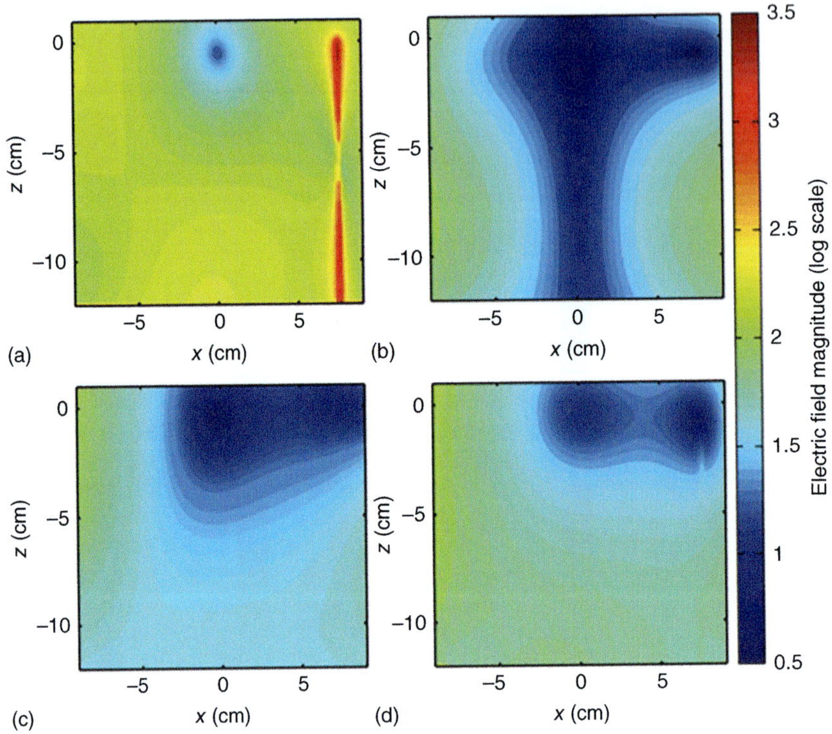

Figure 23.12. Contour plots of *E*-field magnitude on a log scale in the plane parallel to the wire for (a) 16-rung birdcage coil operating in quadrature mode, and optimized (b) 2-element pTx, (c) 4-element pTx, and (d) 8-element pTx. (Source: McElcheran *et al.* [48], https://journals.plos.org/plosone/article?id=10.1371/journal.pone.0134379. Licensed under CC BY 4.0)

technique. It is mentioned that the forward polarized magnetic field is produced by the birdcage body coil. The excited spins' fields are received by a tuned quadrature receive coil. Ideally, if a birdcage coil is physically reversed or used in the reverse polarized mode, the nuclear spins do not get excited. If linear polarization mode of the coil is used, however, the coil does not have a preferred direction, the spins will be excited in both directions. This concept can be applied to the receive coils as well. If a coil is designed to pick-up only the circularly polarized component of the magnetic field, no MR signal will be picked up if it is used in the reverse direction.

The above concept changes in the presence of metallic wires. In the vicinity of the wires, as discussed in Ref. 54, the field polarization becomes linear even if a reverse polarized birdcage coil is used. In this case, the spins near the wires get excited. In this mode of operation, therefore, nothing but only the spins around the wires will be excited and the wires become visible.[56] One other way is to use this concept in the receive mode. In the same study, the investigators picked up signals with a dual channel birdcage coil and computed to generate images in forward polarized and reverse polarized mode to visualize the background and the signal generated by the scattered magnetic field from the wire.

The above technique was later improved by Overall *et al.* to assess the safety of implanted devices.[57] The authors implemented reverse polarization in a scanner's hardware. In addition to transmitter, the receiver polarization was reversed in the experiments. Figure 23.15 shows a pacemaker lead image in the phantom. The lead can be distinguished relatively more easily in the reverse polarized images (Figure 23.15b and c) compared to in forward polarized images (Figure 23.15a). In the chapter, it is argued that the reverse polarized method can be used as a safety detection method for in vivo imaging of patients with implants.

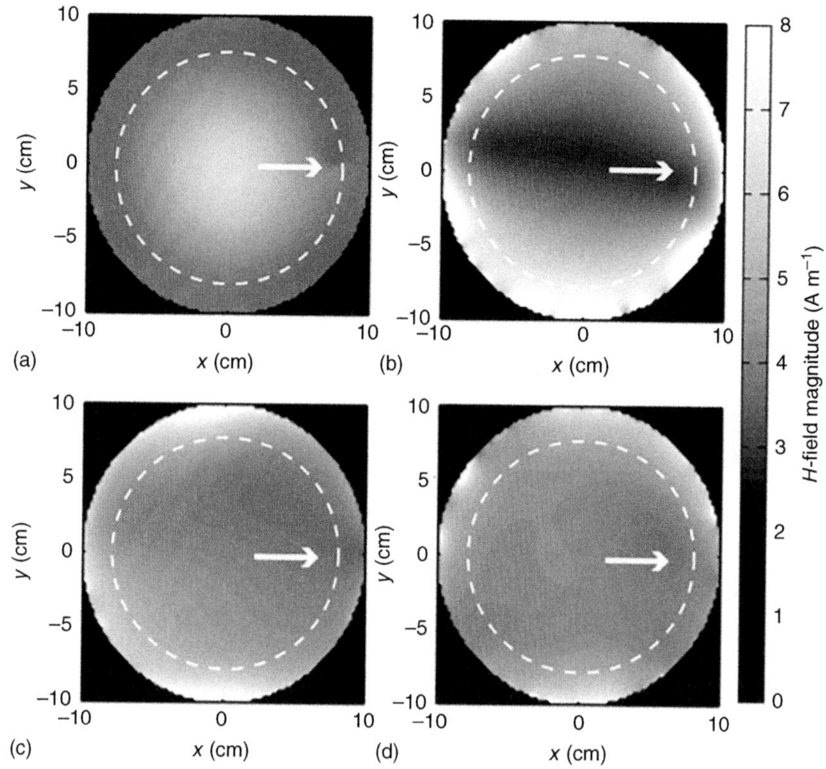

Figure 23.13. (a) Birdcage coil, signal variation = 24%, (b) 2-element pTx, signal variation = 46%, (c) 4-element pTx, signal variation = 17%, and (d) 8-element pTx, signal variation = 9%. Wire is located at $x = 7.5$ cm, $y = 0$ cm, indicated by white arrow. Signal variation is the standard deviation divided by the mean calculated over circular region of interest with radius = 8 cm (dashed line). (Source: McElcheran *et al.* [48], https://journals.plos.org/plosone/article?id=10.1371/journal.pone.0134379. Licensed under CC BY 4.0)

It should be noted, however, that the nonlinear relationship between the B_{1+} and tip angle may lead to errors in predicting the induced currents. The error is, however, limited to the excited volume near the small tip of the implant. Another trade-off may arise from reversing both transmit and reverse signals for the asymmetric loads because the electric field on the wire may not stay the same under the two conditions.[57] A case for this effect was examined using simulations and experiments for a helical wire.[58] The induced current near the free end of the wire of reversed polarized excitation was significantly different than the forward polarized excitation (Figure 23.16). Since the SAR at the tip of the wire is calculated from the induced current on the wire, the tip heating is different in these two cases. The experimental results also agree with the simulations where the SAR ratio at the tip of helical wire is 7–1. The forward polarized tip heating was 3.8 °C and the reverse polarized tip heating was 0.6 °C after 60 s deposition of 4.4 W kg^{-1} whole-body average SAR.[58]

23.5.2 In Vivo Validations

Recent studies have provided solutions to steer the *E*-fields away from the implants[44] and MR conditional AIMDs.[39] However, the problem is not fully characterized in vivo using animal studies. The studies on the phantoms provide only limited information because phantoms are mostly homogeneous and can only be used to simulate mean electrical properties of the human tissue. Similarly, perfusion and blood flow are difficult to model specifically when it is altered by the presence of AIMDs. In vivo validations of these techniques are necessary. One important problem is the

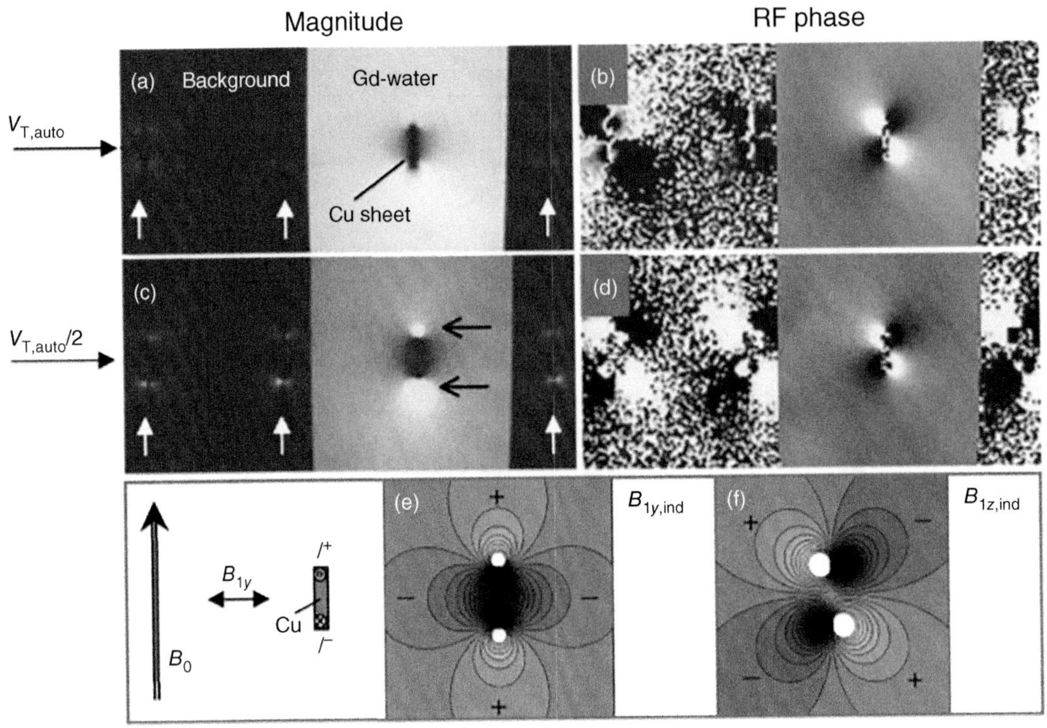

Figure 23.14. Magnitude images (yz slice at $x = 0$) of the Cu sheet obtained at automatically adjusted transmitter amplitude $V_{T,auto}$ (a) and at $V_{T,auto}/2$ (c). Corresponding SE phase images are shown (b) and (d). Calculated polar diagrams of $B_{1y,ind}$ (e) and $B_{1z,ind}$ (f) according to the model of two anti-parallel linear currents I^+ and I^- are depicted (diverging values near the currents are limited to a constant of appropriate sign). At $V_{T,auto}/2$, the SE sequence operates with optimum pulse angles at the location where the RF field from the transmitter and the eddy-current RF field superimpose in phase [+ in the calculated $B_{1y,ind}$ diagram, (e). Bright depiction (c), black arrows] results from increased detection sensitivity (principle of reciprocity). Near the induced currents, rf phase is shifted (b), (d) according to the pattern of $B_{1z,ind}$ (f). For TR = 200 ms, distinct ghosts appeared in the magnitude images (a), (c) white arrows reflecting also the pattern of $B_{1z,ind}$. A small periodic jitter in the rf amplitude of the scanner (B_1) corresponded in frequency to the chosen TR (12.5 Hz = TR/16). (Reproduced with permission from Ref. 54. © John Wiley & Sons, 2006)

difficulties of conducting the animal experiments. The experiments are expensive and multidisciplinary environment is necessary. This is probably the reason for the existence of limited number in vivo animal studies on this subject.

One attempt to model the effect of perfusion in tissue using phantoms is presented in Ref. 59. Related in vivo heating experiments were performed using rabbits. The experiments were repeated on the different types of the tissue and they are performed in acute conditions.

The calculated heating ranges (Figure 23.17) mostly underestimated temperature increases in the experiments. One of the reasons for this underestimation could be the effect of altered thermal, electrical, and thermoregulatory properties of the tissue immediately after surgery or the use of the simplified Pennes model.

Luechinger *et al.* measured in vivo temperature increases during MRI of a pacemaker under chronic conditions.[60] Thermocouples were used to collect the temperature data from the pacemaker lead screws in the pigs. They reported significant impedance change and minor threshold change in their study. In addition, temperature increases of up to 20 °C were reported. Surprisingly, however, the authors did not observe any tissue damage in the pathology.[60]

Normally, temperature measurements in MRI are performed using fiber-optic temperature sensors for their MRI compatibility. In Luechinger *et al.*'s study, however, thermocouples were chosen probably due to

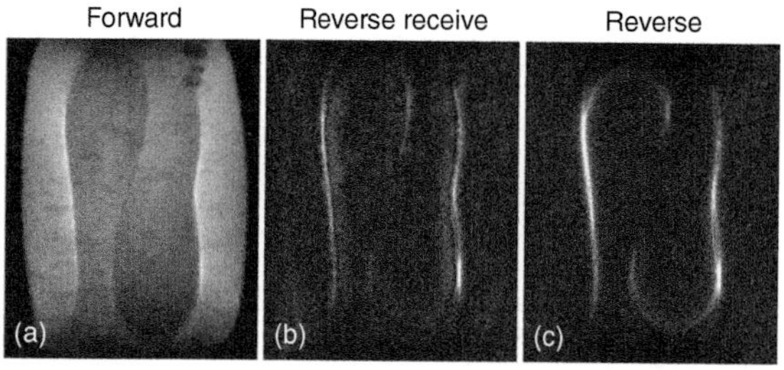

Figure 23.15. Pacemaker lead. Projection images of a pacing lead of 85 cm in a gel phantom of 36 cm. (a) Forward polarization image shows conventional current artifacts. When the receiver polarization is reversed (b) or both transmitter and receiver are reversed in polarization (c), the background signal cancellation in the vicinity of the wire is evident in dually reversed image, along with slightly better background suppression. (Reproduced with permission from Ref. 57. © John Wiley & Sons, 2010)

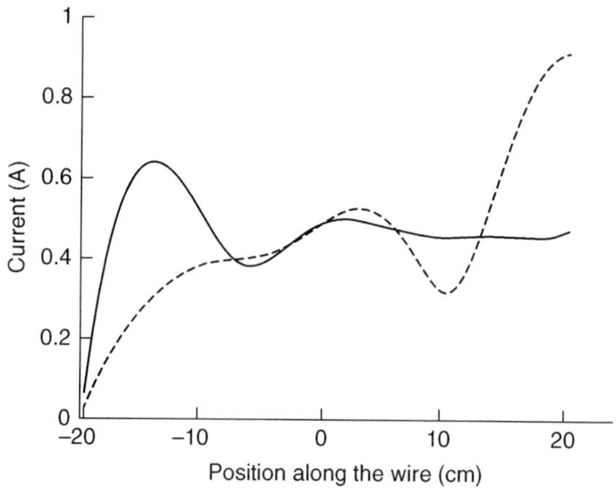

Figure 23.16. The variation of the current along the helical wire is plotted for the reversed (dashed line) and the forward (solid line) polarization. (Reproduced with permission from Ref. 58. © John Wiley & Sons, 2011)

the long-term considerations for the chronic conditions because fiber optic sensors' resilience is much lower than standard wires.[60] This tradeoff might have created temperature measurement bias due to the additional long conductive cables. In addition, the sensor location may have been shifted during the experiment.

It is crucial to perform 'human-relevant' animal experiments to develop a better understanding of the MRI-induced heating in patients with AIMDs. To support such investigation, a test system was developed by Silemek *et al.*[61]. The system mimicked a typical DBS implant in in vivo animal RF heating studies.

Since induced heating near an implant depends on its geometry and materials, a temperature sensor implant (TSI) was developed using the materials and geometry similar to a DBS. It is assumed that the electromagnetic scattering during MRI would be similar in both DBS and TSI.

The home-built TSI was developed with an embedded thermocouple at its electrode providing temperature measurements at the electrode tip. These temperature measurements were transferred to an external computer wirelessly. The proposed device's MRI compatibility and induced heating performance were assessed comparing the temperature increase at the electrode using both fiber optic and TSI measurements. Animal RF heating experiments were done immediately after the implantation of the TSI and 2 weeks after the implantation. The validation of using a dual-drive birdcage coil to reduce the RF-induced heating was shown immediately after the placement of the TSI by measuring the tip temperature during MRI. It was shown that no significant RF-induced heating was produced when a conventional scanning protocol was used. The heating tests were assessed in subacute conditions to reduce the surgery effects due to the implantation. The dual-drive heating reduction method was validated under subacute in vivo conditions. Three heating cases were tested using the same applied SAR ($7\ W\ kg^{-1}$). The in vivo heating was reduced to 1.8 °C even for such high SAR (whole-body average SAR is limited to $4\ W\ kg^{-1}$ for clinical conditions). The worst-case maximum heating for this condition was measured as 12.8 °C and finally, in quadrature mode, the heating was measured as 4.1 °C (Figure 23.18).

Further in vivo studies should be done to understand surgery related effects on the RF heating related studies for the AIMDs. Moreover, commercial AIMDs can be considered when testing them under MRI. The electrical parameters of a specific commercial AIMD can be calculated using implant models such as the one in Ref. 10. Desired testing can be done by constructing a suitable TSI with the same electrical parameters.

As can be understood from the discussion above, in vivo testing is difficult and more research on this topic is needed.

23.6 CLINICAL RESEARCH

While biomedical engineers are trying to understand the risks of MRI scanning in patients with AIMDs and trying to find methods to minimize the risks, a

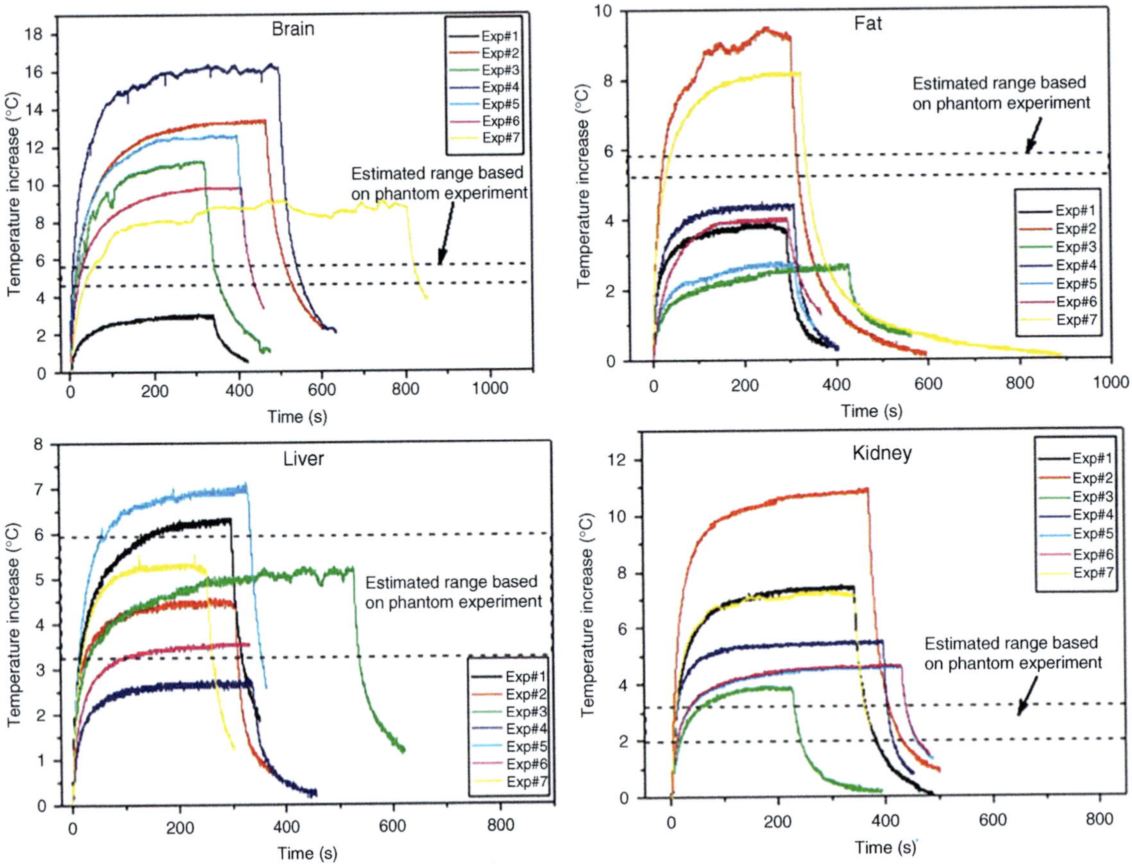

Figure 23.17. Temperature increase versus time graphs for four tissues of rabbit. The regions shown by dashed lines are estimated ranges based on the phantom experiment. Phantom data scaled by heat capacity and applied power of corresponding tissues. (Reproduced with permission from Ref. 59. © John Wiley & Sons, 2007)

significant number of patients with both the MRI conditional and MRI unsafe AIMDs are being scanned. The current data are puzzling, in the sense that other than a few case studies,[6,29] thermal injuries to patients implanted with AIMDs and undergoing MRI are not reported. In addition, there are controlled studies in limited number patients who show no significant problem. One of the largest studies is MagnaSafe Registry which is a prospective study for nonthoracic MRI of patients with ICDs and implanted pacemakers.[62] The study aims to determine the risks of 1.5 T MRI on patients with non-MRI compatible ICDs and pacemakers. In this study, 500 patients with cardiac pacemaker and 500 patients with ICDs were examined.[63] The investigators recorded the device parameter (battery level, lead threshold, and lead impedance) changes pre- and post-MRI examination. During the MRI examination, a cardiologist or a qualified physician on ICD/pacemaker function and trained personnel on advanced cardiac life support were present. In addition, continuous cardiac rhythm and patient oxygen level were recorded. Patient's blood pressure was measured pre- and post-MRI examination. The implants were turned off before the scan and their initial settings were restored after the exam. No significant problem associated with MRI observed in any of the patients in the study. The lead impedance change exceeded 3 Ω for 16.4% of the cases. The conclusion of the study was that MRI can be used in these patients under controlled conditions even if the devices have been labeled as MRI unsafe. The US food drug administration strongly opposes this recommendation.[64]

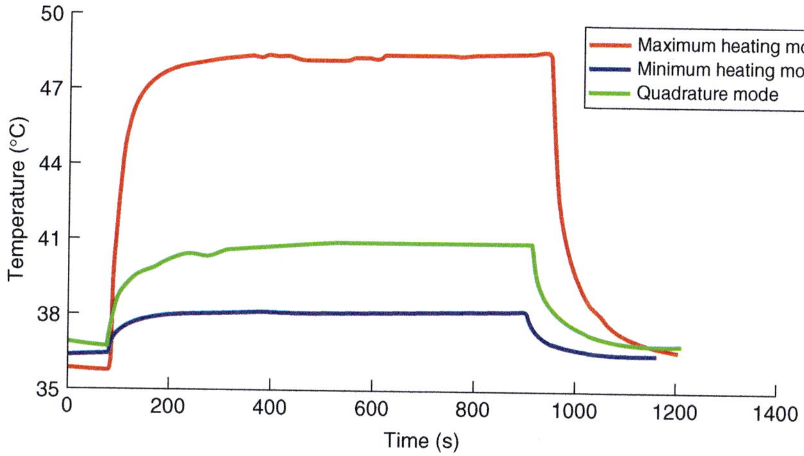

Figure 23.18. Tip temperature measurements during the heating experiments. The temperature rise around the electrode is shown for the maximum coupling (red), implant-friendly (blue), and quadrature modes. (Reproduced with permission from Ref. 61. © John Wiley & Sons, 2018)

Phantom studies show that significant heating occurs only under very specific conditions. It is possible that during the examination of these 1000 patients, these conditions may have not been met. The study does not conclusively rule out the possibility of excessive, clinically harmful induced heating near conductive devices during MRI. Obviously better understanding of the problem is necessary to offer safe and effective MRI to every patient with AIMDs.

Abandoned implant leads pose an additional safety problem. One solution to this is performing lead extraction before MRI for diminishing RF-induced heating. However, the lead extraction processes have their own risks.[65–68] One study concludes that lead extraction for the MRI of a patient can be considered if MRI is the only imaging option and the clinical outcome is significant.[69]

The clinical research on imaging patients with AIMDs has a broad literature. The readers of this book are recommended to investigate them for much more detail.

23.7 CONCLUSION

MRI is widely used because of its high soft tissue contrast. It is noninvasive, very versatile and provides detailed information on the tissue deep inside the body. Although MR imaging method is known to be very safe to use, there is undesired interaction between the leads of the AIMDs with the electromagnetic field generated inside MRI scanners, which may result in a risk of thermal tissue damage at the location of the pacing of the patients. MRI may be the only imaging alternative for some patients who have these implants in their body. As we learn more of the risks of MRI scanning of patients with AIMDs, methods to reduce these risks are being developed. Clinicians may order the scans if they know these risks by weighing against benefits. As discussed in this chapter, there is already a good understanding of the extent of the problem based on the studies on tissue mimicking phantoms and computer simulations. While engineers and scientists are working on finding possible solutions to reduce the risks associated with the implant heating during MR imaging and improve the safety profiles of AIMDs, physicians are collecting data on patients with AIMDs to understand the clinical consequences of the heat generated near the implants during MRI. AIMDs which enable safe MRI scanning under some specified conditions are becoming commercially available. There are also some studies on making MRI scanners AIMD friendly. With new developments, the growing number of patients with AIMDs will be able to benefit from the high diagnostic quality of MRI.

DISCLAIMER

The subject matter, content, and views presented do not represent the views of the Department of Health and Human Services (HHS), US Food and Drug Administration (FDA), and/or the United States.

RELATED ARTICLES IN EMAGRES

Bioeffects and Safety of Radiofrequency Electromagnetic Fields

Birdcage Resonators: Highly Homogeneous Radiofrequency Coils for Magnetic Resonance

Health and Safety Aspects of Human MR Studies

Radiofrequency Fields: Interactions, Biological Effects, and Safety Issues

Safety Regulation in MR

RF Device Safety and Compatibility

Radiofrequency Fields and SAR for Bird Cage Coils

Radiofrequency Heating Models and Measurements

Safety Considerations in MRI

Effects of Hip Prostheses In Situ Exposed to 64 and 128 MHz RF Fields

MRI for Noninvasive Thermometry

REFERENCES

1. IEC, Medical Electrical Equipment-Part 2-33: Particular Requirements for the Basic Safety and Essential Performance of Magnetic Resonance Equipment for Medical Diagnosis; 60601-2-33, 2010.
2. R. Kalin and M. S. Stanton, *Pacing Clin. Electrophysiol.*, 2005, **28**, 326.
3. W. Pavlicek, M. Geisinger, L. Castle, G. P. Borkowski, T. F. Meaney, B. L. Bream, and J. H. Gallagher, *Radiology*, 1983, **147**, 149.
4. J. M. Fontaine, F. B. Mohamed, C. Gottlieb, D. J. Callans, and F. E. Marchlinski, *Pacing Clin. Electrophysiol.*, 1998, **21**, 1336.
5. J. R. Gimbel, *Europace*, 2009, **11**, 1241.
6. J. M. Henderson, J. Tkach, M. Phillips, K. Baker, F. G. Shellock, and A. R. Rezai, *Neurosurgery*, 2005, **57**, E1063, discussion E1063.
7. V. Acikel, A. Uslubas, and E. Atalar, *Med. Phys.*, 2015, **42**, 3922.
8. C. J. Yeung, R. C. Susil, and E. Atalar, *Magn. Reson. Med.*, 2002, **47**, 187.
9. C. Armenean, E. Perrin, M. Armenean, O. Beuf, F. Pilleul, and H. Saint-Jalmes, *Magn. Reson. Med.*, 2004, **52**, 1200.
10. V. Acikel and E. Atalar, *Med. Phys.*, 2011, **38**, 6623.
11. R. W. P. King and C. W. Harrison Jr., Antennas and Waves: A Modern Approach, MIT Press: Cambridge, MA, 1969.
12. V. Açıkel, Analysis of Current Induction on Thin Conductors Inside the Body During MRI Scan, Bilkent University: Ankara, 2014.
13. S.-M. Park, R. Kamondetdacha, and J. A. Nyenhuis, *J. Magn. Reson. Imaging*, 2007, **26**, 1278.
14. S. Feng, R. Qiang, W. Kainz, and J. Chen, *IEEE Trans. Microw. Theory Tech.*, 2015, **63**, 305.
15. J. P. Tokaya, A. J. E. Raaijmakers, P. R. Luijten, J. F. Bakker, and C. A. T. van Den Berg, *Magn. Reson. Med.*, 2017, **78**, 2449.
16. H. H. Pennes, *J. Appl. Physiol.*, 1948, **1**, 93.
17. D. Shrivastava, Theory and Applications of Heat Transfer in Humans, John Wiley & Sons: Hoboken, NJ, 2018.
18. R. Vyas and M. L. Rustgi, *Med. Phys.*, 1992, **19**, 1319.
19. B. Gao, S. Langer, and P. M. Corry, *Int. J. Hyperthermia*, 1995, **11**, 267.
20. C. J. Yeung and E. Atalar, *Med. Phys.*, 2001, **28**, 826.
21. C. J. Yeung, R. C. Susil, and E. Atalar, *Magn. Reson. Med.*, 2002, **48**, 1096.
22. E. Mattei, M. Triventi, G. Calcagnini, F. Censi, W. Kainz, G. Mendoza, H. I. Bassen, and P. Bartolini, *Biomed. Eng. Online*, 2008, **7**, 11.
23. A. R. Rezai, D. Finelli, J. A. Nyenhuis, G. Hrdlicka, J. Tkach, A. Sharan, P. Rugieri, P. H. Stypulkowski, and F. G. Shellock, *J. Magn. Reson. Imaging*, 2002, **15**, 241.
24. J. Kahan, A. Papadaki, M. White, L. Mancini, T. Yousry, L. Zrinzo, P. Limousin, M. Hariz, T. Foltynie, and J. Thornton, *PLoS One*, 2015, **10**, e0129077.
25. M. E. Ladd and H. H. Quick, *Magn. Reson. Med.*, 2000, **43**, 615.
26. W. R. Nitz, A. Oppelt, W. Renz, C. Manke, M. Lenhart, and J. Link, *J. Magn. Reson. Imaging*, 2001, **13**, 105.

27. B. Bhusal, P. Bhattacharyya, T. Baig, S. Jones, and M. Martens, *Magn. Reson. Med.*, 2018, **80**, 1676.
28. G. C. Van Rhoon, T. Samaras, P. S. Yarmolenko, M. W. Dewhirst, E. Neufeld, and N. Kuster, *Eur. Radiol.*, 2013, **23**, 2215.
29. J. Spiegel, G. Fuss, M. Backens, W. Reith, T. Magnus, G. Becker, J.-R. Moringlane, and U. Dillmann, *J. Neurosurg.*, 2003, **99**, 772.
30. W. Greatbatch, V. Miller, and F. G. Shellock, *J. Magn. Reson. Imaging*, 2002, **16**, 97.
31. P. A. Bottomley, W. A. Edelstein, A. Kumar, J. M. Allen, and P. Karmarkar, In *Proceedings of the International Society for Magnetic Resonance in Medicine*, 2009, Vol. 17, p 4805.
32. P. A. Bottomley, A. Kumar, W. A. Edelstein, J. M. Allen, and P. V. Karmarkar, *Med. Phys.*, 2010, **37**, 3828.
33. O. Ocali and E. Atalar, *Magn. Reson. Med.*, 1997, **37**, 112.
34. X. Yang and E. Atalar, *Radiology*, 2000, **217**, 501.
35. B. Qiu, P. Karmarkar, C. Brushett, F. Gao, R. Kon, S. Kar, E. Atalar, and X. Yang, *Magn. Reson. Med.*, 2005, **53**, 986.
36. ASTM-F2503-05, Standard Practice for Marking Medical Devices and Other Items for Safety in the Magnetic Resonance Environment, 2005.
37. R. Sutton, E. Kanal, B. L. Wilkoff, D. Bello, R. Luechinger, I. Jenniskens, M. Hull, and T. Sommer, *Trials*, 2008, **9**, 68.
38. B. L. Wilkoff, D. Bello, M. Taborsky, J. Vymazal, E. Kanal, H. Heuer, K. Hecking, W. B. Johnson, W. Young, B. Ramza, N. Akhtar, B. Kuepper, P. Hunold, R. Luechinger, H. Puererfellner, F. Duru, M. J. Gotte, R. Sutton, T. Sommer, and EnRhythm MRI SureScan Pacing System Study Investigators, *Heart Rhythm*, 2011, **8**, 65.
39. M. Mitka, *JAMA*, 2011, **305**, 985.
40. E. M. Cronin and B. L. Wilkoff, *Indian Pacing Electrophysiol. J.*, 2012, **12**, 204.
41. C. H. Kwon, J. H. Choi, J. Kim, U. Jo, J. H. Lee, W. S. Lee, Y. R. Kim, S. Y. Lee, K. W. Whang, J. Yang, S. H. Kim, Y. S. Oh, K. M. Park, G. B. Nam, K. J. Choi, and Y. H. Kim, *J. Korean Med. Sci.*, 2016, **31**, 1397.
42. S. Nazarian, R. Hansford, A. Roguin, D. Goldsher, M. M. Zviman, A. C. Lardo, B. S. Caffo, K. D. Frick, M. A. Kraut, I. R. Kamel, H. Calkins, R. D. Berger, D. A. Bluemke, and H. R. Halperin, *Ann. Intern. Med.*, 2011, **155**, 415.
43. C. E. Hayes, W. A. Edelstein, J. F. Schenck, O. M. Mueller, and M. Eash, *J. Magn. Reson.*, 1985, **63**, 622.
44. Y. Eryaman, B. Akin, and E. Atalar, *Magn. Reson. Med.*, 2011, **65**, 1305.
45. Y. Eryaman, E. A. Turk, C. Oto, O. Algin, and E. Atalar, *Magn. Reson. Med.*, 2013, **69**, 845.
46. L. Golestanirad, M. I. Iacono, B. Keil, L. M. Angelone, G. Bonmassar, M. D. Fox, T. Herrington, E. Adalsteinsson, C. LaPierre, A. Mareyam, and L. L. Wald, *Neuroimage*, 2017, **147**, 577.
47. G. H. Glover, C. E. Hayes, N. J. Pelc, W. A. Edelstein, O. M. Mueller, H. R. Hart, C. J. Hardy, M. O'Donnell, and W. D. Barber, *J. Magn. Reson.*, 1985, **64**, 255.
48. C. E. McElcheran, B. Yang, K. J. T. Anderson, L. Golenstani-Rad, and S. J. Graham, *PLoS One*, 2015, **10**, e0134379.
49. M. I. Iacono, N. Makris, L. Mainardi, L. M. Angelone, and G. Bonmassar, *Comput. Math. Methods Med.*, 2013, **2013**, 694171.
50. B. Guerin, P. Serano, M. I. Iacono, T. M. Herrington, A. S. Widge, D. D. Dougherty, G. Bonmassar, L. M. Angelone, and L. L. Wald, *Phys. Med. Biol.*, 2018, **63**, 095015.
51. M. G. Zanchi, R. Venook, J. M. Pauly, and G. C. Scott, *IEEE Trans. Med. Imaging*, 2010, **29**, 169.
52. P. Nordbeck, I. Weiss, P. Ehses, O. Ritter, M. Warmuth, F. Fidler, V. Herold, P. M. Jakob, M. E. Ladd, H. H. Quick, and W. R. Bauer, *Magn. Reson. Med.*, 2009, **61**, 570.
53. M. Etezadi-Amoli, P. Stang, A. Kerr, J. Pauly, and G. Scott, *Magn. Reson. Med.*, 2015, **74**, 1790.
54. H. Graf, G. Steidle, P. Martirosian, U. A. Lauer, and F. Schick, *Med. Phys.*, 2006, **33**, 124.
55. M. R. van den Bosch, M. A. Moerland, J. J. W. Lagendijk, L. W. Bartels, and C. A. T. van den Berg, *Med. Phys.*, 2010, **37**, 814.
56. H. Celik, A. Ulutürk, T. Tali, and E. Atalar, *Magn. Reson. Med.*, 2007, **58**, 1224.
57. W. R. Overall, J. M. Pauly, P. P. Stang, and G. C. Scott, *Magn. Reson. Med.*, 2010, **64**, 823.
58. Y. Eryaman, S. Hersek, and E. Atalar, *Magn. Reson. Med.*, 2011, **66**, 1515; author reply 1517.
59. I. B. Akca, O. Ferhanoglu, C. J. Yeung, S. Guney, T. O. Tasci, and E. Atalar, *J. Magn. Reson. Imaging*, 2007, **26**, 1228.
60. R. Luechinger, V. A. Zeijlemaker, E. M. Pedersen,

P. Mortensen, E. Falk, F. Duru, R. Candinas, and P. Boesiger, *Eur. Heart J.*, 2005, **26**, 376, discussion 325–327.

61. B. Silemek, V. Acikel, C. Oto, A. Alipour, Z. G. Aykut, O. Algin, and E. Atalar, *Magn. Reson. Med.*, 2018, **79**, 2824.

62. The MagnaSafe Registry. http://magnasafe.org/aboutmagnasafe.html (accessed October 23, 2018).

63. R. J. Russo, H. S. Costa, P. D. Silva, J. L. Anderson, A. Arshad, R. W. W. Biederman, N. G. Boyle, J. V. Frabizzio, U. Birgersdotter-Green, S. L. Higgins, R. Lampert, C. E. Machado, E. T. Martin, A. L. Rivard, J. C. Rubenstein, R. H. M. Schaerf, J. D. Schwartz, D. J. Shah, G. F. Tomassoni, G. T. Tominaga, A. E. Tonkin, S. Uretsky, and S. D. Wolff, *N. Engl. J. Med.*, 2017, **376**, 755.

64. J. G. Delfino, I. Viohl, and T. O. Woods, *N. Engl. J. Med.*, 2017, **376**, 2495.

65. R. G. Hauser, W. T. Katsiyiannis, C. C. Gornick, A. K. Almquist, and L. M. Kallinen, *Europace*, 2010, **12**, 395.

66. S. O. Jones IV, R. E. Eckart, C. M. Albert, and L. M. Epstein, *Heart Rhythm*, 2008, **5**, 520.

67. O. Wazni, L. M. Epstein, R. G. Carrillo, C. Love, S. W. Adler, D. W. Riggio, S. S. Karim, J. Bashir, A. J. Greenspon, J. P. DiMarco, J. M. Cooper, J. R. Onufer, K. A. Ellenbogen, S. P. Kutalek, S. Dentry-Mabry, C. M. Ervin, and B. L. Wilkoff, *J. Am. Coll. Cardiol.*, 2010, **55**, 579.

68. B. L. Wilkoff, C. L. Byrd, C. J. Love, D. L. Hayes, T. D. Sellers, R. Schaerf, V. Parsonnet, L. M. Epstein, R. A. Sorrentino, and C. Reiser, *J. Am. Coll. Cardiol.*, 1999, **33**, 1671.

69. B. L. Wilkoff, C. J. Love, C. L. Byrd, M. G. Bongiorni, R. G. Carrillo, G. H. Crossley, L. M. Epstein, R. A. Friedman, C. E. H. Kennergren, P. Mitkowski, R. H. Schaerf, O. M. Wazni, Heart Rhythm Society, and American Heart Association, *Heart Rhythm*, 2009, **6**, 1085.

Chapter 24

An Analysis of Factors Influencing MRI RF Safety for Patients with AIMDs

Jingshen Liu[1], Jianfeng Zheng[2], Qingyan Wang[2], and Ji Chen[2]

[1]*IEEE, Calabasas, CA, USA*
[2]*IEEE, Houston, TX, USA*

24.1 INTRODUCTION

An active implantable medical device (AIMD) usually includes an implantable pulse generator (IPG) and implantable lead(s). When a patient with an AIMD undergoes the magnetic resonance imaging (MRI) procedure, the lead can act as an antenna that receives radio-frequency (RF) power generated by the MRI RF coil, which raises the safety issues. The two major concerns are MRI RF-induced heating on the distal end of the lead, which can cause severe tissue injury,[1] and MRI RF-induced voltage on the proximal end of the lead that is connected to the IPG, which can cause the device malfunction or damage.[2] There are two important topics about the MRI safety for patients with AIMDs. One is to evaluate the MRI safety, and the other is to improve the MRI safety. Both of them require the understanding of the factors that influence the MRI RF-induced heating and voltage.

For the first topic, to evaluate the MRI safety for AIMDs, both numerical simulation and experimental approaches were applied.[2–10] Each approach has its limitations. Since AIMD leads often have complex designs such as coradial and coaxial submillimeter coils,[11] it is very difficult to simulate an AIMD simultaneously with an RF coil and an anatomical human model. Also, it is often not feasible to perform in vivo MRI safety measurements. Therefore, for both numerical simulation and experimental approaches, a phantom with tissue-simulating medium is often used. Several standard tissue-simulating media with different relative permittivities and conductivities were proposed in.[12] However, due to the complexity of the implantable pathways, using homogeneous media to simulate the human tissues is often not accurate. Understanding the influence of media surrounding different portions of an AIMD to the MRI safety problem is important in determining tissue-simulating media.

For the second topic, to improve the MRI safety for AIMDs, understanding what factors of the AIMD and how these factors can influence the MRI RF-induced

Safety and Biological Effects in MRI.
Edited by Devashish Shrivastava and J. Thomas Vaughan
 ISBN: 978-1-118-82130-5
Also published in eMagRes (online edition)
DOI: 10.1002/9780470034590.emrstm1641

heating and voltage is also very important. It can help the design of MRI conditionally safe AIMDs.

Researches have been performed to investigate these factors. Influences of implantable lead length and pathway are investigated in.[13] Measurements for implants with different lengths, insulation thicknesses, and paths in phantoms were performed in.[14] However, these investigations did not fit these factors into a general model, and the results might not be able to be applied to different AIMDs.

In this chapter, the influences of different factors, such as the AIMD-surrounding medium, the IPG inner circuit impedance, and the lead tip structure, to the MRI RF-induced heating and voltage are analyzed. The analysis is based on the transfer function method[15] and the transmission line model.[16] The contribution of each factor is analyzed in the form of transmission line coefficients and impedances.

24.2 THEORETICAL AND NUMERICAL ANALYSIS

Figure 24.1(a) shows a human body with an implanted AIMD under the MRI RF coil emission. Schematic of the MRI RF safety problem is shown in Figure 24.1(b). The AIMD includes an IPG and an implantable lead. One end of the lead is connected to the IPG, and the other end of the lead is the lead tip which contains electrodes contacting human tissues. The lead body contains an insulator and a conductor. $\vec{E}_{\text{inc}}, \vec{H}_{\text{inc}}$ are incident electric and magnetic fields in human tissues generated by the RF coil. The fields can interact with the AIMD, which can lead to the RF-induced voltage on the IPG and the RF-induced heating in tissues near the lead tip.

A simplified schematic of the MRI RF safety problem is shown in Figure 24.2(a). An implantable lead in a medium, which can be either human tissues or a phantom, is under incident electromagnetic field emissions. The induced voltage on the IPG end can cause RF-induced voltage, and the induced energy near the device tip end can cause RF-induced heating.

To evaluate the MRI RF-induced field, a transfer function method is proposed.[15] According to the transfer function method,

$$|\vec{E}_{\text{total}} \cdot \hat{J}^{i}| = \left| \int_{l} \left(\vec{E}_{\text{inc}}(l) \cdot \hat{l} \right) T(l) \mathrm{d}l \right| \tag{24.1}$$

where $\hat{l}$ is a unit vector along the lead direction, and $\hat{J}^{i}$ is a unit vector with the direction of the infinitesimal dipole $\vec{J}^{i}$ shown in Figure 24.2(b). $T(l)$ is the transfer function, which transfers the incident electric field $\vec{E}_{\text{inc}}$ along the lead to the total electric field $\vec{E}_{\text{inc}}$ at the lead end.

To extract $T(l)$, a reciprocal problem is created as shown in Figure 24.2(b). The incident fields $\vec{E}_{\text{inc}}, \vec{H}_{\text{inc}}$ are removed, and a unit dipole source $\vec{J}^{i}$ is placed at the lead end where $\vec{E}_{\text{total}}$ is to be evaluated. A current $I(l)$ is induced on the lead, and

$$T(l) = I(l) \tag{24.2}$$

$I(l)$ on an implantable lead in human tissues can be modeled as the current $I(l)$ on a coaxial transmission line.[16] The lead conductor acts as the inner conductor, and human tissues act as the outer conductor. As shown in Figure 24.3, the transmission line is characterized by propagation wavenumber k_z and characteristic impedance Z_0. Two ends of the lead are modeled as lumped impedances Z_s and Z_L. A unit current source $I_s = 1$ A is placed at the end of the transmission line.

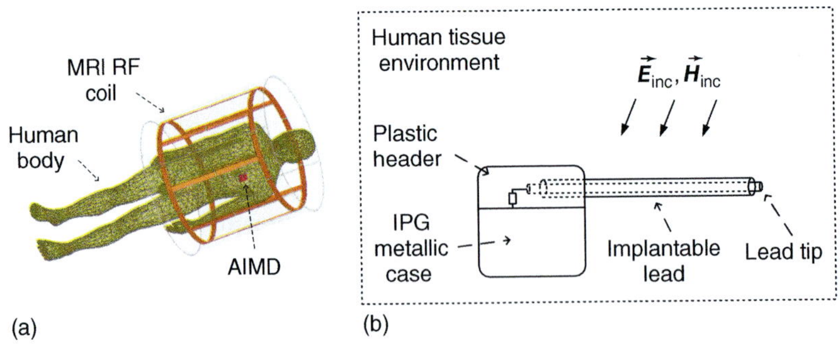

Figure 24.1. (a) Human body with an AIMD in an MRI RF coil. (b) Schematic of the MRI RF safety problem

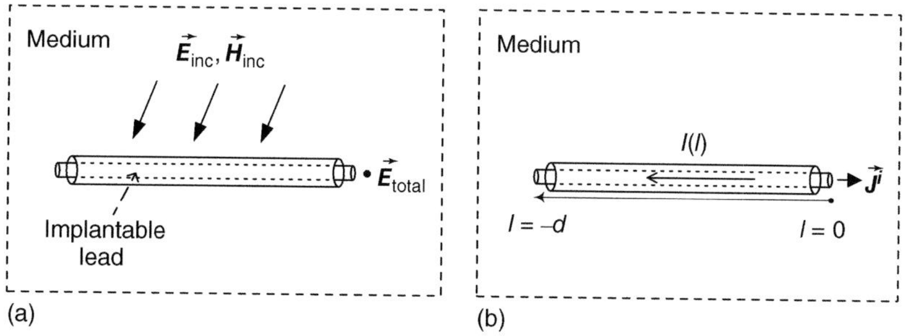

Figure 24.2. (a) The forward problem of the transfer function method. (b) The reciprocal problem of the transfer function method

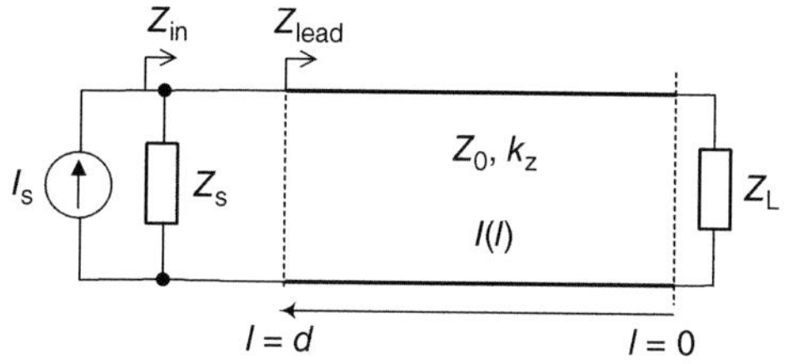

Figure 24.3. The transmission line model for an AIMD in a medium

If the source is placed at the IPG end (the RF-induced voltage problem), Z_s is the IPG impedance Z_{IPG}, and Z_L is the tip impedance Z_{tip}. If the source is placed at the lead tip end (the RF-induced heating problem), Z_s is Z_{tip}, and Z_L is Z_{IPG}.

According to the transmission line model,

$$I(l) = I_s \frac{Z_s}{Z_s + Z_{lead}} e^{jk_z(d-l)} \frac{1 - \Gamma_L e^{j2k_z l}}{1 - \Gamma_L e^{j2k_z d}} \tag{24.3}$$

where Γ_L is the voltage reflection coefficient given by

$$\Gamma_L = (Z_L - Z_0)/(Z_L + Z_0) \tag{24.4}$$

and Z_{lead} can be calculated as

$$Z_{lead} = Z_0 \frac{1 + \Gamma_L e^{j2k_z d}}{1 - \Gamma_L e^{j2k_z d}} \tag{24.5}$$

Substituting (24.3) to (24.1), $\vec{E}_{total}$ can be calculated as

$$|\vec{E}_{total} \cdot \hat{J}^i| = \left| \int_l \left(\vec{E}_{inc}(l) \cdot \hat{l} \right) I_s \frac{Z_s}{Z_s + Z_{lead}} e^{jk_z(d-l)} \frac{1 - \Gamma_L e^{j2k_z l}}{1 - \Gamma_L e^{j2k_z d}} dl \right|. \tag{24.6}$$

Equation (24.6) shows that the transmission line model parameters can fully characterize the MRI RF-induced field by determining the transfer function $T(l)$.

According to (24.3) and (24.4), as shown in Figure 24.4, different transmission line parameters have different influences on $T(l)$. The real part of k_z determines the wavelength, and the imaginary part of k_z determines the attenuation. Therefore, k_z can influence both the $T(l)$ profile and the $T(l)$ magnitude. Z_L mainly influences the $T(l)$ profile by Γ_L and also contributes to the $T(l)$ magnitude. As shown in Figure 24.4(d), Z_s only influences $T(l)$ magnitude and have no influence on $T(l)$ profile.

We denote the parameters in Figure 24.1(b) as physical parameters. These physical parameters can be categorized into two sets: physical parameters of the AIMD itself (e.g., the lead tip structure, IPG circuit impedance, and lead body configuration) and physical parameters of the environment (e.g., conductivity and dielectric constant of medium surrounding the lead tip, IPG, and lead body).

Similarly, we denote the transmission line parameters in Figure 24.3 as model parameters. The model parameters include excitation-end impedance Z_s, load impedance Z_L, and the lead body transmission line parameters (propagation wavenumber k_z and characteristic impedance Z_0).

In the following sections, the influences of physical parameters to model parameters are analyzed numerically. The analysis is performed by varying the physical parameters and observing the variation of the model parameters. The analysis is performed at 64 MHz, which is the operating frequency of the 1.5 T MRI RF coil. ANSYS HFSS is used in numerical simulations.

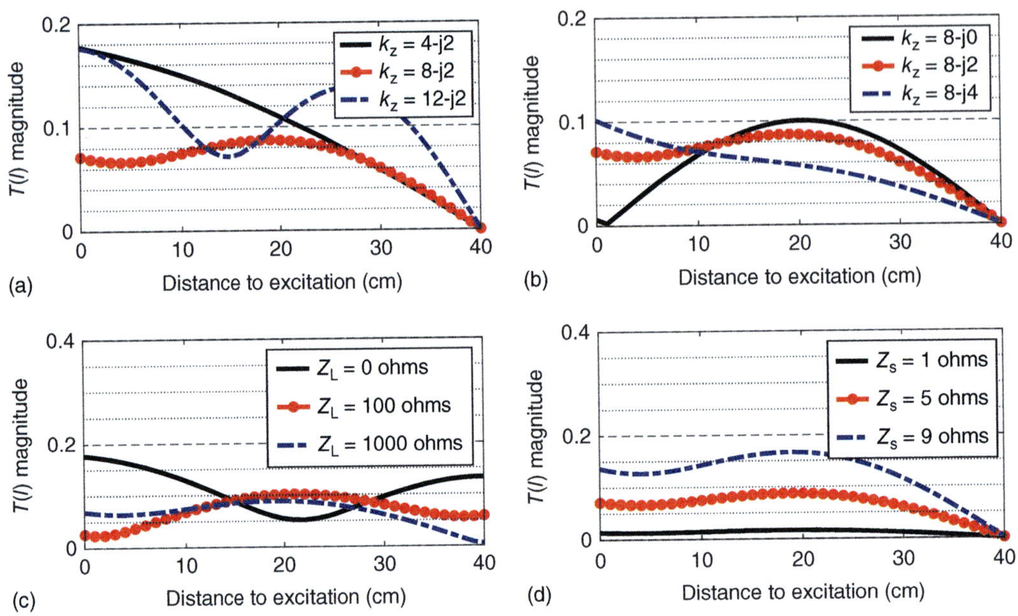

Figure 24.4. (a, b) $T(l)$ with different real and imaginary parts of k_z. (c) $T(l)$ with different Z_L. (d) $T(l)$ with different Z_s

24.2.1 Lead Body Transmission Line Parameters

A practical implantable lead usually includes conductors and a layer of dielectric insulation. The insulation can be silicone rubber or polyurethane, and the conductors can be straight conductors or coiling conductors with different configurations such as coaxial coil, coradial coil, and multifilar coil.[11] Also, different AIMDs are implanted in human bodies with different paths, and the tissues surrounding the lead body are of different kinds.

As discussed previously, two sets of physical parameters were analyzed. For the physical parameters of the AIMD, dielectric constant and dielectric loss tangent of the lead insulator were investigated. For the physical parameters of the environment, dielectric constant and conductivity of the medium were investigated. The lead conductor configuration was not investigated in this chapter, and leads with solid conductors were used to simplify the analysis. Lead body parameters of insulated solid leads can be extracted analytically.[17]

24.2.1.1 Physical Parameters of AIMDs

A lead with a 0.7 mm radius insulator and a 0.2 mm radius conductor was used in the analysis. The lead was submerged in saline with conductivity of 0.47 S m^{-1}, which is a typical phantom medium. We denote $k_z = (k_z' - jk_z'')$, $Z_0 = (Z_0' - jZ_0'')$, dielectric constant of the insulator as ε_{ri}, and loss tangent as $\tan\delta$.

As shown in Figure 24.5, k_z' increases as ε_{ri} increases, and it is not sensitive to the change of $\tan\delta$. k_z'' increases as ε_{ri} and $\tan\delta$ increase. Z_0 is not sensitive to the change of $\tan\delta$. Both Z_0' and Z_0'' decrease as ε_{ri} increases.

24.2.1.2 Physical Parameters of the Medium

Two leads with different dimensions were used in this investigation: a thick insulation lead with insulator radius of 0.7 mm and conductor radius of 0.2 mm and a thin insulation lead with insulator radius of 0.3 mm and conductor radius of 0.2 mm. The insulator had $\varepsilon_{ri} = 3$ and $\tan\delta = 0$. The lead lengths were both 52 cm.

As shown in Figure 24.6, both k_z and Z_0 are more sensitive to medium parameters change in low σ_m and ε_{rm} medium. The thin insulation lead is more sensitive to the medium parameters change than the thick insulation lead.

To visualize this, Figure 24.7 shows the magnitude of current profiles on these two leads when excited at one end in three different media. The lead was insulated at the load end. The three media

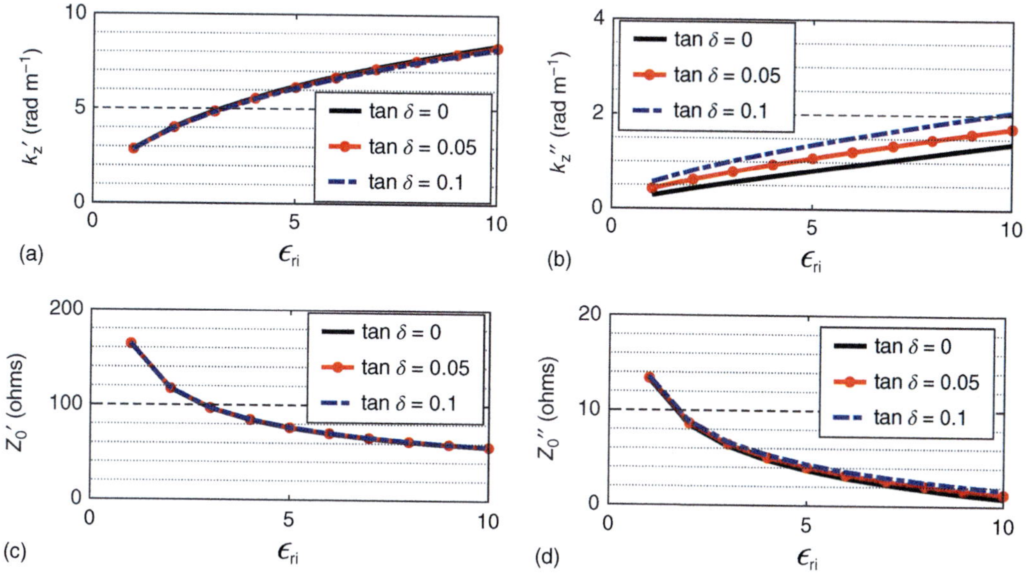

Figure 24.5. (a, b) Real and imaginary parts of k_z for lead with different ε_{ri} and tan δ. (c, d) Real and imaginary parts of Z_0 for lead with different ε_{ri} and tan δ

were chosen to be fat ($\varepsilon_{rm} = 13.6$, $\sigma_m = 0.066$ S m^{-1}), muscle ($\varepsilon_{rm} = 72.2$, $\sigma_m = 0.688$ S m^{-1}), and blood ($\varepsilon_{rm} = 86.4$, $\sigma_m = 1.207$ S m^{-1}).[18]

It can be shown that in low ε_{rm} and low σ_m medium such as fat, $T(l)$ tends to be different than that in other media. Also, for lead with thick insulation, the medium parameters have less influence on $T(l)$.

It needs to be pointed out that the thickness of the insulation is relative. According to the analytical equation given in,[17] if we denote the radius of the lead conductor to be a, and thickness of the insulator to be t, the larger the $(a + t)/a$ is, the less sensitive the model parameters is to the medium change.

24.2.2 Load Impedance

In this section, the lead tip impedance Z_{tip} and the IPG impedance Z_{IPG} are discussed. The method to extract Z is given in.[16]

Similar to the previous section, two sets of physical parameters were analyzed. The parameters of the AIMD include the lead tip structure and the IPG inner circuit impedance, and the parameters of the medium include the conductivity σ_m and dielectric constant ε_{rm} of the medium.

24.2.2.1 Lead Tip Impedance Z_{tip}

As shown in Figure 24.8(a) and (b), two lead tips with different electrode dimensions were used in the analysis. The two lead tips were submerged in the media with variant σ_m and ε_{rm}.

We denote $Z_{tip} = (Z_{tip}' - jZ_{tip}'')$. Figure 24.9 shows the variation of Z_{tip}' and Z_{tip}'' for the two lead tips in the media with different σ_m and ε_{rm}. Z_{tip} is more sensitive to media parameter changes when σ_m and ε_{rm} are small. It also shows that the size of the electrode, and thus the contact area of the electrode to the medium, will also influence Z_L. The increase of the size of the electrode results in the decrease of both Z_{tip}' and Z_{tip}''.

24.2.2.2 IPG Impedance Z_{IPG}

Similar to Z_{tip}, Z_{IPG} was analyzed for IPGs with different inner circuit impedances in media with variant σ_m and ε_{rm}.

Figure 24.10 shows the details of the IPG model. The lead inner conductor was connected to the IPG metallic case via a connecting wire and a lumped element. The lumped element was set to be 5 and 50 ohms to simulate different IPG inner circuit impedances.

Figure 24.11 shows the variation of Z_{IPG}' and Z_{IPG}'' for the two IPGs in media with different

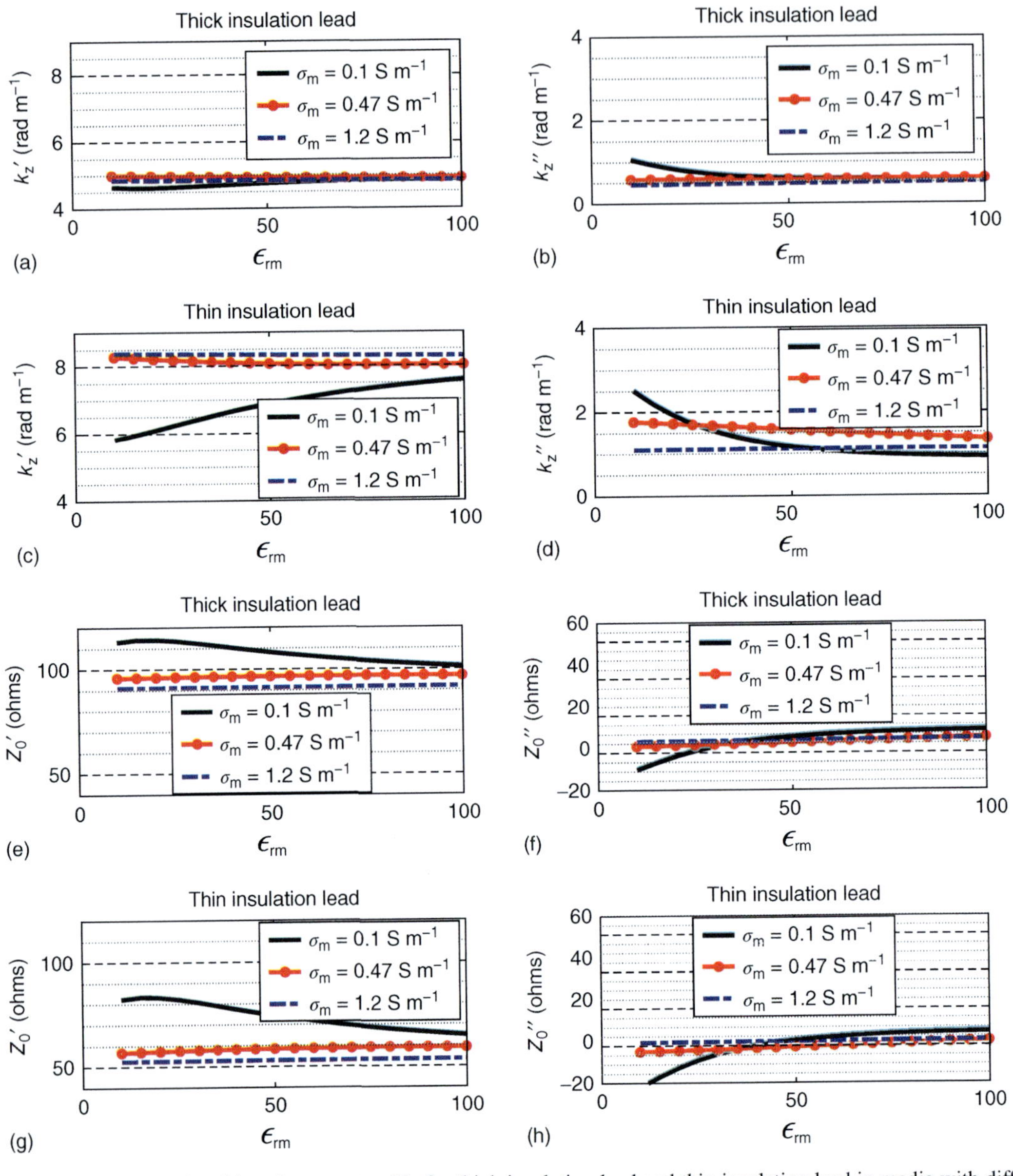

Figure 24.6. (a–d) Real and imaginary parts of k_z for thick insulation lead and thin insulation lead in media with different σ_m and ε_{rm}. (e–h) Real and imaginary parts of Z_0 for thick insulation lead and thin insulation lead in media with different σ_m and ε_{rm}

σ_m and ε_{rm}. Z_{IPG} is more sensitive to media parameters change in small σ_m and ε_{rm} media. It also shows that Z_{IPG} is largely dependent on the IPG inner circuit impedance. The higher σ_m and ε_{rm} are, the closer Z_{IPG} is to the IPG inner circuit impedance.

24.3 EXPERIMENTAL STUDIES

In this section, experimental studies were performed for one of the setups in the previous section, and the extracted parameters from experimental studies were compared with numerical simulations.

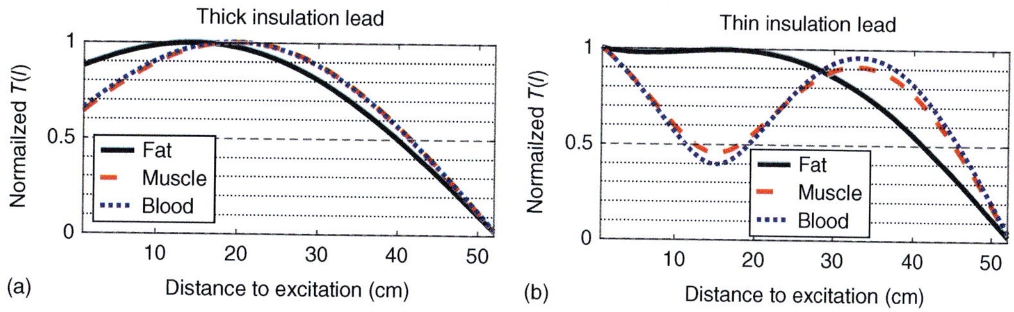

Figure 24.7. (a) Magnitude of $T(l)$ profiles of thick insulation lead in fat, muscle, and blood. (b) Magnitude of $T(l)$ profiles of thin insulation lead in fat, muscle, and blood

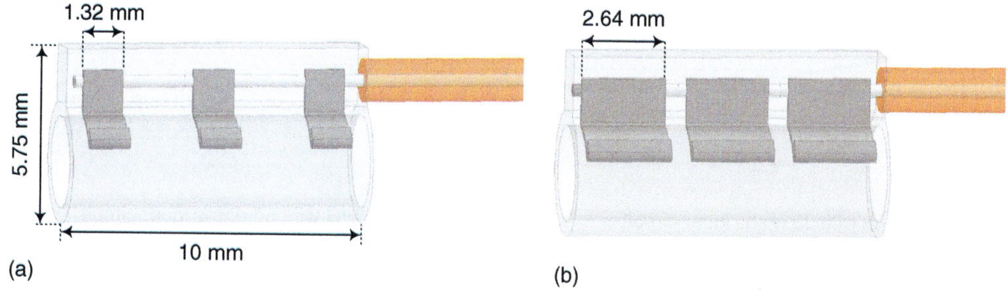

Figure 24.8. Lead tips with different dimensions. (a) Lead tip with small electrodes. (b) Lead tip with large electrodes

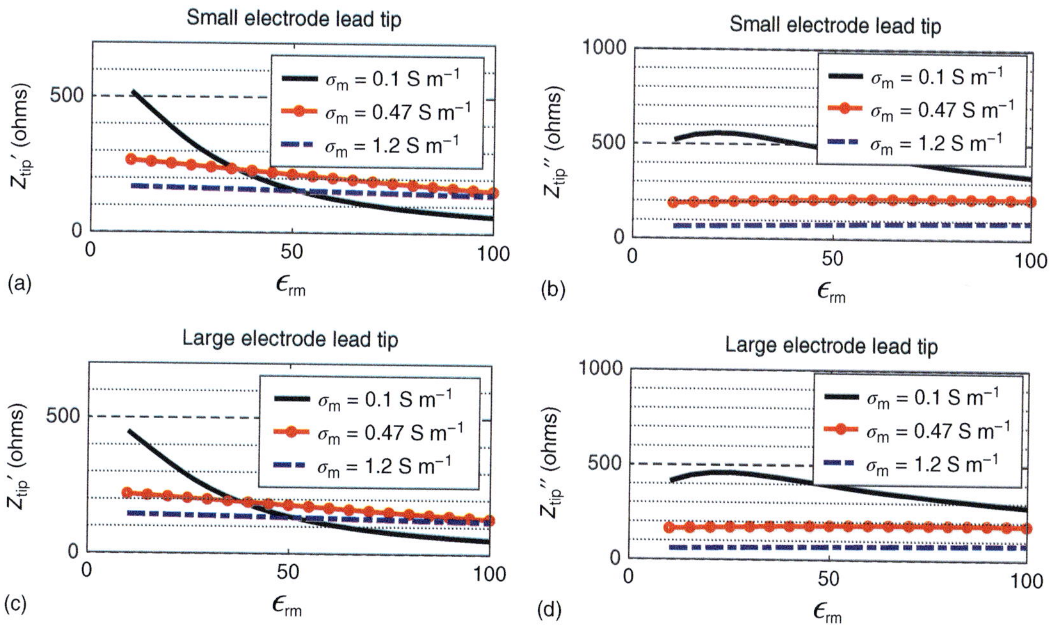

Figure 24.9. (a, b) Real and imaginary parts of Z_{tip} of the small electrode lead tip in media with different σ_{m} and $\varepsilon_{\mathrm{rm}}$. (c, d) Real and imaginary parts of Z_{tip} of the large electrode lead tip in media with different σ_{m} and $\varepsilon_{\mathrm{rm}}$

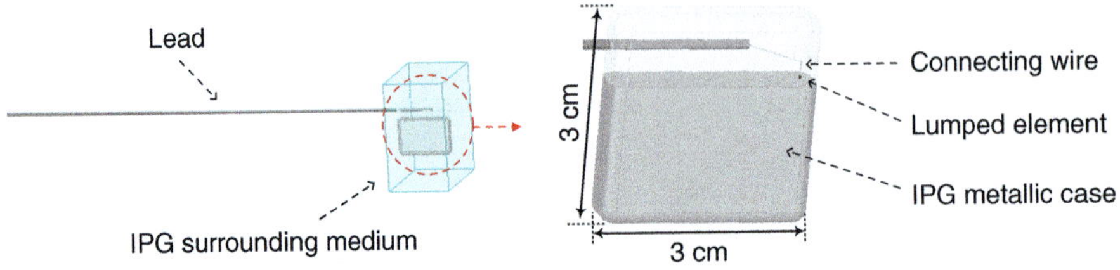

Figure 24.10. Illustration of the details of the IPG model

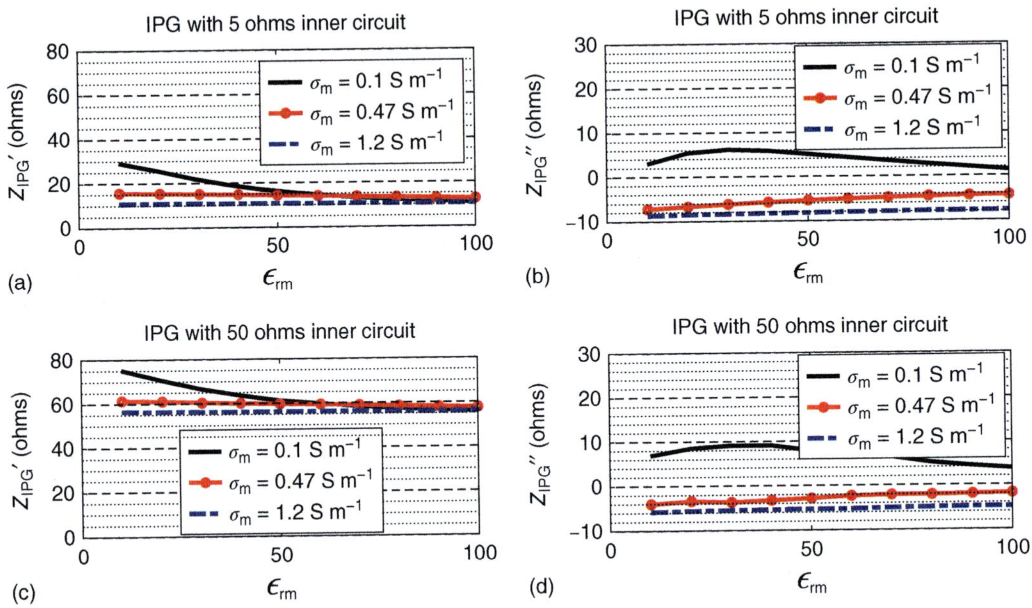

Figure 24.11. (a, b) Real and imaginary parts of Z_{IPG} of the 5 ohms IPG in media with different σ_m and ε_{rm}. (c, d) Real and imaginary parts of Z_{IPG} of the 50 ohms IPG in media with different σ_m and ε_{rm}

An insulated solid lead with a dummy IPG as shown in Figure 24.12 was used in measurements. The insulated solid leads had a 30 cm length. The radius of the lead conductor was 0.4064 mm. The lead insulator was polyvinyl chloride (PVC) with dielectric constant of 3. The thickness of the insulator was 0.4064 mm. One end of the lead (lead tip) was a 5 mm bare conductor, and the other end of the lead was connected to a dummy IPG. The dummy IPG was two pieces of copper pad with a resistor in between as a connection. The upper pad simulated the connecting wire inside the IPG, and it had a dimension of 1 cm by 3 cm. The lower pad simulated the metallic case of an IPG, and it had a dimension of 3 cm by 3 cm. The upper pad and the resistor were sealed with hot glue.

An automatic transfer function measurement system as shown in Figure 24.13 was used to measure the current profile along the lead. A National Instrument PXIe-5630 vector network analyzer (VNA), a Pearson current probe, a stepper motor, and an Arduino microcontroller were used in the system.

In order to measure Z_{IPG}, an excitation was placed at the lead tip. The lead was submerged in saline ($\varepsilon_{rm} = 78$) with σ_m of 0.47 S m^{-1}, which is the human average value. Two dummy IPGs with resistors of 2.2 and 50 ohms were used in the measurements.

The extracted Z_{IPG} was $15.8 + j0.3$ ohms for the 2.2 ohms dummy IPG and $45.4 - j14.9$ ohms for the 50 ohms dummy IPG. It shows that Z_{IPG} is largely dependent on the impedance of the resistor

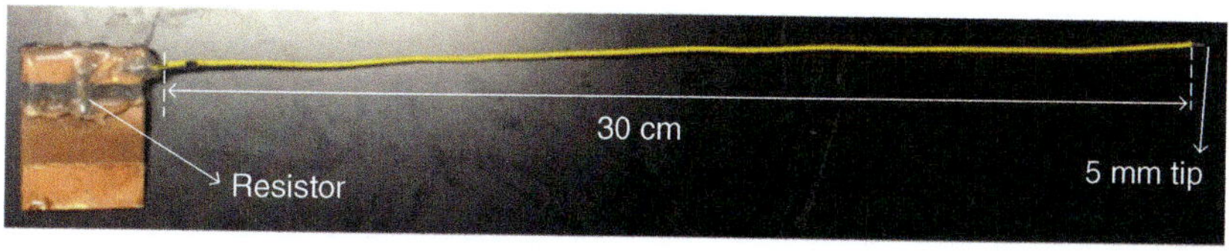

Figure 24.12. Photo of a dummy IPG with an insulated solid lead with bare tip. (Jingshen Liu)

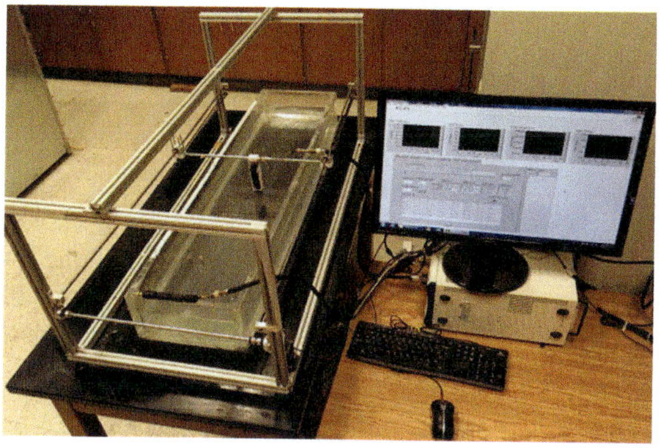

Figure 24.13. Photo of the automatic transfer function measurement system. (Jingshen Liu)

of dummy IPGs, or the inner circuit impedance of practical IPGs.

In addition, the same setup was built in HFSS as a reference. From numerical simulations, the extracted Z_{IPG} was $11.0 - j1.0$ ohms for the 2.2 ohms dummy IPG and $50.0 - j14.3$ for the 50 ohms dummy IPG. Also, the comparison of current profiles between simulations and measurements is shown in Figure 24.14. The good agreement validates the numerical simulations.

24.4 DISCUSSION

As mentioned in the previous sections, there are two important topics about AIMD MRI safety. One is to evaluate the AIMD MRI safety, and the other one is to improve the AIMD MRI safety. We discuss the relations of the analysis in this chapter with these two topics.

First, for the evaluation of the AIMD MRI safety, the analysis results show that the media surrounding the lead body, the lead tip, and the IPG have different contributions to Z_{IPG}, Z_{tip}, and transmission line Z_0, k_z. Consequently, they have different contributions to the MRI RF-induced heating and voltage. Therefore, using a homogeneous medium as the tissue-simulating medium as proposed in Ref. 12 to evaluate MRI safety is not accurate. For example, a pacemaker usually has the IPG implanted in fat tissues, the lead going through fat tissues and blood tissues, and the lead tip implanted in cardiac muscle tissues. A homogeneous high-conductivity and high-permittivity medium can simulate the blood tissues along the lead, but it can give incorrect tip impedances and IPG impedances, which can result in wrong heating and voltage estimations. Inhomogeneous media, such as the one proposed in Ref. 19, can give more accurate estimations. Furthermore, the analysis in this chapter gives the sensitivity of $T(l)$ to different physical medium parameters. It can be used to simplify the inhomogeneous tissue-simulating medium in Ref. 19.

Second, for the improvement of the AIMD MRI RF safety, attention can be paid to the IPG inner circuit impedance and lead tip structures. The proper design of Z_{IPG} or Z_{tip} can result in a reduction of MRI RF-induced voltage or heating for different implanted lead paths.

24.5 CONCLUSION

In this chapter, factors that influence the MRI RF-induced heating and voltage are analyzed in the form of transmission line parameters and impedances based on the transfer function method and the transmission line model. The analysis gives insights into the selection of best tissue-simulating medium and can help the design of MRI conditional safe AIMDs.

DISCLAIMER

The mention of commercial products, their sources, or their use in connection with material reported herein is not to be construed as either an actual or suggested endorsement of such products by the Department of Health and Human Services.

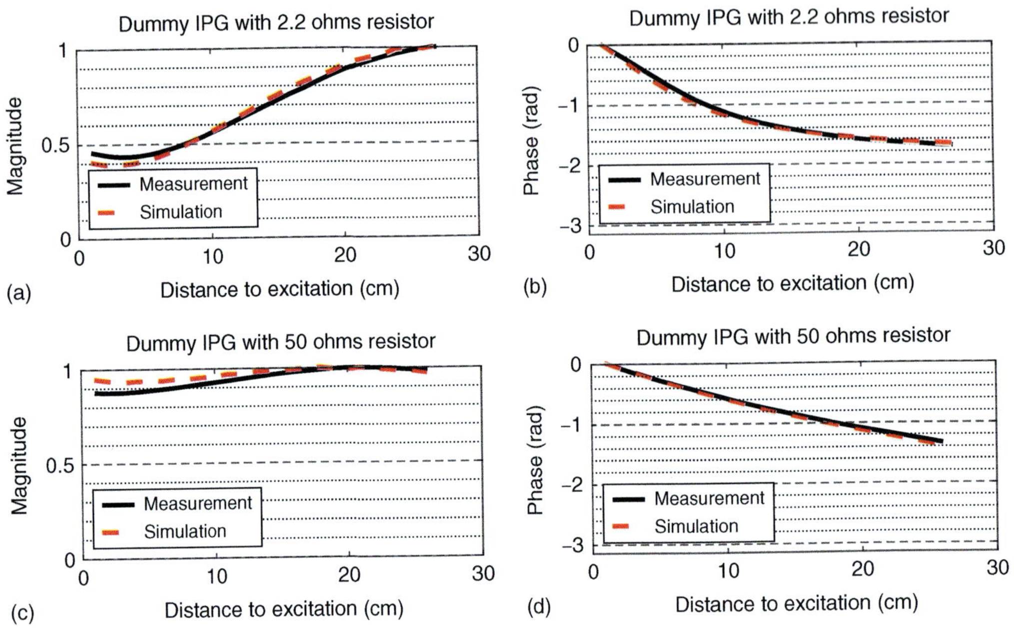

Figure 24.14. (a, b) Normalized magnitude and phase of $T(l)$ profiles of an insulated solid lead connected to a dummy IPG with 2.2 ohms resistor, simulation compared with measurement. (c, d) Normalized magnitude and phase of $T(l)$ profiles of an insulated solid lead connected to a dummy IPG with 50 ohms resistor, simulation compared with measurement

RELATED ARTICLES IN EMAGRES

Birdcage Resonators: Highly Homogeneous Radiofrequency Coils for Magnetic Resonance

Coils for Insertion into the Human Body

Design and Use of Internal Receiver Coils for Magnetic Resonance Imaging

Multifrequency Coils for Whole Body Studies

Radiofrequency Systems and Coils for MRI and MRS

Refrigerated and Superconducting Receiver Coils in Whole Body Magnetic Resonance

Spatial Encoding Using Multiple rf Coils: SMASH Imaging and Parallel MRI

Surface Coil NMR: Detection with Inhomogeneous Radiofrequency Field Antennas

Surface and Other Local Coils for In Vivo Studies

Whole Body Machines: NMR Phased Array Coil Systems

TEM Transceiver Head Array Coils for Ultra High Magnetic Fields

TEM Arrays, Design and Implementation

Quadrature Surface Coils

Double-Tuned Surface Coils

Quadrature Transverse Electromagnetic (TEM) Surface Coils

Radiofrequency Fields and SAR for Transverse Electromagnetic (TEM) Surface Coils

Double-Tuned Birdcage Coils: Construction and Tuning

Radiofrequency Fields and SAR for Bird Cage Coils

TEM Body Coils

Transverse Electromagnetic (TEM) Surface Coils for Extremities

Receiver Loop Arrays

Coil Array Design for Parallel Imaging: Theory and Applications

Millipede Coils

Microcoils

Catheter Coils

Radiofrequency Heating Models and Measurements

Characterization of Multichannel Coil Arrays on the Benchtop

A Standard Procedure for Analyzing Radio Frequency MRI Coils

Litz Coils for High Resolution and Animal Probes, Especially for Double Resonance

RF Field Modeling for Double-Tuned Volume Coils

An Historical Introduction to Surface Coils: The Early Days

Transceiver Loop Arrays

Radiofrequency Coils for NMR: A Peripatetic History of Their Twists and Turns

Nested Surface Coils for Multinuclear NMR

Birdcage Volume Coil Design

Bioeffects and Safety of Radiofrequency Electromagnetic Fields

Radiofrequency Fields: Interactions, Biological Effects, and Safety Issues

RF Device Safety and Compatibility

Safety Considerations in MRI

REFERENCES

1. R. Luechinger, *Eur. Heart J.*, 2005, **26**, 376.
2. O. Anfinsen, R. Berntsen, H. Aass, E. Kongsgaard, and J. Amlie, *Pacing Clin. Electrophysiol.*, 2002, **25**, 1400.
3. E. Mattei, G. Calcagnini, F. Censi, M. Triventi, and P. Bartolini, *IEEE Trans. Biomed. Eng.*, Aug. 2010, **57**, 2045.
4. Y. Liu, J. Chen, F. G. Shellock, and W. Kainz, *J. Magn. Reson. Imaging*, 2012, **37**, 491.
5. P. Nordbeck, I. Weiss, P. Ehses, O. Ritter, M. Warmuth, F. Fidler, V. Herold, P. M. Jakob, M. E. Ladd, H. H. Quick, and W. R. Bauer, *Magn. Reson. Med.*, 2009, **61**, 570.
6. S. Oh, A. G. Webb, T. Neuberger, B. Park, and C. M. Collins, *Magn. Reson. Med.*, 2009, **63**, 218.
7. E. Mattei, M. Triventi, G. Calcagnini, F. Censi, and P. Bartolini, *Am. J. Biomed. Sci.*, 2009, **1** (4), 373. DOI: 10.5099/aj090400373.
8. J. Powell, A. Papadaki, J. Hand, A. Hart, and D. Mcrobbie, *Magn. Reson. Med.*, 2011, **68**, 960.
9. L. M. Angelone, J. Ahveninen, J. W. Belliveau, and G. Bonmassar, *IEEE Trans. Med. Imaging*, 2010, **29**, 1029.
10. S. Pisa, G. Calcagnini, M. Cavagnaro, E. Piuzzi, E. Mattei, and P. Bernardi, *IEEE Trans. Electromagn. Compat.*, 2008, **50**, 35.
11. H. G. Mond and D. Grenz, *Pacing Clin. Electrophysiol.*, 2004, **27**, 887.
12. ISO/TS 10974:2018(E). Assessment of the safety of magnetic resonance imaging for patients with an active implantable medical device, 2018.
13. J. A. Nyenhuis, P. Sung-Min, R. Kamondetdacha, A. Amjad, F. G. Shellock, and A. R. Rezai, *IEEE Trans. Device Mater. Reliab.*, 2005, **5**, 467.
14. E. Mattei, M. Triventi, G. Calcagnini, F. Censi, W. Kainz, G. Mendoza, H. I. Bassen, and P. Bartolini, *Biomed. Eng. Online*, 2008, **7**, 11.
15. S. Feng, R. Qiang, W. Kainz, and J. Chen, *IEEE Trans. Microw. Theory Tech.*, 2015, **63**, 305.
16. J. Liu, J. Zheng, Q. Wang, W. Kainz, and J. Chen, *IEEE Trans. Microw. Theory Tech.*, 2018, **66**, 4271.
17. R. W. P. King and G. S. Smith, Antennas in Matter: Fundamentals, Theory and Applications, MIT Press: Cambridge, MA, 1981.
18. P. A. Hasgall, F. Di Gennaro, C. Baumgartner, E. Neufeld, B. Lloyd, M. C. Gosselin, D. Payne, A. Klingenböck, and N. Kuster, IT'IS database for thermal and electromagnetic parameters of biological tissues, 2015. www.itis.ethz.ch/database, 3.0.
19. J. Liu, J. Zheng, Q. Zeng, Q. Wang, J. Rondoni, J. Olsen, W. Kainz, and J. Chen, *IEEE Trans. Electromagn. Compat.*, 2019, **61**, 1091 DOI: 10.1109/TEMC.2018.2847909.

Chapter 25

On Using Fluoroptic Thermometry to Measure Time-varying Temperatures in MRI

Devashish Shrivastava, Mykhaylo Nosovskyy, and Charles A. Lemaire

In Vivo Temperatures, LLC, Burnsville, MN, USA

25.1 INTRODUCTION

Fluoroptic temperature probes are used widely to measure spatiotemporal temperature distribution in magnetic resonance imaging (MRI) applications (e.g., measuring heating due to MRI and measuring heating near implants or other conductive devices during MRI). This is because these probes are known to be not significantly affected by either the static magnetic field or the time-varying electromagnetic fields encountered in scanners with field strengths of up to 3 T. It should be noted, however, that fluoroptic temperature probes, like other temperature probes, are engineering machines with a finite response time. In other words, these probes take finite amount of time to respond to temperature changes and accurately measure true temperatures.[1,2] In this chapter, we investigate the time it may take for a fluoroptic probe to reach a 'set' temperature, the implication of such measurement behavior in measuring 'true' temperatures, and possible solutions to measure and/or estimate true temperatures.

25.2 METHODS

25.2.1 Theory

In order to characterize the temperature performance of a fluoroptic probe, let us hypothesize that the rate of change of the measured temperature is a function of the temperature difference between the 'true' temperature and the measured temperature. We test our hypothesis using measurements. It is possible that such hypothesis may not hold for the probe investigated herein or other probes, and in such case, one will need to come up with another hypothesis to be able to accurately model the measurement performance of a probe. For now, assuming that the hypothesis holds, the generic relationship between the measured and true temperatures can be

Safety and Biological Effects in MRI.
Edited by Devashish Shrivastava and J. Thomas Vaughan
 ISBN: 978-1-118-82130-5
Also published in eMagRes (online edition)
DOI: 10.1002/9780470034590.emrstm1637

written as follows:

$$\frac{dT_m}{dt} = \sum_1^n \beta_n (T_T - T_m)^n \tag{25.1}$$

where T_m is the measured temperature, T_T is the 'true' temperature, t is time, and β_n is a constant (that can vary with time and temperature). Assuming, for simplicity, that $n = 1$ and β_1 does not vary in time or with temperature, equation (25.1) can be solved to obtain the following equation (25.2) relating the T_m and T_T:

$$T_m = e^{-\beta_1 t} \int \beta_1 e^{\beta_1 t} T_T dt \tag{25.2}$$

Equation (25.2) can be solved for any time-varying T_T to predict the relationship between the T_m and T_T and expected error. The relationship may help estimate the true temperature from the measured temperature for probes for which the assumptions hold. For example, for a step temperature change, equation (25.2) can be solved to provide the following relationship between the T_m and T_T:

$$\theta_m = (1 - e^{-\beta_1 t}) \tag{25.3}$$

where $\theta_m = (T_m - T_i)/(T_T - T_i)$, and T_i is the initial or baseline temperature. Equation (25.3) can be used to estimate the unknown true step temperature using the measured temperature, baseline temperature, and proportionality constant β_1. The error can be expressed as follows:

$$\varepsilon = T_T - T_m = (T_T - T_i)e^{-\beta_1 t} \tag{25.4}$$

Next, please note that equation (25.3) has only one unknown variable (i.e., β_1) for a known true step temperature change. Therefore, to characterize our probe of interest, we expose the probe to a step temperature change and evaluate whether the measurements can be modeled using equation (25.3). Further, we investigate whether the proportionality constant β_1 is a function of the set temperature.

25.2.2 Experimental Method

To better understand the measurement performance of the fluoroptic temperature probe of interest, temperature measurements were made using the probe, a water bath with temperature control, and two glass beakers filled with water (one set in the water bath and another set outside in the room air). Measurements were made by switching the probe between the water in the beaker set at the room temperature (~22 °C) and the water in the beaker in the bath, as quickly as possible, to expose the probe to a step temperature change. The temperature in the water bath was set to ~35, ~55, and ~82 °C to study the measurement performance of the probe as a function of temperature and temperature difference between the set and initial temperatures. Water was used for ease of use and since the measurement performance may be affected by the thermal capacity of the surrounding medium. Measurements were made in a glass beaker filled with water and set in the water bath to minimize the effect of the convective currents on the measurements. Measurements were made once the beaker water in the bath attained thermal equilibrium with the bath water and at least three times for each set temperature.

25.3 RESULTS AND DISCUSSION

Several interesting results are noted, and observations are made. First, fluoroptic probes may take several seconds to reach a 'set' temperature (Figure 25.1). The result is interesting since it suggests that the measured temperature may not always be the 'true' temperature, and additional analysis may be needed to estimate the true temperature from the measured temperature. This is important since thermal effects such as thermal damage are a function of the absolute temperature–time history that the tissue experiences – and not what a probe measures.[3–9]

Second, for the investigated probe, the time taken to reach a 'set' temperature from an initial temperature is independent of the difference between the 'set' and initial temperatures (Figures 25.1 and 25.2). This result suggests that independent of the difference between the true and measured temperatures, the measured temperature value from the probe will always lag behind the instantaneous, time-varying true temperature. Such response is expected to underestimate heating as well as cooling. Therefore, the effect of such measurement error on the correlation between thermal effects such as damage and thermal parameters such as absolute temperature and weighted integrals of absolute temperature–time history (e.g., CEM43-based thermal dose and Arrhenius equation-based cell survivability threshold) may need to be carefully investigated.[3–9]

Also, the measurement error may not be obvious and needs to be determined for a given probe, medium, and the transient nature of the true temperature. This is so since the measured temperature is expected to

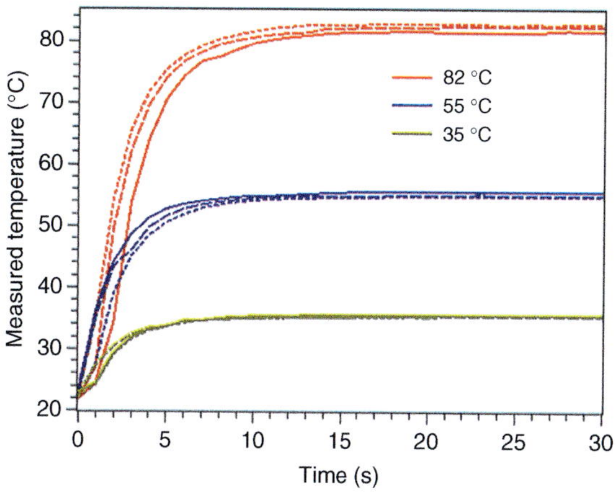

Figure 25.1. Absolute temperatures measured by a fluoroptic temperature probe as a function of time in response to a set step temperature

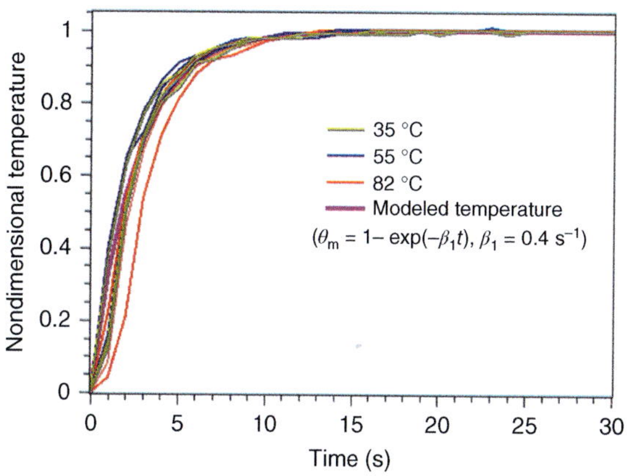

Figure 25.2. Nondimensional temperatures measured by a fluoroptic temperature probe together with the modeled measured temperature (per equation (25.3)) as a function of time in response to a set nondimensional step temperature of 1.0

be a function of the probe, the medium, and the transient nature of the true temperature (or of the source inducing the temperature change). For 'fast' transient temperatures, the temperature probes such as the one under investigation may introduce unacceptable underestimation errors near the source (Figure 25.3), and additional methods (e.g., measuring heating farther away from the source where the transients are not as fast and using these measurements together with the validated bioheat transfer models, such as the generic bioheat transfer model,[3,10–12] to estimate the source term) may need to be employed to estimate the true temperature.

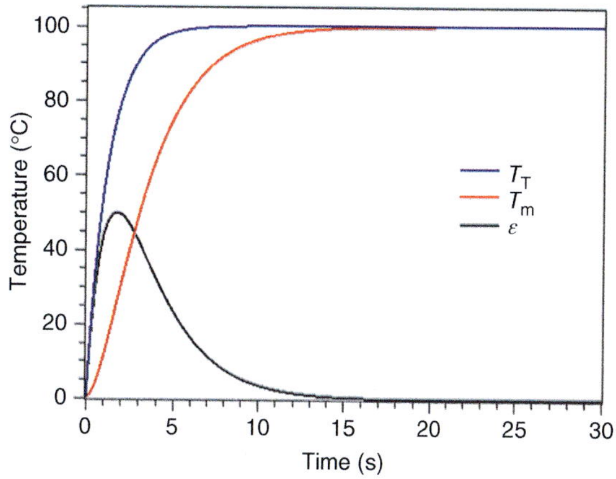

Figure 25.3. Expected probe measurement response and measurement error for a true exponential temperature as a function of time for $M = 100$ and $\gamma = 0.8$

Third, for the investigated probe, the probe response could be modeled successfully as proportional to the difference between the set and measured temperatures and with $n = 1$ alone. Further, the proportionality constant β_1 was found to be ~0.4 s^{-1}, independent of time and the set temperature (Figure 25.2, also see equation (25.3)). For such probes (where $n = 1$ and β_1 is independent of the set temperature), the relationship between the measured and true temperatures and expected error could easily be estimated by solving equation (25.2) for a representative true transient temperature. For example, for a linearly varying true temperature $T_T = \gamma t$ (expected temperature response for a relatively short duration of heating in unperfused or normally perfused tissue with a time-invariant source), the relationship between the true and measured temperatures for such probes can be presented as follows:

$$T_m = T_T - \frac{\gamma}{\beta_1}(1 - e^{-\beta_1 t}) \qquad (25.5)$$

The corresponding error can be presented as follows:

$$\varepsilon = \frac{\gamma}{\beta_1}(1 - e^{-\beta_1 t}) \qquad (25.6)$$

Equation (25.6) suggests that the measurement error for a linearly varying temperature is expected to be proportional to the rate of true temperature change. Likewise, for an exponentially varying true temperature $T_T = M(1 - e^{-\gamma t})$ (expected temperature response for a relatively long duration of heating in unperfused or normally perfused tissue with a time-invariant source and negligible regional/systemic heating), the relationship between the true and measured temperatures for such probes can be presented as follows:

$$T_{\mathrm{m}} = \frac{\beta_1}{\beta_1 - \gamma} T_{\mathrm{T}} - \frac{M\gamma}{\beta_1 - \gamma}(1 - \mathrm{e}^{-\beta_1 t}), \text{when } \beta_1 \neq \gamma \qquad (25.7)$$

$$T_{\mathrm{m}} = M(1 - \{1 + t\beta_1\}\mathrm{e}^{-\beta_1 t}), \text{when } \beta_1 = \gamma \qquad (25.8)$$

The corresponding error can be presented as follows:

$$\varepsilon = \frac{M\gamma}{\beta_1 - \gamma}(\mathrm{e}^{-\gamma t} - \mathrm{e}^{-\beta_1 t}), \text{when } \beta_1 \neq \gamma \qquad (25.9)$$

$$\varepsilon = Mt\beta_1 \mathrm{e}^{-\beta_1 t}, \text{when } \beta_1 = \gamma \qquad (25.10)$$

It can be noted from equations (25.9) and (25.10) that in contrast to the case of linear temperature change where the maximum error was γ/β_1 and the error decreases as the time progresses, in the case of exponential temperature change, the error first increases before decreasing as a function of time (Figure 25.3). Results such as these provide valuable insights into the relationship between the measured and true temperatures and may be useful in analyzing the effect of the error on correlating temperature–time history with thermal effects. For probes, where the measurement performance needs to be modeled with $n > 1$ and/or when β_n is a function of temperature, the relationship between the measured and true temperatures and error should be investigated by solving equation (25.1) directly.

Finally, regarding the proportionality constant β_1, please note that the value of this constant was obtained using water for simplicity. Since thermal capacity may alter the results, interested readers are encouraged to adapt the methodologies presented herein to obtain suitable value for β_n for their probe and measurement medium to estimate true temperature and error.

25.4 SUMMARY

Fluoroptic temperature probes may take several seconds to reach the true temperature. Thus, use of such probes in measuring time-varying temperatures is expected to introduce a time-varying error in the measurements. Additional analysis may be needed to estimate the true temperature and develop correlations between thermogenic hazards and true temperature–time history.

ACKNOWLEDGMENTS

The authors would like to thank Mr. Alexander Lemaire for making preliminary measurements.

DISCLAIMER

The subject matter, content, and views presented in this chapter are mine do not represent the views of the Department of Health and Human Services (HHS), US Food and Drug Administration (FDA), and/or the United States.

RELATED ARTICLES IN EMAGRES

Radiofrequency Heating Models and Measurements

REFERENCES

1. L. Michalski, K. Eckersdorf, and J. McGhee, Temperature Measurement, John Wiley & Sons, Ltd: West Sussex, 1991.
2. J. F. Schooley, Thermometry, CRC Press: Boca Raton, FL, 1986.
3. D. Shrivastava (ed), Theory and Applications of Heat Transfer in Humans, John Wiley & Sons, Ltd: West Sussex, 2018.
4. S. A. Sapareto and W. C. Dewey, *Int. J. Radiat. Oncol. Biol. Phys.*, 1984, **10**, 787.
5. F. C. Henriques and A. R. Moritz, *Am. J. Pathol.*, 1947, **23**, 531.
6. A. R. Moritz and F. C. Henriques, *Am. J. Pathol.*, 1947, **23**, 695.
7. A. R. Moritz, *Am. J. Pathol.*, 1947, **23**, 915.
8. S. A. Sapareto, L. E. Hopwood, W. C. Dewey, M. R. Raju, and J. W. Gray, *Cancer Res.*, 1978, **38**, 393.
9. J.A. Pearce, Relationship between Arrhenius models of thermal damage and the CEM43 thermal dose, SPIE 7181, Energy-based Treatment of Tissue and Assessment V, 718104, 2009.

10. D. Shrivastava and J. T. Vaughan, *J. Biomech. Eng.*, 2009, **131**, 074506.
11. D. Shrivastava, L. Utecht, J. Tian, J. Hughes, and J. T. Vaughan, *Magn. Reson. Med.*, 2014, **72**, 1141.
12. D. Shrivastava, T. Hanson, J. Kulesa, J. Tian, A. Gregor, and J. T. Vaughan, *Magn. Reson. Med.*, 2011, **66**, 255.

Chapter 26

On Using Magnetic Resonance Thermometry to Measure 'Strong' Spatio-temporal Tissue Temperature Variations and Compute Thermal Dose

Devashish Shrivastava
In Vivo Temperatures, LLC, Burnsville, MN, USA

26.1 INTRODUCTION

In this chapter, first, we discuss the thermodynamic challenges of magnetic resonance thermometry (MRT) in measuring 'strong' spatio-temporal temperature variation in tissue. Second, we discuss the effects of such measurements on the computation of thermal dose to predict tissue effects such as thermal damage. Third and finally, we compare the values of two frequently used thermal dose metrics, the cumulative equivalent minutes at 43 °C (*CEM43*) and the Arrhenius equation based approach, for the same spatio-temporal temperature input and thermal damage.[1]

The MRT is used to determine in vivo temperatures to evaluate the safety and/or efficacy of several therapeutic as well as diagnostic applications. Examples of therapeutic applications are tissue destruction using electromagnetic (such as laser, radiofrequency, microwave) or sound (e.g., high-intensity focused ultrasound or HIFU) energy, where the application of energy may raise the temperature locally or in a bulk of tissue. Examples of diagnostic applications are MRIs of patients with and/or without conductive devices, where the interaction between the patient and MR environment may produce local 'hot-spots,' 'hot-regions' of tissue, and/or systemic heating.

The MRT is performed by, first, acquiring an MR signal from a 'finite' three-dimensional volume called voxel (not an infinitesimally small point) in 'finite' time (not instantaneously) at baseline and at the temperature or time of interest. Later, the difference between the two MR signals (i.e., one acquired at the temperature or time of interest and the other at baseline) is scaled against a known signal change over a given temperature difference. The known signals are obtained in the tissue of interest maintained at given, uniform and steady-state temperatures. Thus,

Safety and Biological Effects in MRI.
Edited by Devashish Shrivastava and J. Thomas Vaughan
 ISBN: 978-1-118-82130-5
Also published in eMagRes (online edition)
DOI: 10.1002/9780470034590.emrstm1578

such scaling, intrinsically, fails to take into account the effect of spatially and temporally changing temperatures within a voxel on the MR signal. Consequently, MRT of such voxels (i.e., voxels experiencing spatio-temporal temperature variations) introduces an unknown amount of underestimation error in an MRT parameters dependent way. For more on how to measure temperatures using MRI, please refer to materials presented elsewhere in the book.

26.2 METHODS

26.2.1 Evaluation of Spatio-temporal Temperature Variation due to a Heat Source

To evaluate the expected error of MRT in voxels experiencing spatio-temporal temperature variation, tissue heating is simulated by solving the generic bioheat transfer model (GBHTM) (In Vivo temperatures, LLC, Burnsville, MN) for a given local heat source.[1,2] The GBHTM is used since it is a first principles based, validated bioheat transfer model that has been shown to predict in vivo tissue heating more accurately compared to the traditional, 'simplified' Pennes bioheat transfer model.[3,4] For simplicity, it is assumed that (i) the tissue is uniform and normally perfused, (ii) the baseline tissue temperature is 37 °C, (iii) the local perfusion is irreversibly interrupted when the local tissue temperature exceeds 50 °C, (iv) the peak tissue temperature stays at or below 100 °C and no phase change occurs in the tissue (i.e., no tissue boiling), and (v) thermal properties do not change with temperature. The length and the diameter of the heat source are assumed as 10 and 2 mm, respectively.

Tissue heating is simulated for the following peak source temperatures: 60, 80, and 100 °C. Heating durations are considered as follows: 60, 120, 180, 240, 480, and 960 s. The ramp time (i.e., the time it takes for the tissue next to the source to get to the peak source temperature from the baseline, normal core body temperature of 37 °C) is considered equal to 1 s (simulating fast temporal temperature gradient) or the total heating duration (simulating slow temporal temperature gradient). Tissue is assumed to return to near baseline temperatures naturally due to diffusion and perfusion assisted advection. Resultant spatio-temporal temperature distributions are used to approximate the range of underestimation that MR thermometry may produce for a finite voxel and signal acquisition time.

26.2.2 Evaluation of Thermal Dose

Accumulated thermal dose is computed using the following two approaches: (i) cumulative equivalent minutes at 43 °C (*CEM*43) and (ii) Arrhenius equation. The *CEM*43 is computed using equation (26.1), given below

$$CEM43 = \int_0^{\tau} R^{43-T}\mathrm{d}t \tag{26.1}$$

where T is temperature (°C), t is time (minutes), τ is total time (minutes), and the weighting factor R is equal to 0.5 for $T \geq 43$ °C, and 0.25 for $T < 43$ °C. R is independent of the tissue type.[5]

Arrhenius equation based nondimensional thermal dose (Ω) is computed using equation (26.2), given below

$$\Omega = \int_0^{\tau} A e^{\frac{-E_a}{RT(t)}}\mathrm{d}t \tag{26.2}$$

where T is absolute temperature (K), t is time (s), τ is total time (s), A is the frequency factor (s^{-1}), E_a is an activation energy barrier (J mol^{-1}), and R is the universal gas constant (8.3143 J mol^{-1} K^{-1}). The value of the frequency factor A and activation energy barrier E_a is chosen as 3.1×10^{98} s^{-1} and 6.28×10^5 J mol^{-1}, respectively. These values were proposed originally in 1947 by Henriques and Moritz in their seminal papers investigating the effect temperature and time on the induced thermal damage.[6–8] Since then, several values of A and E_a have been published for various tissue types and with significant variation. To explain these variations, it has been shown that A and E_a are, in fact, dependent on each other and not independent. For more information on different ways to compute thermal dose, and the evaluation of those methods, please refer to materials presented in Ref. 1.

26.2.3 Estimation of Thermal Damage

The dimensions of thermal damage are computed by taking *CEM*43 of ≥60 min. The *CEM*43 of 60 min is chosen since this threshold has been shown to reduce cell survivability by 90% in in vitro studies[9] and is used frequently in literature to determine thermal damage. The dimensions of damage predicted by *CEM*43 of ≥60 min are compared to the dimensions predicted by Ω of ≥1. Ω of ≥1 is chosen for comparison since Ω of ≥1 or higher has, also, been used frequently in literature to determine the dimensions of thermal damage.

26.3 RESULTS

26.3.1 Thermodynamic Challenges: Spatial Temperature Variation Near the Source

Tables 26.1–26.3 present the drop in temperature (T_{drop}), at the end of the heating duration, as a function of the radial distance from the center of the surface of the source, heating duration (HD), and ramp time (RT), for the peak source temperature of 60, 80, and 100 °C, respectively. The results can be used to estimate the lower bound of the spatial temperature variation in a voxel near the source. For example, the temperature drop of ≥4.8 and 7.8 °C occurs in a cubical voxel with the side of 0.7 mm next to the source, for the peak source temperature of 60 °C, total heating duration of 60 s, and ramp time of 1 and 60 s, respectively (Table 26.1, row 1, columns 2 and 3). In comparison, the temperature drop of ≥23.6 and 32.5 °C occurs in a cubical voxel with the side of 3.5 mm next to the source, for the peak source temperature of 100 °C, total heating duration of 960 s, and ramp time of 1 and 960 s, respectively (Table 26.3, last row, columns 8 and 9).

26.3.2 Thermodynamic Challenges: Spatial Temperature Variation Near the Minor Radius of Thermal Damage

Tables 26.4–26.6 present the increase in temperature (T_{gain}) from the temperature at the minor thermal damage radius (per *CEM43*), at the end of the heating duration, as a function of the radial distance from the minor radius toward the center of the source, heating duration (HD), and ramp time (RT), for the peak source temperature of 60, 80, and 100 °C, respectively. The results can be used to estimate the lower bound of the spatial temperature variation in a voxel near the minor thermal damage radius. $T_{gain} > 0$ since the temperature between the source term and minor radius is greater than the temperature at the minor radius. The results can be

Table 26.1. Temperature drop (T_{drop}) at the end of the heating, from the peak source temperature of 60 °C, as a function of the distance away from the source, heating duration (HD), and ramp time (RT)

HD (s)	T_{drop} (°C)							
	1 mm away		2 mm away		3 mm away		5 mm away	
	1 s RT	HD RT	1 s RT	HD RT	1 s RT	HD RT	1 s RT	HD RT
60	−4.8	−7.8	−9.3	−13.5	−13.2	−17.3	−18.6	−21.1
120	−3.7	−6.0	−7.3	−10.9	−10.7	−14.6	−15.9	−19.1
180	−3.3	−5.2	−6.5	−9.6	−9.6	−13.2	−14.5	−17.9
240	−3.1	−4.7	−6.1	−8.9	−9.0	−12.3	−13.8	−17.0
480	−2.7	−3.9	−5.4	−7.4	−7.9	−10.5	−12.5	−15.2
960	−2.6	−3.3	−5.1	−6.4	−7.5	−9.2	−11.8	−13.8

Table 26.2. Temperature drop (T_{drop}) at the end of the heating, from the peak source temperature of 80 °C, as a function of the distance away from the source, heating duration (HD), and ramp time (RT)

HD (s)	T_{drop} (°C)							
	1 mm away		2 mm away		3 mm away		5 mm away	
	1 s RT	HD RT	1 s RT	HD RT	1 s RT	HD RT	1 s RT	HD RT
60	−8.7	−14.4	−16.9	−24.9	−24.1	−32.1	−34.5	−39.5
120	−6.7	−11.0	−13.1	−19.9	−19.0	−26.7	−28.8	−35.6
180	−5.8	−9.5	−11.4	−17.4	−16.6	−23.8	−25.7	−33.0
240	−5.3	−8.5	−10.4	−15.8	−15.2	−22.0	−23.8	−31.1
480	−4.3	−6.7	−8.6	−12.8	−12.6	−18.1	−20.0	−26.8
960	−3.7	−5.5	−7.4	−10.6	−10.9	−15.2	−17.4	−23.2

Table 26.3. Temperature drop (T_{drop}) at the end of the heating from the peak source temperature of 100 °C, as a function of the distance away from the source, heating duration (HD), and ramp time (RT)

HD (s)	T_{drop} (°C)							
	1 mm away		2 mm away		3 mm away		5 mm away	
	1 s RT	HD RT	1 s RT	HD RT	1 s RT	HD RT	1 s RT	HD RT
60	−12.7	−21.1	−24.7	−36.4	−35.1	−46.8	−50.4	−57.8
120	−9.7	−16.0	−19.0	−28.9	−27.5	−38.8	−41.6	−51.8
180	−8.4	−13.7	−16.4	−25.2	−24.0	−34.5	−37.0	−47.8
240	−7.6	−12.3	−14.9	−22.9	−21.9	−31.7	−34.0	−44.9
480	−6.1	−9.6	−12.1	−18.3	−17.8	−25.9	−28.0	−38.2
960	−5.1	−7.7	−10.0	−14.9	−14.8	−21.4	−23.6	−32.5

Table 26.4. T_{gain} at the end of the heating, for the peak source temperature of 60 °C, as a function of the distance from the edge of the minor radius of the thermal damage (per $CEM43 \geq 60$ min) toward the source, heating duration (HD), and ramp time (RT) of 1 s and HD

HD (s)	T_{gain} (°C)							
	1 mm away		2 mm away		3 mm away		5 mm away	
	1 s RT	HD RT	1 s RT	HD RT	1 s RT	HD RT	1 s RT	HD RT
60	3.9	5.7	8.4	13.5	13.2	—	—	—
120	3.2	4.3	6.6	9.8	10.3	—	—	—
180	2.7	3.6	5.8	8.0	9.0	13.2	—	—
240	2.4	3.4	5.2	7.6	8.1	12.3	—	—
480	2.0	2.6	4.2	5.7	6.7	9.2	12.0	—
960	1.6	2.3	3.6	5.0	5.8	7.9	10.6	—

Table 26.5. T_{gain} at the end of the heating, for the peak source temperature of 80 °C, as a function of the distance from the edge of the minor radius of the thermal damage (per $CEM43 \geq 60$ min) toward the source, heating duration (HD), and ramp time (RT) of 1 s and HD

HD (s)	T_{gain} (°C)							
	1 mm away		2 mm away		3 mm away		5 mm away	
	1 s RT	HD RT	1 s RT	HD RT	1 s RT	HD RT	1 s RT	HD RT
60	2.6	2.2	6.4	5.8	11.7	11.5	26.0	32.7
120	2.2	2.1	5.2	5.2	8.9	9.6	18.7	23.4
180	2.3	2.1	5.1	5.0	8.6	9.0	17.1	20.6
240	2.1	2.0	4.8	4.7	8.0	8.3	15.7	18.5
480	1.7	2.0	3.8	4.4	6.3	7.6	12.0	15.6
960	1.5	1.9	3.4	4.2	5.5	7.0	10.4	13.7

Table 26.6. T_{gain} at the end of the heating, for the peak source temperature of 100 °C, as a function of the distance from the edge of the minor radius of the thermal damage (per *CEM43* ≥ 60 min) toward the source, heating duration (HD), and ramp time (RT) of 1 s and HD

HD (s)	T_{gain} (°C)							
	1 mm away		2 mm away		3 mm away		5 mm away	
	1 s RT	HD RT	1 s RT	HD RT	1 s RT	HD RT	1 s RT	HD RT
60	1.0	0.5	2.5	1.5	5.1	3.4	14.7	11.9
120	1.3	0.9	3.1	2.3	5.6	4.4	13.4	12.2
180	1.4	1.2	3.2	2.8	5.6	5.1	12.6	12.8
240	1.5	1.2	3.4	2.9	5.9	5.2	12.6	12.6
480	1.5	1.3	3.3	3.0	5.5	5.2	11.1	11.4
960	1.3	1.4	2.9	3.0	4.8	5.1	9.5	10.7

Table 26.7. Peak temporal temperature gradient (°C s^{-1}) as a function of the peak source temperature and ramp time (RT)

HD (s)	Peak T (°C) = 60		Peak T (°C) = 80		Peak T (°C) = 100	
	1 s RT	HD RT	1 s RT	HD RT	1 s RT	HD RT
60	23	0.38	43	0.72	63	1.05
120	23	0.19	43	0.36	63	0.53
180	23	0.13	43	0.24	63	0.35
240	23	0.10	43	0.18	63	0.26
480	23	0.05	43	0.09	63	0.13
960	23	0.02	43	0.05	63	0.07

used to estimate the minimum spatial temperature variation in a voxel near the minor radius. For example, the temperature variation of ≥3.9 and 5.7 °C is expected to occur in a cubical voxel with the side of 0.7 mm next to the minor radius, for the peak source temperature of 60 °C, total heating duration of 60 s, and ramp time between 1 and 60 s, respectively (Table 26.4, row 1, columns 2–3). In comparison, the temperature variation of ≥9.5 and 10.7 °C is expected to occur in a cubical voxel with the side of 3.5 mm next to the minor radius, for the peak source temperature of 100 °C, total heating duration of 960 s, and ramp time between 1 and 960 s, respectively (Table 26.6, last row, columns 8–9). For the minor thermal damage radius determined per Ω ≥ 1, the T_{gain} is larger since the radius is smaller than the one predicted per *CEM43* ≥ 60 min.

26.3.3 Thermodynamic Challenges: Temporal Temperature Variation Near the Source

Table 26.7 presents the peak temporal temperature gradient (°C s^{-1}) as a function of the peak source temperature and ramp time. The results when multiplied by the MR signal acquisition time help estimate the peak temporal change within a voxel near the source. For example, for an acquisition that takes 10 s, the maximum temporal temperature change within a voxel near the source is expected to be 10 s × 1.05 °C s^{-1} = 10.5 °C for the peak source temperature change of 63 °C (i.e., for the absolute peak source temperature of 100 °C with the baseline core temperature is 37 °C) and ramp time of 60 s (Table 26.7, row 1, last column).

26.3.4 Comparison of Thermal Damage Predicted by *CEM43* and Arrhenius Approaches

Tables 26.8–26.10 present the dimensions of the thermal damage (TD) predicted based upon the thermal dose of *CEM43* ≥ 60 min and Ω ≥ 1, as a function of the heating duration (HD) and ramp time (RT), for the peak source temperatures of 60, 80, and 100 °C, respectively. Value of Ω corresponding to the dimensions of the thermal

Table 26.8. Thermal damage (TD) (minor radius, major radius), for the peak source temperature of 60 °C, as a function of the heating duration (HD), and ramp time (RT)

HD (s)	TD (mm) per *CEM43* ≥ 60 min		TD (mm) per Ω ≥ 1		Ω corresponding to TD per *CEM43* ≥ 60 min	
	1 s RT	HD RT	1 s RT	HD RT	1 s RT	HD RT
60	3.0, 8.0	2.0, 7.0	1.0, 6.0	0.5, 5.0	0.02, 0.03	0.04, 0.03
120	3.5, 9.5	2.5, 8.0	1.5, 6.5	0.5, 5.5	0.04, 0.02	0.04, 0.02
180	4.0, 10.0	3.0, 8.5	2.0, 7.0	1.0, 6.0	0.04, 0.03	0.03, 0.02
240	4.5, 10.5	3.0, 8.5	2.0, 7.5	1.0, 6.0	0.03, 0.03	0.04, 0.04
480	5.5, 12.5	4.0, 9.5	3.0, 8.5	1.5, 7.0	0.03, 0.02	0.03, 0.03
960	6.5, 13.0	4.5, 10.5	3.5, 9.5	2.0, 7.5	0.03, 0.03	0.03, 0.03

Note that the major radius is determined from the center of the source term and thus, includes ½ of the 10 mm long source (i.e., 5 mm).

Table 26.9. Thermal damage (TD) (minor radius, major radius) for the peak source temperature of 80 °C, as a function of the heating duration (HD), and ramp time (RT)

HD (s)	TD (mm) per *CEM43* ≥ 60 min		TD (mm) per Ω ≥ 1		Ω corresponding to TD per *CEM43* ≥ 60 min	
	1 s RT	HD RT	1 s RT	HD RT	1 s RT	HD RT
60	6.5, 13.5	5.5, 12.0	4.0, 10.0	3.5, 9.0	0.03, 0.02	0.03, 0.02
120	8.0, 15.0	6.5, 13.0	5.0, 11.5	4.0, 10.0	0.02, 0.02	0.02, 0.02
180	8.5, 16.0	7.0, 14.0	6.0, 12.5	4.5, 10.5	0.03, 0.03	0.03, 0.02
240	9.0, 17.0	7.5, 14.5	6.5, 13.5	5.0, 11.0	0.03, 0.02	0.02, 0.02
480	11.0, 19.0	8.5, 16.0	8.0, 15.5	5.5, 12.5	0.02, 0.03	0.03, 0.02
960	12.5, 21.5	9.5, 17.5	9.0, 17.5	7.0, 14.0	0.02, 0.03	0.03, 0.03

Note that the major radius is determined from the center of the source term and thus, includes ½ of the 10 mm long source (i.e., 5 mm).

Table 26.10. Thermal damage (TD) (minor radius, major radius) for the peak source temperature of 100 °C, as a function of the heating duration (HD), and ramp time (RT)

HD (s)	TD (mm) per *CEM43* ≥ 60 min		TD (mm) per Ω ≥ 1		Ω corresponding to TD per *CEM43* ≥ 60 min	
	1 s RT	HD RT	1 s RT	HD RT	1 s RT	HD RT
60	9.5, 17.5	8.5, 16.0	7.0, 14.0	6.0, 12.5	0.03, 0.02	0.03, 0.02
120	11.0, 19.5	9.5, 17.0	8.0, 15.5	6.5, 13.5	0.03, 0.02	0.02, 0.03
180	12.0, 20.5	10.0, 18.0	9.0, 17.0	7.0, 14.5	0.02, 0.03	0.03, 0.03
240	12.5, 22.0	10.5, 18.5	9.5, 18.0	7.5, 15.0	0.03, 0.02	0.03, 0.03
480	14.5, 24.5	12.0, 21.0	11.5, 20.5	9.0, 17.0	0.03, 0.03	0.03, 0.02
960	17.0, 28.0	13.5, 23.0	13.5, 24.0	10.5, 19.5	0.02, 0.02	0.03, 0.03

Note that the major radius is determined from the center of the source term and thus, includes ½ of the 10 mm long source (i.e., 5 mm).

Table 26.11. Underestimation of thermal damage (TD) (minor radius, major radius) due to the error of 20 °C in the measured peak source temperature (T_{peak}), as a function of the true, peak source temperature, heating duration (HD), and ramp time (RT)

HD (s)	True T_{peak} = 80 °C, measured T_{peak} = 60 °C		True T_{peak} = 100 °C, measured T_{peak} = 80 °C	
	1 s RT	HD RT	1 s RT	HD RT
60	3.5, 5.5	3.5, 5.0	3.0, 4.0	3.0, 4.0
120	4.5, 5.5	4.0, 5.0	3.0, 4.5	3.0, 4.0
180	4.5, 6.0	4.0, 5.5	3.5, 4.5	3.0, 4.0
240	4.5, 6.5	4.5, 6.0	3.5, 5.0	3.0, 4.0
480	5.5, 6.5	4.5, 6.5	3.5, 5.5	3.5, 5.0
960	6.0, 8.5	5.0, 7.0	4.5, 6.5	4.0, 5.5

Thermal damage is evaluated per *CEM43* ≥ 60 min.

Table 26.12. Peak temperature at the end of the heating vs the peak temperature during the complete temperature–time history, at the edge of the minor radius of the thermal damage (per CEM43 ≥ 60 min), for the peak source temperature of 60 °C

HD (s)	Peak *T* (°C) after heating		Peak *T* (°C)	
	1 s RT	HD RT	1 s RT	HD RT
60	46.8	46.5	47.5	48.3
120	47.8	47.1	48.1	48.2
180	47.7	46.8	47.9	47.7
240	47.3	47.7	47.4	48.3
480	46.6	46.9	46.7	47.3
960	45.6	47.2	45.6	47.4

damage determined per *CEM43* ≥ 60 min is also presented, for comparison.

26.3.5 Underestimation of Thermal Damage

Table 26.11 presents the underestimation of the thermal damage (per *CEM43*) when the peak source temperature is underestimated by 20 °C, as a function of the 'true' peak source temperature, heating duration, and ramp time. The underestimation increases as the heating duration increases or the ramp time decreases. Similar results can be obtained for the thermal damage predicted per Ω ≥ 1 by comparing the results presented in Tables 26.8–26.10.

26.3.6 Peak Temperature Near the Minor Radius of Thermal Damage

Tables 26.12–26.14 present the peak temperature at the end of the heating duration and the peak temperature during the complete temperature–time history, at the edge of the minor radius of the thermal damage (per *CEM43* ≥ 60 min), as a function of the heating duration (HD) and ramp time (RT), for the peak source temperature of 60, 80, and 100 °C, respectively. The results show that the temperatures may continue to grow after the heating, away from the source term. Similar results can be produced at the edge of the minor radius of the thermal damage determined per Ω ≥ 1.

26.4 DISCUSSION

Several observations are made from the results presented in Tables 26.1–26.14. First, temperatures may drop significantly near a source term as a function of the peak source temperature, distance from the source term, heating duration, and ramp time. The difference between the peak source temperature and the temperature at a given location increases with an increase in the peak source temperature, the distance between the source and the location, and/or the ramp

Table 26.13. Peak temperature at the end of the heating vs the peak temperature during the complete temperature–time history, at the edge of the minor radius of the thermal damage (per $CEM43 \geq 60$ min), for the peak source temperature of 80 °C

HD (s)	Peak T (°C) after heating		Peak T (°C)	
	1 s RT	HD RT	1 s RT	HD RT
60	41.1	39.6	46.9	47.2
120	42.3	40.9	46.0	46.5
180	43.8	42.0	46.4	46.5
240	44.6	42.5	46.5	46.3
480	44.7	43.9	45.6	46.3
960	45.1	45.0	45.3	46.4

Table 26.14. Peak temperature at the end of the heating vs the peak temperature during the complete temperature–time history, at the edge of the minor radius of thermal damage (per $CEM43 \geq 60$ min), for the peak source temperature of 100 °C

HD (s)	Peak T (°C) after heating		Peak T (°C)	
	1 s RT	HD RT	1 s RT	HD RT
60	38.0	37.5	46.3	46.2
120	39.5	38.5	45.8	45.9
180	40.5	39.4	45.6	46.1
240	41.6	40.1	45.8	46.0
480	43.2	41.5	45.5	45.7
960	43.9	42.8	44.9	45.6

time. The difference between the peak source temperature and temperature at a location decreases as the heating duration increases (Tables 26.1–26.3). For example, for the peak source temperature of 100 °C, the minimum spatial temperature drop, within 1 mm from the source, is estimated to be between ~12.7 and ~5.1 °C, for the heating duration between 60 and 960 s, and ramp time of 1 s. The spatial temperature is estimated to drop further to between ~50.4 and ~23.6 °C within 5 mm from the source (Table 26.3).

Second, the rate of temperature drop decreases as the distance between the source and the measurement location increases (Tables 26.1–26.3 vs Tables 26.4–26.6). For example, in comparison to the spatial temperature drops near the source noted above, the minimum temperature drop, within 1 and 5 mm from the edge of the minor radius of the thermal damage (per $CEM43 \geq 60$ min), is estimated to be between 1–1.5 °C and 14.7–9.5 °C, respectively (Table 26.6).

Third, regarding the temporal temperature gradient, temporal temperature gradient is directly related to the power density deposited by the source in the tissue. As the power density increases, temporal rate of change of temperature in tissue increases (Table 26.7).

Relating these observations to MRT, the observations suggest that relatively larger voxels are expected to have larger intra-voxel spatial temperature variations compared to smaller voxels. The spatial temperature variation of ≥~5.1, 10.0, 14.8, and 23.6 °C is estimated for a voxel within 1, 2, 3, and 5 mm, respectively, from the source term for the peak source temperature of 100 °C, heating duration ≤960 s, and ramp time of ≥1 s. Likewise, relatively larger acquisition times are expected to have larger intra-voxel temporal temperature variations compared to smaller acquisition times for the same input power density. The effect of such spatial and temporal intra-voxel temperature variation on the MR signal needs to be carefully studied to improve MRT. One can imagine that for such voxels the 'temperature' may need to be redefined as well. From the results presented in Tables 26.1–26.3, and ignoring the effect of temporal variation, the peak error of ≥~5.1, 10.0, 14.8, and 23.6 °C (and the average error of ≥~2.6, 5.0, 7.4, and 11.8 °C) is expected for a voxel within 1, 2, 3, and 5 mm, respectively, from the source term for the peak source temperature of 100 °C, heating duration ≤960 s, and ramp time of ≥1 s. The effect of such underestimation on the underprediction of thermal damage is presented in Table 26.11 for the error of 20 °C between the measured peak temperature and the true peak temperature near the source.

Fourth, the dimensions of the thermal damage predicted by $CEM43 \geq 60$ min are greater than the dimensions of the thermal damage predicted by $\Omega \geq 1$, for the same input temperature–time history, for all cases (Tables 26.8–26.10). The difference in radial dimension lies in between 1.5 and 4.0 mm. Thermal damage comparable to those predicted by $CEM43 \geq 60$ min were obtained for $\Omega \geq 0.02$. Thus, suitability of a thermal dose metric in predicting thermal damage needs to be carefully evaluated as a function of the temperature–time history and tissue.[1,10]

Fifth, the peak temperature away from the source term at the end of the heating duration may not be the maximum temperature at the location since the temperature may keep rising for some time after the heating duration due to the continuous diffusion/advection of the thermal energy from the relatively warmer tissue near the source (Tables 26.12–26.14). For example, for the peak source temperature of 100 °C, the temperature at the minor radius of the thermal damage (per $CEM43 \geq 60$ min), at the end of the heating, is estimated to be only 38 °C for the heating duration of 60 s and ramp time of 1 s. Once the heating stops, the continuous diffusion/advection of the thermal energy from the relatively warmer tissue near the source results in raising this temperature from 38 to 46.3 °C. Thus, caution is warranted if, in a therapeutic or diagnostic application, the goal is to restrict the temperature of the tissue farther away from the source to a given value to prevent thermal damage. In such applications, the temperature should be restricted by considering appropriate parameters affecting the complete spatio-temporal temperature distribution in the tissue of interest.

Finally, regarding the limitations of the study, the results presented herein are computed using constant thermal properties of tissue (i.e., density, specific heat, thermal conductivity, and blood-tissue heat transfer rate) and for a given source term. Interested readers are encouraged to perform similar analyses for different source terms and by including the temperature dependence of thermal properties to develop a deeper understanding of the thermodynamic challenges of MRT and the effect thereof on the computation of thermal dose to predict tissue effects.

26.5 SUMMARY

The accuracy and precision of magnetic resonance imaging-based thermometry on determining temperature changes in tissue experiencing strong spatial and temporal temperature gradients are unexplored. Significant temperature variation, both spatial as well as temporal, within a voxel is expected to introduce an unknown amount of underestimation error in thermometry in an MR parameters dependent way. Future studies to carefully correlate the spatio-temporal temperature variation within a voxel on the MR signal are needed to develop reliable MR thermometry in tissues experiencing strong spatio-temporal temperature distribution.

DISCLAIMER

The subject matter, content, and views presented in this chapter are mine do not represent the views of the Department of Health and Human Services (HHS), US Food and Drug Administration (FDA), and/or the United States.

REFERENCES

1. D. Shrivastava (ed), Theory and Applications of Heat Transfer in Humans, John Wiley and Sons: Hoboken, NJ, 2018.
2. D. Shrivastava and J. T. Vaughan, *J. Biomech. Eng.*, 2009, **131**, 074506.
3. D. Shrivastava, L. Utecht, J. Tian, J. Hughes, and J. T. Vaughan, *Magn. Reson. Med.*, 2014, **72**, 1141.
4. D. Shrivastava, T. Hanson, J. Kulesa, J. Tian, A. Gregor, and J. T. Vaughan, *Magn. Reson. Med.*, 2011, **66**, 255.
5. S. A. Sapareto and W. C. Dewey, *Int. J. Radiat. Oncol. Biol. Phys.*, 1984, **10**, 787.
6. F. C. Henriques and A. R. Moritz, *Am. J. Pathol.*, 1947, **23**, 531.
7. A. R. Moritz and F. C. Henriques, *Am. J. Pathol.*, 1947, **23**, 695.
8. A. R. Moritz, *Am. J. Pathol.*, 1947, **23**, 915.
9. S. A. Sapareto, L. E. Hopwood, W. C. Dewey, M. R. Raju, and J. W. Gray, *Cancer Res.*, 1978, **38**, 393.
10. J. A. Pearce, in 'SPIE 7181, Energy-based Treatment of Tissue and Assessment V', 2009, Vol. 718104.

Chapter 27

The Use and Safety of Iron-Oxide Nanoparticles in MRI and MFH

Hattie L. Ring, John C. Bischof, and Michael Garwood

University of Minnesota, Minneapolis, MN, USA

27.1 INTRODUCTION

In recent decades, iron oxide nanoparticles (IONPs) have been demonstrated as a versatile platform with multiple applications within the clinic. IONP synthesis can result in a broad range of sizes (3–100 nm), shapes, and crystalline structures.[1–3] The adaptability of IONPs has resulted in the establishment of many acronyms (magnetic nanoparticle (MNP), magnetic iron oxide nanoparticle (MION), ferromagnetic iron oxide nanoparticle (FION), superparamagnetic iron oxide nanoparticle (SPION), etc.). Herein, we use the broad acronym IONP referring to any nanoparticle composed of iron oxide.

IONPs were first clinically used as a treatment for anemia in 1980.[4] Since then, IONPs have been introduced to the clinic to aid in cancer diagnosis through their ability to enhance visualization (i.e. create contrast) in magnetic resonance imaging (MRI).[5,6] Recently, IONPs have been implemented to treat glioma through magnetic fluid hyperthermia (MFH).[7–9] A thorough discussion regarding clinical applications of IONPs is provided within the first section of this chapter.

Safety concerning the clinical application of IONPs ranges from known side effects from administration of IONPs to special considerations given the applications of MRI and MFH. The second section of this chapter focuses on the known safety profile of IONPs within the clinic. Safety considerations specific to IONPs, such as the relationship between IONPs within the iron cycle, the impact of iron overload, and allergic responses to IONPs are examined. The impact of IONPs for diagnostic MRI and the potential negative health impacts of MFH are also covered.

MFH clinical applications are improved through the development of an IONP platform which provides image-guided MFH. The final section describes emerging options for noninvasive quantification of IONPs, covering quantitative susceptibility mapping (QSM), magnetic particle imaging (MPI), and echoless MRI. Recent demonstrations with echoless MRI toward image-guide MFH will also be discussed.[10]

Safety and Biological Effects in MRI.
Edited by Devashish Shrivastava and J. Thomas Vaughan

ISBN: 978-1-118-82130-5
Also published in eMagRes (online edition)
DOI: 10.1002/9780470034590.emrstm1606

27.2 IONPS IN THE CLINIC

Clinical use of IONPs can be broken into three applications: treatment of anemia, MRI contrast agent, and treatment of cancer with MFH. The differences between these applications result in a range of administration methods and doses. The focus of this section will be the current clinical application of IONPs. In addition, IONPs undergoing clinical trials and off-label uses of clinically approved IONPs will be discussed.

27.2.1 Anemia Treatments

Iron deficiency, or anemia, is a common medical issue typically remedied through oral iron replacement. Oral iron replacement can be problematic because approximately one-third of treated patients experience adverse effects, which increases patient noncompliance.[11] Even when patients are compliant, poor intestinal absorption can often fail to compensate for conditions with ongoing blood losses, such as chronic renal failure, chronic heart failure, and cancer.[4,11] For cases in which oral iron replacement is inadequate, intravenous (IV) iron is prescribed.

Intravenous iron has been an available anemia treatment in the United States for over 50 years.[12] Owing to severe allergic reactions, some of which have been fatal, clinicians are reluctant to use IV iron unless treatment with oral iron replacement is unsuccessful.[4,11,13] Several formulations of IV iron are currently available (see Table 27.1), each consisting of an IONP core with a surrounding carbohydrate. Dexferrum, INFeD, and Feraheme have all had adverse effects involving severe allergic reactions, and therefore, test doses and preparation for an allergic reaction are recommended before the application of an entire dose.[4,14–16] Recently, Feraheme has had several fatalities associated with it resulting in a black box warning from the Food and Drug Administration (FDA).[17] Ferrlecit, Ferinject, and Venofer have had allergic responses which are less severe and occur less frequently, therefore, test doses are unnecessary.[4,18,19] Ferinject was approved for clinical use in the United States under the name Injectafer.[20]

27.2.2 MRI Contrast Agents

MRI is a well-established tool for medical diagnosis. Nearly one-third of MRI procedures include the use of contrast agents for improving diagnosis.[21] Currently, gadolinium-based contrast agents (GBCAs) dominate the MRI contrast agent market. GBCAs have demonstrated utility for the diagnosis and characterization of cancer lesions, angiography, and organ/lesion perfusion.[22] As a heavy metal, free gadolinium is extremely toxic; however, when chelated with ligands, gadolinium is less toxic and is quickly excreted out of the body via renal clearance.[22] Kidney function is a major consideration in the clinical application of GBCAs. Specifically, nephrogenic systemic fibrosis (NSF) is a disease triggered by GBCAs which causes thickening and scarring of skin and internal organs are known to occur in patients with moderate to severe renal failure.[23,24] This issue has been mitigated by avoiding use on patients with moderate or severe renal failure and testing for acute renal failure before the use of GBCAs.[24–26] However, new concerns have emerged with the recent discovery that GBCAs can remain in the body after use and are deposited in the brain.[27] The European Medicines Agency has responded by removing all linear GBCAs from the market.[28] The FDA has recommended continued use of all GBCAs but required additional human

Table 27.1. IONP clinical applications

Application	Anemia	MRI contrast agent	MFH cancer treatment
IONP-based drug	DexFerrum[a], INFeD[a] (CosmoFer[b]), Venofer[a,b], Ferrlecit[a,b], Ferinject[a,c] (Injectafer), Feraheme[a] (Ferumoxytol), Monofer[b]	Feridex[a] (Endorem, Fermoxide), Resovist[b] (Ferucarbotran, Ferrixan, Cliavist), Combidex[b] (Sinerum, Ferumoxtran-10), GastroMARK[a], Feraheme[c], Magtrace[a,d]	NanoTherm[b,c]

[a]FDA approved.
[b]EMA approved.
[c]FDA clinical trial.
[d]Magtrace is used for diagnostic assessment with Sentimag device rather than MRI contrast detection.

and animal safety studies.[29] With the most recent safety concerns, there has been increased interest in alternatives to GBCAs.

IONPs are an appealing alternative to GBCAs because iron's metabolic pathway is well understood. In addition, IONPs were demonstrated as potential MRI contrast agents as far back as the 1980s.[30] However, GBCAs and IONPs create distinctly different contrast. GBCAs are often referred to as 'positive contrast' agents, because GBCAs produce increased image brightness (hyperintensity) in the tissues that accumulate them; IONPs, on the other hand, are typically referred to as 'negative contrast' agents, because their uptake leads to decreased image intensity (see Figure 27.1).[31] Several IONP based contrast agents have been approved for clinical use; however, production has been discontinued[32,33] (see Table 27.1).

Liver scans represent 5% of MRI examinations.[6] Feridex and Resovist have been approved for the diagnosis of liver cancer. Once administered by IV injection, healthy liver tissue takes up the IONPs causing a rapid loss of image intensity. This results in 'negative' contrast at the location of the cancerous tissue.[6] Feridex caused a high incidence of severe back pain during administration (4% of patients), which led to its diminished clinical use.[6] Resovist did not have the same adverse effects as Feridex and could be administered as a bolus. Administration as a bolus provides vascular information in addition to IONP macrophage uptake.[32] In addition, new GBCAs such as OptiMARK™ OmniScan™, and MultiHance were introduced to the market. The diagnostic images from GBCAs were of similar quality but required less complicated administration, and a bolus injection could be performed without concerns about side effects.[6,34] Since liver images only represented 5% of MRI examinations and there were competing products, the market for IONP-based contrast agents for liver imaging was small.[6] As a result, Feridex was discontinued in 2008 and Resovist is currently only marketed in Japan and some locations in Europe.[33,35] Resovist continues to be developed for additional applications, such as the localization of metastatic breast cancer tumors in lymph nodes.[36]

GastroMARK followed a similar fate. It was FDA approved as an orally administered contrast agent for identifying masses within the gastrointestinal tract. However, there were several imaging methods [computed tomography (CT), Fluorescence, and MRI] and contrast agents available for enterography.[37,38] Ultimately, multiphasic MRI contrast agents, such

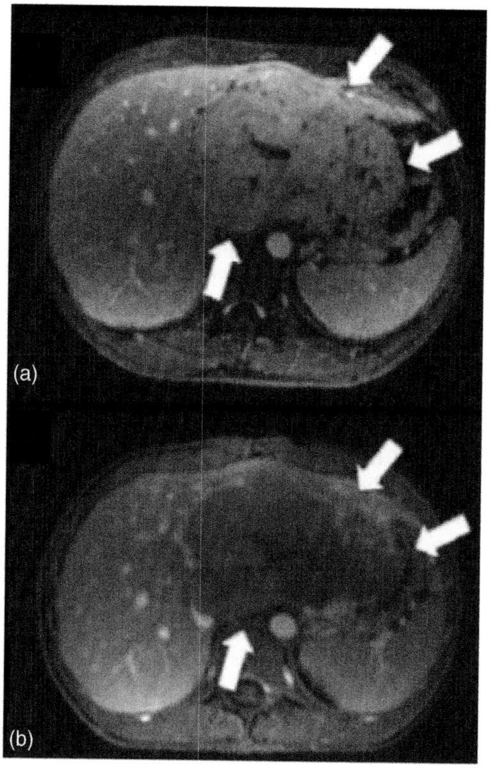

Figure 27.1. (a) Axial *T*1-weighted liver acquisition with volume acquisition image of a hepatocellular carcinoma (arrows) in a 15-year-old patient after intravenous injection of gadolinium chelate shows marked increase in signal intensity of both liver and tumor. (b) Corresponding MRI after intravenous injection of ferumoxytol (obtain 1 day after Gd image) shows a decrease in signal intensity at the tumor site (arrows). (This image has been reproduced from Radiology, volume 284, Daldrup-Link, Heike E. *et al.*, 'Ten Things You Might Not Know about Iron Oxide Nanoparticles' Copyright 2017, with permission from the Radiological Society of North America[31])

as dilute barium with sorbitol, became the preferred contrast agents[38] and low usage of GastroMARK led to its eventual discontinuation.[39]

Since few IONP-based contrast agents remain in active clinical use, off-label use of IONP anemia treatments, such as Feraheme, has been explored. Many of these clinical studies have focused around the application of Feraheme as a contrast agent alternative to GBCAs for cardiac and central nervous system MRI.[40] In addition, the uptake of IONPs into macrophages provides unique imaging opportunities for the assessment of inflammation to provide contrast to diagnose brain tumors, arterial plaque stability, and lymph node tumors.[39,40] In March of 2015, the strongest warning from the FDA was issued related to severe allergic reactions and deaths, halting off-label clinical use.[17] This product was removed from the European Market.[39] However, clinical studies are ongoing for applications in central nervous system,[41] angiography,[42] pancreatic cancer,[43] bone cancer,[44] as well as metastatic spread.[33,40,45] The high promise of this contrast agent has still resulted in many ongoing pre-clinical studies despite safety concerns.

Combidex (Sinerem) initially had very promising results for the detection of lymph node metastasis in prostate cancer.[39] However, FDA approval was never received due to the small number of clinical patients within the studies addressing the safety and efficacy of the drug.[46] Furthermore, Combidex was also removed from the EMA submission process.[39] While the development of Combidex was abandoned by AMAG Pharmaceuticals, the licensing has been purchased by a spin-off company from Radboud University Medical Center, SPL Medical, and is still administered in the Netherlands for diagnosis of metastatic spread related to prostate cancer.[47] Currently, the use of Combidex is undergoing clinical trials for diagnosing lymph node metastasis in patients with rectal, breast, cervical, uterine, and prostate cancer.[48]

Sienna Plus is another encouraging IONP-based contrast agent for diagnosing cancerous lymph nodes.[33] Sienna Plus is injected subcutaneously near the tumor site, where it drains through the lymphatics and accumulates in the sentinel lymph node. The localization of the sentinel lymph node can be determined by using the SentiMag® magnetic probe or the visual brown discoloration of the tissue.[39] Sienna+® has been approved for sentinel lymph node diagnosis in the EU. The Magtrace™ and Sentimag® Magnetic Localization System has been approved by the US FDA and is indicated to assist in localizing lymph nodes draining a tumor site, as part of a sentinel lymph node biopsy procedure, in patients with breast cancer undergoing a mastectomy.[39,49]

27.2.3 Cancer Treatments

MFH exploits the heat produced by the forced change in the IONPs magnetic moment when exposed to an alternating magnetic field operating in the tens to hundreds of kilohertz range. The heat generated is often referred to as the specific absorption rate (SAR) or the specific loss power (SLP). Demonstrated applications of MFH include organ preservation, neuromodulation, and cancer therapy.[7–9,50,51] To date, however, only MFH of cancer has reached the clinic.

Cancer treatment with MFH requires that a baseline temperature of ≥43 °C be produced at the tumor site over time to accumulate a lethal thermal dose.[7,52] NanoTherm® was approved in conjunction with the NanoActivator® thermoablation system by the EMA in 2012 for treatment of glioblastoma with radiation therapy and remains the only clinically used IONP cancer therapeutic.[7] Clinical studies have demonstrated that combinatorial therapies, such as radiation with hyperthermia are more effective than radiation alone. For example, the median survival rate for primary diagnosis changed from 14.6 to 23.2 months and reoccurrence diagnosis from 6.2 to 11.2 months when including hyperthermia in the treatment plan.[8] Additional promising results have been demonstrated with the application of this treatment to prostate cancer.[53] Clinical trials for the application of NanoTherm with prostate cancer recently began in the United States.[54]

27.3 SAFETY CONCERNS

IONPs, MRI, and MFH all have inherent safety concerns related to them. This section focuses on the safety concerns unique to IONPs and MFH. There are several risks which are inherent to the use of iron preparations. Several initial concerns, such as increase infections and negative impact on heart health, have been demonstrated to not be a concern.[11] Iron overload and allergic reactions continue to be a concern for IONPs and therefore will be discussed in further detail below. In addition, precautions related to the presence of ferromagnetic materials, such as IONPs in tattoos during an MRI, warrant additional examination. Finally, the clinical application of MFH has produced several unique safety precautions.

27.3.1 Iron Metabolism and IONPs

Some background on the iron cycle within the human body is necessary to better understand the concerns related to iron overload and allergic reactions. IONPs are considered safe, biocompatible, and nontoxic materials, largely because once they are degraded, the

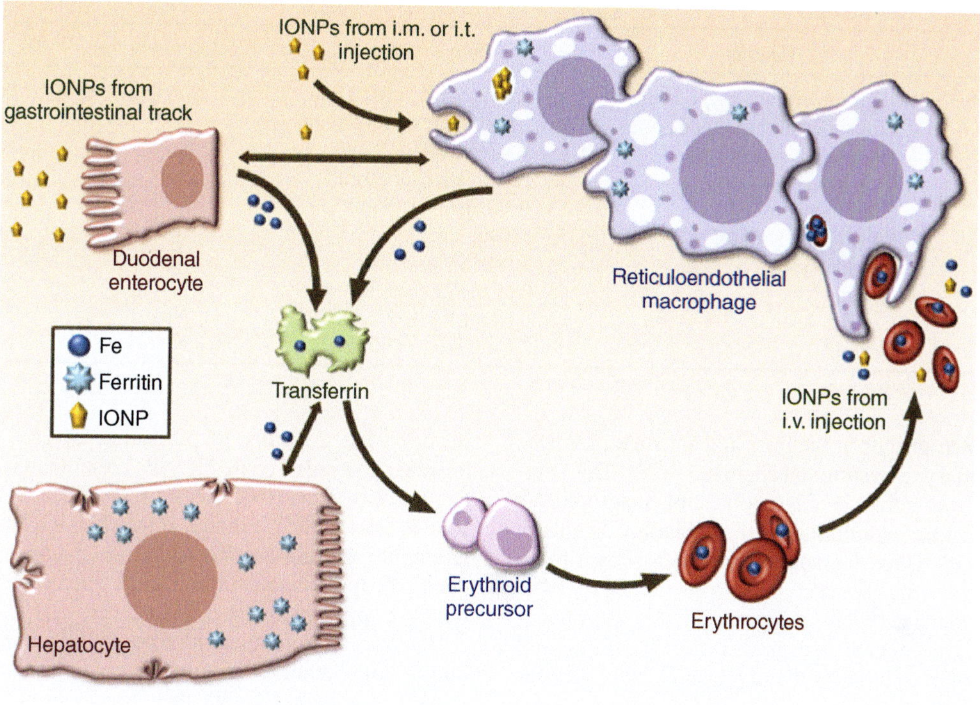

Figure 27.2. Iron cycle with IONP degradation. (Adapted from Robert E. Fleming, M.D. and Prem Ponka, M.D., Ph.D (2012) Mechanisms of Disease Iron Overload in Human Disease N Engl J Med 2012;366:348–359)

iron ions follow the metabolic pathways for iron (see Figure 27.2).[55,56] Unlike dietary iron, IONPs have several routes of exposure within the body.

Ingested dietary iron is broken down into its ionic form and taken into the bloodstream with the duodenum in the small intestine. In order to survive in the gastrointestinal tract, ingested IONPs must have a coating which can survive the harsh acidic environment. GastroMARK®'s poly [*N*-(2-aminoethyl)-3-aminopropyl] siloxane coating allows the IONPs to maintain structure for imaging in the intestinal tract.[57] Several coatings are being investigated for their stability within the gastrointestinal track such as casein and poly(lactide-*co*-glycolide acid).[58,59] Once taken up through the intestinal lining, IONPs are speculated to undergo the same interaction with the reticuloendothelial system (RES) as intravenously injected IONPs.[60] However, further research is necessary to establish these pathways.

In addition to ingestion, IONPs are often administered through injection. IONPs administered subcutaneously, intramuscularly, or intratumorally are taken up within the tissue and then by macrophages within the lymphatics system.[15,61–63] Intravenous injection results in the IONPs being directly administered to the bloodstream. Once within the bloodstream, the iron becomes bound to transferrin where it can be used to form erythrocytes within the bone marrow. Once the free iron concentration reaches a level that saturates the transferrin in the blood, non-transferrin bound iron (NTBI) is produced. NTBI can be taken up by hepatocytes and cardiomyocytes. Excess iron is stored as ferritin within macrophages and hepatocytes.[55] IONPs are treated differently than iron ions because IONPs are similar in size to viruses and bacteria. Therefore, IONPs undergo opsonization, the process where plasma proteins are deposited on the surface of the IONP. The plasma proteins signal the response from the rest of the body. Often the result is macrophage uptake; however, an allergic response can also be elicited.

The exact biodistribution of IONPs is highly dependent on the size, shape, coating, and charge of the IONP. Ultra-small IONPs (<10 nm) are rapidly cleared via renal clearance.[64] However, most IONPs are taken

Table 27.2. Clinical IONPs

IONP	Coating	Administration	Black box warning	Test dose
Dexferrum®	High-molecular weight dextran	i.v. 100 mg day^{-1} over 2 min	Yes[14]	Yes[14]
INFeD®	Low-molecular weight dextran	i.v. 100 mg day^{-1} over 2 min	Yes[15]	Yes[15]
Venofer	Sucrose	i.v. 100 mg over 3–10 min	No[19]	No[19]
Ferrlecit	Gluconate	i.v. 125 mg Fe over 10 min	No[18]	No[18]
Ferinject	Carboxymaltose	i.v. 1000 mg over 15 min	No[20]	No[20]
Feraheme	Polyglucose sorbitol	i.v. 510 mg day^{-1}	Yes[17]	Yes[16]
Monofer	Isomaltoside	i.v. 20 mg Fe/kg bolus	No[70]	No[70]
Feridex	Dextran	i.v. 0.56 mg/kg over 30 min	No[5]	No[5]
Resovist	Carboxydextran	i.v. 0.89 mg/kg over 2.5 min	N/A	No[71]
Combidex	Dextran	i.v. 2.6 mg/kg over 30 min	N/A	No[47]

up by macrophages in the liver and spleen and follow hepatobiliary excretion mechanisms.[4,39,56] Degradation occurs within the lysosomes of macrophages within acidic conditions with chelating agents.[65] The rate of IONP degradation has been shown to be impacted by the presence of ferritin proteins within the macrophage.[66] Once degraded, ^{59}Fe radiotracer studies have shown iron degraded from IONPs is used in a similar fashion to dietary iron.[56] This process and the subsequent excretion of excess iron can take several months.[16] However, IONPs with a highly negative charge have been demonstrated to undergo rapid hepatobiliary excretion, where IONPs leave the body within hours after injection.[10]

27.3.2 Iron Overload

Iron overload occurs when free iron in the blood has saturated the transferrin and high concentrations of NTBI are present.[39] NTBI acts as a catalyst in the formation of reactive oxygen species (ROS), resulting in cellular injury and organ malfunction.[55,67] The expected lethal iron dose for an adult (~70 kg or 150 lbs.) is 2–4 g of iron; however, toxic symptoms are known to appear when doses contain iron in mg concentrations.[68,69] The toxic effects observed from iron overload include increased body temperature, hypotension, peripheral edema, metallic taste, tachycardia, palpitations, diarrhea, nausea, vomiting, chills, and back pain.[67,68]

The risk of iron overload is dependent on the route of administration and iron concentration. Orally administered IONPs are the least likely formulation to cause iron overload because iron uptake is regulated by homeostatic mechanisms.[55] Iron administered by injection has a history of producing adverse effects; however, the use of coated IONPs rather than iron salts has decreased many of the adverse effects related to iron overload.[4,68,69] Finally, injectable IONP formulations for anemia are most likely to cause this issue due to the high concentrations used when compared to imaging applications (see Table 27.2).

The rate of iron released from IONPs can be reduced with changes in surface coating. Slow iron release is associated with decreased toxicity caused by free iron.[4,67] For commercially available IONPs, the pharmacokinetics, such as iron release rate and transferrin uptake, have been directly compared. The rate of iron release based on surface coating for IONP anemia treatments is known to be sodium ferric gluconate (Ferrlecit®) > iron sucrose (Venofer®) > ferric carboxymaltose (Ferinject®) > polyglucose sorbitol (Feraheme®) > Iron dextran (INFeD®).[67] Feridex, Resovist, and Combidex are anticipated to have similar kinetic release with dextran-coated iron formulations (INFeD®).

A major route of toxicity caused by iron overload is the production of ROS, which can also be produced by the surface coatings. Zager *et al.* compared the production of ROS and cytotoxic potentials between several clinically used IONPs providing the following order for cytotoxic potentials: iron sucrose (Venofer) ≫ iron glucose (Ferrlecit) > iron dextran (INFeD).[72] This result matches other studies which have shown that Venofer could cause renal damage due to the production of ROS.[73]

27.3.3 IONP Allergic Reactions

The recent (2015) FDA warning for Feraheme related to fatal anaphylactic response has obtained

Table 27.3. MRI impact of clinical IONPs

IONP	Post-administration	Contrast type	Location
Venofer[80]	3–24 h	T_2/T_2^*	Liver, kidney, spleen
Feraheme[16,40,81]	1–3 days	T_1	Blood pool agent[40]
	Hours–10 days	T_2/T_2^*	Inflammation/brain/lymph nodes/arterial plaques[40]
	1 day to 11 months	T_2/T_2^*	Liver[16,81]
Feridex[82]	30 s	T_1	Vasculature
	10 min–6 h	T_2/T_2^*	Liver legions[a]
Resovist[34]	40 min after injection	T_2/T_2^*	Liver legions[a]
Combidex[47]	24–36 h	T_2/T_2^*	Lymph nodes[a]
NanoTherm[8]	Unknown	T_2/T_2^*	Tumor progression monitoring inhibited
GastroMARK[57]	30–45 min	T_2/T_2^*	Stomach and small intestine
	7 h	T_2/T_2^*	Large intestine

[a]FDA or EU approved use.

considerable attention.[17,74] This warning was released after 18 fatalities occurred between 2009 and 2014 from serious hypersensitivity reactions despite immediate medical intervention.[17] Hypersensitivity reactions are a risk with several IONP formulations and have been an adverse effect since the early formulations of dextran-coated IONPs (see Table 27.2).[4] IONPs with severe allergic responses which have resulted in fatalities require a test dose before administration and should only be administered where resuscitation equipment is readily available.[14–16] Overall, the rate of fatalities from IV administered IONPs is 0.007%.[75,76]

The chemical composition of the surface coating on the IONP strongly influences the immune system response. Dextran, in particular, is known to induce anaphylactic responses due to a reaction with endogenous dextran-reactive immunoglobulin (Ig) G antibodies.[77] However, not all dextran coatings elicit the same response, with high molecular weight dextran inducing an allergic response at a rate 8.1x higher than low molecular weight (LMW) dextran.[4,12,78] Newer formulations of anemia IONPs, such as gluconate and sucrose, were designed to avoid coating-related allergic reactions.[12] Polyethylene glycol is currently used in many emerging IONP formulations; however, it can produce an immune response.[79]

The details of the injection are known to impact the severity of the allergic reaction. Although hypersensitive reactions are noted as a risk with Feridex, neither a test dose or resuscitation equipment are deemed necessary for administration.[5] When compared to the doses used in the treatment of anemia (e.g., using DexFerrum), Feridex requires a lower dose.[5,14] The rate of injection can also have a major impact on adverse reactions. For instance, the fast infusion rate initially used with Combidex had an increased risk of severe hypersensitive reactions as compared to later optimized protocols with slower infusion rates.[47]

27.3.4 IONP MRI Impact

Unintentionally altered MRI contrast can be an issue related to clinical use of IONPs (see Table 27.3). Feraheme specifically warns that effects may be observed in MRI up to 3 months following the last Feraheme dose[16,83] (see Figure 27.3). In addition, clinical studies with NanoTherm note that MRI scans cannot be used for measurement of tumor progression after the injection of the IONP due to obstruction of the tumor in the image.[8] While there have been some preclinical studies on IONP anemia formulations, such as Venofer, none of the anemia-based treatments appear to be used as an MRI contrast agent or even warn against any issues with MRI scanning after administration.

Black and dark brown tattoo ink is also known to contain IONPs. Image artifacts have been observed with patients with tattoos.[84] The ink itself does not appear to produce heat when exposed to MRI conditions; however, loops are theoretically capable of creating a voltage within the tattoo.[85,86] Several case studies have reported burns caused in black and dark brown tattoos.[87–90] However, burns from tattoos have an extremely low rate of incidence (1.5% for permanent cosmetics) and the current recommendation is the application of a cold compress over the tattoo site.[91,92]

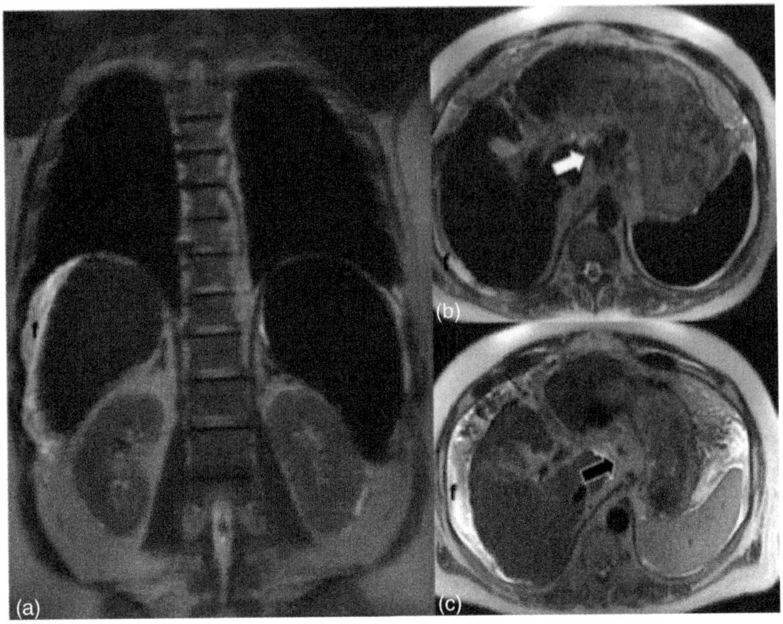

Figure 27.3. The change in contrast produced by Feraheme on the liver, spleen, and lymph nodes (white arrow) postinjection axial (a) and coronal view (b) and the same patient 15 months preinjection (c). The decreased signal intensity obscures the liver, spleen, and lymph nodes obstructing the assessment of tumor progression. (Nicola Schieda, Perenteral ferumoxytol interaction with magnetic resonance imaging: a case report, review, of the literature and advisory warning. Insights into Imaging, 2013. 4(4): p. 509-512)

27.3.5 MFH Safety

Precautions need to be followed to avoid unintentional heating of surrounding tissue during the application of MFH. Similar to MRI, unintentional heating can be produced through eddy currents created by the oscillating magnetic field used in MFH.[93,94] The strength of the electric field created is proportional to the product of the magnetic field strength and frequency. The upper limits reported (450–850 kA $(\text{m kHz})^{-1}$) have been defined based on the heating dose that could be administered to a patient for over an hour without major complications.[95] Preclinical studies have demonstrated the severe issues that can occur when IONP localization is not taken into consideration and collateral damage occurs within the RES organs.[96] Clinically, the localization of IONPs is controlled by using an inter-tumoral injection of IONPs.[8] However, the lack of controlled diffusion/spread of IONPs in vivo after the injection and the possible dependence of the induced heating on the concentration of IONPs makes the image-based determination of the shape and concentration of IONPs critical for tumor destruction with minimal collateral damage. Finally, clinical studies have included the precaution of ensuring that all metal within 40 cm of the affected area is removed. For the application with glioblastoma, the removal of dental implants is necessary.[8]

27.4 IONP IMAGING

Many methods can be used to assess the concentration of iron or IONPs within a sample. Prussian blue staining is often used for histological assessment. Spectroscopic methods, such as atomic emission spectroscopy, and colorimetric assays (Ferrozine and Ferene) allow for quantitative analysis of iron within the sample.[97,98] However, these methods are impractical in the clinical setting, because they are invasive.

As clinically established noninvasive imaging methods, CT and conventional echo-based MRI methods are natural choices for imaging IONPs. CT relies on having a high density of IONPs, and therefore, is most effective at high IONP concentrations (>89 mM_{Fe}, 5 mg Fe mL^{-1}), although IONP concentrations as low as 18 mM_{Fe} (1 mg Fe mL^{-1}) have been detected.[99] Conventional echo-based MRI methods, such as spin echo (SE) or gradient echo (GRE) pulse sequences, have demonstrated utility with IONPs as negative contrast agents; however, they are only effective at quantifying low (<1.8 mM_{Fe}, 1 mg Fe mL^{-1}) IONP concentrations.[99,100] This section presents many of the emerging imaging techniques that enable noninvasive IONP imaging, along with an overview of recent work focused on MRI guided MFH.

27.4.1 Quantitative Susceptibility Mapping (QSM)

Quantitative susceptibility mapping (QSM) is a method still in development for IONP detection but has many already demonstrated clinical uses. QSM uses phase information obtained from GRE images to estimate a material's magnetic susceptibility.[101] Heterogeneity in magnetic susceptibility (e.g., due to changing levels of IONPs in different tissues) causes the image phase to vary spatially when image acquisition is performed with a GRE sequence. Specifically, after a radiofrequency (RF) pulse is used to excite transverse magnetization, the magnetization accumulates phase until the time of signal detection; this time interval is an adjustable parameter in GRE and SE imaging called echo time (TE). When using a GRE sequence, the time constant describing the transverse magnetization decay during TE is denoted as T_2*. Spatial variation of the magnetic susceptibility in the tissues (e.g. due to nonuniform IONP distributions) leads to varying rates of magnetization evolution during TE and thus to spatial phase variation at the time of signal detection. Large variations in phase occurring across small spatial scales similar in dimension to the image pixels are responsible for the negative contrast in T_2*-weighted GRE imaging. However, phase variation occurring at lower spatial frequencies can still be measured in GRE images. In QSM, changes in image phase caused by IONPs are considered to provide greater accuracy and a higher quantitative limit of IONP detection as compared to standard T_2*-weighted GRE imaging.[102] QSM has been utilized for cell tracking and quantification in vivo and for the localization of IONPs throughout the body.[102–104] Although most applications focus on qualitative changes caused by the presence of IONPs, quantifiable signals have been demonstrated up to 11 mM_{Fe} (0.62 mg Fe mL^{-1}).[105] Recently, Lu *et al.* demonstrated quantification of IONPs in agarose at concentrations as high as 22 mM_{Fe} (1.2 mg Fe mL^{-1}) using a QSM echoless MRI sequence hybrid.[106]

27.4.2 Echoless MRI

Conventional echo-based MRI sequences are problematic at high IONP concentrations, due to the destructive interference (negative contrast) caused by variable rates of magnetization evolution during TE (Figure 27.4). In GRE and SE sequences, for technical reasons, the minimum achievable TE is typically

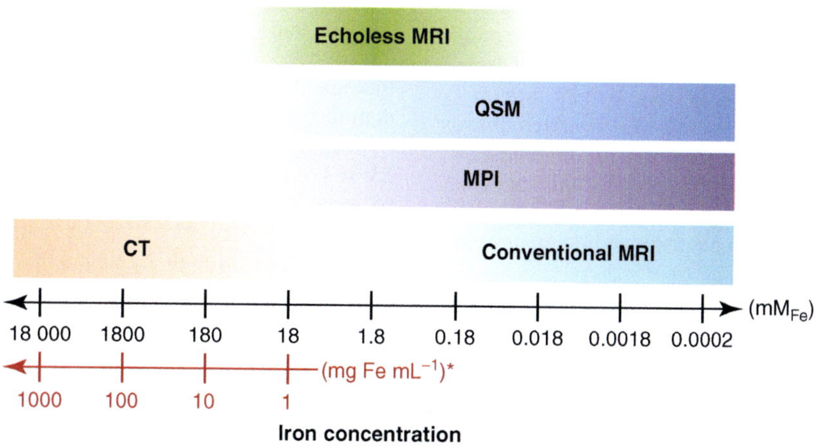

Figure 27.4. IONP quantitative range with noninvasive imaging methods, computed tomography (CT), conventional MRI such as GRE and SE, magnetic particle imaging (MPI), quantitative susceptibility mapping (QSM), and echoless MRI such as SWIFT or UTE.[99,100,106–108] (*Note: mg Fe mL^{-1} is the typical iron concentration unit used in MFH)

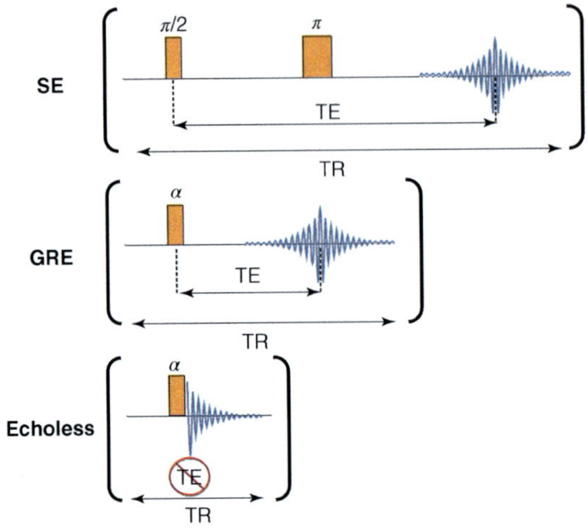

Figure 27.5. Schematic of spin echo (SE), gradient echo (GRE), and echoless pulse sequences, demonstrating the decrease in time between the excitation pulse (orange block) and the ensuing MRI signal (blue) that is recorded. Both SE and GRE sequences have an echo time (TE), whereas echoless sequences do not. TR denotes the repetition time

on the order of milliseconds, which is too long to avoid destructive interferences at high IONP concentrations. More recently, echoless MRI sequences have been developed for imaging tissues with ultrashort T_2 or T_2*, such as bones, tendons, or the lung.[109–114] A key feature of echoless sequences is the lack of the time interval, TE in which the transverse magnetization evolves, thereby mitigating signal loss from ultrashort T_2 or T_2* (see Figure 27.5). With no TE period, image contrast is a function of the spin density (i.e., water concentration) and the degree of recovery of the longitudinal magnetization following each RF excitation pulse. The time constant describing this recovery of longitudinal magnetization is called T_1. IONPs shorten T_1 of the surrounding water protons. T_1-weighted images are produced by using a short repetition time (TR) together with an RF pulse that tips a significant fraction of the longitudinal magnetization per TR. Maps of IONP concentrations can be generated by quantifying T_1 in images.

Specific echoless sequences that have been utilized to visualization the distributions of IONPs include ultrashort time echo (UTE) and sweep imaging with Fourier transformation (SWIFT).[100,115–122] UTE minimizes destructive interferences (negative contrast) by using a short RF pulse and acquiring signal during the gradient ramp up, although the latter can cause image artifacts due to eddy currents or gradient switching delays.[111,123,124] SWIFT is based on a radically different excitation and acquisition scheme. The SWIFT sequence splits the excitation pulse into sub-pulses and performs signal acquisition between those sub-pulses. In addition, SWIFT exploits frequency-modulated excitation, which allows excitation of a large tip angle over a large bandwidth.[125] Example images of a tumor injected with IONPs, comparing positive T_1-weighted contrast of SWIFT to negative T_2*-weighted contrast of GRE, are shown in Figure 27.6.

The positive contrast created through the T_1-weighted acquisition from echoless sequences affords the capability to quantify IONPs within biological systems. Quantification of IONPs was demonstrated in vivo in blood using UTE at concentrations ranging from 0.54 to 2.9 mM_{Fe}.[126] Furthermore, SWIFT has been used to demonstrate a correlation between R_1 ($=1/T_1$), iron concentration, and the SAR produced by MFH.[10,120–122,127,128] In particular, iron quantification through R_1 mapping with SWIFT has demonstrated an overlap at lower concentrations with mapping of R_2 ($=1/T_2$) using echo-based sequences.[100]

27.4.3 Magnetic Particle Imaging (MPI)

Magnetic particle imaging directly detects IONPs allowing for an extensive concentration range (150 nM_{Fe} to 189 mM_{Fe}; 8.4 ng Fe mL^{-1} to 10.6 mg

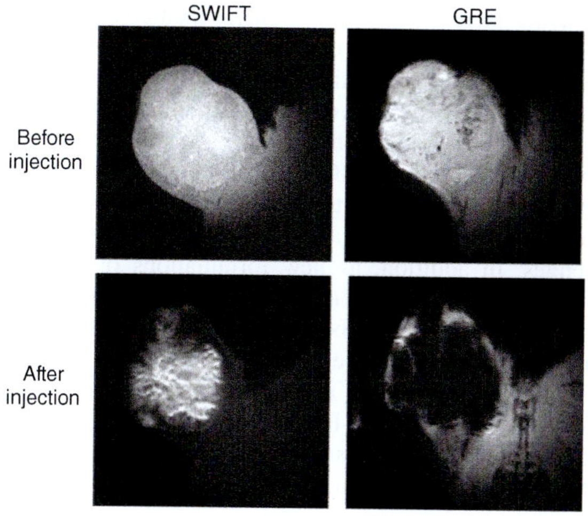

Figure 27.6. LNCaP tumor before and after intratumoral injection of 18 mM_{Fe} (1 mg Fe mL^{-1}) tumor volume with IONPs. LNCaP tumor before and after intratumoral injection of IONPs at 18 mM_{Fe} (1 mg Fe mL^{-1}) tumor volume. With the gradient echo (GRE) sequence, IONPs produce decreased image intensity which extends beyond the actual IONP locations (i.e., blooming effect). With the echoless sequence (SWIFT), IONPs produce increased image intensity, which required reducing the image intensity scale to visualize IONP locations. All animal procedures and care were approved by the University of Minnesota Institutional Animal Care and Use Committee. (Courtesy of Dr. Jinjin Zhang and Prof. P. Jack Hoopes)

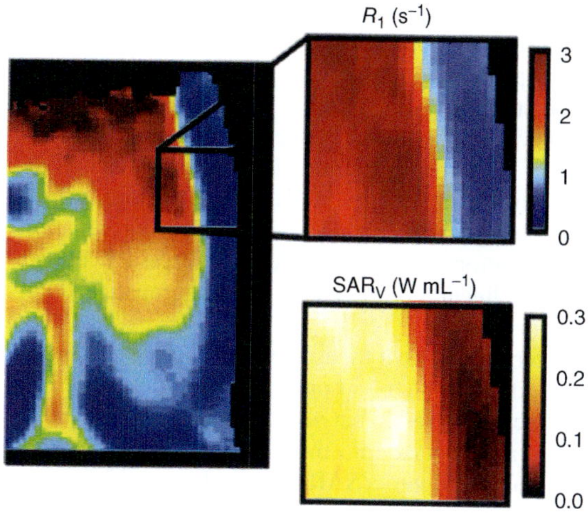

Figure 27.7. The ex vivo specific absorption rate (SAR_v) with the in vivo R_1. Using the calibration from the liver, a section of the R_1 map including nearby tissue without IONP uptake is converted to a SAR_v map. (Zhang, J., Ring, H. L., Hurley, K. R., Shao, Q., Carlson, C. S., Idiyatullin, D., ... Garwood, M. (2017). Quantification and biodistribution of iron oxide nanoparticles in the primary clearance organs of mice using T_1 contrast for heating. Magnetic resonance in medicine, 78(2), 702-712. https://doi.org/10.1002/mrm.26394. Reproduced with permission from John Wiley & Sons)

Fe mL^{-1}).[107,108] MPI takes advantage of the magnetic response in IONP magnetization when the background magnetic field is below magnetic saturation. Similar to MRI, the sample is exposed to a background magnetic field above the magnetic saturation of the IONP. A field-free region (FFR) is created and moved across the sample. Within the FFR, a magnetic pulse (kHz) is applied and the nonlinear IONP magnetization response is detected.[129] MPI is synergistic when used with MFH because the same equipment used to create the FFR allows for controlled heating of the IONP.[130] Controlled heating has been demonstrated within a preclinical model with resolution of a 7 mm diameter circle throughout the tissue.[131] MPI has also been demonstrated to have utility for IONP imaging related to traumatic brain injuries, cell tracking, angiography, and assessing IONP distributions.[108,132–134] The recent advancement of MPI toward clinical application is due to the availability of commercial MPI scanners[132]. MPI shows exceptional promise for IONP imaging applications, however, is still under development.

27.4.4 MRI Guided MFH

Although CT is the clinically used method to quantify IONPs before MFH therapy, quantification of IONPs between 1.8 and 18 mM_{Fe} (0.1 – 1 mg Fe mL^{-1}) are still desired for newly developed methods and applications. Newly developed IONPs provide more heat than commercially available IONPs at a lower concentration and therefore will require MRI-based methods to avoid unintentional heat injuries.[2,135] Much recent progress has been made on advancing echoless MRI sequences to assist in guiding MFH. SWIFT-based MRI is better suited than some other echoless sequences due to certain technical limitations that constrain the flip angle below the optimum for signal-to-noise ratio (SNR) and T_1 contrast.[124]

SWIFT MRI has demonstrated a linear correlation between R_1 and SAR. Initial studies established a linear correlation within simplified agarose systems with several IONPs.[121,127,128] Further models were developed to demonstrate the impact of aggregation by first placing IONPs in a solution in which they are known to be unstable, such as phosphate buffered saline, and measuring the impact on heating and imaging characteristics.[127] However, heating effects can change dramatically with IONP aggregation, and therefore further research is necessary to validate a linear correlation within aggregated IONP systems.[136]

Later studies have focused on the complex milieu of the body. One study, in particular, demonstrated how the linear correlation between R_1 and SAR_v was maintained after uptake into the liver and spleen.[10] An R_1 map converted into a SAR_v map in Figure 27.7 shows the capability of image guidance for predicting heating dose. A challenge observed with R_1 IONP quantification in vivo was that the R_1 relaxivity changed depending on the organ and IONP degradation. Therefore, a calibration curve would be required for each individual organ and depending on the organ, the desired timeframe of measurement. The variations in the calibration curve create a limitation on the utility of R_1 IONP quantification to biodistribution of IONPs within the body; however, with a well-characterized tissue and IONP, R_1 IONP quantification might be used clinically in the future.

A recently explored complex biological system is that of cryopreserved tissue. It has recently been demonstrated that surrounding tissue with IONPs can create the uniform and rapid heating necessary to heat tissues from cryogenic temperatures without injury.[50] The technological advancement makes cryopreservation a possibility for the use of larger volume tissues, such as organs.[137] The capability to quantify IONPs within a cryopreserved tissue was demonstrated with an R_1 map.[50] Cryopreserved tissues provide a potential simplification of the water diffusion, since many of the biological processes, which would cause cellular uptake of the IONPs, are not occurring. There is still much to explore regarding the water diffusion within cryopreserved tissues, including the linear correlation between R_1 and SAR_v.

27.5 CONCLUSION AND OUTLOOK

This chapter provided an overview of the current clinical applications of IONPs with a focus on relevant safety concerns. IONPs show great potential for playing increasing roles in clinical medicine, as well as in biomedical research. Newly emerging methods, such as neuromodulation, organ preservation, cell tracking, and drug delivery provide additional motivation for the development of IONPs. Within the current clinical landscape of IONP use, we understand the potential hazards to human subjects, complications to diagnosis, and mitigation strategies for these challenges. In addition, as new formulations of IONPs demonstrate a reduction in the allergic and overload side effects which had been prevalent within early formulations, clinical acceptance has increased. Finally, in understanding the clinically observed concerns with IONPs, emerging IONPs can be designed around these known limitations producing improved solutions for MRI and MFH clinical use.

ACKNOWLEDGMENTS

The authors are grateful to Dr. Jinjin Zhang for MRI sequence development and the acquisition of images shown in Figure 27.6. We are also grateful to Prof. P. Jack Hoopes for initiating the study and providing technical expertise, animals, and IONPs to obtain the results shown in Figure 27.6. This work was supported by NIH grants R01 HL135046, R01 DK117425, and P41 EB015894.

RELATED ARTICLES IN EMAGRES

James, Thomas L.: Time for Preparation and Evolution. But what is the Mechanism for Relaxation?

Koenig, Seymour H.: I. I. Rabi, F. Bloch, E. M. Purcell, and the History of NMR and Relaxometry

Bioeffects and Safety of Radiofrequency Electromagnetic Fields

Contrast Agents in Magnetic Resonance: Operating Mechanisms

Contrast Agents in MRI: Superparamagnetic Iron Oxide

Contrast Agents in Whole Body Magnetic Resonance: An Overview

Gadolinium Chelate Contrast Agents in MRI: Clinical Applications

Gadolinium Chelates: Chemistry, Safety and Behavior

Radiofrequency Fields: Interactions, Biological Effects, and Safety Issues

Relaxation Measurements in Imaging Studies

Relaxation Measurements in Whole Body MRI: Clinical Utility

Safety Regulation in MR

Contrast Agents for MRI: Recent Advances

Garwood, Michael: Frequency-Modulated Pulses in the Early Days of Biomedical NMR

Safety Considerations in MRI

Centric SPRITE MRI of Biomaterials with Short T_2^*

Quantitative Ultrashort TE (UTE) Imaging of Short T_2 Tissues

Imaging of Short and Ultrashort T_2 and T_2^* Components of Tissues, Fluids, and Materials in the Body Using Clinical Magnetic Resonance Systems

Mechanisms for Short T_2 and $T_2{}^*$ in Collagen-Containing Tissue

MRI with Zero Echo Time

Overview of Short and Ultrashort $T_2/T_2{}^*$ Echo Time (UTE) Imaging

Adiabatic RF Pulses

REFERENCES

1. C. L. Dennis, K. L. Krycka, J. A. Borchers, R. D. Desautels, J. van Lierop, N. F. Huls, A. J. Jackson, C. Gruettner, and R. Ivkov, *Adv. Funct. Mater.*, 2015, **25**, 4300.
2. J. Mohapatra, A. Mitra, M. Aslam, and D. Bahadur, *IEEE Trans. Magn.*, 2015, **51**, 1.
3. W. Wu, Z. Wu, T. Yu, C. Jiang, and W.-S. Kim, *Sci. Technol. Adv. Mater.*, 2015, **16**, 023501.
4. M. Auerbach and H. Ballard, *ASH Educ. Progr. Book*, 2010, **2010**, 338.
5. Feridex I.V. [package insert]. Bayer HealthCare Pharmaceuticals Inc., Whippany, NJ, 2008. United States Food and Drug Administration. https://dailymed.nlm.nih.gov/dailymed/drugInfo.cfm?setid=82ceb312-3aaa-4a5c-9849-7f246cc06ded&audience=consumer.
6. O. Clement, N. Siauve, C.-A. Cuénod, and G. Frija, *Top. Magn. Reson. Imaging*, 1998, **9**, 167.
7. K. Mahmoudi, A. Bouras, D. Bozec, R. Ivkov, and C. Hadjipanayis, *Int. J. Hyperthermia*, 2018, 1.
8. K. Maier-Hauff, F. Ulrich, D. Nestler, H. Niehoff, P. Wust, B. Thiesen, H. Orawa, V. Budach, and A. Jordan, *J. Neuro-Oncol.*, 2011, **103**, 317.
9. A. C. Silva, T. R. Oliveira, J. B. Mamani, S. M. F. Malheiros, L. Malavolta, L. F. Pavon, T. T. Sibov, E. Amaro, A. Tannús, E. L. G. Vidoto, M. J. Martins, R. S. Santos, and L. F. Gamarra, *Int. J. Nanomed.*, 2011, **6**, 591.
10. J. Zhang, H. L. Ring, K. R. Hurley, Q. Shao, C. S. Carlson, D. Idiyatullin, N. Manuchehrabadi, P. J. Hoopes, C. L. Haynes, J. C. Bischof, and M. Garwood, *Magn. Reson. Med.*, 2017, **78**, 702.
11. T. Avni, A. Bieber, A. Grossman, H. Green, L. Leibovici, and A. Gafter-Gvili, *Mayo Clinic Proc.*, 2015, **90**, 12.
12. S. B. Silverstein and G. M. Rodgers, *Am. J. Hematol.*, 2004, **76**, 74.
13. FDA Safety Announcement Feraheme (ferummoxytol). United States Food and Drug Administration. https://www.fda.gov/downloads/Drugs/DrugSafety/UCM440336.pdf
14. Dexferrum [package insert]. Vifor Inc., Shirley, NY, 2008. United States Food and Drug Administration. https://www.accessdata.fda.gov/drugsatfda_docs/label/2009/040024s022lbl.pdf
15. INFeD. Watson Pharmaceuticals, Inc., Parsippany-Troy Hills, NJ, 2009. U.S.F.A.D. Administration, Editor.
16. Feraheme (ferumoxytol) [package insert]. AMAG Pharmaceuticals, Waltham, MA, 2015. U.S.F.A.D. Administration, Editor. http://www.accessdata.fda.gov/drugsatfda_docs/label/2015/022180s011s013lbl.pdf
17. FDA Safety Announcement Feraheme (ferumoxytol), 2015. United States Food and Drug Administration. https://www.fda.gov/downloads/Drugs/DrugSafety/UCM440336.pdf
18. Ferrlecit [package insert]. Sanofi-Aventis US, LCC., Bridgewater, NJ, 2011. United States Food and Drug Administration. https://www.accessdata.fda.gov/drugsatfda_docs/label/2011/020955s013s015lbl.pdf

19. Venofer [package insert]. American Reagent, Inc., Shirley, NY, 2006. United States Food and Drug Administration. https://www.accessdata.fda.gov/drugsatfda_docs/label/2011/021135s020lbl.pdf
20. Injectafer [package insert]. American Reagent, Inc., Shirley, NY, 2013. U.S.F.A.D. Administration, Editor. https://www.accessdata.fda.gov/drugsatfda_docs/label/2013/203565s000lbl.pdf
21. M. Rohrer, H. Bauer, J. Mintorovitch, M. Requardt, and H.-J. Weinmann, *Invest. Radiol.*, 2005, **40**, 715.
22. D. A. Bluemke and S. Liu, in 'Principles and Practice of Clinical Research', 3rd edn, eds J. I. Gallin and F. P. Ognibene, Academic Press: Boston, 2012, p 597.
23. W. W. Ting, M. Stone, K. C. Madison, and K. Kurtz, *Arch. Dermatol.*, 2003, **139**, 903.
24. J. Perez-Rodriguez, S. Lai, B. D. Ehst, D. M. Fine, and D. A. Bluemke, *Radiology*, 2009, **250**, 371.
25. E. Altun, D. R. Martin, R. Wertman, A. Lugo-Somolinos, E. R. Fuller, and R. C. Semelka, *Radiology*, 2009, **253**, 689.
26. M. R. Prince, H. Zhang, M. Morris, J. L. MacGregor, M. E. Grossman, J. Silberzweig, R. L. DeLapaz, H. J. Lee, C. M. Magro, and A. M. Valeri, *Radiology*, 2008, **248**, 807.
27. E. Kanal and M. F. Tweedle, *Radiology*, 2015, **275**, 630.
28. Restriction of Linear Gadolinium Agents in Body Scans, European Medicines Agency, 2017. http://www.ema.europa.eu/docs/en_GB/document_library/Referrals_document/gadolinium_contrast_agents_31/European_Commission_final_decision/WC500240575.pdf
29. FDA Drug Safety Communication: No harmful effects to date with brain retention of gadolinium-based contrast agents for MRIs; review to continue, 2017. US Food and Drug Administration. https://www.fda.gov/downloads/Drugs/DrugSafety/UCM589442.pdf
30. M. H. M. Dias and P. C. Lauterbur, *Magn. Reson. Med.*, 1986, **3**, 328.
31. H. E. Daldrup-Link, *Radiology*, 2017, **284**, 616.
32. Y.-X. J. Wang, *World J. Gastroenterol.*, 2015, **21**, 13400.
33. A. C. Anselmo and S. Mitragotri, *AAPS J.*, 2015, **17**, 1041.
34. P. Reimer and T. Blazer, *Eur. Radiol.*, 2003, **13**, 1266.
35. A. L. Cortajarena, D. Ortega, S. M. Ocampo, A. Gonzalez-García, P. Couleaud, R. Miranda, C. Belda-Iniesta, and A. Ayuso-Sacido, *Nanobiomedicine*, 2014, **1**, 2.
36. M. Sekino, A. Kuwahata, T. Ookubo, M. Shiozawa, K. Ohashi, M. Kaneko, I. Saito, Y. Inoue, H. Ohsaki, H. Takei, and M. Kusakabe, *Sci. Rep.*, 2018, **8**, 1195.
37. M. S. Gee and M. G. Harisinghani, *J. Magn. Reson. Imag. JMRI*, 2011, **33**, 527.
38. A. Kilcoyne, J. L. Kaplan, and M. S. Gee, *World J. Gastroenterol.*, 2016, **22**, 917.
39. Y. X. J. Wáng and J.-M. Idée, *Quant. Imag. Med. Surg.*, 2017, **7**, 88.
40. M. R. Bashir, L. Bhatti, D. Marin, and R. C. Nelson, *J. Magn. Reson. Imag.*, 2015, **41**, 884.
41. Feraheme central nervous system clinical trials: NCT00659776, NCT03270059, NCT02549898, NCT01674257, NCT03084523.
42. Feraheme angiography clinical trials: NCT03266848, NCT01995799, NCT00707876, NCT02997046, NCT02752191, NCT02954510, NCT03173066.
43. Feraheme pancreatic cancer clinical trial: NCT02070705.
44. Feraheme bone cancer clinical trial: NCT01336803.
45. Feraheme metastatic cancer clinical trials: NCT0181533, NCT01770353, NCT02857218, NCT03280277, NCT03084523, NCT03325166, NCT03264300 NCT00659126, NCT0347617, NCT03234309, NCT00978562, NCT01895829, NCT00103038, NCT02359097.
46. M. J. Fromer, *Oncol. Times*, 2005, **27**, 7.
47. A. S. Fortuin, R. Brüggemann, J. Linden, I. Panfilov, B. Israël, T. W. J. Scheenen, and J. O. Barentsz, *Wiley Interdiscip. Rev. Nanomed. Nanobiotechnol.*, 2017, **10**, e1471.
48. Combidex clinical trials: NCT02751606, NCT02751606, NCT00416455, NCT03223064.
49. SiennaPlus sentinel lymph node diagnosis clinical trial: NCT02445456, NCT03036475.
50. N. Manuchehrabadi, Z. Gao, J. Zhang, H. L. Ring, Q. Shao, F. Liu, M. McDermott, A. Fok, Y. Rabin, K. G. M. Brockbank, M. Garwood, C. L. Haynes, and J. C. Bischof, *Sci. Trans. Med.*, 2017, **9**, 379.
51. R. Chen, G. Romero, M. G. Christiansen, A. Mohr, and P. Anikeeva, *Science*, 2015, **347**, 1477.
52. S. A. Sapareto and W. C. Dewey, *Int. J. Radiat. Oncol. Biol. Phys.*, 1984, **10**, 787.
53. M. Johannsen, B. Thiesen, P. Wust, and A. Jordan, *Int. J. Hyperthermia*, 2010, **26**, 790.

54. NanoTherm pancreatic cancer clinical trial: NCT03604562.
55. R. E. Fleming and P. Ponka, *New England J. Med.*, 2012, **366**, 348.
56. R. Weissleder, D. D. Stark, B. L. Engelstad, B. R. Bacon, C. C. Compton, D. L. White, P. Jacobs, and J. Lewis, *Am. J. Roentgenol.*, 1989, **152**, 167.
57. GastroMARK [package insert]. AMAG Pharmaceuticals Inc., Cambridge, MA, 2010. U.S.F.a.D. Administration, Editor. https://dailymed.nlm.nih.gov/dailymed/archives/fdaDrugInfo.cfm?archiveid=101519
58. J. Cheng, B. A. Teply, S. Y. Jeong, C. H. Yim, D. Ho, I. Sherifi, S. Jon, O. C. Farokhzad, A. Khademhosseini, and R. S. Langer, *Pharmaceut. Res.*, 2006, **23**, 557.
59. J. Huang, Q. Shu, L. Wang, H. Wu, A. Y. Wang, and H. Mao, *Biomaterials*, 2015, **39**, 105.
60. H. Arami, A. Khandhar, D. Liggitt, and K. M. Krishnan, *Chem. Soc. Rev.*, 2015, **44**, 8576.
61. L. Johnson, S. E. Pinder, and M. Douek, *Histopathology*, 2012, **62**, 481.
62. J. J. Pouw, M. R. Grootendorst, R. Bezooijen, C. A. H. Klazen, W. I. De Bruin, J. M. Klaase, M. A. Hall-Craggs, M. Douek, and B. ten Haken, *Br. J. Radiol.*, 2015, **88**, 20150634.
63. K. Motomura, T. Izumi, S. Tateishi, H. Sumino, A. Noguchi, T. Horinouchi, and K. Nakanishi, *BMC Med. Imag.*, 2013, **13**, 32.
64. H. Wei, O. T. Bruns, M. G. Kaul, E. C. Hansen, M. Barch, A. Wiśniowska, O. Chen, Y. Chen, N. Li, S. Okada, J. M. Cordero, M. Heine, C. T. Farrar, D. M. Montana, G. Adam, H. Ittrich, A. Jasanoff, P. Nielsen, and M. G. Bawendi, *Proc. Natl. Acad. Sci. USA*, 2017, **114**, 2325.
65. M. Lévy, F. Lagarde, V.-A. Maraloiu, M.-G. Blanchin, F. Gendron, C. Wilhelm, and F. Gazeau, *Nanotechnology*, 2010, **21**, 395103.
66. J. Volatron, F. Carn, J. Kolosnjaj-Tabi, Y. Javed, Q. L. Vuong, Y. Gossuin, C. Ménager, N. Luciani, G. Charron, M. Hémadi, D. Alloyeau, and F. Gazeau, *Small*, 2016, **13**, 1602030.
67. P. Geisser and S. Burckhardt, *Pharmaceutics*, 2011, **3**, 12.
68. J. Nissim, *Lancet*, 1947, **250**, 49.
69. C. W. Heath, M. B. Strauss, and W. B. Castle, *J. Clin. Invest.*, 1932, **11**, 1293.
70. P. A. Kalra and S. Bhandari, *Int. J. Nephrol. Renovasc. Dis.*, 2016, **9**, 53.
71. H. Onishi, T. Murakami, T. Kim, M. Hori, S. Hirohashi, M. Matsuki, Y. Narumi, Y. Imai, K. Sakurai, and H. Nakamura, *J. Magn. Reson. Imag.*, 2008, **29**, 106.
72. R. A. Zager, A. C. M. Johnson, S. Y. Hanson, and H. Wasse, *Am. J. Kidney Dis.*, 2002, **40**, 90.
73. R. Agarwal, N. Vasavada, N. G. Sachs, and S. Chase, *Kidney Int.*, 2004, **65**, 2279.
74. L. McCulley, K. Gelperin, S. Bird, S. Harris, C. Wang, and P. Waldron, *Am. J. Hematol.*, 2016, **91**, E496.
75. M. Auerbach and J. Adamson, *Am. J. Hematol.*, 2016, **91**, E497.
76. C. Wang, D. J. Graham, R. C. Kane, D. Xie, M. Wernecke, M. Levenson, M. C. TE, M. Houstoun, Q. Ryan, S. Wong, K. Mott, T. C. Sheu, S. Limb, C. Worrall, J. A. Kelman, and M. E. Reichman, *JAMA*, 2015, **314**, 2062.
77. C. E. Zinderman, L. Landow, and R. P. Wise, *J. Vasc. Surg.*, 2006, **43**, 1004.
78. G. M. Rodgers, M. Auerbach, D. Cella, G. M. Chertow, D. W. Coyne, J. A. Glaspy, and D. H. Henry, *J. Am. Soc. Nephrol.*, 2008, **19**, 833.
79. D. Boraschi and A. Duschl, Nanoparticles and the Immune System: Safety and Effects, Academic Press, 2013, p 1.
80. K. Span, E. H. E. Pieters, W. E. Hennink, A. van der Toorn, V. Brinks, R. M. Dijkhuizen, and G. A. F. van Tilborg, *Pharmaceut. Res.*, 2018, **35**, 88.
81. P. Varallyay, G. Nesbit, L. L. Muldoon, R. R. Nixon, J. Delashaw, J. I. Cohen, A. Petrillo, D. Rink, and E. A. Neuwelt, *Am. J. Neuroradiol.*, 2002, **23**, 510.
82. Y.-X. J. Wang, *Quant. Imag. Med. Surg.*, 2011, **1**, 35.
83. N. Schieda, *Insights Imag.*, 2013, **4**, 509.
84. Sacco, D.C., Steiger, D. A., Bellon, E. M., Coleman, P. E., Haacke, E. M., *Am. J. Roentgenol.*, 1987. **148**(5): 1001.
85. K. K. Alsing, H. H. Johannesen, R. Hvass Hansen, M. Dirks, O. Olsen, and J. Serup, *Skin Res. Technol.*, 2017, **24**, 278.
86. T. Nakamura, K. Fukuda, K. Hayakawa, I. Aoki, Kazuyamatsumoto, T. Sekine, H. Ueda, and Y. Shimizu, *Front. Med. Biol. Eng.*, 2001, **11**, 117.
87. J. R. Ross and M. J. Matava, *Sports Health*, 2011, **3**, 431.

88. M. L. Kreidstein, D. Giguere, and A. Freiberg, *Plastic Reconstr. Surg.*, 1997, **99**, 1717.

89. W. A. Wagle and M. Smith, *Am. J. Roentgenol.*, 2000, **174**, 1795.

90. M. Vahlensieck, *Eur. Radiol.*, 2000, **10**, 197.

91. W. D. Tope and F. G. Shellock, *J. Magn. Reson. Imag.*, 2002, **15**, 180.

92. E. Kanal and F. G. Shellock, *Plastic Reconstr. Surg.*, 1998, **101**, 1150.

93. Z. Wang and C. M. Collins, *Concept Magn. Reson. B: Magn. Reson. Eng.*, 2010, **37B**, 215.

94. R. Hergt and S. Dutz, *J. Magn. Magn. Mater.*, 2007, **311**, 187.

95. R. V. Stigliano, F. Shubitidze, J. D. Petryk, L. Shoshiashvili, A. A. Petryk, and P. J. Hoopes, *North Am. Hyperthermia Group*, 2016, **32**, 735.

96. C. Kut, Y. Zhang, M. Hedayati, H. Zhou, C. Cornejo, D. Bordelon, J. Mihalic, M. Wabler, E. Burghardt, C. Gruettner, A. Geyh, C. Brayton, T. L. Deweese, and R. Ivkov, *Nanomedicine (London England)*, 2012, **7**, 1697.

97. M. Hedayati, B. Abubaker-Sharif, M. Khattab, A. Razavi, I. Mohammed, A. Nejad, M. Wabler, H. Zhou, J. Mihalic, C. Gruettner, T. DeWeese, and R. Ivkov, *Int. J. Hyperthermia*, 2017, 1.

98. H. L. Ring, Z. Gao, N. D. Klein, M. Garwood, J. C. Bischof, and C. L. Haynes, *ChemRxiv*, 2018, (Pre print).

99. U. Gneveckow, A. Jordan, R. Scholz, V. Brüss, N. Waldöfner, J. Ricke, A. Feussner, B. Hildebrandt, B. Rau, and P. Wust, *Med. Phys.*, 2004, **31**, 1444.

100. H. L. Ring, J. Zhang, N. D. Klein, L. E. Eberly, C. L. Haynes, and M. Garwood, *Magn. Reson. Med.*, 2017, **79**, 1420, DOI: 10.1002/mrm.26800.

101. A. Deistung, F. Schweser, and J. R. Reichenbach, *NMR Biomed.*, 2017, **30**, e3569.

102. J. Klohs, A. Deistung, G. D. Ielacqua, A. Seuwen, D. Kindler, F. Schweser, M. Vaas, A. Kipar, J. R. Reichenbach, and M. Rudin, *J. Cerebral Blood Flow Metab.*, 2016, **36**, 1614.

103. R. Wong, X. Chen, Y. Wang, X. Hu, M. M. Jin, *Ann. Biomed. Eng.*, 2012. **40**(6): 1328.

104. R. Di Corato, F. Gazeau, C. Le Visage, D. Fayol, P. Levitz, F. Lux, D. Letourneur, N. Luciani, O. Tillement, and C. Wilhelm, *ACS Nano*, 2013, **7**, 7500.

105. T. Liu, P. Spincemaille, L. de Rochefort, R. Wong, M. Prince, and Y. Wang, *Magn. Reson. Imag.*, 2010, **28**, 1383.

106. X. Lu, Y. Ma, E. Y. Chang, Q. He, A. Searleman, A. Drygalski, and J. Du, *Magn. Reson. Med.*, 2018, **79**, 2315.

107. D. Hensley, Z. W. Tay, R. Dhavalikar, B. Zheng, P. Goodwill, C. Rinaldi, and S. Conolly, *Phys. Med. Biol.*, 2017, **62**, 3483.

108. T. Knopp, S. M. Conolly, and T. M. Buzug, *Phys. Med. Biol.*, 2017, **62**, E4.

109. D. Idiyatullin, C. Corum, S. Moeller, H. S. Prasad, M. Garwood, and D. R. Nixdorf, *J. Endodontics*, 2011, **37**, 745.

110. N. Kobayashi, D. Idiyatullin, C. Corum, J. Weber, M. Garwood, and D. Sachdev, *Magn. Reson. Med.*, 2015, **73**, 1812.

111. D. M. Grodzki, P. M. Jakob, and B. Heismann, *Magn. Reson. Med.*, 2012, **67**, 510.

112. Y. Qiao, H.-Y. Tao, K. Ma, Z.-Y. Wu, J.-X. Qu, and S. Chen, *BioMed Res. Int.*, 2017, **2017**, 2729807.

113. P. D. Gatehouse, R. W. Thomas, M. D. Robson, G. Hamilton, A. H. Herlihy, and G. M. Bydder, *Magn. Reson. Imag.*, 2004, **22**, 1061.

114. C. J. Bergin, J. M. Pauly, and A. Macovski, *Radiology*, 1991, **179**, 777.

115. C. A. Gharagouzloo, P. N. McMahon, and S. Sridhar, *Magn. Reson. Med.*, 2015, **74**, 431.

116. O. M. Girard, J. Du, L. Agemy, K. N. Sugahara, V. R. Kotamraju, E. Ruoslahti, G. M. Bydder, and R. F. Mattrey, *Magn. Reson. Med.*, 2011, **65**, 1649.

117. W. Liu, H. Dahnke, J. Rahmer, E. K. Jordan, and J. A. Frank, *Magn. Reson. Med.*, 2009, **61**, 761.

118. L. Wang, X. Zhong, W. Qian, J. Huang, Z. Cao, Q. Yu, M. Lipowska, R. Lin, A. Wang, L. Yang, and H. Mao, *J. Magn. Reson. Imag.*, 2014, **40**, 1071.

119. P. J. Hoopes, A. A. Petryk, B. Gimi, A. J. Giustini, J. B. Weaver, J. Bischof, R. Chamberlain, and M. Garwood, *Proc. SPIE*, 2012, **8317**, 83170R.

120. L. Wang, C. A. Corum, D. Idiyatullin, M. Garwood, and Q. Zhao, *Magn. Reson. Med.*, 2013, **70**, DOI: 10.1002/mrm.24831.

121. J. Zhang, R. Chamberlain, M. Etheridge, D. Idiyatullin, C. Corum, J. Bischof, and M. Garwood, *Magn. Reson. Med.*, 2014, **71**, 1982.

122. R. Zhou, D. Idiyatullin, S. Moeller, C. Corum, H. Zhang, H. Qiao, J. Zhong, and M. Garwood, *Magn. Reson. Med.*, 2010, **63**, 1154.

123. M. D. Robson, P. D. Gatehouse, M. Bydder, and G. M. Bydder, *J. Comput. Assist. Tomogr.*, 2003, **27**, 825.

124. M. Garwood, *J. Magn. Reson.*, 2013, 6.

125. D. Idiyatullin, C. Corum, J.-Y. Park, and M. Garwood, *J. Magn. Reson.*, 2006, **181**, 342.

126. C. Sun, C. Fang, Z. Stephen, O. Veiseh, S. Hansen, D. Lee, R. G. Ellenbogen, J. Olson, and M. Zhang, *Nanomedicine (London, England)*, 2008, **3**, 495.

127. M. L. Etheridge, K. R. Hurley, J. Zhang, S. Jeon, H. L. Ring, C. Hogan, C. L. Haynes, M. Garwood, and J. C. Bischof, *Technology*, 2014, **02**, 214.

128. K. R. Hurley, H. L. Ring, M. Etheridge, J. Zhang, Z. Gao, Q. Shao, N. Klein, V. M. Szlag, C. Chung, T. M. Reineke, M. Garwood, J. Bischof, and C. L. Haynes, *Mol. Pharm.*, 2016, **13**, 2172.

129. B. Gleich and J. Weizenecker, *Nature*, 2005, **435**, 1214.

130. K. Murase, H. Takata, Y. Takeuchi, and S. Saito, *Phys. Med.*, 2013, **29**, 624.

131. Z. W. Tay, P. Chandrasekharan, A. Chiu-Lam, D. W. Hensley, R. Dhavalikar, X. Y. Zhou, E. Y. Yu, P. W. Goodwill, B. Zheng, C. Rinaldi, and S. M. Conolly, *ACS Nano*, 2018, **12**, 3699.

132. P. Chandrasekharan, Z. W. Tay, X. Y. Zhou, E. Yu, R. Orendorff, D. Hensley, Q. Huynh, K. L. B. Fung, C. C. VanHook, P. Goodwill, B. Zheng, and S. Conolly, *Br. J. Radiol.*, 2018, 20180326.

133. X. Y. Zhou, K. E. Jeffris, E. Y. Yi, B. Zheng, P. W. Goodwill, P. Nahid, and S. M. Conolly, *Phys. Med. Biol.*, 2017, **62**, 3510.

134. E. Y. Yu, P. Chandrasekharan, R. Berzon, Z. W. Tay, X. Y. Zhou, A. P. Khandhar, R. M. Ferguson, S. J. Kemp, B. Zheng, P. W. Goodwill, M. F. Wendland, K. M. Krishnan, S. Behr, J. Carter, and S. M. Conolly, *ACS Nano*, 2017, **11**, 12067.

135. S. Tong, C. A. Quinto, L. Zhang, P. Mohindra, and G. Bao, *ACS Nano*, 2017.

136. S. M. Cassim, A. J. Giustini, I. Baker, and P. J. Hoopes, *Proc. SPIE*, 2011, **7901**, 790115.

137. G. M. Fahy, B. Wowk, J. Wu, J. Phan, C. Rasch, and A. Chang, *Cryobiology*, 2004, **48**, 157.

Chapter 28

Numerical Simulation for MRI RF Coils and Safety

Julie M. Kabil[1] and Anand Gopinath[2]

[1]*Columbia University, New York, NY, USA*
[2]*University of Minnesota, Minneapolis, MN, USA*

28.1 INTRODUCTION

With the progress made over the past decades in computation power and resources, numerical simulation became an invaluable tool for many industries and research areas,[1] and magnetic resonance imaging (MRI) is no exception. The advent of parallel computing with GPU and the overall improvement in speed and performance of CPU allowed for calculations that were previously prohibitively expensive in terms of time and hardware resources.[2] From coil design and prototyping to safety, simulation provides a means to reduce costs and explore phenomena sometimes hardly accessible in real-life experiments.

In MRI, numerical simulation is used for every part of the MRI machine: magnet design and evaluation,[3] gradient coil studies,[4] and of course radio-frequency (RF) coils and safety in general.[5,6] In particular, medical devices safety in MRI often requires insights brought by simulation, to study the device behavior in the MRI environment[7]; indeed, international safety standards describe the process to evaluate and label a medical device for MRI use, involving numerical simulation.[8]

In this chapter, we cover some electromagnetic theory, different solvers principles, and also more practical matters such as a practical workflow, the need and means of validating a simulation, and a nonexhaustive list of simulation software (open source and commercial).

The unifying equations of electromagnetics were formalized by Maxwell.[9] These four equations link together the electric field and magnetic field in time and space, along with the medium's dielectric properties (permittivity, conductivity, and permeability). A particularity of Maxwell's equations is that they can be written in different forms: frequency or

Safety and Biological Effects in MRI.
Edited by Devashish Shrivastava and J. Thomas Vaughan

ISBN: 978-1-118-82130-5
Also published in eMagRes (online edition)
DOI: 10.1002/9780470034590.emrstm1568

time-domain and differential or integral form. We give below, for reference, these relations in differential form:

Maxwell–Gauss:

$$\nabla \cdot \boldsymbol{E} = \frac{\rho}{\varepsilon} \tag{28.1}$$

Maxwell–Gauss for magnetism:

$$\nabla \cdot \boldsymbol{B} = 0 \tag{28.2}$$

Maxwell–Faraday:

$$\nabla \times \boldsymbol{E} = -\frac{\partial \boldsymbol{B}}{\partial t} \tag{28.3}$$

Maxwell–Ampère:

$$\nabla \times \boldsymbol{B} = \mu \left(\boldsymbol{J} + \varepsilon \frac{\partial \boldsymbol{E}}{\partial t} \right) \tag{28.4}$$

where ρ is the charge density, ε is the medium permittivity (with $\varepsilon = \varepsilon_0 \varepsilon_r$), μ is the medium permeability ($\mu = \mu_0 \mu_r$), and $\boldsymbol{J}$ is the current density.

Each equation has a clear signification: Maxwell–Gauss' equation shows the relationship between an electric charge and the electric field it generates. Maxwell–Gauss' equation for magnetism means that the magnetic field does not diverge; in other words, the magnetic field lines form a loop – the corollary is that there are no magnetic monopoles that would be analogous to single electric charges. Maxwell–Faraday's equation reflects Faraday's law of induction: an electric field is associated with a time-varying magnetic field. Finally, Maxwell–Ampère's equation shows how a magnetic field can be created: either by an electrical current or by a time-varying electric field.

Overall, it is interesting to note that Maxwell–Faraday's and Maxwell–Ampère's equations show that the electric and magnetic fields are intrinsically coupled, which is the reason we use the term 'electromagnetic' fields. The principle of electromagnetic simulations is to discretize Maxwell's equations and solve them in a defined environment such as an RF coil model. We see in the next parts that there are several ways to do this, each with their own pros and cons.

Finally, it is noteworthy that different equations may be used to solve electromagnetic problems, such as the Biot–Savart's law for static magnetic field calculation in a magnet model (which can itself be derived from Maxwell equations applied to a magnetostatic situation).

The need for simulations is twofold: we need to consider the need for modeling and calculation first, which can either be numerical or analytical, and the reason to choose specifically the numerical method.

First of all, solving a physical problem's equations allows bringing insights into situations when the data or phenomenon considered is not readily accessible or measurable. This is of tremendous importance, for example when we need to find an explanation for something observed experimentally. Second, it allows us to reduce costs, both in money and time, that would be associated with experiments or prototyping. Indeed, calculations allow us to design and predict a coil's behavior without having to build it and modify it to test each parameter or modification. Finally, when we consider the efficiency and safety of a medical procedure (such as an MRI scan or the behavior of a medical device), calculating the relevant equations inside a human model is of great importance – provided that this model is reliable enough.

Now that we established the necessity for these calculations, a choice has to be made between analytical and numerical resolutions. Although Maxwell's equations can be solved analytically in many simple cases, when introducing more advanced systems such as MRI coils with phantoms or numerical human models, the calculations become much more challenging to do 'by hand'. Realistically, analytical models are limited by the model complexity, and at a certain point, the numerical methods are more efficient timewise – of course, provided that the numerical accuracy is ensured.

28.2 FINITE ELEMENT METHOD (FEM)

The finite element method (FEM) is a numerical method for the solution of boundary value problems, described by partial differential equations by converting them into linear algebraic equations. The FEM process obtains the approximate solution of the differential operator. This was first described by Courant[10] and subsequently expanded by Duffin.[11] The early work on finite elements was in structural and continuum mechanics[12] and then led to applications in electrical engineering.[13,14] It is currently widely used for various kinds of calculations: mechanics, thermal, fluidics, and of course, electromagnetics, to solve partial differential equations. The FEM can, for example, be applied to RF simulations by writing Maxwell's equations in the frequency domain:

$$\nabla \times \boldsymbol{H} = j\omega\varepsilon \boldsymbol{E} + \boldsymbol{J} \quad (28.5)$$

$$\nabla \times \boldsymbol{E} = -j\mu\omega \boldsymbol{H} \quad (28.6)$$

In particular, this method allows to easily conform to any geometry and to set a variable element size, in order to solve differentials equations coupled to boundary conditions. This characteristic can be especially useful when considering a complex geometric model such as thin wires or curved surfaces.

The name of the method comes from the discretization of the structure to be analyzed. After modeling the object, it will be discretized into a finite number of small, tessellated elements, hence the 'finite elements' term. These elements can be of different geometries: for example, line segments in case of a one-dimension problem, triangles or quadrilaterals in a 2D system, and tetrahedrons or rectangular/cubic bricks for a 3D structure.[15] Each of these elements has interconnected common nodes. The fields to be solved for, for example in the 2D triangle, are approximated in the first order as linear functions of x and y, and the nodal values are obtained from this linear approximation. Simply put, the FEM aims to make approximations locally inside single elements and then to connect all these elements at the nodes.

Let us illustrate the principle on a simple example: our simulation space Ω is represented in Figure 28.1. Let $F(x, y)$ be a field whose value is to be calculated on every point of Ω. We discretize this space using triangular elements, as represented in Figure 28.1; only one is shown here for the sake of simplicity.

We can now define the field inside the nth triangular element, based on the field values at the nodes and on interpolation functions I_i (also called *basis functions*) which are predetermined[16]:

$$F^n(x,\ y) = a + bx + cy \quad (28.7)$$

The nodal vertex values $F_1^n,\ F_2^n,\ F_3^n$ are obtained from the equations:

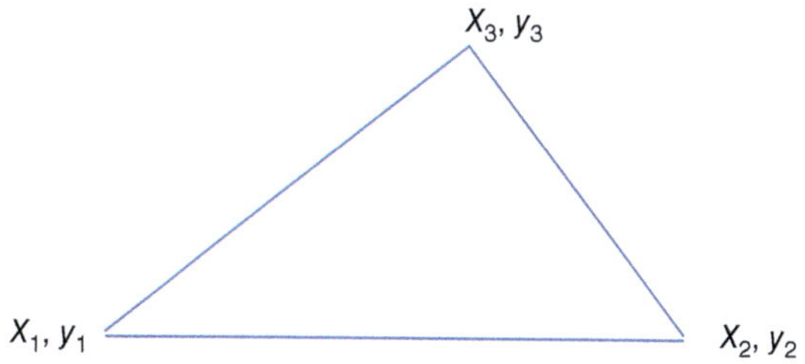

Figure 28.1. Single triangular element in the simulation space

$$\begin{aligned} F_1^n &= a + bx_1 + cy_1 \\ F_2^n &= a + bx_2 + cy_2 \\ F_3^n &= a + bx_3 + cy_3 \end{aligned} \quad (28.8)$$

from which

$$F^n = N_1^n(x,\ y)F_1^n + N_2^n(x,\ y)F_2^n + N_3^n(x,\ y)F_3^n \quad (28.9)$$

where

$$\begin{aligned} N_1^n &= \frac{1}{2A}[(x_2y_3 - x_3y_2) + (y_2 - y_1)x + (x_3 - x_2)y] \\ N_2^n &= \frac{1}{2A}[(x_3y_1 - x_1y_3) + (y_3 - y_2)x + (x_1 - x_3)y] \\ N_3^n &= \frac{1}{2A}[(x_1y_2 - x_2y_1) + (y_1 - y_3)x + (x_2 - x_1)y] \end{aligned} \quad (28.10)$$

where A is the area of the triangle. Note that N_i^n are the interpolating functions at the three vertices of the triangle; each function vanishes at all vertices except one and has unity value at that vertex node:

$$\begin{aligned} N_i^n(x_i,\ y_j) &= 0 \quad i = j \\ &= 1 \quad i \neq j \end{aligned} \quad (28.11)$$

Consider the wave equation in a source-free region as an example. The Maxwell's equations are

$$\nabla \times \boldsymbol{E} = -j\omega\mu \boldsymbol{H} \quad (28.12)$$

$$\nabla \times \boldsymbol{H} = j\omega\epsilon \boldsymbol{E} \quad (28.13)$$

Take the curl of equation (28.12), and substituting from equation (28.13)

$$\nabla \times \nabla \times \boldsymbol{E} = -j\omega\mu\nabla \times \boldsymbol{H} = \omega^2\mu\epsilon \boldsymbol{E} \quad (28.14)$$

Using the vector identity, this equation becomes

$$\nabla \times \nabla \times \boldsymbol{E} = \nabla(\nabla \cdot \boldsymbol{E}) - \nabla^2 \boldsymbol{E} = k^2 \boldsymbol{E} \quad (28.15)$$

where the propagation constant $k = \omega\sqrt{\mu\epsilon} = \omega/v$, and the velocity is $v = 1/\mu\varepsilon$.

Since the equations are for a source-free region, $\nabla \cdot \boldsymbol{E} = 0$ equation (28.15) becomes

$$\nabla^2 \boldsymbol{E} + k^2 \boldsymbol{E} = 0 \quad (28.16)$$

Consider the application to a rectangular waveguide: the boundaries are perfect conductors where the tangential electric field is zero. Note that the vector $\boldsymbol{E}$ in Cartesian coordinates has three components: E_x, E_y, E_z.

Let us examine the transverse magnetic (TM) mode of this guide where $H_z = 0$, and $E_z \neq 0$ and the other four components of the field can be derived from the curl equations (28.12) and (28.13). Assume also that the guide has no dielectric or magnetic filling so that $\mu = \mu_0$ and $\varepsilon = \varepsilon_0$ at a given frequency k^2 may be evaluated. The vector wave equation now becomes a scalar equation in E_z. The E_z field in the guide is of the form $E_z(x,y)e^{-j\beta z}$, substituting in the wave equation:

$$\nabla^2 E_z e^{-j\beta z} + k^2 E_z e^{-j\beta z} = \left(\frac{\partial^2}{\partial x^2} + \frac{\partial^2}{\partial y^2} + \frac{\partial^2}{\partial z^2}\right) E_z e^{-j\beta z} + k^2 E_z e^{-j\beta z} = 0 \quad (28.17)$$

which simplifies to, assuming that $e^{-j\beta z}$ is implicit,

$$\left(\frac{\partial^2}{\partial x^2} + \frac{\partial^2}{\partial y^2}\right) E_z + (\omega^2 \mu_0 \epsilon_0 - \beta^2) E_z = \nabla^2_{x,y} E_z + K^2 E_z = 0 \quad (28.18)$$

where $K^2 = (\omega^2 \mu_0 \epsilon_0 - \beta^2)$.

The guide is sectioned into triangle elements, and the field in the nth triangle is given in equation (28.9) replacing F^n by $E_z^{\ n}$:

$$E_z^n = N_1^n(x, y)E_{z1}^n + N_2^n(x, y)E_{z2}^n + N_3^n(x, y)E_{z3}^n \quad (28.19)$$

Hence

$$E_z = \sum_{i=1}^{N} N_i E_z^i \quad (28.20)$$

excluding the nodes on the perfect boundaries which are zero. This expansion in terms of the interior nodes will now be substituted in equation (28.18) to determine the nodal field values by the method of weighted residuals.

Consider the vector identity:

$$\nabla \cdot (w\boldsymbol{F}) = w\nabla \cdot \boldsymbol{F} + \nabla w \cdot \boldsymbol{F}$$

where w is the weighting factor satisfying all the boundary conditions. Now replacing $\boldsymbol{F}$ by ∇E_z, the identity becomes, with the integration over the problem domain Ω:

$$\int_\Omega \nabla \cdot (w\nabla E_z)\mathrm{d}S = \int (w\nabla^2 E_z + \nabla w \cdot \nabla E_z)\mathrm{d}S \quad (28.21)$$

The left-hand side of this equation in two dimensions becomes

$$\int_\Omega \nabla \cdot (w\nabla E_z)\mathrm{d}S = \oint_C \left(w\frac{\partial E_z}{\partial n}\right) \mathrm{d}C \quad (28.22)$$

If the boundary condition has either $w = 0$ or $\partial E_z/\partial n = 0$, then the product of the weighting factor w and equation (28.18) becomes

$$\int_\Omega w(\nabla^2 E_z + K^2 E_z)\mathrm{d}S = \int_\Omega (-\nabla w \cdot \nabla E_z + K^2 w E_z)\mathrm{d}S = 0 \quad (28.23)$$

Choose the weighting function $w_j = N_j$ for $j = 1, 2, \ldots, N$, N is the number of nodes excluding the nodes at the boundaries where E_z is zero.

Substituting from equation (28.18) in (28.23):

$$\sum_{j=1}^{N} E_z^j \int_\Omega (\nabla N_i \cdot \nabla N_j - K^2 N_i N_j)\mathrm{d}\Omega = 0 \quad (28.24)$$

which leads to the eigenvalue matrix equation

$$[A]\{E_z\} = K^2[B]\{E_z\} \quad (28.25)$$

$$\text{where} \quad [A] = \int_\Omega (\nabla N_i \cdot \nabla N_j)\mathrm{d}\Omega$$

$$\text{and} \quad [B] = \int_\Omega (N_i N_j)\mathrm{d}\Omega$$

When the eigenvalue of zero is obtained, $K^2 = 0$, which gives $\beta_c = k_0$, the cutoff frequency of the mode is determined.

It can be shown that the integrations over the nth planar triangle are

$$\int_{\Delta^n} (N_1^n)^i (N_2^n)^j (N_3^n)^k \mathrm{d}\Delta^n = \frac{i!j!k!}{(i+j+k+2)!} 2A^n \quad (28.26)$$

where A^n is the area of the nth triangle.

It follows that

$$\int_{\Delta^n} \nabla N_i^n \cdot \nabla N_j^n \mathrm{d}\Delta^n = \frac{1}{4A^2} \sum_i \sum_j (b_i b_j + c_i c_j) \quad (28.27)$$

where

$$b_i = y_{i+1} - y_{i-1}, \ \text{modulo } 3 \quad (28.28)$$

$$c_i = x_{i-1} - x_{i+1}, \ \text{modulo } 3 \quad (28.29)$$

With these formulae, the modified wave equation in (28.24) is evaluated for each triangle. Adjacent triangles have a common side and two common nodes, and these are assembled in the matrices $[A]$ and $[B]$, which are both symmetric and real; the eigenvalues should be real.

Similarly, the transverse electric (TE) modes of the guide are determined for $E_z = 0$, and $H_z \neq 0$ with the Neumann boundary condition $\partial H_z/\partial n = 0$. From equation (28.22) it follows that no further provisions be made to satisfy the boundary conditions. The wave equation to be solved is

$$\int_{\Omega}(\nabla^2 H_z - K^2 H_Z^2)\,\mathrm{d}\Omega = 0 \tag{28.30}$$

The domain Ω in this case also is the rectangular waveguide which is divided into triangles, and the strategy discussed above is repeated.

The scalar elements are not used in MRI modeling due to the computational domain having mixed materials, and vector elements are used, and these are discussed below.

28.2.1 Vector Fields

The nodal technique works well for scalar fields as discussed above for the air-filled rectangular waveguide. If the filling is mixed dielectric regions when both the TE and TM modes are present, resulting in hybrid modes, then the scalar approach results in spurious modes, and all kinds of techniques have been used to eliminate these spurious modes. The alternative is to use vector basis functions[17] while retaining the triangle elements in 2D and tetrahedral elements in 3D. In this section, the approach is briefly discussed, and interested readers should refer to books and papers listed in the reference section.

Consider a source-free inhomogeneous rectangular waveguide filled with mixed dielectric media. From equations (28.12) and (28.13), the following wave equation is derived:

$$\nabla \times \left(\frac{1}{\mu_r}\nabla \times \boldsymbol{E}\right) - k_0^2\epsilon_r \boldsymbol{E} = 0 \tag{28.31}$$

where $\mu = \mu_0\mu_r$, $\varepsilon = \varepsilon_0\varepsilon_r$, and $k_0{}^2 = \omega^2\mu_0\varepsilon_0$. The boundary condition at the boundary Γ_D of the rectangular waveguide: $\boldsymbol{a}_n \times \boldsymbol{E} = 0$.

The vector edge elements in the present 2D discussion are in the transverse plane for $\boldsymbol{E}$ and for all the propagating modes have the transverse vector function $\boldsymbol{e}_t$ in x and y and a scalar exponential function e_z in the $\boldsymbol{a}_z$ directions:

$$\boldsymbol{E}(x,\ y,\ z) = \left[\frac{1}{\beta}\boldsymbol{e}_t(x,\ y) + j\boldsymbol{a}_z e_z(x,\ y)\right] \mathrm{e}^{-j\beta z} \tag{28.32}$$

and the weight function is

$$\boldsymbol{W}(x,\ y,\ z) = \left[\frac{1}{\beta}\boldsymbol{w}_t(x,\ y) - j\boldsymbol{a}_z w_z(x,\ y)\right] \mathrm{e}^{j\beta z} \tag{28.33}$$

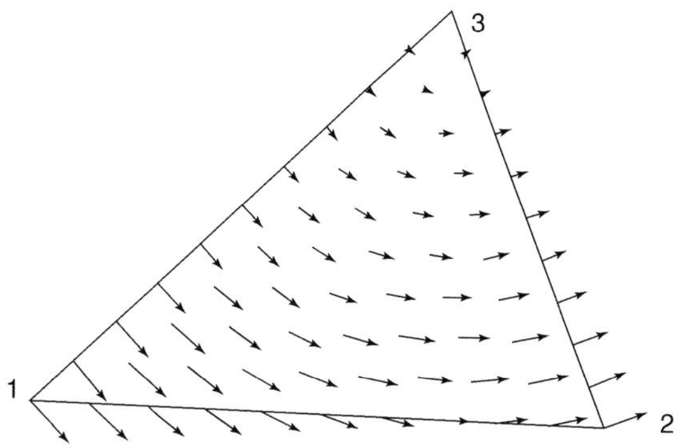

Figure 28.2. Sketch of the edge element $\boldsymbol{N}_{12}$ field in equation (28.35). (Jian-Ming Jin. Theory and Computation of Electromagnetic Fields, John Wiley-IEEE Press, 2010)

The wave equation in (28.31) after dot product with $\boldsymbol{W}$ and further simplification becomes

$$\int_{\Omega}\left\{\frac{1}{\mu_r}(\nabla_t \times \boldsymbol{w}_t)\cdot(\nabla_t \times \boldsymbol{e}_t) = k_0^2\epsilon_r \boldsymbol{w}_t \cdot \boldsymbol{e}_t + \beta^2\left[\frac{1}{\mu_r}(\boldsymbol{w}_t + \nabla_t w_z)\cdot(\boldsymbol{e}_t + \nabla_t e_z) - k_0^2\epsilon_r w_z \cdot e_z\right]\right\}\mathrm{d}\Omega = 0 \tag{28.34}$$

where Ω is the computational domain, the cross section of the waveguide and ∇_t the transverse del operator.

The finite element transverse vector operator of the nth triangle is defined as the edge element between vertex 1 and vertex 2 as

$$\boldsymbol{N}_{12}^n(\boldsymbol{r}) = [N_1^n \nabla N_2^n - N_2^n \nabla N_1^n]\ell_{12}^n \quad \text{and} \quad \boldsymbol{N}_{12}^n = \boldsymbol{N}_1^n \tag{28.35}$$

where the scalars N_1 and N_2 are defined in equation (28.10), and l_{12} is the length of the triangle side between vertices 1 and 2. The other edge elements for the nth triangle follow with the interchange of the subscripts, modulo 3 (Figure 28.2).

The computational domain Ω is subdivided into small triangles and the transverse field $\boldsymbol{e}_t$ are in terms of the vector elements $\boldsymbol{N}_j$ and the longitudinal field e_z in terms of the nodal elements N_j:

$$\boldsymbol{e}_t(x,\ y) = \sum_{j=1}^{N_e\mathrm{dges}} \boldsymbol{N}_j(x,\ y)\boldsymbol{e}_{tj} \tag{28.36}$$

$$e_z(x,\ y) = \sum_{j=1}^{N} N_j(x,\ y)\, e_{zj} \tag{28.37}$$

Substituting $\boldsymbol{W}_t = \boldsymbol{N}_t$ and $W_z = N_z$ in equation (28.34) and simplifying reduces the equation to

$$\begin{bmatrix} A_{tt} & 0 \\ 0 & 0 \end{bmatrix} \begin{bmatrix} e_t \\ e_z \end{bmatrix} = \beta^2 \begin{bmatrix} B_{tt} & B_{tz} \\ B_{zt} & B_{zz} \end{bmatrix} \begin{bmatrix} e_t \\ e_z \end{bmatrix} \quad (28.38)$$

where

$$\boldsymbol{A}_{tt\,ij} = \int_\Omega \left[\frac{1}{\mu_r} (\nabla_t \times \boldsymbol{N}_i) \cdot (\nabla_t \times \boldsymbol{N}_j) - k_0^2 \epsilon_r \boldsymbol{N}_i \cdot \boldsymbol{N}_j \right] d\Omega \quad (28.39)$$

$$B_{tt\,ij} = \int_\Omega \left[\frac{1}{\mu_r} \boldsymbol{N}_i \cdot \boldsymbol{N}_j \right] d\Omega \quad (28.40)$$

$$B_{tz\,ij} = \int_\Omega \left[\frac{1}{\mu_r} \boldsymbol{N}_i \cdot \nabla_t N_j \right] d\Omega \quad (28.41)$$

$$B_{zt\,ij} = \int_\Omega \left[\frac{1}{\mu_r} \nabla_t N_i \cdot \boldsymbol{N}_j \right] d\Omega \quad (28.42)$$

$$B_{tt\,ij} = \int_\Omega \left[\frac{1}{\mu_r} (\nabla_t N_i \cdot \nabla_t N_j) - k_0^2 \epsilon_r N_i N_j \right] d\Omega \quad (28.43)$$

Note that the second equation in (28.38) is

$$[B_{zt}]\{e_t\} + [B_{zz}]\{e_z\} = 0 \quad (28.44)$$

and may be used to eliminate $\{e_z\}$ from the first equation of (28.38):

$$[A_{tt}]\{e_t\} = \beta^2 [B_{tt}^t]\{e_t\} \quad (28.45)$$

where

$$[B_{tt}^t] = [B_{tz}][B_{zz}]^{-1} - [B_{tt}] \quad (28.46)$$

The matrix equation (28.45) is usually solved by standard methods, provided the number of unknowns are not too large! An example of an enclosed image guide results with vector elements is shown in Figure 28.3.

The 3D version of the edge element may use tetrahedron or the brick elements, depending on the data provided. For the human body, the standard models are usually in Cartesian mesh of 2×2×2 mm spacing with about 36 permittivities and conductivities, and standard CAD programs choose their elements.

28.2.2 Meshing

As mentioned before, the FEM can use triangular/tetrahedral mesh to resolve a geometry: such mesh cells are better able to resolve curved boundaries in objects, rather than a cubic mesh.[18] The more elements we add, i.e., the finer we discretize our

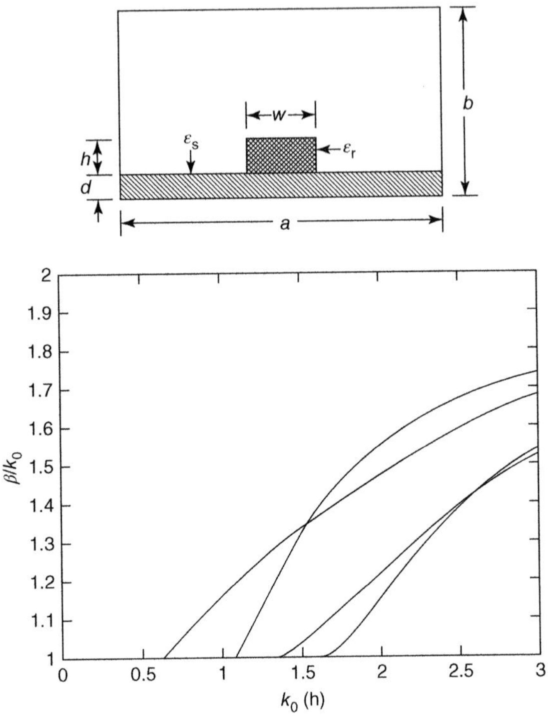

Figure 28.3. Dispersion characteristics of the insulated image guide ($w/h = 2.25$, $d/h = 0.5$, $a/h = 13.5$, $b/h = 8.0$, $\varepsilon_r = 3.8$, and $\varepsilon_s = 1.5$). (J. H. Jin, permission of John Wiley)

object, the closer our calculations will be to the exact solution. Of course, this accuracy comes with a price in terms of computational cost: the higher the number of elements or the smaller the elements are, the longer the simulation will take.

However, it is possible to refine the mesh only for some specific parts or areas of the model, particularly with adaptive meshing techniques.[19] This is especially interesting when considering curved geometries and eventual high-field gradients areas (as examples shown in Figure 28.4).

Adaptive mesh methods work, for example, by obtaining fields calculated with a coarse mesh, then with a finer mesh, comparing the results, and reducing the mesh in areas of interest until successive mesh sizes produce steady enough results. The convergence is established based on a user-defined threshold, always keeping in mind the accuracy/computational cost balance.

Overall, the goal of these interpolation functions is to be smooth enough to correctly represent and approximate the physical problem at hand[20]; of course,

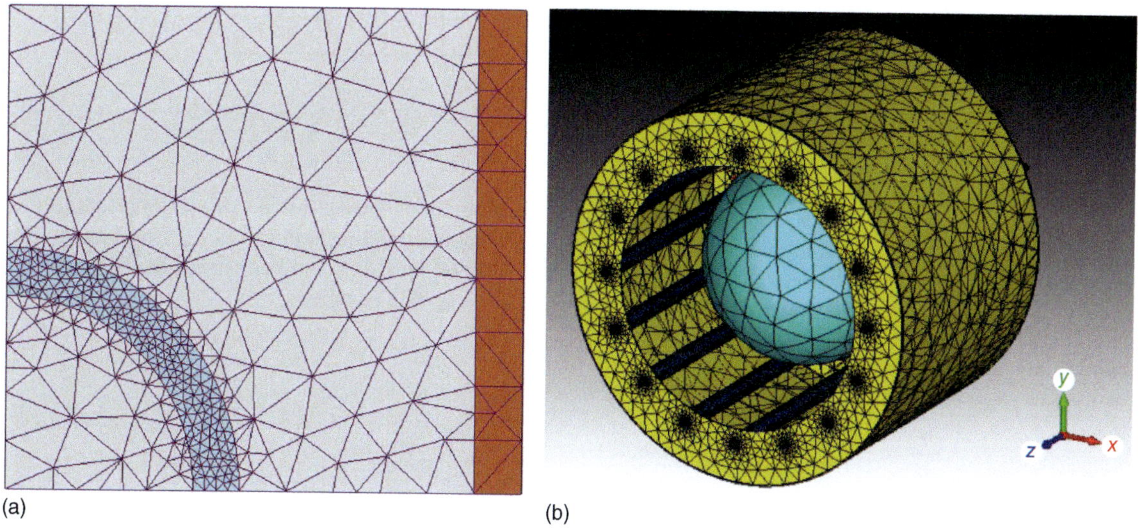

Figure 28.4. (a) Illustration of the mesh refinement in areas of interest in a simple case. (By I, Zureks, CC BY-SA 3.0, https://commons.wikimedia.org/w/index.php?curid=2358783) (b) FEM mesh on a TEM coil with a spherical, homogeneous phantom after mesh adaptation

as we mentioned for the mesh size, there is also a balance to find between the order of the polynomial (i.e., its smoothness and flexibility) and the computational time.

28.2.3 Pros and Cons of the FEM

The FEM has several advantages, which makes it one of the most widely used method in many physics problems and electromagnetic simulation in particular: its mesh is flexible and able to conform to complex geometries, such as spheres and curves, where a rigid cubic mesh – used in other simulations techniques as we will see later in this chapter – will either have to make coarse approximation by *staircasing* or require a very large number of mesh cells to properly resolve the geometry. This is very useful for MRI coil simulations which very often present curved, complex geometries. Furthermore, adaptive mesh techniques can be used to reduce the size of mesh cells only in regions that require it, allowing for a gain both in accuracy and simulation time.

However, FEM calculations require a large matrix inversion: when considering a large and/or complex problem, for example an RF coil with a whole-body numerical human model, many mesh cells will be required and the calculation time can rapidly become prohibitive. Thus, important hardware resources may have to be engaged. Additionally, and contrary to the finite-difference time-domain (FDTD) method, the FEM solver cannot be accelerated by GPU and primarily relies on RAM. It is also noteworthy that for MRI simulation, in particular for coil design and safety, human voxel models are widely used: these models are more straightforward to use directly with a simple hexahedral mesh, such as the FDTDs. Finally, the FEM typically allows solving for one frequency at a time; therefore, when a broadband analysis is required, the FDTD or finite-integration technique (FIT) method may be more suitable. It is, however, noteworthy that interpolation methods to realize a frequency sweep are also available.[21]

28.3 THE FINITE-DIFFERENCE TIME-DOMAIN (FDTD) METHOD

28.3.1 Introduction

Proposed by Yee,[22] the FDTD solver is based – as its name suggests – on the finite-difference discretization to approximate differential equations. It has a wide range of applications in electromagnetics, such as microwaves and visible light applications such as photonics. Its conceptual simplicity and other advantages, such as being suitable for GPU acceleration, make it one of the most largely used technique for electromagnetic calculations and in particular for RF coil and safety simulations. Therefore, we describe in detail below the theory and also give practical advice.

Let us consider a cuboid-shaped space defined by three orthogonal axes x, y, and z, which will be our simulation space. To have a closer look at the principle, the starting point is the fundamental equations that are at the core of the Yee algorithm: Maxwell–Faraday and Maxwell–Ampère equations. For clarity purposes, to describe the algorithm we consider here the equations without any conductive current or free charges with $\varepsilon = \varepsilon_0 \varepsilon_r$ and $\mu = \mu_0 \mu_r$ (characteristics of the medium):

$$\frac{\partial \boldsymbol{E}}{\partial t} = \frac{1}{\varepsilon} \nabla \times \boldsymbol{H} \tag{28.47}$$

$$\frac{\partial \boldsymbol{H}}{\partial t} = -\frac{1}{\mu} \nabla \times \boldsymbol{E} \tag{28.48}$$

Note that the two other Maxwell's equations (Maxwell–Gauss and Maxwell flux), in the absence of charges, both lead to the divergence of the electric and magnetic fields being null at all times. For clarity in developing the equations, we consider here one-dimension equations with a plane wave traveling along z, but the principle can be extended very easily to three dimensions following the same principle:

$$\frac{\partial E_x}{\partial t} = -\frac{1}{\varepsilon} \frac{\partial H_y}{\partial z} \tag{28.49}$$

$$\frac{\partial H_y}{\partial t} = -\frac{1}{\mu} \frac{\partial E_x}{\partial z} \tag{28.50}$$

Now that we have written the fundamental equations, we can use Yee's method. It consists in considering E_x and H_y with a shift of half a time step for E_x and half a spatial step for H_y, using an approximation of the central differences of the derivatives, which ultimately leads to the explicit FDTD equations. This choice of staggered grid for $\boldsymbol{E}$ and $\boldsymbol{H}$, or Yee grid, is an elegant way to represent the curl equations (this is particularly visible when switching to a three-dimension grid). It also ensures the validity of the two other Maxwell's equations in a source-free region by ensuring divergence-free fields.

At $t = 0$, all the fields are supposed to be initialized to zero.

$$\frac{E_x^{n+\frac{1}{2}}(k) - E_x^{n-\frac{1}{2}}(k)}{\Delta t} = -\frac{1}{\varepsilon} \frac{H_y^n\left(k+\frac{1}{2}\right) - H_y^n\left(k-\frac{1}{2}\right)}{\Delta z} \tag{28.51}$$

$$\frac{H_y^{n+1}\left(k+\frac{1}{2}\right) - H_y^n\left(k+\frac{1}{2}\right)}{\Delta t} = -\frac{1}{\mu} \frac{E_x^{n+\frac{1}{2}}(k) - E_x^{n+\frac{1}{2}}(k+1)}{\Delta z} \tag{28.52}$$

The notations are as follows: $E_x^{n+\frac{1}{2}}(k)$ refers to the E_x component at the point k, at the time $n + \frac{1}{2}$. Finally, these equations can be rearranged to obtain the so-called update equations:

$$E_x^{n+\frac{1}{2}}(k) = E_x^{n-\frac{1}{2}}(k) + \frac{\Delta t}{\varepsilon\, \Delta z}\left(H_y^n\left(k-\frac{1}{2}\right) - H_y^n\left(k+\frac{1}{2}\right)\right) \tag{28.53}$$

$$H_y^{n+1}\left(k+\frac{1}{2}\right) = H_y^n\left(k+\frac{1}{2}\right) + \frac{\Delta t}{\mu\, \Delta z}\left(E_x^{n+\frac{1}{2}}(k) - E_x^{n+\frac{1}{2}}(k+1)\right) \tag{28.54}$$

E_x is defined at every integer step in space and every half time step, and H_y is defined at every half-step in space and every integer step in time. The quantity $\frac{\Delta t}{\varepsilon\, \Delta z}$ is referred to as the update coefficient.

When extended to a three-dimensional space, these equations can be solved in the representation of the solid model considered (e.g., a numerical human voxel model) discretized in cells, called the Yee cells (Figure 28.5).

This is the core of the FDTD algorithm. This type of algorithm is called a *leap-frog* algorithm, as it alternately calculates the current electric field component from the previous electric field value and the

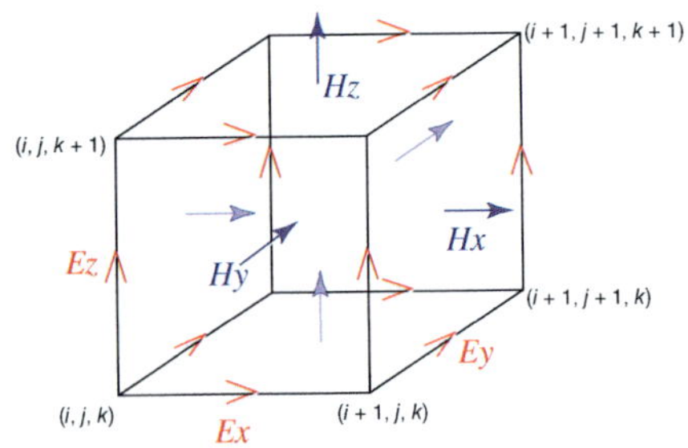

Figure 28.5. Yee cell representation. (By Steven G. Johnson [GFDL (http://www.gnu.org/copyleft/fdl.html) or CC-BY-SA-3.0 (http://creativecommons.org/licenses/by-sa/3.0/)], from Wikimedia Commons)

previous magnetic field value, then calculates the current magnetic field value from the previous magnetic field value and the previous electric field value, and so on.

Thanks to its conceptual simplicity and efficiency, this method is currently widely used to solve various problems. It is indeed relatively easy to implement in different programming languages such as Matlab, Python, or Julia.

28.3.2 Spatial Resolution of the Grid: Cell Size

The question that now arises is how to choose the size of the cell, i.e., grid spatial resolution. As a general rule of thumb and with λ being the smallest wavelength considered in the model, a cell should be at least of size $\frac{\lambda}{10}$.[23,24] In the presence of specific materials as will be described below, the smallest of all the wavelengths in the materials has to be considered to determine the cell size.

However, when considering the features in complex models, this choice of cell size might be too coarse if these characteristic dimensions are small compared to the wavelength in the material.[24] In such a case and with d being the smallest dimension in the model, having at least three or four cells per d would be more suitable.

28.3.3 Temporal Resolution of the Grid: Time Step

To ensure the stability of the algorithm, the time step Δt has to be defined appropriately. Indeed, the nature of the algorithm makes the propagation happen only one cell at a time; therefore, the physical propagation distance cannot be bigger than the numerical spatial step:

$$\underbrace{c\Delta t} \leq \underbrace{\Delta z} \tag{28.55}$$

Based on this limit, the Courant–Friedrich–Lewy (CFL) stability criterion can be introduced as follows in three dimensions[25]:

$$\Delta t \leq \frac{1}{c\sqrt{\frac{1}{(\Delta x)^2} + \frac{1}{(\Delta y)^2} + \frac{1}{(\Delta z)^2}}} \tag{28.56}$$

We note that the quantity $\frac{c\Delta t}{\Delta x}$ is often referred to as the Courant number Sc. Therefore, the stability condition expressed in (28.55) can be summed up by $Sc \leq 1$.

28.3.4 Addition of a Source

To actually see a field propagation, if the fields are not initialized to zero (which would be unusual), a source has to be introduced at some point in the simulation space. One advantage of the FDTD is to allow to get a system response to a wide range of frequencies in only one simulation, instead of computing only one frequency at a time as it is the case for frequency-domain solvers. The excitation should be preceded by a temporal offset in order to avoid abrupt variations and consequently large field gradients. One simple way to do so is to have the source value at zero for a defined time and a smooth source function afterward.

A Gaussian pulse is commonly used for the FDTD solver source, described by the following function:

$$g(t) = \mathrm{e}^{\frac{-t^2}{\tau\tau}} \tag{28.57}$$

In this equation, τ represents the pulse duration. To design a pulse source, the first step is to determine the maximum frequency $f_{\max}$ that will be considered and then calculate the pulse duration τ using the following relation:

$$f_{\max} = \frac{1}{\pi\tau} \tag{28.58}$$

To inject the source in the FDTD code, this source must be added to the field at the desired position in space.

28.3.5 Number of Time Steps and Total Simulation Time

The simulation time is an important parameter to keep in mind. Indeed, the finer the mesh, the greater the accuracy, but the simulation time will also increase accordingly. This trade-off between accuracy and time will be especially important for highly resonant structures, as it is necessary to wait until the excitation has decayed enough to ensure the accuracy of the results.

With N being the number of time steps, and T being the total simulation time for the wave to propagate and decay, we have the following relation:

$$N = \frac{T}{\Delta t} \tag{28.59}$$

T will depend on three factors: the pulse duration τ, the offset before the pulse effectively starts, and the number of 'rebounds' the wave may experience across the grid (which will themselves depend on how resonant the considered structure is).

28.3.6 Frequency Resolution

To ensure the resolution of the Gaussian pulse, the size of the time step must be sufficiently small; this is to avoid missing any important spectral behavior if the temporal resolution was too coarse. The Nyquist theorem on sampling gives the following relation, f_{max} being the highest resolvable frequency:

$$f_{max} = \frac{1}{2\Delta t} \tag{28.60}$$

Then, the frequency resolution Δf is given by

$$\Delta f = \frac{f_{max}}{N/2} = \frac{1}{N \times \Delta t} \tag{28.61}$$

We notice that this equation gives another way to calculate Δt, other than the CFL criterion. Typically, the way to proceed is to follow the CFL criterion which will give a value of Δt. Then, the desired frequency resolution will lead to another value for Δt: the smallest of the two can be chosen as the Δt value that will be used.

28.3.7 Materials

The FDTD solver can handle different types of materials, which is necessary to include the structure to simulate. For example, perfect electric conductor (PEC) materials are represented by setting the electric field inside specific cells to zero.

For dielectric materials, it requires including their characteristic properties (relative permittivity ε_r, relative permeability μ_r, and conductivity σ) in Maxwell's equations at the desired location in space:

$$\frac{\partial \boldsymbol{E}}{\partial t} = \frac{1}{\varepsilon_0 \varepsilon_r} \nabla \times \boldsymbol{H} - \frac{\sigma}{\varepsilon_0 \varepsilon_r} \tag{28.62}$$

$$\frac{\partial \boldsymbol{H}}{\partial t} = -\frac{1}{\mu_0 \mu_r} \nabla \times \boldsymbol{E} \tag{28.63}$$

In other words, to include the particular geometry of an object made of a particular material, the material properties of the cells included in the geometry have to be changed in these equations to represent the object.

28.3.8 Preventing Reflections: Boundary Conditions and Impedance Matching

As the computer cannot handle an infinite simulation space, some boundaries conditions have to be set up to specify how the fields will behave when arriving at the space limit. A specific kind of boundary conditions is called the absorbing boundary condition (ABC). As the name suggests, this type of boundary aims to fully absorb the incoming wave.

Another popular method is the perfectly matched layer (PML), formulated by Bérenger,[26] aiming to artificially absorb the incoming wave and to avoid any reflection back to the calculation domain from any incident wave.

The idea behind the PML is to bound the simulation domain by an artificial layer of material that would perfectly absorb any incoming wave without any reflection. The layer has to be perfectly matched to the impedance Z (given below) of the material on the inner side of the boundary, meaning that both impedances must be equal.

$$Z = \sqrt{\frac{\mu}{\varepsilon}} \tag{28.64}$$

28.3.9 A Fast-solving Approach for Specific Problems: the Huygens Box

When trying to solve specific problems involving different geometric scales, for example, a very small implant inside a large phantom, the computation time can become burdensome. Indeed, if we consider a pacemaker lead, it will require a very fine mesh to resolve the small diameter of the structure (in the order of millimeters) while the overall phantom dimensions will be in the order of tens of centimeters.

The Huygens box method can be used to overcome this issue, which is based on the Love–Schelkunoff theorem of equivalent surface currents (i.e., equivalence between sources inside and outside a surface and the tangential field on that surface).[27] In practice, it consists of running a first simulation with the coil and empty phantom, 'recording the fields' applied to the phantom with a box surrounding the area where the implant is supposed to be. In this situation, only the phantom and the coil need to be resolved, which allows us to use a coarser mesh. Then, in a second time, we place our implant model inside the phantom and run the simulation without the coil, only using the field recorded with the imaginary Huygens box. This allows us to use a smaller computation space, and the fine mesh required to resolve the implant is not detrimental to the calculation time anymore (Figure 28.6).

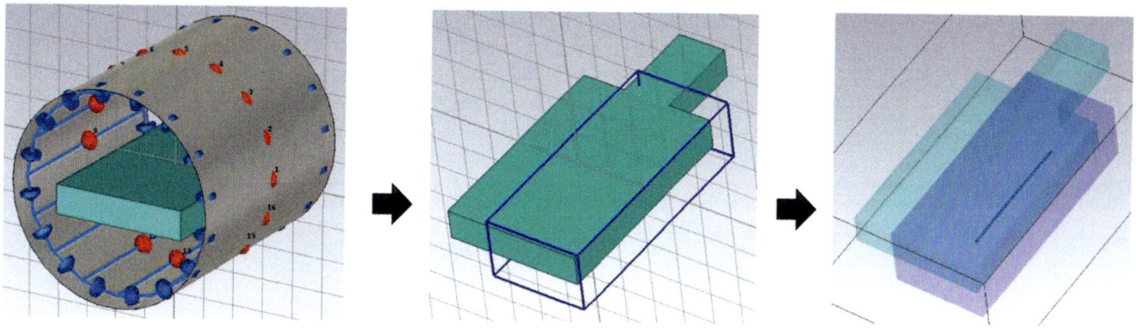

Figure 28.6. Illustration of the Huygens box method

28.3.10 Code Implementation

After describing the algorithm, it can be useful to know how to implement it in detail. There are many open-source codes available on the Internet in various languages,[28–30] and an example of the steps to follow is given below.

First, after introducing the fundamental constants, the grid parameters have to be defined, which include the size of the grid, the size of the cells, the time step, and the total number of steps. Then, a source can be included; its parameters and location have to be defined. A geometric model may be introduced, the correct material parameters assigned to the correct positions on the grid, and the boundary conditions defined. Finally, the fields have to be initialized (usually set to zero), and the update equations can be written before running the algorithm. The fields can be recorded as desired, and then the postprocessing steps can be written to visualize the propagation of the fields over time.

The diagram in Figure 28.7 summarizes these steps.

28.3.11 Pros and Cons of the FDTD Method

Since its introduction and popularization by Yee in 1966, the FDTD method has found a large success due to its possibility of implementation for different physics problems. The main reasons are its simplicity of implementation and its modularity. Indeed, the FDTD allows getting a system response to a wide range of frequencies using only one simulation. This solver is also parallelizable; with the advance in computing over the past few years, GPU-accelerated calculations are getting more and more available and can speed up simulations to an extent that was not possible before. This can be a major advantage compared to an FEM, which is not parallelizable and demands important RAM resources.

However, despite all these advantages, the FDTD method suffers from some drawbacks: it requires to mesh the entire simulation space. Due to the cell's hexahedral shape, it is also not optimal for curved structure and will induce a *staircasing* effect on the rounded geometry. Therefore, to accurately model curved, complex structures, a very fine mesh can be necessary, which will have a significant impact on the simulation time (Figure 28.8). Finally, the nature of the algorithm makes it converge only once all fields have decayed enough. When considering highly resonant structures, this can lead to proportionally long simulation times.

To offer a solution to these problems, Weiland[31] introduced the FIT in 1977. This technique, as will be

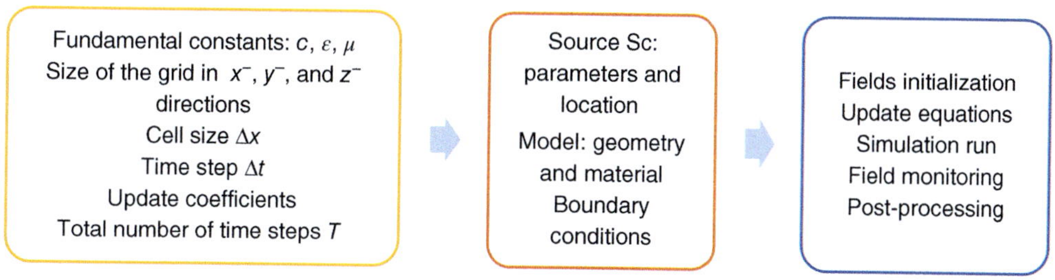

Figure 28.7. Code structure example to implement the FDTD algorithm

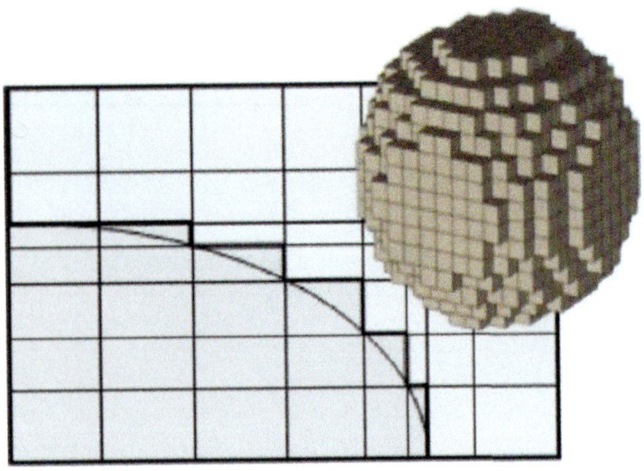

Figure 28.8. Representation of the staircasing issue when modeling curved geometries. (Adapted from CST Microwave Studio, 'Understanding Time Domain Meshing', 2010. © 2010 Dassault Systèmes)

detailed in the following section, provides the advantages of the FDTD while addressing the staircasing issue.

28.4 THE FINITE-INTEGRATION TECHNIQUE (FIT)

28.4.1 Principle

This technique was developed by Weiland[31,32] and a proprietary solver used in the CST multiphysics software. As for the FDTD, the FIT uses cubic mesh cells and a staggered Yee grid for electric field and magnetic field computation. However, instead of writing Maxwell's equations in a differential form, the FIT involves their integral form:

$$\oiint_{\partial\Omega} \boldsymbol{E}.\mathbf{d}\boldsymbol{S} = \iiint_{\Omega} \rho \mathrm{d}V \tag{28.65}$$

$$\oiint_{\partial\Omega} \boldsymbol{B}.\mathbf{d}\boldsymbol{S} = 0 \tag{28.66}$$

$$\oint_{\partial\Sigma} \boldsymbol{E}.\mathbf{d}\boldsymbol{l} = -\frac{\mathrm{d}}{\mathrm{d}t}\iint_{\Sigma} \boldsymbol{B}.\mathbf{d}\boldsymbol{S} \tag{28.67}$$

$$\oint_{\partial\Sigma} \boldsymbol{B}.\mathbf{d}\boldsymbol{l} = \mu_0\left(\iint_{\Sigma} \boldsymbol{J}.\mathbf{d}\boldsymbol{S} + \varepsilon_0\frac{\mathrm{d}}{\mathrm{d}t}\iint_{\Sigma} \boldsymbol{E}.\mathbf{d}\boldsymbol{S}\right) \tag{28.68}$$

As with the other discretization methods, the simulation space will be delimited by a set of boundaries. We consider here a Cartesian mesh (Figure 28.9) for

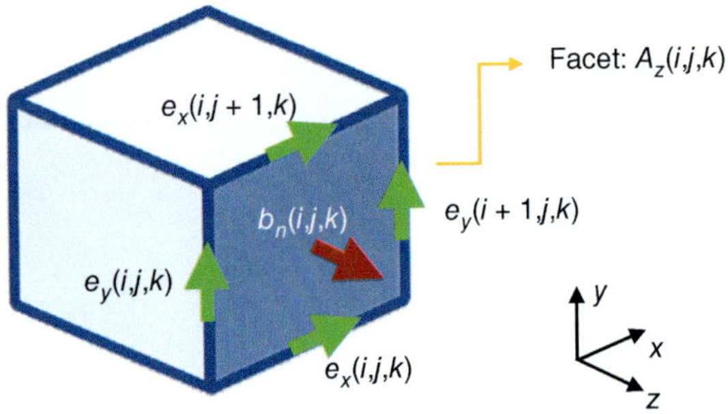

Figure 28.9. FIT cubic mesh cell for the Maxwell–Faraday equation reformulation

clarity sake; however, the FIT can be extended to all types of meshes.[33]

Let us consider first the Maxwell–Faraday equation:

$$\oint_{\partial\Sigma} \boldsymbol{E}.\mathbf{d}\boldsymbol{l} = -\frac{\mathrm{d}}{\mathrm{d}t}\iint_{\Sigma} \boldsymbol{B}.\mathbf{d}\boldsymbol{S} \tag{28.69}$$

We can rewrite the Maxwell–Faraday equation on the blue facet $A_z(i,j,k)$ accordingly:

$$e_x(i,j,k) + e_y(i+1,j,k) - e_x(i,j+1,k) - e_y(i,j,k) = -\frac{\mathrm{d}}{\mathrm{d}t}b_n(i,j,k) \tag{28.70}$$

with

$e_x(i,j,k) = \int_{(x_i,y_j,z_k)}^{x_{i+1},y_j,z_k} \vec{E}$ representing the electrical voltage along one edge of the facet.

$b_n(i,j,k) = \iint_{A_z(i,j,k)} \vec{B}\cdot\vec{\mathrm{d}A}$ representing the magnetic flux density through the cell facet.

This can be extended to all the facets considered in the simulation space, giving the following matrix form:

$$\begin{pmatrix} \cdots & \cdots & \cdots\cdots \\ 1 & 1 & -1\ -1 \\ \cdots & \cdots & \cdots\cdots \end{pmatrix}\begin{pmatrix} \vdots \\ e_{n1} \\ e_{n2} \\ e_{n3} \\ e_{n4} \\ \vdots \end{pmatrix} = -\frac{\mathrm{d}}{\mathrm{d}t}\begin{pmatrix} \vdots \\ b_n \\ \vdots \end{pmatrix} \tag{28.71}$$

Rewritten using simpler matrix notations:

$$\boldsymbol{Ce} = -\frac{\mathrm{d}}{\mathrm{d}t}\boldsymbol{b} \tag{28.72}$$

This is our first FIT equation. Then, we now consider the Maxwell–Gauss equation for magnetism (Figure 28.10):

$$\oiint_{\partial\Omega} B.\mathrm{d}S = 0 \tag{28.73}$$

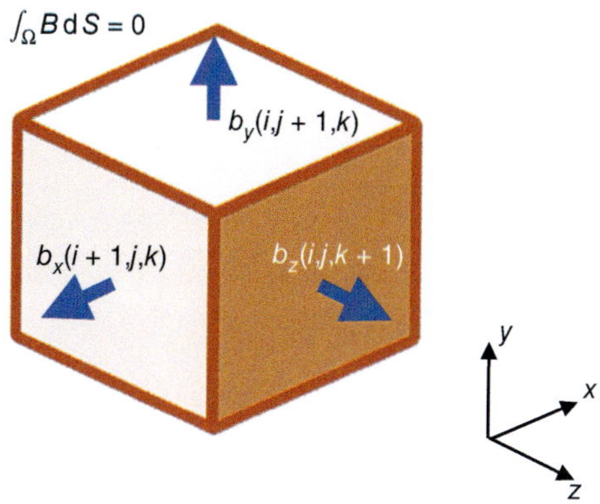

Figure 28.10. FIT cubic mesh cell for the reformulation of the Maxwell–Gauss equation for magnetism

The three other magnetic fluxes are similarly defined on the three other hidden facets and yield

$$-b_x(i,j,k) + b_x(i+1,j,k) - b_y(i,j,k) + b_y(i,j+1,k) - b_z(i,j,k) + b_x(i,j,k+1) = 0 \quad (28.74)$$

As before, the matrix form of the Maxwell–Gauss equation for magnetism can be derived as follows:

$$\begin{pmatrix} \cdots & \cdots & \cdots & \cdots & \cdots\cdots \\ -1 & 1 & -1 & 1 & -1\;\;1 \\ \cdots & \cdots & \cdots & \cdots & \cdots\cdots \end{pmatrix} \begin{pmatrix} \vdots \\ b_{m1} \\ b_{m2} \\ b_{m3} \\ b_{m4} \\ b_{m5} \\ b_{m6} \\ \vdots \end{pmatrix} = 0 \quad (28.75)$$

Rewritten using simpler notations, we obtain our second FIT equation:

$$\boldsymbol{Sb} = 0 \quad (28.76)$$

To discretize the last two Maxwell equations, it is necessary to introduce a secondary grid $\tilde{G}$, dual to the primary grid G previously considered.[31] The center of the cell of the dual grid is the grid point of the primary grid (Figure 28.11).

This new grid allows us to rewrite the remaining Maxwell's equations in a matrix form, leading to a set of four matrix equations to be solved:

$$\boldsymbol{Ce} = -\frac{\mathrm{d}}{\mathrm{d}t}\boldsymbol{b} \quad (28.77)$$

$$\boldsymbol{Sb} = 0 \quad (28.78)$$

$$\tilde{\boldsymbol{C}}\boldsymbol{h} = -\frac{\mathrm{d}}{\mathrm{d}t}\boldsymbol{d} + \boldsymbol{j} \quad (28.79)$$

$$\tilde{\boldsymbol{S}}\boldsymbol{d} = \boldsymbol{q} \quad (28.80)$$

28.4.2 A Solution to Material Approximations: the Perfect Boundary Approximation (PBA)

When considering two cells from the primary and dual grids, such as in Figure 28.11, the direction associated with the facet and the direction associated with the penetrating edge are the same. Material relations will be expressed in matrix form:

$$\boldsymbol{d} = \boldsymbol{M}_\varepsilon \boldsymbol{e} + \boldsymbol{p} \quad (28.81)$$

$$\boldsymbol{j} = \boldsymbol{M}_\kappa \boldsymbol{e} \quad (28.82)$$

with $\boldsymbol{M}_\varepsilon$ being the permittivity matrix, $\boldsymbol{M}_\kappa$ the conductivity matrix, and $\boldsymbol{p}$ the permanent electric polarization.

Let us illustrate the approximation made on material parameters by considering an edge belonging to the primary grid, coupled to a facet flux allocated on a dual-grid cell. For the facet area, the four-cell corner permittivities and conductivities will be averaged. The constitutive relations then yield an averaged current density and electric field intensity; thus, the discretization errors arise from the constitutive material equations.[33]

When filling cells with materials, problematic staircase approximations can arise on curved surfaces, as with the FDTD method. To avoid this, methods such as the perfect boundary approximation (PBA) – CST's proprietary method – can be used.[34] As we saw in the FDTD method, a typical Yee grid allows for only one type of material per cell, resulting in the staircase approximation illustrated in our FDTD part. The PBA consists of allowing the path of integration of Maxwell's equations to follow the geometry of the object considered, rather than the edges of the cell itself. This way, different materials can be distinguished inside the same cell, even for curved geometries.

28.4.3 Pros and Cons of the FIT

The FDTD and FIT methods are similar, in the sense that both will typically use Yee's dual grid, will take into consideration Courant's stability criterion, allow for GPU acceleration, etc. Similar to the FDTD method, no matrix inversion is required meaning that the memory requirement is not a major obstacle,

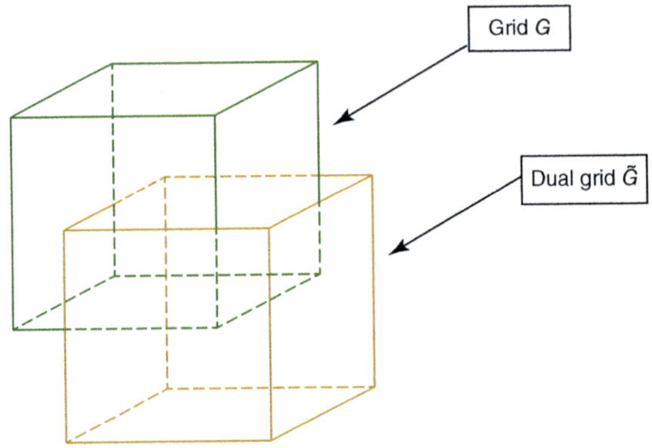

Figure 28.11. Dual-grid diagram

as this can be the case for the FEM. However, a crucial difference is in the consideration of material for staircasing. The FIT indeed has the potential to better approximate geometries, either by applying a nonorthogonal mesh (not necessarily straightforward) or using the PBA technique. This allows solving one of the major issues of FDTD, the staircasing effect on curved geometries.[21,35]

However, the FIT method also suffers from some drawbacks similar to the FDTD: in particular, the need for the fields to decay enough before converging, which, in the case where a high-quality factor coil is considered, can lead to very long simulation times.

28.5 WORKFLOW EXAMPLE

When performing simulations for MRI purposes, be it safety or coil performance, a few steps are typically followed (Figure 28.12). We describe below a typical workflow for RF coil simulations.

28.5.1 Coil Model

- First, the global geometry has to be defined. The coil structure is modeled: end rings, rods, and shield are created following some user-specified parameters such as coil length, diameter, and number of rods/legs. Some space may have to be left available to later place the capacitors. Finally, material properties are attributed to the coil (e.g., copper).
- The feeding ports are positioned with their phase/location set up accordingly, e.g., 90° difference both in space and in phase for a circularly polarized mode.
- Then, the capacitors need to be implemented: to do so, we have two choices. The most straightforward way is to place lumped capacitors with values obtained from a first guess – analytical calculation, previous experience, or tools such as the Birdcage Builder.[36] Then, we run the electromagnetic

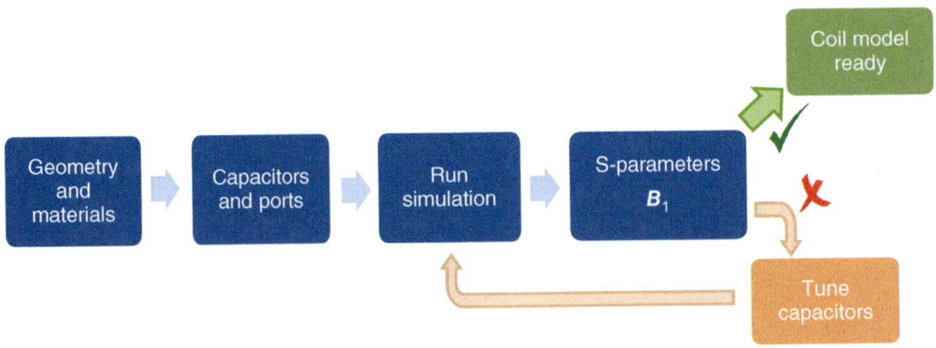

Figure 28.12. Example of steps to realize a coil simulation

simulation, adjusting the capacitance value and repeating the simulation.

This is a simple, trial-and-error approach; however, many simulations may be required before finding a satisfying capacitance value. Thus, it may be more efficient to use a circuit-based approach. This method, thoroughly described by Kozlov[28] and implemented in several commercial simulation software, allows adjusting the capacitance value with only one electromagnetic simulation. All capacitors are replaced by 50 Ω ports, and the 3D simulation is run. Then, based on the S-matrix obtained, circuit capacitors are connected to each port and tuned, and the 3D-circuit combined fields can be obtained without having to rerun the simulation. This is particularly interesting with array coils.

- To validate a coil model, we look at the $\boldsymbol{B}_1$ field maps and the S-parameters: if the field pattern and the S-parameter spikes are achieved at the desired frequency, we can move on to the next steps.

Below is an example of a TEM head coil model (Figure 28.13a) and its $\boldsymbol{B}_1$-field map (Figure 28.13b) at the desired resonance frequency. The pattern achieved is the one expected for such a coil, which is an indicator that the coil model behaves as desired. On top of the S-parameters graphs that help to check the coil behavior, it is also a good practice to check the field uniformity along the three different axes, to ensure there is no glitch in the model that could be overlooked.

28.5.2 Phantoms and Numerical Human Models

Once the coil is properly set up, we can include a load if we want to perform further calculations: for example, the effect of a load on the S-parameters or safety purposes. Depending on these goals, we will use either a phantom or a numerical human model.

- For a phantom, it is rather straightforward: we simply have to define and model its geometry, along with its physical properties (e.g., conductivity, permittivity, and thermal properties). A well-known phantom for MRI safety purposes is the ASTM phantom. This roughly humanoid phantom's dimensions and physical properties are described in an ASTM standard,[37] widely used by medical device manufacturers to test and label their products for MRI use. Figure 28.14(a) shows a modeled ASTM phantom.
- For a numerical human model (Figure 28.14b), we have several choices: simulation software companies may directly provide models compatible with their software, such as CST's Voxel Family[38] and Sim4Life's Virtual Population.[39] In general, several models are available, varying in age, gender, morphology, etc. The IT'IS Foundation also proposes for a fee some models which can be used in any software accepting the CAD file's type, and these models are directly downloadable from their website.

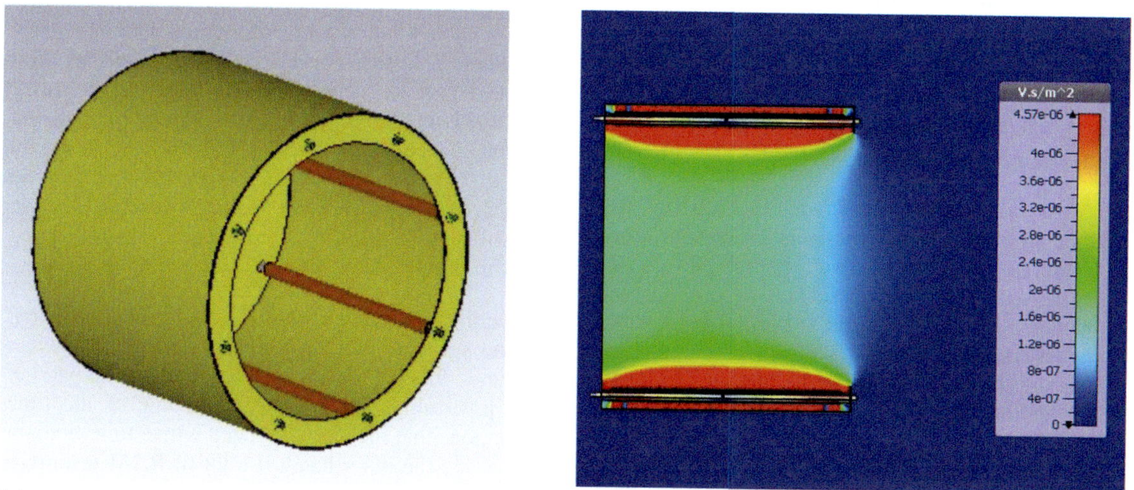

(a) (b)

Figure 28.13. (a) TEM head coil model. (b) $\boldsymbol{B}_1$ field map from this coil model

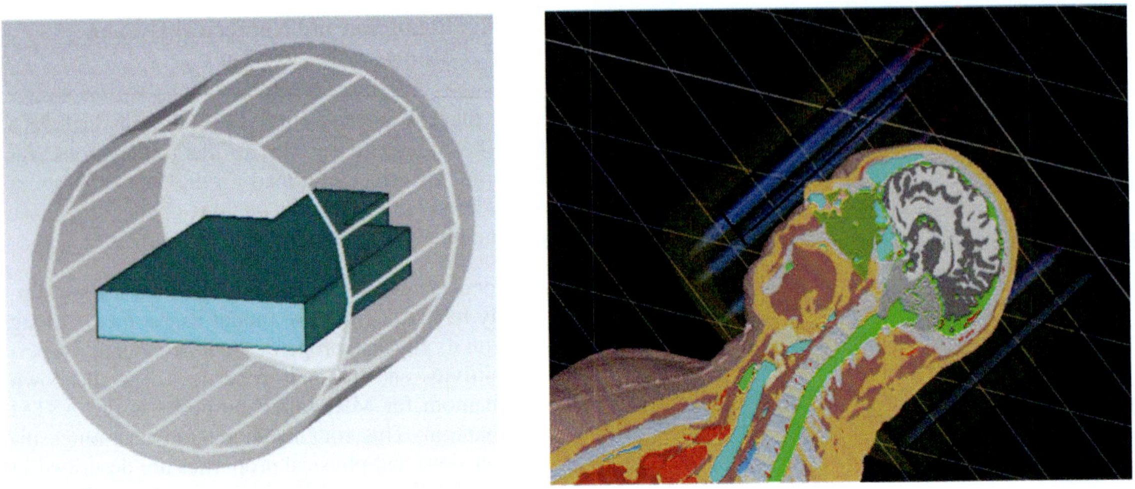
(a) (b)

Figure 28.14. (a) ASTM phantom in birdcage coil. (b) Human model in TEM head coil

One important note about these numerical human models is that depending on how they are built, they may not support all kinds of mesh: voxel models are staircased, with a fixed voxel resolution, while surface models are smoother and allow to be meshed at the user's convenience. Their typically high resolution is very useful when fine body structures are studied. But as always, there is a trade-off between model resolution and detail and simulation speed.

28.5.2.1 *Which Solver for Which Purpose?*

Depending on the problem at hand or on the phase of the project (prototyping and safety testing on loads), different solvers may work more efficiently: if available, it may be more interesting in some cases to use one solver instead of another.

- An unloaded coil with a very high-quality factor may require a very long simulation time when using a time-domain solver. This is because, as discussed in the FDTD section of this chapter, we need to wait for the initial excitation to have faded enough to achieve a steady state and finish the simulation. The higher the quality factor, the longer the simulation would take; in this case, a frequency-domain solver might allow a significant gain in simulation time.
- When considering a solver, we must also consider the geometry of the coil we are working with: when cylindrical or spherical geometries are involved, in some cases a lot of cubic mesh cells are required to resolve them accurately enough (unless using techniques such as the PBA described in the FIT part of this chapter). In these situations, a frequency-domain solver such as FEM may be more suitable.
- The type of load is also to be considered: many numerical human phantoms are voxel models, whose use is more straightforward with a cubic mesh.
- The number of frequencies considered is also an important factor: if we only need one frequency, then the frequency-domain solver may be a better choice than the time-domain solver. However, when we need to observe the coil and load behavior on a large frequency band, the time-domain solver can be more appropriate, given that it is able to get the coil behavior for a large frequency band with only one simulation. There still exist some ways to interpolate frequencies with a frequency-domain solver, to 'reconstruct' the frequency band only by simulating only a few frequency samples.

Overall, the choice of solver will be dependent on the software available and also on the hardware at hand. Indeed, if using several GPUs in parallel is a possibility, it can overcome some of the time limitations that may be associated with a time-domain solver. On the other hand, if a lot of RAM resources are provided, it can help significantly speeding up an FEM solver. It is noteworthy that nowadays, with the advent of cloud computing, one does not necessarily have to purchase expensive hardware to keep on-site; instead, it is possible to only purchase computing time on the cloud to run simulations. This solution is particularly interesting when simulation is not run on an everyday basis. To assess whether this choice is the best in practice, cost, convenience, and frequency of the simulation work will have to be considered.

28.6 VALIDATION OF NUMERICAL SIMULATIONS

Simulations are an invaluable tool for research and experimental design, which is part of breakthrough research in MRI and RF safety.[40] However, to ensure their reliability, validation through real-world experiments is essential. There are indeed several sources of errors that should not be disregarded when simulating: the size and number of mesh cells, model approximations, material/tissue properties, etc.[41] For example, it may often be challenging to know the exact dielectric properties of an object, which can in certain situations have a significant impact on the results obtained.

Experiments are therefore crucial before making definitive conclusions solely based on simulation results, especially when considering safety matters.[42] On the other hand, simulation is a very useful tool to gain insight into phenomena experienced in practice; it allows access to countless useful information such as the electric field in a particular area or the current in specific parts of a coil. In short, simulation and experiments can (and should) work hand-in-hand. At any stage of a project, some methods can be used to ensure that the simulations correspond to what is observed in practice.

28.6.1 Validation Methods

Depending on the problem at hand, there are several ways to validate a simulation.

28.6.1.1 Intravalidation: Different Solvers on the Same Problem

A useful step is, if possible, to run the exactly same simulation with a different solver.[21] For example, a time-domain simulation should be run again in frequency domain; if both simulations give the same results, it is an indication that the simulation is set up correctly. Of course, the purpose of this method is only to validate the parameter settings in simulation, and it should not be exclusively used to the detriment of the experimental validation method proposed below.

28.6.1.2 Field Maps

$\boldsymbol{B}_1$ mapping is a widely used experimental method that allows to obtain the $\boldsymbol{B}_1$ field distribution generated by a coil. A way of verifying the correlation between simulation and experiments is to acquire a $\boldsymbol{B}_1$ map and compare it to the one obtained in simulation. For safety studies, it is also very important to check the correlation between experimental and numerical $\boldsymbol{E}$-field maps; indeed, similar $\boldsymbol{B}_1$ maps do not necessarily imply exactly similar $\boldsymbol{E}$-field maps, and it is also very important to check the model on the entire volume, not only on one slice.[43,44] To obtain $\boldsymbol{E}$-field maps, cartography can be realized with $\boldsymbol{E}$-field probes, using mechanical support to help displace the probe precisely along the three spatial axes.

28.6.1.3 Thermal Data

When working on RF safety studies, comparing EM/thermal simulations can be achieved by getting thermal measurements from the phantom, for example by setting up fiber optic temperature probes in specific positions and comparing the data with the results obtained numerically.[42,45]

28.6.1.4 S-parameters and Local B_1 *Probes*

When building and validating a coil, S-parameter measurements are a proper method to ensure that the modes of a coil are located at the expected frequencies in simulation.[46] Most commercial software allows plotting the S-parameters directly in the graphical interface, without requiring any specific postprocessing. Additionally, $\boldsymbol{B}_1$ field probes can be used to ensure the homogeneity of the field and its correlation at specific locations.[47]

28.7 NONEXHAUSTIVE LIST OF SIMULATION SOFTWARE

To perform electromagnetic simulations, it is either possible to develop one's own code from the scratch (Matlab, Python, C/C++, …), for example as we described in the FDTD part, or to use the existing software.

We report below a *nonexhaustive* list of free/open-source and commercial software.[36] The pros of using free software are obviously that it is available at no cost and allows to get started right away with a simple download. On the other hand, it may not provide user support as readily available as commercial software. Another advantage of commercial software is that it should have been rigorously tested and thus should provide extensive proof of its reliability. However, before committing to a commercial software, it is recommended to test it on different projects, to check the user-friendliness of the interface, the available tutorials, and the quality of the results obtained. For reference, we also list here some available publications for some free/open-source software.[28,37,38] Additionally, a thermal solver is available for MRI safety applications,[39] to help solve for the temperature change based on Pennes bioheat equation as well as the Generic BioHeat Transfer Model (GBHTM).

28.7.1 Free/Open-source Software

Software	Solver	Scripts/interface
MEEP	FDTD	Python
openEMS	FDTD	Matlab, Octave
gprMax	FDTD	–
MaxFEM	FEM	–

28.7.2 Commercial Software

Software	Example of available EM solvers	Scripts/interface
CST studio suite	FIT, FEM, and MoM	VBA
REMCOM XFDTD	FDTD	Matlab and Xtend (Java)
Ansys HFSS	FEM	Matlab
COMSOL Multiphysics	FEM	Java and Matlab
Altair FEKO	MoM, FEM, and FDTD	Lua
ZMT Sim4Life	FDTD and FEM	Python

28.8 SUMMARY

With the advent of supercomputing, GPU calculations, and the development of hardware technologies, numerical simulation became a very powerful tool over the past decades for various applications in many industries. In MRI, it is used for several design stages for various parts of the machine (magnet, gradients, and RF coils) and also for research, including safety studies. Numerical human models are indeed useful to have insights on the potential risks associated with an MRI scan, for example, heating effects.

Different solvers are available to solve Maxwell's equations. Depending on the stage and type of the project, one solver may be better than another in terms of simulation time – accuracy balance. Many commercial software proposes several solvers (time domain and frequency domain); whenever available, it is always a good idea to take advantage of those, be it to run a more efficient simulation or to verify the similarity of results between different solvers. Some simulation software is also available online for free, and it is always possible to develop one's own code, especially with the many examples to be found online in various programming languages.

Although simulation is an extremely useful tool for design and prototyping and is rightfully so part of international safety standards for MRI, it should not be overlooked that it may potentially be prone to errors. Indeed, incorrect modeling, mesh, or other settings may lead to inaccurate or misleading results. Another source of errors would be unknown parameters, for example, dielectric or geometric properties, which can be critical in some situations. Therefore, as much as possible, definitive conclusions should not be made solely on a numerical simulation basis but should rely on experimental validations as well. Simulations and experiments can work well together and benefit from each other; numerical modeling can help the design of a prototype and bring insights to experimental phenomena, while well-designed and rigorous experiments will provide real-world results and conclusions.

RELATED ARTICLES IN EMAGRES

Birdcage Resonators: Highly Homogeneous Radiofrequency Coils for Magnetic Resonance

Coils for Insertion into the Human Body

Design and Use of Internal Receiver Coils for Magnetic Resonance Imaging

Multifrequency Coils for Whole Body Studies

Radiofrequency Systems and Coils for MRI and MRS

Refrigerated and Superconducting Receiver Coils in Whole Body Magnetic Resonance

Spatial Encoding Using Multiple rf Coils: SMASH Imaging and Parallel MRI

Surface Coil NMR: Detection with Inhomogeneous Radiofrequency Field Antennas

Surface and Other Local Coils for In Vivo Studies

Whole Body Machines: NMR Phased Array Coil Systems

TEM Transceiver Head Array Coils for Ultra High Magnetic Fields

TEM Arrays, Design and Implementation

Quadrature Surface Coils

Double-Tuned Surface Coils

Quadrature Transverse Electromagnetic (TEM) Surface Coils

Radiofrequency Fields and SAR for Transverse Electromagnetic (TEM) Surface Coils

Double-Tuned Birdcage Coils: Construction and Tuning

Radiofrequency Fields and SAR for Bird Cage Coils

TEM Body Coils

Transverse Electromagnetic (TEM) Surface Coils for Extremities

Receiver Loop Arrays

Coil Array Design for Parallel Imaging: Theory and Applications

Millipede Coils

Microcoils

Catheter Coils

Radiofrequency Heating Models and Measurements

Characterization of Multichannel Coil Arrays on the Benchtop

A Standard Procedure for Analyzing Radio Frequency MRI Coils

Litz Coils for High Resolution and Animal Probes, Especially for Double Resonance

RF Field Modeling for Double-Tuned Volume Coils

An Historical Introduction to Surface Coils: The Early Days

Transceiver Loop Arrays

Radiofrequency Coils for NMR: A Peripatetic History of Their Twists and Turns

Nested Surface Coils for Multinuclear NMR

Birdcage Volume Coil Design

Bioeffects and Safety of Radiofrequency Electromagnetic Fields

Radiofrequency Fields: Interactions, Biological Effects, and Safety Issues

RF Device Safety and Compatibility

Safety Considerations in MRI

REFERENCES

1. J. P. Durbano, J. R. Humphrey, F. E. Ortiz, P. F. Curt, D. W. Prather, and M. S. Mirotznik, In *IEEE Antennas and Propagation Society Symposium*, 2004.
2. N. Goodnight, R. Wang, and G. Humphreys, *IEEE Comput. Graph. Appl.*, 2005, **25**, 12.
3. Z. Yue, Z. Sun, and Z. Liu, *IEEE Trans. Appl. Supercond.*, 2019, **29**, 4901106.
4. Y. Hu, Q. Wang, X. Hu, X. Zhu, S. Crozier, Y. Wang, and F. Liu, *Meas. Sci. Technol.*, 2017, **28**, 035402.
5. X. Wu, J. Tian, S. Schmitter, J. T. Vaughan, K. Uğurbil, and P. F. Van de Moortele, *Magn. Reson. Med.*, 2016, **75**, 2464.
6. C. M. Collins, *NMR Biomed.*, 2009, **22**, 919. DOI: 10.1002/nbm.1251.
7. J. Kabil, L. Belguerras, S. Trattnig, C. Pasquier, J. Felblinger, and A. Missoffe, *Yearb. Med. Inform.*, 2016, **2016**, 152.
8. ASTM F2182-11a, Standard Test Method for Measurement of Radio Frequency Induced Heating On or Near Passive Implants During Magnetic Resonance Imaging, ASTM International: West Conshohocken, PA, 2011, www.astm.org.

9. J. C. Maxwell, *Philos. Trans. R. Soc. Lond.*, 1865, **155**, 459.
10. R. L. Courant, *Bull. Am. Math. Soc.*, 1943, **49**, 1.
11. R. J. Duffin, *J. Math. Mech.*, 1959, **8**, 796.
12. O. C. Zienkiewicz, The Finite Element Method in Structural and Continuum Mechanics, McGraw-Hill: London, 1967.
13. S. Ahmed and P. Daly, *Radio Electron. Eng.*, 1969, **38**, 217.
14. P. Silvester, *Alta Frequenza*, 1969, **38**, 313.
15. S. P. Venkateshan and P. Swaminathan, in 'Computational Methods in Engineering', eds S. P. Venkateshan and P. Swaminathan, Academic Press: Oxford, 2014, p 255 Chapter 6.
16. P. P. Silvester and R. L. Ferrari, Finite Elements for Electrical Engineers, 2nd edn, Cambridge University Press: Cambridge, 1990.
17. J.-M. Jin, Theory and Computation of Electromagnetic Fields, John Wiley-IEEE Press: Hoboken, NJ, 2010.
18. E. Wang, T. Nelson, and R. Rauch, In *2004 International ANSYS Conference*, 2004.
19. COMSOL Multiphysics Cyclopedia, Finite element mesh refinement, 2017. https://www.comsol.com/multiphysics/mesh-refinement
20. A. Ern and J. L. Guermond, Theory and Practice of Finite Elements. Part I, Chapter 1, Springer Science & Business Media: New York, 2004.
21. T. Weiland, M. Timm, and I. Munteanu, *IEEE Microw. Mag.*, 2008, **9**, 62.
22. K. S. Yee, *IEEE Trans. Antennas Propag.*, 1966, **14**, 302.
23. R. C. Dorf, The Electrical Engineering Handbook, 2nd edn, CRC Press: Boca Raton, FL, 1997, p 2640.
24. T. W. Hertel and G. S. Smith, *IEEE Trans. Antennas Propag.*, 2003, **51**, 1771.
25. R. Courant, K. O. Fredrichs, and H. Lewy, *Math. Ann.*, 1928, **100**, 32.
26. J. P. Bérenger, *J. Comput. Phys.*, 1994, **114**, 185.
27. H. Rogier, *URSI Radio Sci. Bull.*, 2003, **2003**, 22–29.
28. A. Oskooi, D. Roundy, M. Ibanescu, P. Bermel, J. D. Joannopoulos, and S. G. Johnson, *Comput. Phys. Commun.*, 2010, **181**, 687.
29. J. B. Schneider, Understanding the finite-difference time-domain method, 2010. www.eecs.wsu.edu/~schneidj/ufdtd
30. C. Meyer, Simple FDTD solver in Julia, 2018. http://github.com/cmey/uFDTD.jl
31. T. Weiland, *Electron. Commun.*, 1977, **31**, 116.
32. T. Weiland, *Int. J. Numer. Model.*, 1996, **9**, 295.
33. M. Clemens and T. Weiland, *Prog. Electromagn. Res.*, 2001, **32**, 65.
34. CST Microwave Studio, Understanding time domain meshing, White Paper, 2010.
35. B. Krietenstein, R. Schuhmann, P. Thoma, and T. Weiland. In *Proceedings of the XIX International Linear Accelerator Conference (LINAC)*, Chicago, USA, 1998, 860–862.
36. K. Y. You, C. W. Lee, and C. Y. Lee, *Int. J. Adv. Microw. Technol.*, 2017, **2**.
37. T. Liebig, A. Rennings, S. Held, and D. Erni, *Int. J. Numer. Model.*, 2013, **26**, 680.
38. C. Warren, A. Giannopoulos, and I. Giannakis, *Comput. Phys. Commun.*, 2016, **209**, 163.
39. D. Shrivastava, Theory and Applications of Heat Transfer in Humans, John Wiley & Sons: Chichester, West Sussex, UK, 2018.
40. D. Shrivastava, J. Tian, J. Hughes, and J. T. Vaughan,In *Frontiers in Biomedical Devices Conference Proceedings*, 2014.
41. M. Kozlov and R. Turner, *PIERS Online*, 2010, **6**, 395.
42. D. Shrivastava, L. Utecht, J. Tian, J. Hughes, and J. T. Vaughan, *Magn. Reson. Med.*, 2014, **72**, 1141.
43. E. Lucano, M. Liberti, G. G. Mendoza, F. Apollonio, E. Lucano, T. Lloyd, S. Wedan, M. I. Iacono, W. Kainz, and L. M. Angelone, *IEEE Trans. Biomed. Eng.*, 2016, **63**, 1591. DOI: 10.1109/TBME.2015.2506680.
44. L. Angelone, In *Talk Given at the ISMRM Workshop on Ensuring RF Safety in MRI: Current Practices & Future Directions*, 2017. https://cds.ismrm.org/protected/Safety17/program/program.htm
45. Y. Liu, J. Chen, F. G. Shellock, and W. Kainz, *J. Magn. Reson. Imaging*, 2013, **37**, 491.
46. N. Li, S. Liu, X. Hu, C. Luo, X. Zhang, and Y. Li, *IEEE Trans. Magn.*, 2018, **54**, 5100504 DOI: 10.1109/TMAG.2017.2758518.
47. S. Kühn, N. Kuster, and B. Kochali, In *2014 International Symposium on Electromagnetic Compatibility*, Tokyo, 2014, 666–669.

Chapter 29

Integral Equation Approach to Modeling RF Fields in Human Body in MRI Systems for Safety

Anand Gopinath

University of Minnesota, Minneapolis, MN, USA

29.1 INTRODUCTION

This chapter discusses the integral equation solution for predicting the radio-frequency (RF) fields in the human body undergoing magnetic resonance imaging.

The modeling of RF fields is based on Maxwell's equations:

$$\nabla \times \mathcal{E} = \frac{\partial \mathcal{B}}{\partial t} \tag{29.1}$$

$$\nabla \times \mathcal{H} = \mathcal{J} + \frac{\partial \mathcal{D}}{\partial t} \tag{29.2}$$

$$\nabla \cdot \mathcal{B} = 0 \tag{29.3}$$

$$\nabla \cdot \mathcal{D} = \rho \tag{29.4}$$

and the constitutive relations are

$$\mathcal{D} = \varepsilon \mathcal{E} \tag{29.5}$$

$$\mathcal{B} = \mu \mathcal{H} \tag{29.6}$$

$$\mathcal{J} = \sigma \mathcal{E} \tag{29.7}$$

where ε, μ, and σ are the permittivity, permeability, and conductivity, respectively. In most biological materials, the permittivity is a function of frequency, and the appropriate value at the frequency concerned is chosen for time harmonic calculations. The permeability μ in these nonmagnetic materials is usually μ_0, and the conductivity is also assumed to be independent of frequency though this may not be the case in all instances.

All the RF phenomena discussed in the integral equation formulation herein are assumed to have a harmonic time variation. This is acceptable because the time variations that modulate these electromagnetic waves are much slower than the RF frequencies, and for all practical purposes, they may be modeled as variants to the harmonic time formulations. For simplicity it may be assumed that the RF is of a single frequency with a time variation given by $e^{j\omega t}$.

Thus, the electric field in Cartesian coordinates is given as

$$\mathcal{E}(x, y, z, t) = \mathrm{Re}[\boldsymbol{E}(x, y, z)e^{j\omega t}] \tag{29.8}$$

Safety and Biological Effects in MRI.
Edited by Devashish Shrivastava and J. Thomas Vaughan

ISBN: 978-1-118-82130-5
Also published in eMagRes (online edition)
DOI: 10.1002/9780470034590.emrstm1567

Note that the bold $\boldsymbol{E}$ represents the time invariant part of the electric field vector, and the usual $\boldsymbol{\mathcal{E}}$ form for the time-dependent vector.

The *real part* qualifier Re is omitted, as well as the $e^{j\omega t}$, both being tacitly understood.

With this convention, Maxwell's equations become

$$\nabla \times \boldsymbol{E} = -j\omega\mu\boldsymbol{H} - \boldsymbol{M} \tag{29.9}$$

$$\nabla \times \boldsymbol{H} = \boldsymbol{J} + j\omega\varepsilon\boldsymbol{E} \tag{29.10}$$

$$\nabla \cdot \boldsymbol{D} = \rho \tag{29.11}$$

$$\nabla \cdot \boldsymbol{B} = 0 \tag{29.12}$$

Note that the magnetic current density has been added to the curl $\boldsymbol{E}$ equation to account for scattering from dielectric objects.

The biological material usually has a conductivity, and the current density is expressed as

$$J = \sigma E \tag{29.13}$$

Assuming that $\varepsilon = \varepsilon_0\varepsilon_r$, where ε_0 is the free space permittivity and ε_r is the relative permittivity of the material at that point

$$\nabla \times \boldsymbol{H} = \boldsymbol{J} + j\omega\varepsilon\boldsymbol{E} \tag{29.14}$$

$$= j\omega\varepsilon_0\varepsilon_{cr}\boldsymbol{E} \tag{29.15}$$

where

$$\varepsilon_{cr} = \varepsilon_r + \frac{\sigma}{j\omega\varepsilon_0} \tag{29.16}$$

In the MRI system, transmit RF coils generate the RF field excitation at the Larmor frequency determined by the background magnetic field $\boldsymbol{B}_0$. For this introductory chapter on integral equation simulations, it is assumed that the RF excitation source is not modeled together with the phantom or the human body, the region being imaged is source free, and the currents generated are due to the incident field on the region of interest (ROI) in the phantom or human head/body. To obtain the wave equation in a source-free region, where $\boldsymbol{J} = \boldsymbol{M} = \rho = 0$, take the curl of equation (29.9)

$$\nabla \times \nabla \times \boldsymbol{E} = -j\omega\mu_0\nabla \times \boldsymbol{H} \tag{29.17}$$

and using the vector identity for the left-hand side and equation (29.10) for the right-hand side

$$\nabla(\nabla \cdot \boldsymbol{E}) - \nabla^2\boldsymbol{E} = -j\omega\mu_0 j\omega\varepsilon_0\varepsilon_{rc}\boldsymbol{E} = \omega^2\mu_0\varepsilon_0\varepsilon_{cr}\boldsymbol{E} \tag{29.18}$$

Since the region is source free, $\nabla \cdot \boldsymbol{E} = 0$, this equation becomes

$$\nabla^2\boldsymbol{E} + \omega^2\mu_0\varepsilon_0\varepsilon_{cr}\boldsymbol{E} = 0 \tag{29.19}$$

or

$$\nabla^2\boldsymbol{E} + k^2\boldsymbol{E} = 0 \tag{29.20}$$

where $k^2 = \omega^2\mu_0\varepsilon_0\varepsilon_{cr}$.

Similarly, it can be shown that

$$\nabla^2\boldsymbol{H} + k^2\boldsymbol{H} = 0 \tag{29.21}$$

The solutions of these equations represent wave propagation in the complex medium which is the human head/body. When the RF coil is modeled, these equations become much more complex.

29.1.1 Vector Potentials

The simulations may also be performed with vector potentials for the electric and magnetic fields as they allow some flexibility, and this approach is outlined below.

Define the magnetic vector potential as

$$\boldsymbol{B} = \mu\boldsymbol{H} = \nabla \times \boldsymbol{A} \tag{29.22}$$

or

$$\boldsymbol{H} = \frac{1}{\mu}\nabla \times \boldsymbol{A} \tag{29.23}$$

Maxwell's first curl equation (29.9) neglecting the magnetic current becomes

$$\nabla \times \boldsymbol{E} = -j\omega\mu\boldsymbol{H} = -j\omega(\nabla \times \boldsymbol{A}) \tag{29.24}$$

or

$$\nabla \times (\boldsymbol{E} + j\omega\boldsymbol{A}) = 0 \tag{29.25}$$

which leads to

$$\boldsymbol{E} + j\omega\boldsymbol{A} = -\nabla\phi_e \tag{29.26}$$

since the curl of the gradient of a scalar is zero.

From equations (29.10) and (29.22)

$$\nabla \times \boldsymbol{H} = \boldsymbol{J} + j\omega\varepsilon\boldsymbol{E} = \frac{1}{\mu}\nabla \times \nabla \times \boldsymbol{A} \tag{29.27}$$

$$-\frac{1}{\mu}\left[\nabla(\nabla \cdot \boldsymbol{A}) - \nabla^2\boldsymbol{A}\right] \tag{29.28}$$

Substituting from equation (29.26):

$$\nabla(\nabla \cdot \boldsymbol{A}) - \nabla^2\boldsymbol{A} = \mu(\boldsymbol{J} + j\omega\varepsilon\boldsymbol{E}) \tag{29.29}$$

$$= \mu\boldsymbol{J} + j\omega\mu\varepsilon\left(-j\omega\boldsymbol{A} - \nabla\phi_e\right) \tag{29.30}$$

Simplifying

$$\nabla^2 \boldsymbol{A} + k^2 \boldsymbol{A} = -\mu \boldsymbol{J} + \nabla(\nabla \cdot \boldsymbol{A} + j\omega\mu\varepsilon\phi_e) \quad (29.31)$$

where $k^2 = \omega^2 \mu$, and to simplify this equation, let

$$\nabla \cdot \boldsymbol{A} + j\omega\mu\varepsilon\phi_e = 0 \quad (29.32)$$

which is termed the *Lorentz gauge* and leads to

$$\nabla^2 \boldsymbol{A} + k^2 \boldsymbol{A} = -\mu \boldsymbol{J} \quad (29.33)$$

and equation (29.27) becomes

$$\boldsymbol{E} = -j\omega \boldsymbol{A} - \nabla\phi_e = j\omega \boldsymbol{A} - j\frac{\nabla\nabla \cdot \boldsymbol{A}}{\omega\mu\varepsilon} \quad (29.34)$$

$$= -j\frac{k^2 + \nabla\nabla\cdot}{\omega\mu\varepsilon}\boldsymbol{A} \quad (29.35)$$

The electric vector potential $\boldsymbol{F}$ also includes the magnetic current $\boldsymbol{M}$ which was omitted in the above derivation. Define

$$\boldsymbol{D} = -\nabla \times \boldsymbol{F} \quad (29.36)$$

and therefore

$$\boldsymbol{E} = -\frac{1}{\varepsilon}\nabla \times \boldsymbol{F} \quad (29.37)$$

Maxwell's curl equation (29.10) for the magnetic field $\boldsymbol{H}$, omitting the current density $\boldsymbol{J}$:

$$\nabla \times \boldsymbol{H} = j\omega\varepsilon \boldsymbol{E} = -j\omega\nabla \times \boldsymbol{F} \quad (29.38)$$

which then results in

$$\boldsymbol{H} = -j\omega \boldsymbol{F} - \nabla\phi_m \quad (29.39)$$

Maxwell's curl equation (29.9) for $\boldsymbol{E}$ is

$$\nabla \times \boldsymbol{E} = -\boldsymbol{M} - j\omega\mu \boldsymbol{H} = -\frac{1}{\varepsilon}\nabla \times \nabla \times \boldsymbol{F} \quad (29.40)$$

$$= -\frac{1}{\varepsilon}\left[\nabla(\nabla \cdot \boldsymbol{F}) - \nabla^2 \boldsymbol{F}\right] \quad (29.41)$$

Simplifying

$$\nabla^2 \boldsymbol{F} + k^2 \boldsymbol{F} = -\boldsymbol{M} + \nabla(\nabla \cdot \boldsymbol{F} + j\omega\mu\varepsilon\phi_m) \quad (29.42)$$

Invoking the *Laurentz gauge*

$$\nabla \cdot \boldsymbol{F} + j\omega\mu\varepsilon\phi_m = 0 \quad (29.43)$$

results in

$$\nabla^2 \boldsymbol{F} + k^2 \boldsymbol{F} = -\boldsymbol{M} \quad (29.44)$$

and also

$$\boldsymbol{H} = -j\frac{k^2 + \nabla\nabla\cdot}{\omega\mu\varepsilon}\boldsymbol{F} \quad (29.45)$$

The $\boldsymbol{E}$ and $\boldsymbol{H}$ fields due to the vector potentials $\boldsymbol{A}$ and $\boldsymbol{F}$ have to be summed. The wave equations for the two vector potentials in equations (29.34) and (29.45) remain valid, but the fields need to be summed

$$\boldsymbol{E} = -j\frac{k^2 + \nabla\nabla\cdot}{\omega\mu\varepsilon}\boldsymbol{A} - \frac{1}{\varepsilon}\nabla \times \boldsymbol{F} \quad (29.46)$$

$$\boldsymbol{H} = \frac{1}{\mu}\nabla \times \boldsymbol{A} - j\frac{k^2 + \nabla\nabla\cdot}{\omega\mu\varepsilon}\boldsymbol{F} \quad (29.47)$$

These equations are used in the integral equation formulations.

29.2 INTEGRAL EQUATION APPROACH

In the integral equation approach, the boundary conditions are automatically satisfied in this formulation by the choice of the basis functions. However, singularities arise in the method of moments approach, but these are evaluated quite accurately.

There are two methods: the first method calculates surface current densities on the surface of the subject that acts as the scatterer and assumes that the subject is a homogeneous phantom or a human head or parts of the body or other dielectric subjects. The second method uses the volumetric integral equations to calculate the fields in inhomogeneous subjects like the human head or body parts. Both methods are discussed briefly below. Interested readers are encouraged to read from the listed references for more details.

29.2.1 Surface Integral Equation Approach

The RF coil creates incident waves characterized by $\boldsymbol{E}^{inc}$ and $\boldsymbol{H}^{inc}$, and these fields in turn create scattered waves, $\boldsymbol{E}^s$ and $\boldsymbol{H}^s$, which penetrate the subject. Instead of calculating the volumetric fields in the inhomogeneous subject, it is assumed that surface current densities $\boldsymbol{J}_1$ and $\boldsymbol{M}_1$ are generated on the surface of the subject, assuming that it is homogeneous, with an average permittivity and conductivity. Then the currents are calculated assuming a vector basis function usually over a triangular mesh by the method of moments. The assumption here is that the interior fields of the inhomogeneous subject may be obtained from these current densities, but none of the papers published[1,2] have performed the interior calculations. The ROI to be investigated, for example, the human head or phantom, assumed to be homogeneous with additional homogeneous islands of different permittivity and conductivity, has been discussed by Wang and Duyn.[2] However,

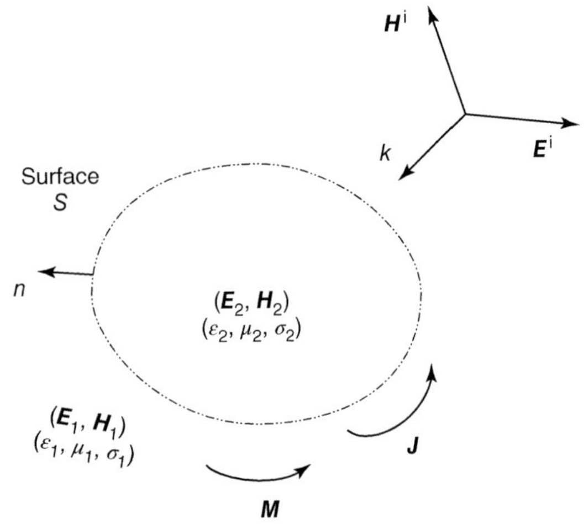

Figure 29.1. The region of interest (ROI) shown with the incident fields ($\boldsymbol{E}^{\mathrm{i}}$, $\boldsymbol{H}^{\mathrm{i}}$), scattered fields ($\boldsymbol{E}_2{}^{\mathrm{s}}$, $\boldsymbol{H}_2{}^{\mathrm{s}}$), the total fields outside the ROI ($\boldsymbol{E}_1$, $\boldsymbol{H}_1$), and the current densities ($\boldsymbol{J}_{\mathrm{s}}$, $\boldsymbol{M}_{\mathrm{s}}$)

in the interest of simplicity, the ROI is assumed to be a single homogeneous region, excited by an incident plane wave ($\boldsymbol{E}^{\mathrm{i}}$, $\boldsymbol{H}^{\mathrm{i}}$), as shown in the Figure 29.1.

The excitation results in forward wave ($\boldsymbol{E}_2$, $\boldsymbol{H}_2$) into the ROI, a scattered signal ($\boldsymbol{E}^{\mathrm{s}}$, $\mathbf{H}^{\mathrm{s}}$) from the ROI, and the current densities $\boldsymbol{J}_1$ and $\boldsymbol{M}_1$ on the surface S.

Since the ROI of the MRI scan is the human head or body part or phantom which is a lossy dielectric, the combined field integral equation is used since both electric and magnetic current densities are present. The magnetic ($\boldsymbol{A}$) and the electric ($\boldsymbol{F}$) vector potentials are used. The electric and magnetic fields corresponding to the magnetic vector potential $\boldsymbol{A}$ are

$$\boldsymbol{H}_A = \frac{1}{\mu}(\nabla\times\boldsymbol{A});\;\; \boldsymbol{E}_A = -j\omega\boldsymbol{A} - j\frac{1}{\omega\mu\varepsilon}\nabla(\nabla\cdot\boldsymbol{A}) = -j\frac{1}{\omega\mu\varepsilon}[\omega^2\mu\varepsilon\boldsymbol{A} + \nabla(\nabla\cdot\boldsymbol{A})] \tag{29.48}$$

The corresponding fields from the electric vector potential $\boldsymbol{F}$ are

$$\boldsymbol{E}_F = -\frac{1}{\varepsilon}(\nabla\times\boldsymbol{F});\;\; \boldsymbol{H}_F = -j\frac{1}{\omega\mu\varepsilon}[\omega^2\mu\boldsymbol{F} + \nabla(\nabla\cdot\boldsymbol{F})] \tag{29.49}$$

The magnetic vector potential $\boldsymbol{A}$ is defined as

$$\boldsymbol{A}(r) = \frac{\mu}{4\pi}\int_S \boldsymbol{J}_{\mathrm{s}}(r')G(r')\mathrm{d}S' \tag{29.50}$$

where

$$G = \mathrm{e}^{-jk_0R}/R \tag{29.51}$$

Similarly

$$\boldsymbol{F}(r) = \frac{\varepsilon}{4\pi}\int_S \boldsymbol{M}_{\mathrm{s}}(r')G(r')\mathrm{d}S' \tag{29.52}$$

In equations (29.50) and (29.52), $\boldsymbol{J}$ is the equivalent current density, and $\boldsymbol{M}$ is the equivalent magnetic current density on the surface of the dielectric head/body or phantom. These equivalent current densities are related to the tangential total surface magnetic and electric fields:

$$\boldsymbol{J}(r') = \boldsymbol{a}_n \times \boldsymbol{H}(r') \tag{29.53}$$

$$\boldsymbol{M}(r') = \boldsymbol{E}(r') \times \boldsymbol{a}_n \tag{29.54}$$

Thus, combining the electric and magnetic sources, the scattered fields in region 1 (external region) are given as ($\boldsymbol{a}_{n1}$ is outward at the surface S, for r on or outside the surface S)

$$\boldsymbol{E}_1^s(r) = -j\omega\boldsymbol{A}(r) + \frac{\nabla\nabla\cdot\boldsymbol{A}(r)}{j\omega\mu_1\varepsilon_1} - \frac{1}{\varepsilon_1}\nabla\times\boldsymbol{F}(r) = -j\frac{k_1^2+\nabla\nabla\cdot}{\omega\mu_1\varepsilon_1}\boldsymbol{A}_1(r) - \frac{1}{\varepsilon_1}\nabla\times\boldsymbol{F}(r)_1 \tag{29.55}$$

$$\boldsymbol{H}_1^s(r) = -j\frac{k_1^2+\nabla\nabla\cdot}{\omega\mu_1\varepsilon_1}\boldsymbol{F}_1(r) + \frac{1}{\mu_1}\nabla\times\boldsymbol{A}_1(r) \tag{29.56}$$

The scattered fields in region 2, the ROI, are given as ($\boldsymbol{a}_{n2}$ is inward at the surface S with the changed sign, for r on or inside the surface S)

$$\boldsymbol{E}_2^s(r) = j\frac{k_2^2+\nabla\nabla\cdot}{\omega\mu_2\varepsilon_2}\boldsymbol{A}_2(r) + \frac{1}{\varepsilon_2}\nabla\times\boldsymbol{F}_2(r) \tag{29.57}$$

$$\boldsymbol{H}_2^s(r) = j\frac{k_2^2+\nabla\nabla\cdot}{j\omega\mu_2\varepsilon_2}\boldsymbol{F}_2(r) - \frac{1}{\mu_2}\nabla\times\boldsymbol{A}_2(r) \tag{29.58}$$

Imposing boundary conditions, the tangential fields of both $\boldsymbol{E}$ and $\boldsymbol{H}$ are continuous of the arbitrary dielectric object. Thus, the combined field integral equations in terms of the equivalent surface currents, equations (29.53) and (29.54), are given as

$$\boldsymbol{M}(r') = \left\{ j\left[\frac{k_1^2+\nabla\nabla\cdot}{\omega\mu_1\varepsilon_1}\boldsymbol{A}_1(r) + \frac{k_2^2+\nabla\nabla\cdot}{\omega\mu_2\varepsilon_2}\boldsymbol{A}_2(r)\right] + \nabla\times\left[\frac{\boldsymbol{F}(r)_1}{\varepsilon_1} + \frac{\boldsymbol{F}(r)_2}{\varepsilon_2}\right] + \boldsymbol{E}^{\mathrm{inc}}\right\} \times a_n \quad \text{for } r \text{ on the surface } S \tag{29.59}$$

$$J(r') = a_n \times \left\{ j \left[\frac{k_1^2 + \nabla\nabla\cdot}{\omega\mu_1\varepsilon_1} \boldsymbol{F}_1(r) + \frac{k_2^2 + \nabla\nabla\cdot}{\omega\mu_2\varepsilon_2} \boldsymbol{F}_2(r) \right] + \nabla \times \left[\frac{\boldsymbol{A}(r)_1}{\mu_1} + \frac{\boldsymbol{A}(r)_2}{\mu_2} \right] + \boldsymbol{H}^{\text{inc}} \right\} \quad \text{for } r \text{ on the surface } S \tag{29.60}$$

The vector potentials $\boldsymbol{A}$ and $\boldsymbol{F}$ are in terms of the unknown surface current densities $\boldsymbol{J}$ and $\boldsymbol{M}$, respectively.

29.2.1.1 *Moment Method of Solution*

The surface is subdivided into triangles in a tessellation, and the current densities in each triangle are the unknowns and form the basis functions. The favored vector basis functions are the Rao–Wilton–Gleason (RWG) functions.[1,3] The electrical and magnetic current densities are expanded as

$$\boldsymbol{J}(r') = \sum_{n=1}^{n=N} \boldsymbol{J}_n \boldsymbol{f}_n(r) \tag{29.61}$$

$$\boldsymbol{M}(r') = \sum_{n=1}^{n=N} \boldsymbol{M}_n \boldsymbol{f}_n(r) \tag{29.62}$$

where N is the number of unknown functions being evaluated.

Each triangle on the surface S has three sides, and there are a maximum of six RWG basis functions in each triangle, three representing the electrical current density and the other three representing the magnetic current density, all the currents flowing perpendicular to the sides. These are substituted in equations (29.60) and (29.61), and the exercise is now to evaluate the unknown $\boldsymbol{J}_n$ and $\boldsymbol{M}_n$ values. The gradient, divergence operations in the equations are readily carried out.[3]

To evaluate the unknown magnitudes, testing functions identical to the basis functions are used with the inner products reducing the operators to matrix components

$$\langle f, g \rangle = \int_S g \cdot f \mathrm{d}S \tag{29.63}$$

The solution of the matrix equation provides the required field component distributions.

An example of the results is shown in a paper by Wang and Duyn.[2] This chapter also includes the excitation head surface coils in the formulation with the $\boldsymbol{E}^{\text{inc}}$ and $\boldsymbol{H}^{\text{inc}}$ terms. The chapter also considers the signal-to-noise ratio of RF coils. The details in the head have not been obtained with this approach. The calculation of the SAR at specific locations in the subject which is the human head is not possible with this technique unless further calculations obtain the interior fields. The technique discussed here is most useful for evaluating the performance of RF coils.[4]

29.2.2 Volumetric Integral Equation Approach

The calculation of the interior fields in an inhomogeneous lossy dielectric subject, for example, the human head/body in a MRI system, was first performed in 1996 by Jin *et al.*[5] Since then, two other papers have been published.[6,7] All of these papers use the fast Fourier transform (FFT) algorithm to perform their matrix vector multiplications and use a conjugate gradient method and its variations to solve the large rather full matrix equation. The Polimeridis paper[6] has been used as the basis for the analysis of MRI RF coils as discussed by Villena *et al.*[8] The weak form formulation pioneered by Zwamborn[9] was used by Huang[7] to speed up the solution time to about 7 min for the human head, and the results compare very well with those obtained using a commercial FDTD program. This weak form approach is discussed below.

The assumption is that the MRI object being scanned is an inhomogeneous isotropic lossy dielectric object, also termed the scatterer, which has a permeability $\mu_r = 1$ and a complex permittivity $\varepsilon_{\text{cr}}(r) = \varepsilon_r - j\sigma/(\omega\varepsilon_0)$. The object with a support domain Ω_d is embedded in a homogeneous free space background. The scatterer has an incident electric field E_{inc} generated by the RF coil during MRI. For the present calculation, the assumption is that the incident electric field is a plane wave. Invoking the volumetric equivalence principle,[7] the dielectric domain Ω_d is replaced by a polarizing electric current density

$$J_v(r) = j\omega\varepsilon_0[\varepsilon_{\text{cr}}(r) - 1]E(r) \quad r \in \Omega_d \tag{29.64}$$

The total electric field is given by the superposition of the incident electric field and the secondary scattered field and in the weak form formulation[9] with the magnetic vector potential $\boldsymbol{A}$. The domain integral equation is formulated in terms of the unknown electric flux density $\boldsymbol{D}(r)$, and the incident electric field becomes

$$E^{\text{inc}}(r) = \frac{\boldsymbol{D}(r)}{\varepsilon(r)} - (k_0^2 + \nabla\nabla\cdot)\boldsymbol{A}(r) \tag{29.65}$$

where the vector potential is defined as

$$A(r) = \frac{1}{\varepsilon_0}\int_{\Omega_d} G(r, r')\chi(r')D(r')\mathrm{d}r'' \tag{29.66}$$

where

$$G(r, r') = \frac{\mathrm{e}^{-jk_0(r-r')}}{4\pi|r - r'|} \tag{29.67}$$

and the contrast function χ is given as

$$\chi(r) = 1 - \frac{1}{\varepsilon_r} \tag{29.68}$$

The computational domain Ω is discretized in a uniform grid with contiguous small cuboid voxels Δx, Δy, Δz in size where the permittivity is constant in each voxel. Thus, the dielectric object is totally embedded in the rectangular block $M\Delta x\, N\Delta y\, P\Delta z$. In the cuboid voxel, rooftop basis functions $f^i(r)$, where $i = x, y, z$ are the coordinate directions. The choice of the flux density formulation $D(r)$ enables the continuity of normal flux density across voxel interface boundaries to be preserved. The expansion and the testing functions are identical roof top functions in one direction, with pulse functions repeated for the other two directions. The self-testing singularities are dealt with by taking the spherical average of the vector potential A, which then leads to a weak form of the Green's function. The grad div of the vector potential with the testing function is modified by applying the divergence theorem, and then the convolution integral is speeded up by taking the FFT of the two components, multiplying them, and taking the inverse FFT. The results are quite spectacular for a 7 min computational effort and compare very well with those from the FDTD results as seen in the following figures. Since the electric fields are known, the SAR is readily calculated as required, and then the MRI parameters are set to ensure the safety of the subject.

Note that these calculations assume plane wave excitation, and for the head, this is usually in the vertical downward direction. For calculation with a specific RF coil, please refer to the paper by Villena *et al.*[8]

RELATED ARTICLES IN EMAGRES

Birdcage Resonators: Highly Homogeneous Radiofrequency Coils for Magnetic Resonance

Coils for Insertion into the Human Body

Design and Use of Internal Receiver Coils for Magnetic Resonance Imaging

Multifrequency Coils for Whole Body Studies

Radiofrequency Systems and Coils for MRI and MRS

Refrigerated and Superconducting Receiver Coils in Whole Body Magnetic Resonance

Spatial Encoding Using Multiple rf Coils: SMASH Imaging and Parallel MRI

Surface Coil NMR: Detection with Inhomogeneous Radiofrequency Field Antennas

Surface and Other Local Coils for In Vivo Studies

Whole Body Machines: NMR Phased Array Coil Systems

TEM Transceiver Head Array Coils for Ultra High Magnetic Fields

TEM Arrays, Design and Implementation

Quadrature Surface Coils

Double-Tuned Surface Coils

Quadrature Transverse Electromagnetic (TEM) Surface Coils

Radiofrequency Fields and SAR for Transverse Electromagnetic (TEM) Surface Coils

Double-Tuned Birdcage Coils: Construction and Tuning

Radiofrequency Fields and SAR for Bird Cage Coils

TEM Body Coils

Transverse Electromagnetic (TEM) Surface Coils for Extremities

Receiver Loop Arrays

Coil Array Design for Parallel Imaging: Theory and Applications

Millipede Coils

Microcoils

Catheter Coils

Radiofrequency Heating Models and Measurements

Characterization of Multichannel Coil Arrays on the Benchtop

A Standard Procedure for Analyzing Radio Frequency MRI Coils

Litz Coils for High Resolution and Animal Probes, Especially for Double Resonance

RF Field Modeling for Double-Tuned Volume Coils

An Historical Introduction to Surface Coils: The Early Days

Transceiver Loop Arrays

Radiofrequency Coils for NMR: A Peripatetic History of Their Twists and Turns

Nested Surface Coils for Multinuclear NMR

Birdcage Volume Coil Design

RF Safety of Active Implantable Medical Devices

Bioeffects and Safety of Radiofrequency Electromagnetic Fields

Radiofrequency Fields: Interactions, Biological Effects, and Safety Issues

RF Device Safety and Compatibility

Safety Considerations in MRI

REFERENCES

1. K. Umashankar, A. Taflove, and S. M. Rao, *IEEE Trans. Antennas Propag.*, 1997, **34**, 758.
2. S. Wang and J. H. Duyn, *Phys. Med. Biol.*, 2006, **51**, 3211.
3. S. M. Rao, D. R. Wilton, and A. W. Glisson, *IEEE Trans. Antennas Propag.*, 1982, **30**, 409.
4. S. Wang, J. A. de Zwart, and J. H. Duyn, *Phys. Med. Biol.*, 2011, **56**, 2779.
5. J. M. Jin, J. Chen, W. C. Chew, H. Gan, R. L. Magin, and P. J. Dimbylow, *Phys. Med. Biol.*, 1996, **41**, 2719.
6. A. G. Polimeridis, J. F. Villena, L. Daniel, and J. K. White, *J. Comput. Phys.*, 2014, **269**, 280.
7. S. Y. Huang, Z.-H. Ma, L. Wan, W. Yu, and J. T. Vaughan, *J. Eng.*, 2018, **2018**, 262.
8. J. F. Villena, A. G. Polimeridis, Y. Eryaman, E. Adalsteinsson, L. L. Wald, J. K. White, and L. Daniel, *IEEE Trans. Biomed. Eng.*, 2016, **63**, 2250.
9. P. Zwamborn and P. M. van den Berg, *IEEE Trans. Microw. Theory Tech.*, 1992, **40**, 1757.

Chapter 30

Safety Practices and Protocols in the MR Research Center of the Columbia University in the City of New York

Kathleen Durkin, Dania Elder, and David H. Gultekin

Columbia University, New York, NY, USA

30.1 INTRODUCTION

The development and management of safety programs at a large research university requires multidisciplinary approach and teamwork. At the Columbia Magnetic Resonance Research Center, we have implemented a series of safety practices and protocols to protect participants, researchers, and the magnetic resonance imaging (MRI) systems. This chapter briefly discusses the risks of magnetic resonance (MR) research and the practices we have established to mitigate those risks.

Risks:

- Main Magnetic Field
  - Displacement force
  - Torque
- Radiofrequency Field
  - Induced heating
  - Induced currents interfering with the electronics present in/near the scanner in/on patients
- Gradient Field
  - Peripheral nerve stimulation
  - Acoustic noise
- Mitigation Practices
  - For research participants
  - For attendants (caretaker, parent, and other family member)
  - For support personnel (e.g., MR technologists)
  - For researchers
  - For emergency responders

30.2 MAIN MAGNETIC FIELD RISKS

- Displacement force
- Torque

*Main Magnetic Field (**B0**).* When considering the potential hazards of an MRI machine, we generally think of the main magnetic field, or the static magnetic field. Like most MRIs in research, Columbia University works with superconducting magnets, and their field is associated with a strong magnetic attraction called ferromagnetism. The 'missile effect' describes how metallic objects are affected by a magnetic field: they can move toward the magnet at speeds

Safety and Biological Effects in MRI.
Edited by Devashish Shrivastava and J. Thomas Vaughan

ISBN: 978-1-118-82130-5
Also published in eMagRes (online edition)
DOI: 10.1002/9780470034590.emrstm1565

≥40 mph.[1,2] Imaging centers around the world have been known to have had serious incidents, including patient fatalities, when objects such as ferromagnetic oxygen tanks entered the MRI room. We have implemented many safety practices to minimize the risk of the missile effect. Metallic implants can also cause damage in a magnetic field. If a person with a ferromagnetic metallic implant enters the main magnetic field, the strong magnetic attraction can cause torque, displacement, or completely dislodge implants. The ***B0*** field can also cause the malfunction of components that are located within certain devices. The potential hazards of the main magnetic field must be managed with extreme caution. In our MR safety training courses, we emphasize that the main magnetic field is always on, in comparison to both the RF and gradient fields which are only activated during scanning.

30.3 RADIOFREQUENCY FIELD RISKS

- Induced heating
- Induced currents interfering with the electronics present in/near the scanner in/on patients

Radiofrequency Field (RF). At Columbia MR Research Center, we know users are less familiar with the risks of the RF field, also known as the ***B1*** field, compared to their familiarity with the ***B0***-related risks. This field can induce harmful heating on the surface as well as deep within a patient.[3] For that reason, we decided it was imperative that all users are educated on these RF field risks. According to the Food and Drug Administration (FDA), the most reported incidents within MR have been in relation to heating/burns.[4–7] RF fields can also interfere with the electronics in/near the scanner or in/on patients (e.g., cardiac pacemakers or other implanted electronics).

30.4 GRADIENT FIELD RISKS

- Peripheral nerve stimulation (PNS)
- Acoustic noise

Gradient Field (dB/dt). Users tend to know about the time-varying gradient field because it causes the loud noises people associate with MRI scans. However, noise is not the only concern. The gradient field works by constantly switching gradient coils on and off. This subjects the body to induced electric fields. One main concern with the gradient field is peripheral nerve stimulation, or PNS. This field may cause stimulation of muscles, limbs, and nerves.[8]

Acoustic Noise. The loud noises pose another kind of risk, of course. Acoustic vibrations as loud as 140 dB have been measured during some MR sequences,[9] and participants who lacked hearing protection during scans have reported acoustic injuries.[10] The Columbia MR Research Center requires participants to wear hearing protection with at least a 29 dB noise reduction rating (NRR) specified by American National Standards Institute (ANSI) recommendations.

30.5 MITIGATION PRACTICES

30.5.1 Mitigation Practices for Research Participants: Before the Scan

Institutional ethics approval of the research study. Before a human participant walks into an MR scan room at the Columbia MR Research Center, the researcher's study must have Institutional Review Board (IRB) approval. As per Code of Federal Regulations, Title 21 (21 CFR), a research study that uses MR must have institutional approval from the IRB in place before the first MRI scan. This is the first chance for committee members to assess a study for safety and ethics, by reviewing scanning procedures, recruitment methods, consent forms, screening forms, and staffing. Like many major research facilities, Columbia University has an in-house IRB. Some outside institutions are known to outsource the work of reviewing studies to a private IRB company. An IRB may alternately be referred to as an Independent Ethics Committee (IEC), Ethical Review Board (ERB), or Research Ethics Board (REB).

Similarly, we require all research studies at Columbia University that use live animals to have Institutional Animal Care and Use Committee (IACUC) approval before the study can begin. In fact, every institution that uses animals for federally funded laboratory research must have an IACUC within the organization.

Similar to all medical device investigators, Columbia researchers who are working to determine the safety and effectiveness of a new device must have an FDA investigational device exemption (IDE). If the IRB decides that the device involves significant risk, the FDA will need to approve the IDE.[11]

The principal investigator (PI) is responsible for learning the IRB/IACUC policies for their institution, completing the IRB/IACUC application, obtaining an IDE if applicable, and providing all the information requested. We work with them to provide information and guidance as requested/needed.

We encourage Columbia University PIs to submit their application to the IRB/IACUC committee as soon as they can. Research may not be conducted until after approval is granted, and the approval process can take some time. Columbia also offers expedited IRB/IACUC procedures if the research involves no more than minimal risk to participants/subjects.

Safety screening. Research participants enrolling in any Columbia MRI research study are screened in advance by the PI or their trained research staff. We use an MRI screening form, and researchers work with their participants to complete the form prior to entering Zone III or IV (Zones are explained below). The Columbia MR Research Center uses a five-part screening process:

1. Verbal screening
2. Screening form documentation
3. Metal detector
4. Magnets
5. Ferrodetector

We require all personnel with the intent to enter the magnet room (Zone IV) to complete their own safety screening form in advance. This happens during their initial safety training, and the MR safety officer reviews each form. We instruct them to complete the form again if any of their answers change. They are aware that the static magnetic field (***B0***) is always on, and that the field is strongest in the middle of the bore of the magnet (the isocenter). The magnetic attraction decreases with distance from the magnet. At a certain distance, the magnetic field decreases to 5 G. Five gauss and below are considered 'safe' levels of static magnetic field exposure for the general public. We have placed 5 G line markings on the floors of all the magnet rooms.

We perform safety screening procedures for every person entering the MR suite. This includes researchers, staff, participants, parents/caretakers accompanying a participant, one-time visitors on a tour, short-term interns, maintenance workers who need to enter the room for any reason, vendors installing or maintaining equipment in the MR room, public relations staff taking pictures or making videos (while keeping all cameras outside the 5 G line), and anyone else who needs to enter the room for any reason. Since the magnet is always on, the risk from the static magnetic field (***B0***) is always present.

At our center, we require researchers to complete the prospective participant's safety screening form on two occasions before being scanned. They generally administer the form as part of their initial participant recruitment process. Once, in advance, to obtain any potential contraindication or device safety information. Then, it is completed again on the day of the MRI scan, in case anything has changed since they were initially recruited. The MR technologist or other certified MR operator (the 'reviewer') reviews the completed form, asks questions about any potential problems, and confirms the safety of each participant before proceeding to scan.

If there are any unknowns or other concerns, and the reviewer cannot reasonably guarantee the person's safety in the magnet room, the reviewer requests additional information about the unknown item. If the researcher or participant cannot provide sufficient information, the reviewer denies the person entry to the magnet room and the participant cannot be scanned. An implant, medical device, or other objects may be considered 'unknown', that is, the participant may have an implant but does not know the make, model, and material (Table 30.1).

If there are no concerns, trained personnel validate and approve the screening form. The prospective participant is deemed safe to scan, and they may proceed with preparations. We instruct all participants to change into scrubs or gowns since clothing can contain metallic components such as zippers or metallic threads. We also have participants remove all their personal belongings and devices, including watches, jewelry, and activity trackers such as Fitbits. If the participant's screening form indicated they wear a drug delivery patch, we ask them to remove it. All of their belongings must be stored in a locker, especially items that could be hazardous or damaged in the magnetic field such as cell phones and credit cards. All of these steps are necessary to minimize the likelihood of a metallic object entering the MRI room.

The participant's risks in the scanner include more than those associated with ferrous metal or electronic implants. The reviewer must also be aware of tattoos, markings/makeup, or other implants that could increase the participant's risk for RF burns.

Pregnancy. We developed policies to treat pregnant participants with extra caution. This is so since the effects of the three fields on pregnant people and fetuses

Table 30.1. Unacceptable reasons to make exceptions

Unacceptable reasons to allow an unknown implant or item in the magnet room	Rationale
'My doctor says I can be scanned in an MRI' without accompanying information about an implant's make and model	The doctor may not be qualified to make that determination. The make and model information are needed so the reviewer can look up its safety status on the manufacturer's website or through FDA and learn of its safety status/label
'I've had an MRI since I've gotten this implant'	According to the American College of Radiology Guidance Document on MR Safe Practices: 'prior uneventful MRI examinations do not ensure subsequent uneventful procedures'[4,6]

are unknown (and high temperature, such as the one that can be induced due to RF power deposition during MRI is a known teratogen).[12,13] For clinical scans, the Department of Radiology at Columbia University Irving Medical Center/New York-Presbyterian Hospital scans pregnant people in normal mode whenever possible. However, we have different standard at the Columbia MR Research Center since research provides no clinical benefit for the participant, unlike a clinically recommended MR scan. This means the risk of a research MRI scan for a pregnant person, even in normal mode, may not be justified. Columbia's IRB generally requires urine pregnancy tests on the day of the scan for participants who are able to bear children. Pregnant people are not scanned unless the study's IRB specifically states they can be scanned. If a pregnant person does participate in a research study, there are additional risks if the MRI scan includes administering contrast agent. Administration of gadolinium-based contrast agent (GBCA) to pregnant participants must be evaluated for various risks to the parent and fetus. The primary risk is that gadolinium chelates may accumulate in the amniotic fluid and potentially dissociate into free gadolinium ions, which may present a risk for the development of nephrogenic systemic fibrosis (NSF) in the fetus or parent.[14]

Temperature, humidity, electricity, and ventilation are carefully managed in the scanning spaces in the Columbia MR Center. Participant screening is critical, but environmental controls are also important to minimize risks during an MR scan. Excess humidity and high temperature in the scan room can be detrimental to subjects' normal cooling processes and may increase the risk of burn/heat stress in participants.[12,13] The Columbia MR Research Center partners with Columbia Facilities to maintain appropriate environmental settings:

- Monitoring and adjusting the temperature and humidity in Zone IV is critical. We maintain the temperature (≤22 °C, or 72 °F) and humidity (≤60%) as recommended by the MR manufacturers in the magnet room. We have also established a protocol for users to report deviation from these standards and receive immediate attention.
- We have established a system for uninterrupted power including backup or generator connections.
- With Siemens, we work to manage cryogen and adjacent equipment. Columbia Facilities conduct regular checks of the ventilation system to be prepared in case of a quench.

Our building staffers work to accommodate researchers' requests for structural changes to the rooms or equipment. We have responsive operations workers who are familiar with the unique needs of MR systems, like power requirements and shielded walls.

30.5.2 Mitigation Practices for Research Participants: During the Scan

Missile effect. To minimize the risk of ferromagnetic items entering the magnet room, we have installed ferromagnetic detectors in our MRI control rooms. Unlike a conventional metal detector, ferromagnetic detectors differentiate between ferrous objects and nonferrous objects. The system sounds its alarm if it detects objects that attract to the magnet. ACR states 'the use of ferromagnetic detection systems is recommended as an adjunct to thorough and conscientious screening of persons and devices approaching Zone IV'. This provides a clear warning to anyone entering the MR environment with potentially hazardous medical devices, tools, and metallic objects. If the ferromagnetic detector indicates a hazardous entry, the user

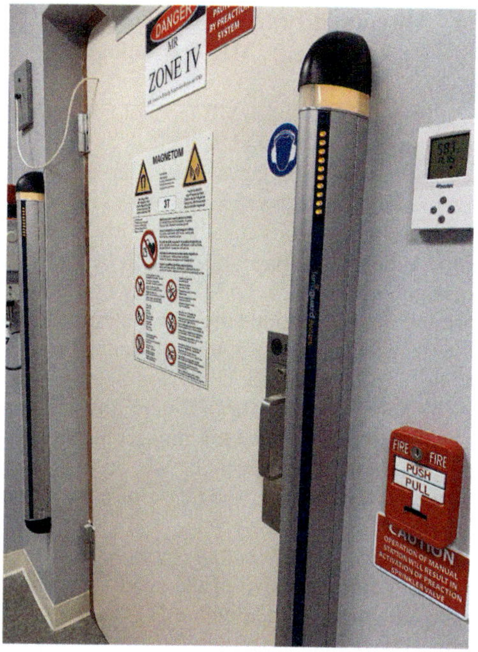

Figure 30.1. Ferromagnetic detectors

is immediately alerted that this object is MR-unsafe, thus reducing the potential for an MR-related incident or injury (Figure 30.1).

Thermal risk. The Columbia MR Research Center takes the following precautions to prevent local thermal risk, damage, pain, or systemic thermal stress during scanning:

- We prevent skin-to-skin contact that can result in loop burns. The participant's body parts should not come in direct contact. Hands are not to be intertwined, and legs should not be crossed. This prevents the formation of conductive loops through adjacent tissue contact with arms or legs.
- We use a minimum of 5 mm padding to separate a participant's limbs and body from the magnet bore, to decrease the risk of proximity and loop burns. A single sheet is not sufficient to create this 5 mm separation. Multiple sheets, blankets, or padding is required.
- We route cables in a straight line. We do not coil cables or allow them to touch the participant.
- We use the lowest possible specific absorption rate (SAR) values in the scanning.
- We communicate with the participant before, during, and after the scan. This is critical to preventing burns. Before the scan, we advise the participant that they should alert us if they feel any heating or tingling of any kind. We explain the communication tools and methods (squeeze ball, microphone in the magnet room, and speaker at the console) and emphasize they should not wait until a sensation is uncomfortable. We check in frequently during the scan. After the scan, we ask if they felt any discomfort while in the scanner.

Acoustic damage risk. We require participants to wear earplugs with sufficient/MR manufacturer's recommended specifications to reduce the risk of hearing damage. Depending on the requirements of the study, they may also wear headphones. The Columbia MR Research Center has incorporated added protection using an audio system with active noise-canceling technology.

Cryogen leak risk. We continuously monitor oxygen levels in the scanning spaces in the Columbia MR Center. A decrease in oxygen can indicate a possible cryogen (helium) leakage. All Columbia University MR suites contain two oxygen monitors in Zone III that display the oxygen level in the MRI magnet room (Zone IV) and the control room. Monitors sound an alarm if levels drop below 19%, and all personnel are trained to evacuate the area immediately (Figure 30.2).

Incidental findings (IFs) can arise in the course of research. The Columbia MR Research Center has a policy of informing research participants of IFs. We have established a system where a Columbia MD contacts participants, discusses the finding and its potential implications, and provides them with resources to pursue additional follow-up care where appropriate. The entire IF follow-up process is managed in a systematic way, and in a way that holds researchers accountable for complying with the guidelines. This makes it easier for our researchers to be in compliance. Our process contains the following components:

- a health insurance portability and accountability act (HIPAA)-compliant procedure for securely transferring images to radiologists for review
- a procedure to obtain reports from radiologist
- guidelines for determining which IFs are sufficiently severe to warrant informing the participant
- a procedure for informing the participant of the IF and referring them to Columbia University Medical Center for further evaluation and consultation.

Details of the Columbia MR Research Center IF policy, process, and documents are provided in the standard operating procedures.

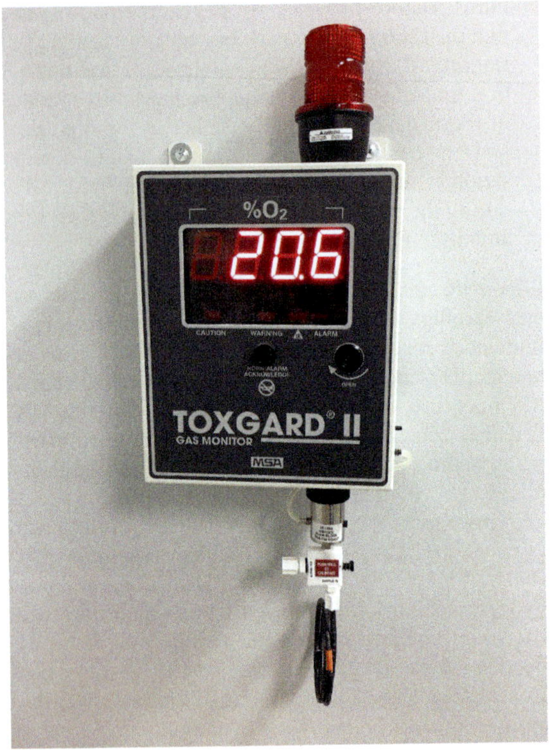

Figure 30.2. Oxygen monitor

30.5.3 Mitigation Practices for Attendants (Caretaker, Parent, and Other Family Member)

Most practices that mitigate risk for research participants also apply to attendants.

IRB approval: The attendants are present at an IRB-approved study, even though they are not participating.

Safety screening: Attendants are screened for safety using the same five-step process as we use with the participant.

Acoustic damage risk: Just as we require participants to wear earplugs and/or headphones with sufficient specifications to reduce the risk of hearing damage, caregivers must also wear hearing protection.

RF field-related risks: Caretakers sit outside of the magnet bore, and therefore have a much lower risk of PNS or RF heating than the participant. For this reason, it is not necessary to implement the same precautions as we do for the participant in the scanner.

30.5.4 Mitigation Practices for Support Personnel (e.g., MR Technologists)

Support personnel includes MR technologists, the MR platform safety officer and technical assistant, and nonresearch staff. They have a number of responsibilities in and around the MR systems. Technologists must acquire high-quality data, keep participants safe, and also keep themselves and their colleagues safe. Nonresearch staff must keep MR safety in mind while performing their job around the MR systems. Safety is our top priority, and our support personnel are given all the resources they need. We have implemented the following safety practices to mitigate risk to support personnel: extensive safety training including annual refreshers, zoning with signage, MR area access restrictions, device labeling, and the same safety screening used for participants.

Risk of magnetic field-related harm. Safety training is the most comprehensive of the safety practices we have implemented. All Columbia MR Research Center support personnel are required to attend MR safety training. This includes all staff members who will be working in the MR systems, if they will be attending the MR scans, bringing research participants or animals into the magnet room, or operating the MR system.

We also train nonresearch staff (security and facilities) in MR safety if they work in any of the Columbia MR Research Center buildings. Educating nonresearch staff in a facility that contains MRI systems helps reduce the likelihood of MR-related incidents. Nonresearch staff may need to enter the magnet room or the scan console room when installing or working with MR-related hardware and software, doing general building maintenance, providing security, or cleaning. Nonresearch staff safety training is a separate training class than the researchers' training class, since the material does not need as much detail and needs no information about working with participants or animals. There is also a separate test for nonresearch staff.

People who do need MR safety training include:

- Employees/technologists/researchers who will need to enter the console room or the magnet room at any time at all, for any reason at all, with or without an accompanying staff member (researchers, research support staff, students, unpaid interns, visiting researchers, and building staff)
- Facilities, security, and janitorial staff who work in buildings with MR systems.

People who do not need MR safety training include:

- Researchers and research support staff who will never attend MR scans
- Visitors on a tour of the MR spaces accompanied by an MR platform staff member (the screening process is required if they enter the magnet room on the tour)
- Facilities, security, and janitorial staff who work in buildings that lack MR systems
- Research participants
- Firefighters and paramedics in emergency situations

Columbia's MR safety training is on-site and in-person. Training includes a tour of the MR rooms (control rooms, magnet rooms, supply areas, animal prep rooms, and participant changing areas), a lecture, and a safety video. We have made annual safety training refreshers (reviewing material and retesting) available online. Online review is more convenient, and this correlates with greater compliance. The Columbia MR Research Center requires in-person safety training every 4 years.

We have implemented a process that allows researchers to train and be certified in scanner operation. This training and certification allow certified personnel to operate the MRI independently, frees them from the limitations of the MR technologist's schedule, and enables them to pay a lower hourly rate for their scan time, compared to researchers who do need the MR technologist's assistance. The training is only available to researchers who have already completed Level II safety training and includes:

1. Hands-on training in scanner operation
2. Running several scans under close observation of the MR technologist or another Level III-certified researcher
3. Hands-on practical exam.

Expedited certification is an option for highly experienced researchers, at the discretion of the MR senior technical director.

Risk of untrained people entering the magnet room. We have implemented three practices to minimize the risk of untrained and unscreened people encountering the magnetic field: zoning, restricted access, and signage (Diagrams 30.1 and 30.2). As per the recommendations of the American College of Radiology, every building that has an MR system has been divided into four safety zones (Zone I, Zone II, Zone III, and Zone IV), which correspond to the level of risk from MR systems. The Columbia MR Research Center restricts access to certain zones using security personnel, ID cards, swipe card-activated turnstiles and elevators, and locked doors. Signs indicate the level of MR risk in a room. The zones are:

1. Zone I: public spaces in the building. Zone I is the area any person may enter before they encounter any security staff or access restriction. The lobbies of the Neurological Institute, the Kolb Annex and Pardes Building of the New York State Psychiatric Institute, the Nathan S. Kline Institute, and the Jerome L. Greene Science Center are the Zone I areas in the Columbia MR Research Center. These buildings have security staff, swipe card-activated turnstiles, or both to restrict access beyond Zone I. A person who wants access into the building to do MR research must first complete MR safety training. Building access beyond the lobby is not automatically granted for all Columbia faculty, staff, and students. The access policy for MR buildings is more restrictive than for other campus or hospital buildings at Columbia University.
2. Zone II: the area past the initial security desk/turnstiles, up to the door to the MR control room (aka Zone III). Some Columbia buildings have additional security features within Zone II (like card swipe access in the elevators or locked MR suite doors). After the users have completed their safety training, we grant them access through these additional security features as well, all the way to the locked control room door at Zone III. Many people have access to Zone II despite having never completed MR safety training, since all Columbia MR Center buildings contain labs and offices for researchers who do not use MR in their work. This is acceptable from a safety point of view because they are still unable to enter Zone III and thus are restricted from accessing the MR systems.
3. Zone III: the MR console room. Access through the MR console room door into Zone III is the most restricted. We grant Level III access to certified MR system operators (Level III certification) only and a select few MR platform staff members who need access to this room to do their jobs. The locked door to Zone III prevents accidental entry by untrained people. Researchers with only Level II safety training can work in Zone III, but they must have a Level III operator present at all times. The Level III person allows them into the

MR control room, operates the MR system during the scan, and oversees all safety procedures during the scan. This means no one can be in Zone III without a Level III-certified person also present.

4. Zone IV: the MR magnet room. At Columbia, the door between the MR console room (Zone III) and the magnet room (Zone IV) is unlocked. This is acceptable because there is adequate security at Zone II and Zone III entry points. The door to Zone IV is kept closed at all times except when people need to enter or exit the room. The Level III-certified person at the scan oversees all safety procedures and ensures that only metal-free and safety screened people can enter Zone IV.

The zones can be visualized with these diagrams (Diagrams 30.1 and 30.2):

The red indicates doors that must be kept locked or secured with some other security measure.

Signage is required to ensure MR users are aware of their MR risk. The required signs are:

We have posted yellow 'Zone III' signs (Figure 30.3) on doors that connect Zone II (like a waiting room or a hallway) to Zone III (the MR console room). The sign is posted on the exterior (that is, the Zone II side) of the door. We keep the door between Zone II and Zone III locked at all times. At the Columbia MR Research Center locations, we grant key card swipe access into Zone III only to people who have completed Level III MR scanner operation training. (There are a select few exceptions: a few staff members such as veterinary technicians and MR administrators who lack Level III certification, but do have Zone III access, since it is necessary for them to do their jobs. All exceptions were discussed by the safety or governance committee in advance. We maintain a record of these exceptions.) This locked door physically restricts access to Zone III because the door in Zone III leading to the Zone IV, the magnet room, is unlocked (Figure 30.4).

Black, white, and red 'Zone IV' signs are posted on the exterior of the door that connects Zone III (the MR control room) with Zone IV (the magnet room). At Columbia, this door is kept unlocked. Access to this unlocked door is physically restricted by the locked door with the yellow 'Zone III' sign, which separates Zone II from Zone III.

Columbia University does not have signage for Zone I and Zone II since those areas make up the vast majority of the building (and the universe).

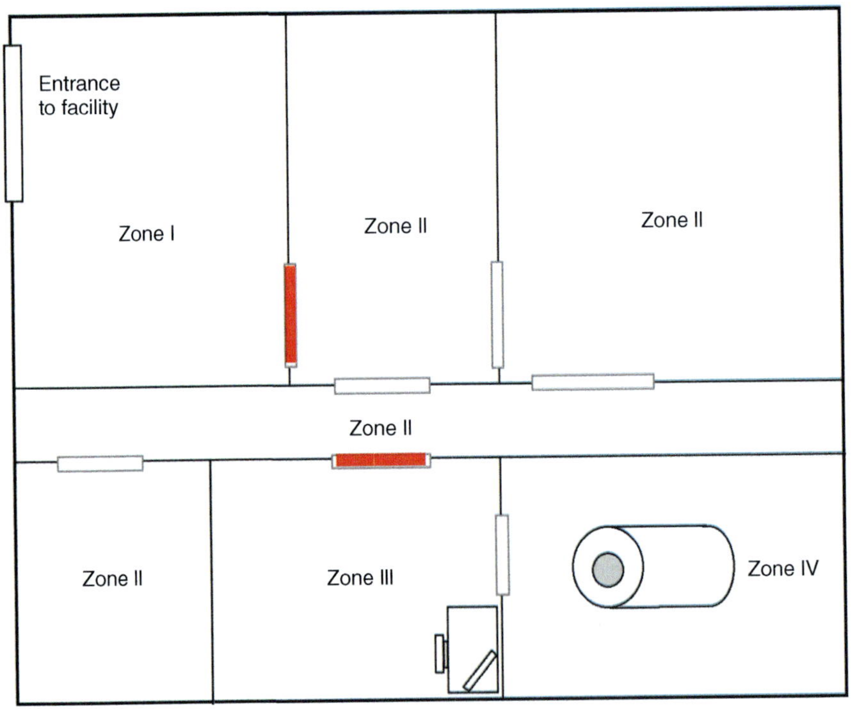

Diagram 30.1. MR zones

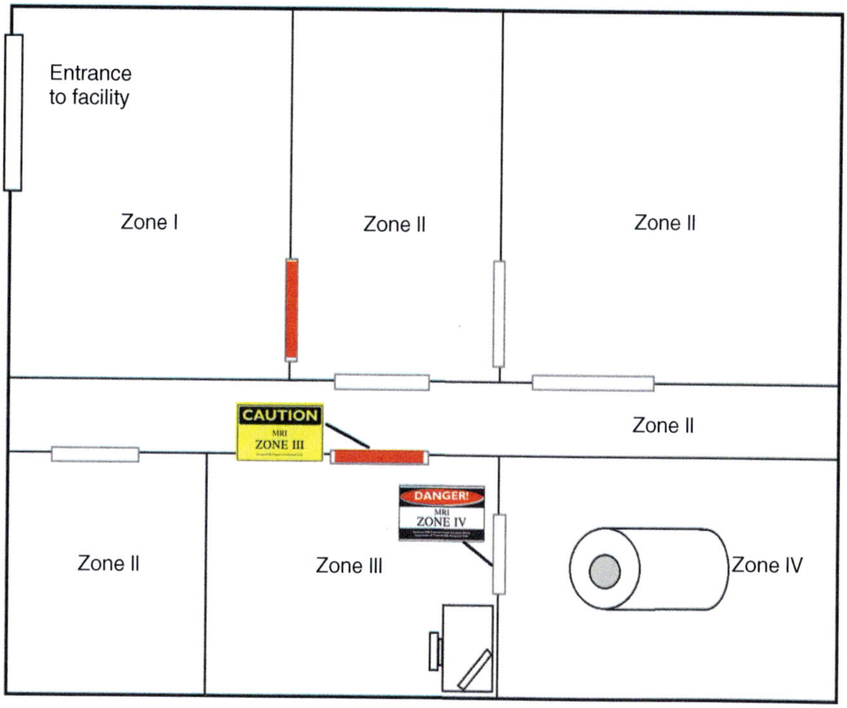

Diagram 30.2. MR zones with signs

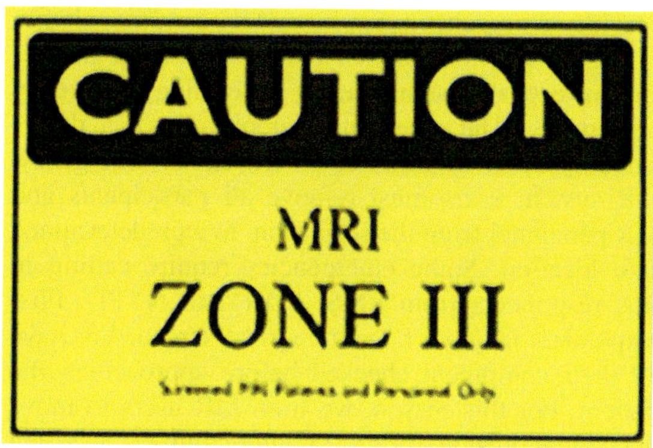

Figure 30.3. Zone III sign

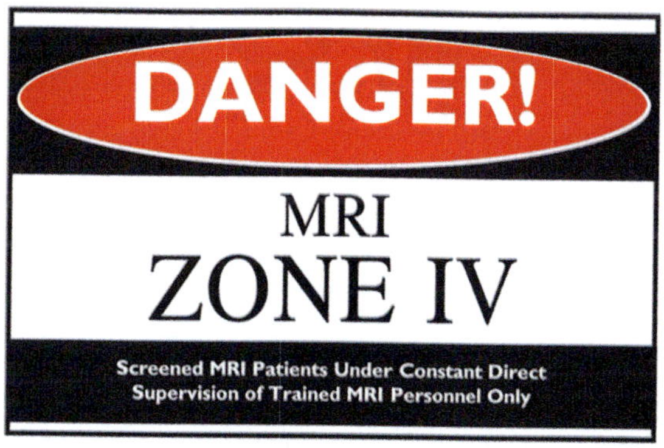

Figure 30.4. Zone IV sign

In the model, the signage would appear in the following locations:

Risks from items entering Zone IV. Devices, equipment, lab supplies, office supplies, and tools can become missiles within a magnetic field and cause severe injury or death. We use the FDA-recognized standards for device labeling, so MR users know which items are safe to bring into Zone IV (MR-safe), which are safe in Zone IV under certain conditions (MR-conditional), and which items must stay out of Zone IV (MR-unsafe).

We test and label all MR platform devices (tools, metal detectors, and research-related equipment such as response devices or physiology monitors) using The American Society for Testing Materials (ASTM) International Standard F2503.[15] Columbia researchers who

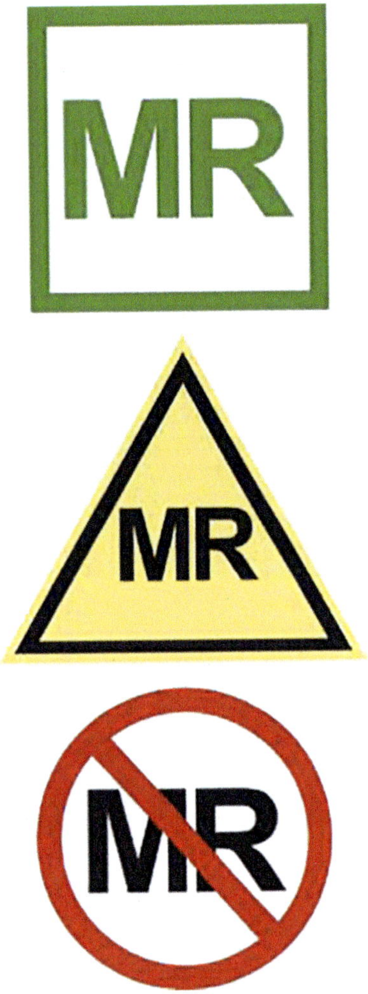

Figure 30.5. Labels to indicate the safety of an item

bring their own items to a scan coordinate with the MR safety officer and MR technologist before the scan to determine the safety of the items and label them accordingly. We perform these tests first using metal detector wands to establish the presence of metal or electronic components. If metal is present, we use small magnets to determine if the metal is ferrous. Testing can occur anywhere outside Zone IV and can take place any time before an item is brought into Zone IV. Columbia MR Research Center safety training (both Level I and Level II) includes information about how to test items, and labels are provided by the center. The labels are:

We use green MR-safe labels to indicate the item is 100% metal free. We do not distinguish between ferrous and nonferrous metals. Examples include paper, glass, plastic, fabric, polyvinyl chloride (PVC), and carbon fiber items. The only way to determine if an item gets a green 'MR-safe' sticker is with a metal detector wand. If the wand indicates the presence of metal, then the item is not MR-safe.

We use yellow MR-conditional labels if the item has a nonferrous metal or conductive components, but the item is safe in Zone IV *under specific conditions*. The MR technologist and MR safety officer work with the user to know what the specific conditions are, but ultimately this is the user's responsibility. For example, an item may be safe only in a specific MR environment (conditional in 1.5 T may not be safe in 3 or 7 T).

We use red MR-unsafe labels when the item contains ferrous metal or unsafe conductive components. MR-unsafe devices can never enter Zone IV.

If any item is unlabeled, users are trained to assume it is MR-unsafe (Figure 30.5).

Risks from serious emergencies including those that require emergency medical services (EMS), Fire Department of the City of New York (FDNY), and New York City Police Department (NYPD). Safety training at the Columbia MR Research Center includes procedures for emergency management. We provide emergency supplies (MR-conditional fire extinguishers, first aid kits, and crash carts) at all sites and have posted signs clearly describing emergency procedures. The emergency supplies have a designated location in Zone II or III. In an emergency, MR system users must remove all participants and MR personnel from the scan room to a predetermined safe location. Some emergencies require calling in first responders from EMS, FDNY, or NYPD. First responders may not have time to be screened or have all their equipment checked before approaching the patient. For this reason, we train MR users to move the patient outside of Zone IV after calling 911. When emergency personnel need to come to Columbia, the MR user strictly monitors access to Zone IV. Emergency personnel are not allowed into Zone IV under any circumstances unless the magnetic field decreases to 5 G. This can only happen with a quench.

As previously discussed, the magnet is always on. However, certain situations may require partial or complete shutdowns: either shutting off the power to the MR system, or in extreme circumstances, shutting down the magnet itself. Natural disasters can affect MR systems, as we saw firsthand in the northeast blackout in 2003 and Hurricane Sandy in 2012. Everyone who attends MR safety training is taught about the use of the emergency power button and the system quench button. The training includes the locations of, and the difference between, these two buttons. The quench button and the power button are sited inside the MRI room in Zone IV, as well as in the control room in Zone III. Each button has an indication of use.

Pressing the power button cuts power to all of the MR systems except the magnet, and the magnetic field is not affected. MR system users are trained to push the MR emergency power button only in these cases:

- Natural disasters: an earthquake, a tornado, and an impending storm/hurricane with likely flooding
- Active flooding the control room (Zone III), the magnet room (Zone IV), or the equipment room (Zone III)
- An electrical accident in Zone IV
- A fire of any size in Zone IV.

MR system users are taught that, after they shut down the power, they must remain in Zone III and keep Zone IV secure. Even with the power down, the magnet is still on in Zone IV.

Two types of quenches exist: spontaneous and intentional. A spontaneous quench is rare and occurs due to a machine malfunction, fire, or natural disaster. An intentional quench happens when MR personnel initiate it during an emergency situation. When a quench occurs, almost all of the helium will escape safely through the quench vents to the outside air, posing no serious danger. However, if there is a failure of the ventilation system, there *is* danger. Helium will accumulate in the magnet room, causing a fog. This can displace oxygen and make temperatures and hardware dangerously cold. Prolonged exposure to helium can result in asphyxiation or frostbite.

We train users that intentional quenches should be avoided at all costs, but an intentional quench is necessary when (Figures 30.6 and 30.7):

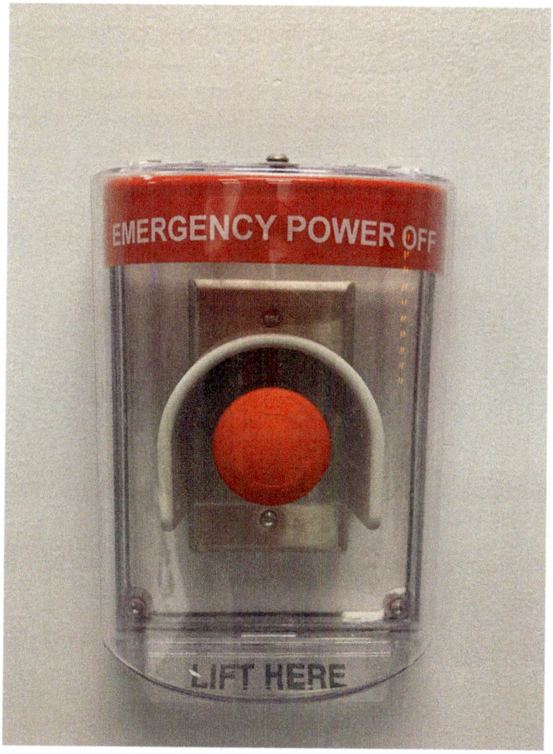

Figure 30.6. MR system power button

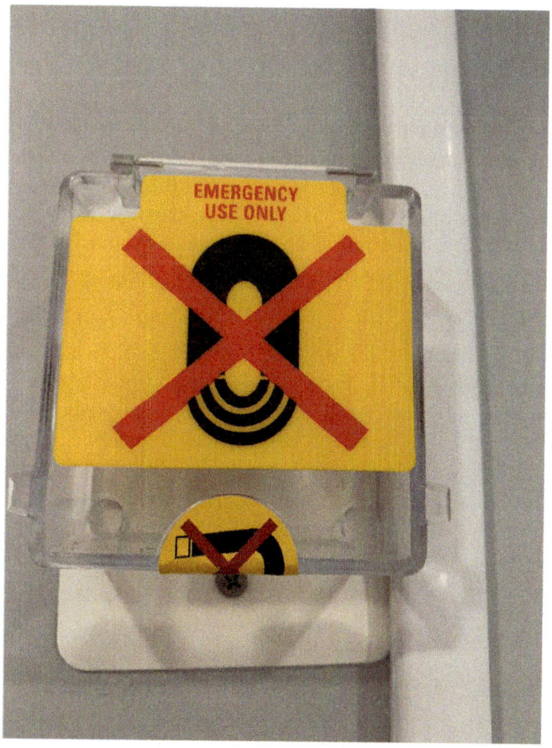

Figure 30.7. MR system quench button

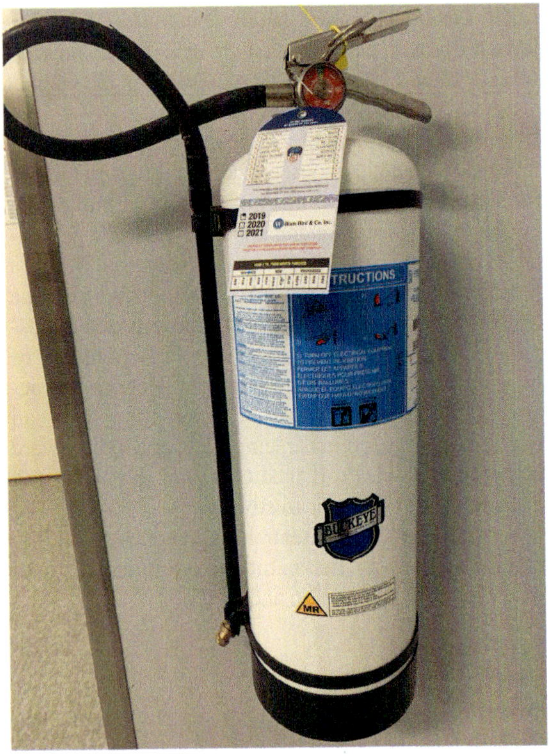

Figure 30.8. MR-conditional fire extinguisher

- The magnetic field is causing a life-threatening emergency or injury (e.g., an oxygen tank is pinning a person to the MRI machine).
- A fire in Zone IV that is too large to extinguish with the MR-conditional fire extinguishers and FDNY responders need to enter the room safely.

Fire Emergency. We provide MR-conditional extinguishers in all the MRI spaces, which are located in Zone III. Extra extinguishers are stationed in the hallways. Smaller fires can be extinguished by safety-trained staffers. Larger, uncontrollable fires will require a quench if emergency responders and the FDNY are needed to contain and extinguish the fire. The only way this can be safe is if the magnet is quenched and the magnetic field decays to 5 G or lower (Figure 30.8).

30.5.5 Mitigation Practices for Researchers

The practices that mitigate risk for research support staff also apply to researchers. A researcher who attends scans or operates the MR system has the same responsibilities as support staff: data acquisition while also safekeeping their participant, colleagues, and themselves. We have implemented the following safety practices to mitigate risk to researchers: extensive safety training including annual refreshers, zoning with signage, MR area access restrictions, device labeling, and the same safety screening used for participants. An exception is for researchers who delegate 100% of the work of MR scanning to their lab members. Those researchers do not need to attend MR safety training if they will never go in Zone III or Zone IV, although they are welcome to attend if they want.

30.5.6 Mitigation Practices for Emergency Responders

We do not offer broad training for emergency responders such as emergency medical technicians, paramedics, firefighters, or police officers. In a situation that requires emergency responders, MR users are trained to call both 911 and Columbia Public Safety. We offer Level I training periodically to the Columbia Public Safety, Facilities Engineering and Operations personnel. The Public Safety team has relationships with the police stations, hospitals, and fire stations nearest to the different Columbia campuses. They coordinate with the first responders when they arrive at the building and bring them where they are needed, while other Public Safety officers help MR users to keep Zone IV secure. All MR users are trained to initiate a quench when necessary to ensure that first responders can enter Zone IV safely.

RELATED ARTICLES IN EMAGRES

Bottomley, Paul A.: The Development of High-Field NMR Imaging: 0.12 T to 1.5 T

Radiofrequency Heating Models and Measurements

REFERENCES

1. J. F. Schenck, *J. Magn. Reson. Imaging*, 2000, **12**, 2.
2. M. W. Carr and M. L. Grey, *Am. J. Nurs.*, 2002, **102**, 26.

3. T. Vaughan, L. DelaBarre, C. Snyder, J. Tian, C. Akgun, D. Shrivastava, W. Liu, C. Olson, G. Adriany, J. Strupp, P. Andersen, A. Gopinath, P. F. van de Moortele, M. Garwood, and K. Ugurbil, *Magn. Reson. Med.*, 2006, **56**, 1274.
4. Expert Panel on MR Safety, E. Kanal, A. J. Barkovich, C. Bell, J. P. Borgstede, W. G. Bradley Jr., J. W. Froelich, J. R. Gimbel, J. W. Gosbee, E. Kuhni-Kaminski, P. A. Larson, J. W. Lester Jr., J. Nyenhuis, D. J. Schaefer, E. A. Sebek, J. Weinreb, B. L. Wilkoff, T. O. Woods, L. Lucey, and D. Hernandez, *J. Magn. Reson. Imaging*, 2013, **37**, 501.
5. T. Gilk and E. Kanal, *J. Magn. Reson. Imaging*, 2013, **37**, 531.
6. ACR Committee on MR Safety, T. D. Greenberg, M. N. Hoff, T. B. Gilk, E. F. Jackson, E. Kanal, M. K. AM, J. G. Och, I. Pedrosa, T. L. Rampulla, S. B. Reeder, J. M. Rogg, F. G. Shellock, R. E. Watson, J. C. Weinreb, and D. Hernandez, *J. Magn. Reson. Imaging*, 2019, **51**, 331. DOI: 10.1002/jmri.26880.
7. J. G. Delfino, D. M. Krainak, S. A. Flesher, and D. L. Miller, *Med. Phys.*, 2019, **46**, 5562.
8. M. Davids, B. Guerin, M. Malzacher, and L. L. Wald, *Sci. Rep.*, **7**, 5316. DOI: 10.1038/s41598-017-05493-9.
9. P. Mansfield, P. Glover, and J. Beaumont, *Magn. Reson. Med.*, 1998, **39**, 539.
10. L. L. Tsai, A. K. Grant, K. J. Mortele, J. W. Kung, and M. P. Smith, *Radiographics*, 2015, **35**, 1722.
11. Food and Drug Administration (FDA), Device advice: investigational device exemption (IDE), Silver Spring, MD, USA, 2018 (www.fda.gov).
12. Food and Drug Administration (FDA), Magnetic resonance imaging, Silver Spring, MD, USA, 2018 (www.fda.gov).
13. D. Grainger, 'Safety Guidelines for Magnetic Resonance Imaging Equipment in Clinical Use', Medicines and Healthcare Products Regulatory Agency: London, UK, 2015.
14. ACR Committee on Drugs and Contrast Media, 'ACR Manual on Contrast Media', American College of Radiology (ACR), Reston, VA, USA, 2020. ISBN: 978-1-55903-012-0 (www.acr.org).
15. ASTM F2503-20, 'Standard Practice for Marking Medical Devices and Other Items for Safety in the Magnetic Resonance Environment', ASTM International, West Conshohocken, PA, 2020.

PART C
Engineering

Chapter 31

History, Physics, and Design of Superconducting Magnets for MRI

Bruce Breneman

Breneman Consulting, Rancho Santa Fe, CA, USA

Safety and Biological Effects in MRI.
Edited by Devashish Shrivastava and J. Thomas Vaughan

ISBN: 978-1-118-82130-5
Also published in eMagRes (online edition)
DOI: 10.1002/9780470034590.emrstm1590

31.1 HISTORICAL REVIEW OF MRI SUPERCONDUCTING MAGNETS

In many ways, the superconducting magnets central to today's magnetic resonance imaging (MRI) systems can trace their roots back to the Ancient World and European Scientists living during the Late Middle Ages through the modern period.

Magnetism was first discovered about 700–500 BC when it was observed that lodestones could attract iron. Thales of Miletus is credited with the first scientific discussion on magnetism (by fellow European philosopher Aristotle), whereas the first literary reference to magnetism is recorded in fourth-century BC China. In the twelfth century, Neckam was the first European to describe the use of a magnetized needle for navigation and in the thirteenth century, Peregrinus de Maricourt wrote about the properties of magnets. Fast forward to 1600 and Gilbert concluded that the Earth was itself magnetic, thus explaining why compass needles 'pointed north'. In the early nineteenth century, famed scientists Oersted and Ampere performed pioneering experiments to understand the relationship between electricity and magnetism. Mathematical equations and experiments describing magnetic fields and electricity quickly followed by such noted mathematicians and scientists as Gauss, Biot, Savart, Faraday, Maxwell, and Einstein. In the late nineteenth century, Tesla made numerous advances in the understanding and application of magnetic fields. Tesla is credited with many fundamental discoveries in physics.

In 1908, Dutch physicist Kamerlingh Onnes first liquefied helium. At standard pressure, the most common isotope of helium, helium-4, exists in a liquid state only at very low temperature, specifically −269 °C, −452 °F or 4.2 K. The ability to study materials at low temperatures led to research in the field of cryogenics, a term later defined by the U.S. Institute of Standards and Technology as involving temperatures below −180 °C, −292 °F or 93 K. In 1911, Professor Onnes' research led to the discovery of zero electrical resistance (superconductivity), the quantum phenomenon which occurs in rare materials when cooled below a critical temperature. At 4.2 K, niobium titanium (NbTi), commonly used in today's MRI magnets, exhibits this magical quality allowing for very large electrical currents to flow in small wires. Low weight and high magnetic field magnets could now be developed.

Turning to NMR, MRI and magnet development, Nobel Prize-winning Professor Rabi observed the quantum phenomenon in 1937, which would be termed nuclear magnetic resonance or NMR. Felix Bloch and Edward Purcell extended NMR to liquids and solids in 1946 ultimately leading both to the cherished 1952 Nobel Prize.

In 1955, Odeblad and Lindstrom published their groundbreaking work on NMR in living cells and excised animal tissue. Many consider Odeblad the most important pioneer in NMR in medicine having laid the foundation for both NMR and MRI. Another notable achievement during this time period was reported by Carr who created the first one-dimensional MR image.

In 1972, Damadian filed for a patent whereby he describes the major components associated with an MRI machine. Damadian's patent was issued in 1974 and in 1977/1978 Dr. Damadian (with the help of Goldsmith and Minkoff) built 'Indomitable' – the first MRI scanner which went on to generate the first MRI human body scan.

Paul Lauterbur, in 1973, published the first nuclear magnetic resonance image and the following year generated images from a living mouse. Peter Mansfield was at that time developing the echo-planar imaging (EPI) technique leading to quick scans requiring seconds and minutes instead of hours. Lauterbur and Mansfield received the Nobel Prize in 2003 for their contributions to applying MRI to medicine as a diagnostic tool.

In 1975, University of California, San Francisco founded the Radiologic Imaging Laboratory (RIL) with Dr. Leon Kaufman and Dr. Lawrence Crooks. Together they published *Nuclear Magnetic Resonance Imaging in Medicine* considered by many to be the authoritative textbook for MRI.

In 1980, Paul Bottomley joined General Electric, purchased a 1.5 T magnet, and developed the very popular 1.5 T GE MRI system which arguably became the de facto standard in the industry.

During the 1990s, John Mallard and his research team obtained the first clinically useful image of a patient's internal tissues using MRI. Mallard is credited with many technological advances leading to the widespread introduction of MRI.

MRI magnet design and commercial fabrication can be traced to the early 1980s. Highlights from a manufacturer's perspective are as follows:

- Early magnet designers came out of the nuclear fusion industry. MRI was seen as the first commercial application of superconductivity. In the early 1980s, magnet design incorporated very long solenoidal coils so as to obtain the required homogeneous central volume.
- The 1980s saw the formation of three main magnet manufacturers – General Atomics' Applied Superconetics (ASC), Intermagnetics General Corporation (IGC), and Oxford Magnet Technologies (OMT).
- In the mid-1980s, ASC designed the first magnets to be used in MRI mobile vans/trailers for Diasonics Corporation.
- The 1980s saw 0.35, 0.60, and 1.5 T magnet field strengths became the de facto standards – however, much debate occurred over the merits of 1.5 T vs 0.5 T.
- In the 1980s superconducting magnets in MRI ran 'open cycle' and consumed liquid nitrogen (LN_2) and liquid helium (LHe).
- In 1986 – high-temperature superconductor (HTS) was discovered.
- In 1986 – the first active (utilizing bucking coils) and first passively (utilizing carbon steel) shielded MRI superconducting magnets were introduced.
- The mid-1980s saw MRI superconducting magnets utilize single stage Gifford-McMahon (GM) cryocoolers to recondense LN_2 thus allowing for zero LN_2 boil-off magnets. Magnets continued to run open cycle LHe systems.
- In the late 1980s, magnets utilized two-stage GM cryocoolers allowing for conductively cooled 80 K thermal shields and reduced LHe boil-off.
- In the latter 1980s, shorter actively shielded magnets were introduced by OMT and GE.

- The early 1990s saw Diasonics and Toshiba develop the 0.064 T access MRI system – the first open geometry MRI with improved handling for obese and pediatric patients and the potential for interventional radiology in MRI.
- In 1996, the recent development of rare-earth two-stage GM cryocoolers and HTS current leads allowed ASC to design the first cryogenless superconducting magnet for MRI (Toshiba America MRI's 0.35 T Opart/Ultra MRI).
- In the mid-2000s, shorter 'open or compact' magnets brought a near halt to the open geometry MRI magnet market.
- In the 2000s, 3 T whole-body MRI magnets become commercially available.
- In the 2000s, 7 T whole-body MRI magnets become popular with those with large budgets.
- In the 2000s to present time, magnets have become lower cost and very short (only limited by the physics associated with creating a homogeneous field within the desired field of view). Actively shielded gradient coils were introduced and shorter image acquisition times became standard.
- Finally, during the 2000s to present time, magnetic resonance spectroscopy (MRS) in humans (up to 9 T) and mice (up to 21 T) has been performed.

31.2 WHY SUPERCONDUCTING MAGNETS FOR MRI?

There are several ways to generate magnetic fields appropriate for an MRI system, but only one that is practical for mid to high field MRI.

A dipole magnet is a device that drives magnetic flux from one magnetic pole to the other finally returning to the original source. MRI magnets must have an opening suitable for a human patient placement (50 cm or greater gap or diameter), be of relatively high magnetic field (≥0.2 T) within a central volume, have a uniform or homogeneous field with no more than a few parts per million (ppm) field difference when comparing maximum and minimum field values within the central volume, have a low field decay rate (<0.1 ppm h^{-1}) and be of practical size, weight, and of course, relative low cost to manufacture.

Early MRI magnets were built as resistive magnets. These had conventional copper wound coils that required dozens of kW of power, water cooling with associated water chillers, were sensitive to central field drift and had weights of 20–100 tons making siting of these magnets very challenging. Resistive MRI magnets are thus typically limited to approximately 0.6 T.

Permanent magnets have also been used in ultra-low and low-field MRI magnets. In the early 1990s, Toshiba America MRI (TAMI) developed and sold the pioneering 0.064 T permanent magnet access open MRI system. Flux was generated by magnetized ferrite and two horizontal pole faces creating a vertical magnetic field. The properties of ferrite, however, do not permit fields much above 0.1 T. Hitachi used rare-earth permanent magnets to develop their very successful Airis and Airis II open MRI system. These magnets operate at 0.3 T. High rare-earth material cost and material property limitations make rare-earth permanent magnets prohibitive much above Airis' 0.3 T.

Another significant disadvantage of permanent magnets is that, by definition, they are 'permanent' – meaning there is no way to discharge the magnet in case of emergency. All modern superconducting magnets used in MRI have an emergency ramp-down capability allowing the field to be brought to near zero in a matter of seconds in case of an emergency. MRI history, unfortunately, has examples of human injury caused by ferromagnetic objects being 'sucked' into the magnet while a patient or system operator is nearby or in the bore of the system. There are times that call for immediate removal of the magnetic field – something permanent magnets cannot do.

Superconducting magnets typically use superconductors comprising of NbTi, although a small minority use niobium tin (Nb_3Sn). Advances in HTS have resulted in magnesium diboride (MgB_2) or rare-earth barium copper oxide (REBCO) magnets. However, cost of materials may keep HTS materials from common use in MRI magnets for now and the near future.

Superconductors exhibit zero electrical resistivity below a certain simultaneous critical temperature (T_c), critical current (I_c), and critical field (B_c). Zero electrical resistivity equates to infinite electrical conductivity thus leading to the name 'superconductivity'. Zero electrical resistance allows for zero ohmic heating when electrical current passes through a wire (unlike resistive copper wire) allowing for extremely high electrical currents to flow within small wires. Typical 12 gauge copper wire found in many households is rated for 20 A whereas the same size NbTi superconducting wire may carry currents approaching 1000 A (limited by many factors such as temperature, peak field, hoop stress, etc.). Superconducting coils within the magnet structure can operate at very high currents (current densities) thus generating large magnetic fields in a relatively small size. In addition, since the field generated by a current loop is inversely proportional to the loop's radius, larger fields are inherently created by these compact coil windings. Finally, as stated above, an MRI system must have a stable field with typical drift rate of <0.1 ppm h^{-1}. Again, superconducting coils uniquely meet this requirement. Superconducting wires themselves have zero resistance when at low temperature resulting in no current decay. Indeed there are superconducting coils that have been energized, disconnected from the power source, and left for years without discharging. The only drift or decay rate in a superconducting MRI magnet is due to resistance in the wire joints between wire segments as well as wire joints made to the internal persistent switch as will be discussed later.

31.3 THE SCIENCES WITHIN SUPERCONDUCTING MAGNET DESIGN

MRI superconducting magnets are complex devices, drawing on a large range of physical sciences and engineering disciplines: superconductivity, cryogenics, vacuum technology, magnetostatics, mechanics, and structures.

31.3.1 Superconductivity

As previously described, MRI magnets are typically superconducting using conductors comprised of NbTi or niobium tin (Nb_3Sn). HTS have been found in research prototypes comprising of MgB_2 or REBCO.

Superconductors exhibit zero electrical resistivity below a simultaneous critical temperature (T_c), critical current (I_c), and critical field (B_c). Zero electrical resistivity equates to infinite electrical conductivity thus leading to the name 'superconductivity'.

31.3.2 Cryogenics

The study and application of materials at very low temperatures is inherent to MRI superconducting magnets due to the use of superconductors near absolute zero temperature. Most MRI magnets operate at the boiling point of the most common helium isotope, helium-4. When in liquid state, and at atmospheric pressure, liquid helium, or LHe, has a temperature of 4.2 K or −269 °C or −452 °F. Besides superconductivity, other interesting and useful phenomena also occur at very low temperatures. Mechanical properties such as yield and tensile strengths for stainless steel and aluminum alloys can increase by upwards of 100%. The resistivity of copper used as stabilizer surrounding the NbTi conductor can decrease by a factor of 100 or more. Thermal conductivity in certain aluminum alloys increases by as much as 50% as temperatures decrease toward 100 K and then abruptly decreases at temperatures below 50 K.

Unwanted phenomena must also be considered at low temperatures. Many materials such as plastics and carbon steels become brittle with inherent poor ability to withstand elongation or deformation. Indeed the lack of ductility at low temperature must be carefully considered when choosing materials.

31.3.3 Vacuum Technology

It is imperative to minimize heat transfer from the room temperature vacuum vessel to the internal thermal shield as well as from thermal shield to helium vessel. By employing a hard vacuum of $<10^{-7}$ Torr or $<10^{-10}$ atm, thermal convection heat transfer is eliminated. Roughing and turbomolecular pumps are employed to initially create vacuum while internally mounted 4 K activated charcoal getters, or molecular sieves, further reduces molecular conduction of remnant gases such as helium within the vacuum space.

31.3.4 Magnetostatics

Magnetostatics is the study of magnetic fields in systems where the current is constant in time. In MRI superconducting magnets, the current is DC and, once energized, the current is in an 'infinite loop' through the coils and internal persistent switch. Knowledge of the famed Maxwell equations, Biot–Savart law as well as Ampere's and Gauss' laws are the foundation of Magnetostatics. Coil design and optimization, Lorentz force, hoop stress calculation, and 2D scalar and 3D vector solutions of coils and circuits are all within the magnet designer's responsibility.

31.3.5 Mechanics and Structures

Mechanical design of the magnet's internal helium pressure vessel, coil former/bobbin, and high strength/low conductivity supports between vacuum vessel, thermal shield, and helium vessel are examples of the complex internal mechanisms and structures comprising an MRI superconducting magnet. A typical MRI magnet may require well over 500 individual drawings to fully describe and define these components.

31.4 BASIC MAGNET THEORY, COILS, AND FLUX LINES

A magnetic field is created when a moving charge (or current) flows through a wire. The magnetic field from an electric current traveling in a straight wire curls around the wire. The 'right-hand rule' is useful to illustrate this phenomenon. Pointing your right thumb in the direction of the current in the wire and curling your fingers, the generated magnetic field curls around the wire in the same direction as your curled fingers (see Ref. 1). Similarly, current flowing around a loop of wire produces a magnetic field.[1]

Grouping a large set of wire turns concentrates the magnetic field. This is the basic principle of most MRI superconducting magnets. The magnetic flux lines travel continuously from one magnetic pole to the opposite pole thus forming a closed loop. A higher concentration of flux lines indicates greater magnetic field (magnetic flux density).

The equation for the magnetic flux density at the center of a group of turns is given by the Biot–Savart law:

$$B = \frac{\mu_0 N I}{2r}$$

where $\mu_0 = 4\pi(10^{-7})$ T m A^{-1} is the permeability of free space or vacuum, N = number of turns, I = current in A, r = radius of turns in m.

Thus magnetic field is proportional to number of turns, current, and permeability of material it passes through and inversely proportional to the turn's radius. Typically, whole-body human MRI superconducting magnets operate at 0.2–10.5 T with 1.5 and 3.0 T being the standards of industry. A Tesla is equivalent to 10 000 G (1.0 T = 10 000 G). As a reference, the earth's magnetic field is approximately 0.5 G thus typical MRI superconducting magnets operate at 30 000–60 000 times the magnetic field as compared to earth.

31.5 SUPERCONDUCTING WIRE (CONDUCTOR)

Superconductivity, as applicable to MRI, occurs in certain materials known as Type-II superconductors such as NbTi or niobium tin (Nb_3Sn) when operating below the three-dimensional threshold of critical temperature, T_c, critical magnetic field, B_c, and critical current density, J_c, as shown in Figure 31.1.

NbTi wires are formed in high purity/high conductivity copper billets with NbTi rods inserted into drilled holes. After vacuum sealing the ends, the billet is extruded, drawn and heat treated multiple times thus reducing the assembly to the required wire gauge and transforming the NbTi rods into filaments. Typical wires diameters range from 0.5 mm to several millimeters with number of filaments ranging from 20 to 100 and continuous lengths of 5–30 km. Often the wire is soldered into a larger copper channel in what is known as 'wire in channel' (WIC) as seen in cross-section in Figure 31.2 (http://www.wstitanium.com/superconducting/NbTi-SUPERCONDUCTING-WIRE.html).

WIC conductors are usually electrically insulated using a Dacron or polyester braid, whereas conventional round conductor typically employs a Formvar/Vinylec thermoplastic resin coating.

Each superconducting wire has a unique performance curve used by the magnet designer

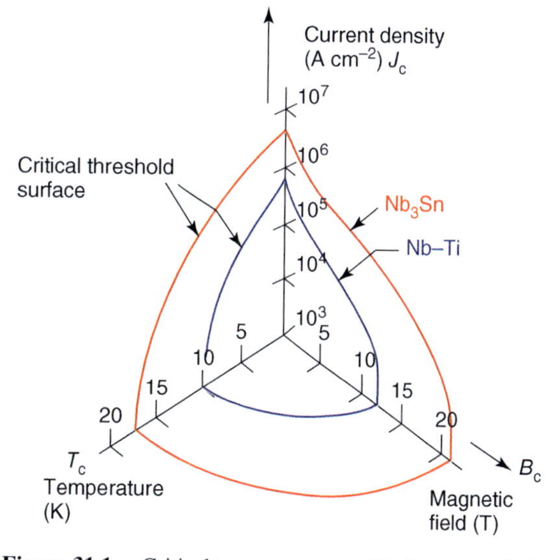

Figure 31.1. Critical temperature vs critical magnetic field vs critical current density

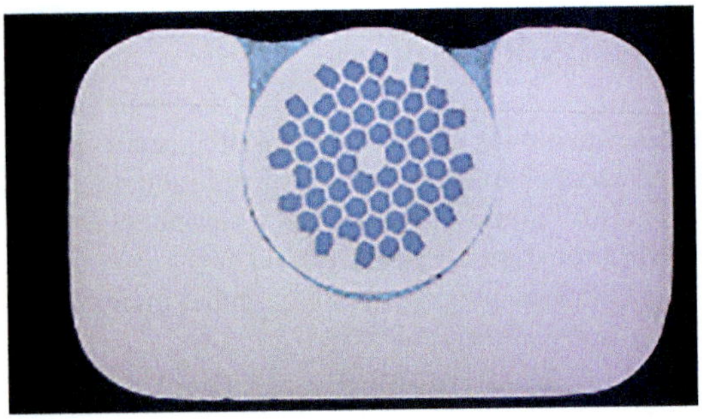

Figure 31.2. Wire in channel cross-section (http://www.wstitanium.com/superconducting/NbTi-SUPERCONDUCTING-WIRE.html)

to understand the operational limits. Typically, a critical current (I_c) versus critical field (B_c) test is performed at 4 K. Figure 31.3 shows the performance for a new generation high-temperature superconducting (HTS) material.[2]

The magnet designer must consider many factors when selecting a conductor and its operating current. The conductor load line shown in Figure 31.4 plots critical current vs peak field using the data in Figure 31.3. An operating current of 50–70% of load line current is typically chosen. In addition, the magnet designer must also consider the implications of operating current on conductor hoop stress, coil module peak fields, coil module 3D stress and coil layer shear stress, axial and radial Lorentz forces, radial pressure acting on coil former/bobbin when energized, and conductor displacement and strain. The following sections discuss these important magnet parameters in detail.

31.6 1.5 AND 3.0 T SUPERCONDUCTING COIL DESIGN

An MRI superconducting magnet is constructed with multiple discrete wire bundles, or modules, that collectively are referred to as the magnet coil. The modules comprise of varying lengths of wire connected in series thus carrying identical current. By definition axisymmetric, the coil must produce a strong and uniform magnetic field within a specified imaging volume. For our 1.5 T example below, the imaging volume is a centrally located 50 cm diameter spherical volume (DSV) with inhomogeneity (maximum to minimum field within DSV) not to exceed a few ppm. In addition, the localized field gradients within the imaging volume must be minimal, the distance from the magnet to the magnet's 5 G fringe field location minimized and the coil's internal forces, stresses, peak fields, current densities, etc. all within limits.

These simultaneous design goals are achieved by utilizing a 2D axisymmetric coil design optimization program using an algorithm such as simulated annealing. These computer programs are generally created

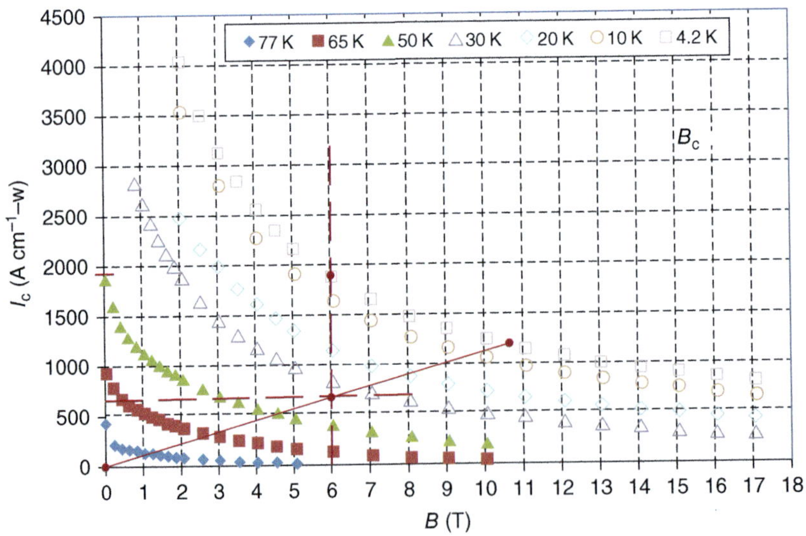

Figure 31.3. HTS superconductor critical current vs magnetic field[2]

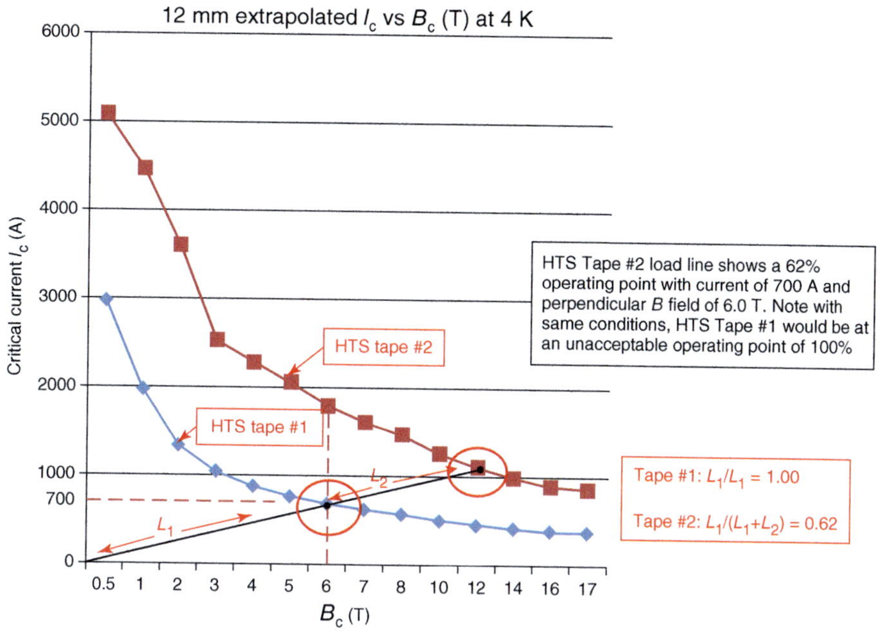

Figure 31.4. HTS superconductor load line

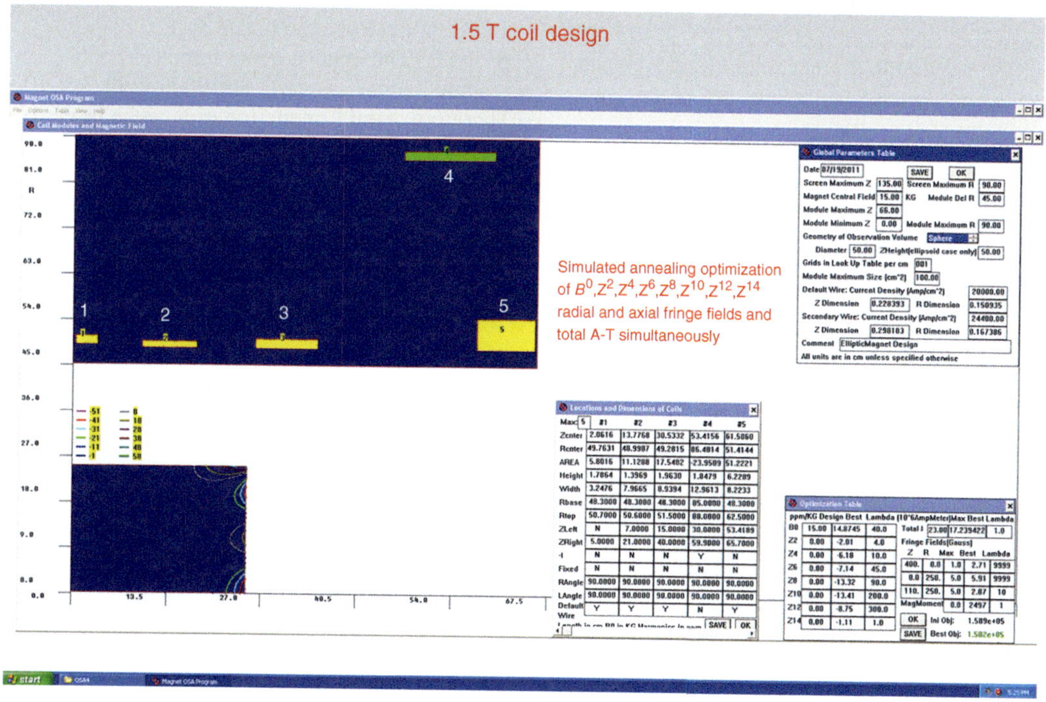

Figure 31.5. 1.5 T coil design

by the magnet manufacturers at great expense over many years of development. This type of program may calculate the exact field distribution in every turn or as distinct coil modules.

A typical 1.5 T coil design is shown in Figure 31.5. As the coil has symmetry about the vertical axis, only half of the coil need be calculated.

In this case, there are four main driver module pairs that are axisymmetric about the horizontal axis with mirror symmetry about the vertical axis. The module pairs are labeled modules 1, 2, 3, and 5. A single symmetric module pair (labeled 4), that is driven with negative polarity current, is also included. This negative current module pair is referred to as a bucking or field cancellation coil and reduces the fields external to the magnet as well as helps to shape the field within the central volume. Each module pair has a width, height, radial position, axial position, limits to axial and radial positions, current polarity and current density that are preliminarily set by the designer and then optimized by the program. Simultaneously the maximum to minimum field differences within the specified 50 cm DSV are minimized as well as the target central field B_0. Finally, all localized field gradients that describe the fields within an axisymmetric coil (known as zonal harmonic coefficients of the Legendre expansion) and quantified as Z^2, Z^4, Z^6, Z^8, Z^{10}, Z^{12}, and Z^{14} are simultaneously minimized. A detailed discussion on Legendre coefficients is found in subsequent sections.

Altogether there are over 22 parameters being optimized simultaneously.

The optimized coil design of a typical 3.0 T MRI magnet is shown in Figure 31.6.

As can be seen, the coil's modules are substantially larger in order to achieve the central field, B_0 of 3.0 T. In addition the number of modules is reduced to four pairs.

As described previously, the radial and axial fringe fields must be reduced to a typical industry standard value of <5 G at a radius = 2.5 m, $Z = 0$ m, and $Z = 4.0$ m, $R = 0$ m with $R = Z = 0$ being magnet isocenter. This is achieved by the coil optimization program adjusting each module's position, size (thus ampere-turns), and location. The bucking coil is simultaneously adjusted.

Experienced coil designers also know that higher aspect ratio coil modules (coil height/coil width) lead to inherently higher peak B fields within the coil's modules. Reducing this aspect ratio lowers peak B fields thus increasing the magnet's operating margin.

Many hundreds of coil optimizations are generally run for a particular coil design as optimization algorithms often find many 'local minimum solutions' where one particular parameter is emphasized over others. For example, the coil's total ampere-turns may be minimized while the Legendre coefficients are higher than desired. Weighting factors can be adjusted to 'jog' the program away from such minimums and search toward a different optimized solution. With over 22 parameters being optimized simultaneously, discretion and judgment by the experienced coil designer is required to yield an overall optimal solution.

31.7 COIL LORENTZ FORCES AND HOOP STRESS

The coil modules in an MRI superconducting magnet experience large forces when the coil is at field or 'energized'. These forces, known as Lorentz forces, are exerted by the magnetic field on a moving electric charge (or current) and can be both axial and radial in direction. An example of the axial Lorentz forces in our 3.0 T example can be seen in Figure 31.7.

Each coil module is subject to these potentially large axial Lorentz forces produced by their respective radial B_r fields. The axial Lorentz force (F_z) acting on coil module 3 alone is nearly 800 000 lbf. or 3 560 000 N. Therefore, axial Lorentz forces must be properly supported by the bobbin (winding former) as well as by shear stresses within the coil modules themselves.

Radial Lorentz forces (F_r) result from axial fields (B_z). In our 3 T example below, the maximum B_z fields shown in Figure 31.8 are 5.8 T near the coil's inner radius and −4.8 T at the coil's outer radius.

Axial field B_z produces radial Lorentz force F_r, which, in turn, produces radial pressure P_r on the coil modules and conductors. A circumferential hoop stress is induced from this radial force. At the coil inner radius, B_z is positive causing a radial outward force while at the coil's outer radius, B_z has a reverse (negative) polarity causing a radial inwards force and pressure. Coil and/or bobbin hoop stress due to energization can be approximated by the simple expression:

$$\text{Hoop stress} = B_z J R$$

where B_z is the axial field at mean coil radius, J is the current density, R is the mean coil radius.

A more accurate and detailed stress analysis comes from considering the hoop stress due to three factors:

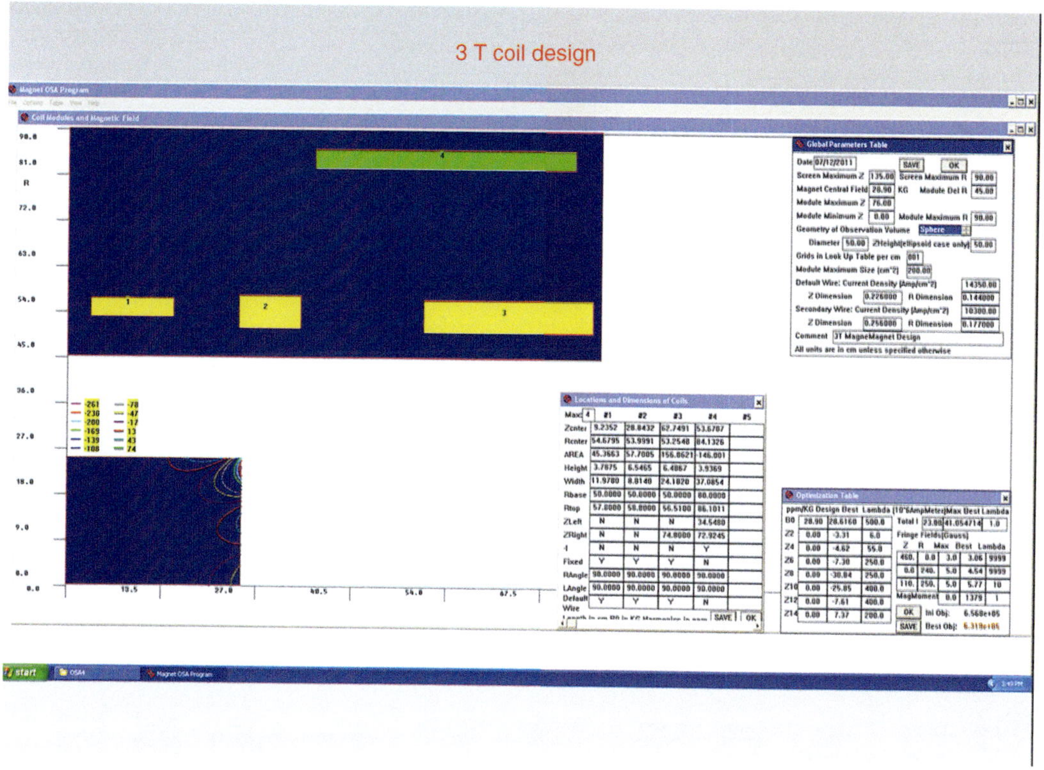

Figure 31.6. 3.0 T coil design

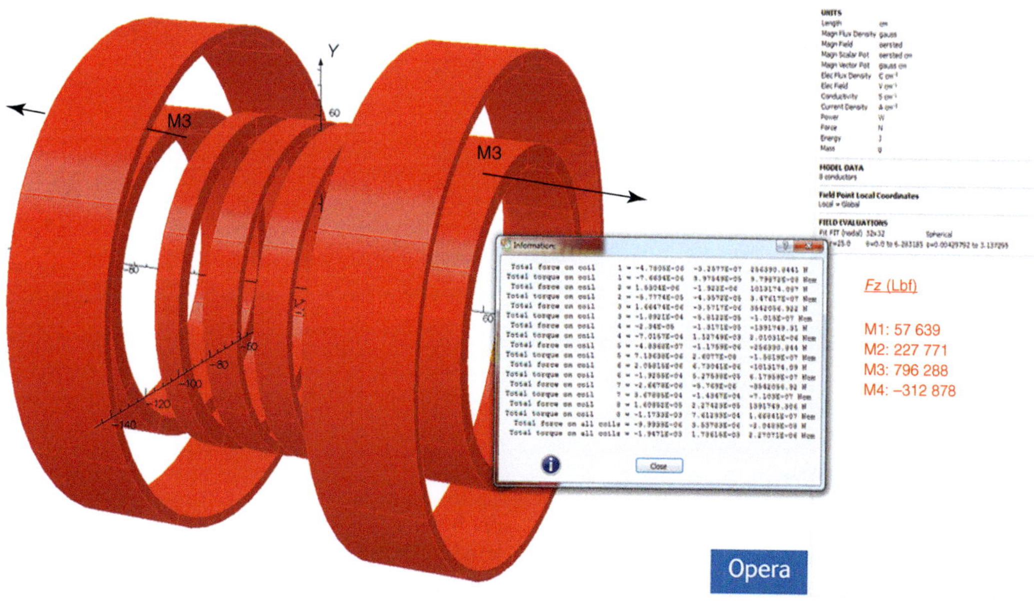

Figure 31.7. 3.0 T coil axial Lorentz forces

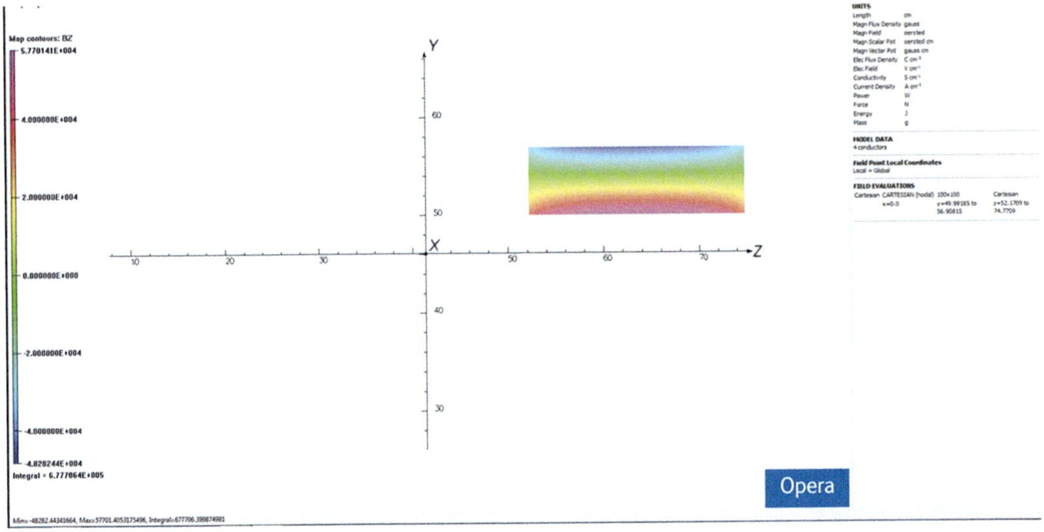

Figure 31.8. B_z peak field in 3.0 T coil

Coil stress analysis M#3
SUS bobbin, 20# winding tension

LAYER NUMBER	INSIDE RADIUS INCHES	LAYER THICKN. INCHES	LAYER WIDTH INCHES	ELASTI MODULUS PSI	POISSONS RATIO LBS	PRETENSION FORCE PSI	INSIDE HOOPSTRESS PSI	OUTSIDE HOOPSTRESS STRESS	INSIDE RADIAL STRESS	OUTSIDE RADIAL STRESS
1	18.5157	0.5000	0.0660	30000000.0000	0.300	0.000	-6922.0	-6742.4	0.0000	-179.6
2	19.0158	0.0200	0.0660	2200000.0000	0.300	0.000	-544.4	-544.1	-179.6260	-180.0
3	19.0358	0.0030	0.0660	1000000.0000	0.200	0.000	-258.8	-258.8	-180.0001	-180.0
4	19.0388	0.0440	0.0660	22000000.0000	0.300	20.000	2377.5	2371.6	-180.0216	-174.1
5	19.0828	0.0030	0.0660	1000000.0000	0.200	0.000	-237.3	-237.3	-174.1316	-174.1
6	19.0858	0.0440	0.0660	22000000.0000	0.300	20.000	2798.7	2791.8	-174.1415	-167.3
7	19.1298	0.0030	0.0660	1000000.0000	0.200	0.000	-216.9	-216.9	-167.3120	-167.3
8	19.1328	0.0440	0.0660	22000000.0000	0.300	20.000	3194.7	3187.0	-167.3197	-159.6
9	19.1768	0.0030	0.0660	1000000.0000	0.200	0.000	-197.6	-197.5	-159.6149	-159.6
10	19.1798	0.0440	0.0660	22000000.0000	0.300	20.000	3568.4	3559.9	-159.6206	-151.1
11	19.2237	0.0030	0.0660	1000000.0000	0.200	0.000	-179.0	-179.0	-151.0982	-151.1
12	19.2267	0.0440	0.0660	22000000.0000	0.300	20.000	3922.0	3912.7	-151.1025	-141.8
13	19.2707	0.0030	0.0660	1000000.0000	0.200	0.000	-161.3	-161.3	-141.8138	-141.8
14	19.2737	0.0440	0.0660	22000000.0000	0.300	20.000	4257.4	4247.4	-141.8168	-131.8
15	19.3177	0.0030	0.0660	1000000.0000	0.200	0.000	-144.2	-144.2	-131.8067	-131.8
16	19.3207	0.0440	0.0660	22000000.0000	0.300	20.000	4576.3	4565.7	-131.8106	-121.1
17	19.3647	0.0030	0.0660	1000000.0000	0.200	0.000	-127.7	-127.7	-121.1258	-121.1
18	19.3677	0.0440	0.0660	22000000.0000	0.300	20.000	4880.2	4868.9	-121.1268	-109.8
19	19.4117	0.0030	0.0660	1000000.0000	0.200	0.000	-111.8	-111.8	-109.8041	-109.8
20	19.4147	0.0440	0.0660	22000000.0000	0.300	20.000	5170.4	5158.4	-109.8044	-97.9
21	19.4587	0.0030	0.0660	1000000.0000	0.200	0.000	-96.5	-96.5	-97.8793	-97.9
22	19.4617	0.0440	0.0660	22000000.0000	0.300	20.000	5447.8	5435.3	-97.8791	-85.4
23	19.5057	0.0030	0.0660	1000000.0000	0.200	0.000	-81.6	-81.6	-85.3845	-85.4
24	19.5087	0.0440	0.0660	22000000.0000	0.300	20.000	5713.6	5700.6	-85.3839	-72.3
25	19.5527	0.0030	0.0660	1000000.0000	0.200	0.000	-67.1	-67.1	-72.3499	-72.3
26	19.5557	0.0440	0.0660	22000000.0000	0.300	20.000	5968.7	5955.1	-72.3491	-58.8
27	19.5997	0.0030	0.0660	1000000.0000	0.200	0.000	-53.0	-53.0	-58.8038	-58.8
28	19.6027	0.0440	0.0660	22000000.0000	0.300	20.000	6213.7	6199.6	-58.8029	-44.8
29	19.6467	0.0030	0.0660	1000000.0000	0.200	0.000	-39.3	-39.3	-44.7723	-44.8
30	19.6497	0.0440	0.0660	22000000.0000	0.300	20.000	6449.4	6434.9	-44.7714	-30.3
31	19.6937	0.0030	0.0660	1000000.0000	0.200	0.000	-25.9	-25.9	-30.2796	-30.3
32	19.6967	0.0440	0.0660	22000000.0000	0.300	20.000	6676.4	6661.5	-30.2789	-15.3
33	19.7407	0.0030	0.0660	1000000.0000	0.200	0.000	-12.8	-12.8	-15.3484	-15.3
34	19.7437	0.0440	0.0660	22000000.0000	0.300	20.000	6895.3	6880.0	-15.3480	0.0
35	19.7877	0.0030	0.0660	1000000.0000	0.200	0.000	0.0	0.0	0.0000	0.0

Figure 31.9. Coil stress analysis

(i) force introduced via the conductors during winding fabrication, (ii) differential contraction between coil modules and bobbin former from cooling of the magnet to 4 K, and (iii) Lorentz forces when energizing. Figure 31.9 is for our 1.5 T example and shows the hoop stress and radial pressure winding layer by winding layer. At the coil inner radius, the winding force (or tension) induces a hoop stress of −6922 psi and a radial pressure of −180 psi. A negative first layer radial stress indicates that the coil module's first layer

Coil stress analysis M#3
SUS bobbin
cooldown to 4 K & energization

(a)

LAYER NUMBER	INSIDE RADIUS INCHES	LAYER THICKN. INCHES	UNIT THERM. EXPAND.	FREE INSIDE RADIUS	START TEMP. K DEGREES	FINAL TEMP. K DEGREES	INSIDE HOOPSTRESS PSI	OUTSIDE HOOPSTRESS PSI	INSIDE RADIAL STRESS	OUTSIDE RADIAL STRESS
1	18.4579	0.4986	0.0030	18.4607	293.000	4.200	-11403.7	-11107.7	[illegible]	-295.9
2	18.9565	0.0199	0.0030	18.9592	293.000	4.200	[illegible]	-896.3	-295.9467	-296.6
3	18.9764	0.0030	0.0069	18.9042	293.000	4.200	3528.5	3527.9	[illegible]	-296.0
4	18.9794	0.0439	0.0033	18.9767	293.000	4.200	5428.9	5415.7	[illegible]	-282.8
5	19.0232	0.0030	0.0069	18.9509	293.000	4.200	3550.3	3549.7	-282.7952	-282.2
6	19.0262	0.0439	0.0033	19.0236	293.000	4.200	5826.9	5812.8	-282.1956	-268.2
7	19.0701	0.0030	0.0069	18.9975	293.000	4.200	3571.0	3570.4	-268.1624	-267.6
8	19.0730	0.0439	0.0033	19.0704	293.000	4.200	6199.9	6185.1	-267.5634	-252.7
9	19.1169	0.0030	0.0069	19.0442	293.000	4.200	3590.7	3590.1	-252.7432	-252.1
10	19.1199	0.0439	0.0033	19.1172	293.000	4.200	6550.7	6535.2	-252.1450	-236.6
11	19.1637	0.0030	0.0069	19.0909	293.000	4.200	3609.5	3606.9	-236.5943	-236.0
12	19.1667	0.0439	0.0033	19.1641	293.000	4.200	6881.6	6865.3	-235.9971	-219.8
13	19.2106	0.0030	0.0069	19.1376	293.000	4.200	3627.6	3627.0	-219.7667	-219.2
14	19.2135	0.0439	0.0033	19.2109	293.000	4.200	7194.4	7177.6	-219.1707	-202.3
15	19.2574	0.0030	0.0069	19.1842	293.000	4.200	3644.9	3644.3	-202.3063	-201.7
16	19.2604	0.0439	0.0033	19.2578	293.000	4.200	7490.9	7473.5	-201.7118	-184.3
17	19.3042	0.0030	0.0069	19.2309	293.000	4.200	3661.6	3661.0	-184.2551	-183.7
18	19.3072	0.0439	0.0033	19.3046	293.000	4.200	7772.5	7754.5	-183.6622	-165.7
19	19.3510	0.0030	0.0069	19.2776	293.000	4.200	3677.8	3677.2	-165.6510	-165.1
20	19.3540	0.0439	0.0033	19.3515	293.000	4.200	8040.5	8022.0	-165.0600	-146.5
21	19.3979	0.0030	0.0069	19.3242	293.000	4.200	3693.4	3692.8	-146.5290	-145.9
22	19.4008	0.0439	0.0033	19.3983	293.000	4.200	8296.1	8277.0	-145.9399	-126.9
23	19.4447	0.0030	0.0069	19.3709	293.000	4.200	3708.5	3708.0	-126.9210	-126.3
24	19.4477	0.0439	0.0033	19.4452	293.000	4.200	8540.0	8520.6	-126.3340	-106.9
25	19.4915	0.0030	0.0069	19.4176	293.000	4.200	3723.3	3722.7	-106.8564	-106.3
26	19.4945	0.0439	0.0033	19.4920	293.000	4.200	8773.4	8753.5	-106.2716	-86.4
27	19.5384	0.0030	0.0069	19.4643	293.000	4.200	3737.6	3737.0	-86.3625	-85.8
28	19.5413	0.0439	0.0033	19.5388	293.000	4.200	8996.8	8976.5	-85.7801	-65.5
29	19.5852	0.0030	0.0069	19.5109	293.000	4.200	3751.5	3750.9	-65.4646	-64.9
30	19.5882	0.0439	0.0033	19.5857	293.000	4.200	9211.2	9190.5	-64.8845	-44.2
31	19.6320	0.0030	0.0069	19.5576	293.000	4.200	3765.1	3764.5	-44.1859	-43.6
32	19.6350	0.0439	0.0033	19.6325	293.000	4.200	9416.9	9395.9	-43.6084	-22.5
33	19.6788	0.0030	0.0069	19.6043	293.000	4.200	3778.3	3777.8	-22.5483	-22.0
34	19.6818	0.0439	0.0033	19.6794	293.000	4.200	9614.7	9593.3	-21.9735	-0.6
35	19.7257	0.0030	0.0069	19.6509	293.000	4.200	3791.3	3790.7	-0.5721	0.0

TOTAL COMPRESS STRAIN ENERGY AT THIS STAGE = 7.87609 INCH-LBS
TOTAL TENSILE STRAIN ENERGY AT THIS STAGE = 10.6445 INCH-LBS
TOTAL STRAIN ENERGY AT THIS STAGE = 18.5206 INCH-LBS

(b) THE DATA LISTED BELOW APPLY AFTER THE AXIAL AND RADIAL FIELDS HAVE BEEN INTRODUCED

LAYER NUMBER	INSIDE RADIUS INCHES	AXIAL FIELD K-GAUSS	RADIAL FIELD K-GAUSS	CURRENT DENSITY A/CMSQ	AXIAL PRESSURE PSI	CONDUCTOR SUPPORT SPACING	INSIDE HOOPSTRESS PSI	OUTSIDE HOOPSTRESS PSI	INSIDE RADIAL STRESS	MAXIUM TENSILE OR COMP
1	18.4621	0.0000	0.0000	0.0000	0.000	0.000	-39584.1	-4490.7	[illegible]	39584.1
2	18.9606	0.0000	0.0000	0.0000	0.000	0.000	-8053287.6	-362.4	-119.6781	8053287.6
3	18.9806	0.0000	0.0000	0.0000	0.000	0.000	-54020685.7	[illegible]	[illegible]	54020685.7
4	18.9835	26.4300	0.0000	23393.7895	0.000	0.000	-883037.7	10500.2	[illegible]	883037.7
5	19.0274	23.8587	0.0000	0.0000	0.000	0.000	-7357181.1	3786.0	-194.6250	7357181.1
6	19.0304	23.6833	0.0000	23393.9751	0.000	0.000	21216.7	10832.0	-194.0023	21216.7
7	19.0742	21.1120	0.0000	0.0000	0.000	0.000	-22724.4	3790.7	-258.0579	22724.4
8	19.0772	20.9367	0.0000	23394.1417	0.000	0.000	-32028.9	11141.7	-257.4261	32028.9
9	19.1211	18.3654	0.0000	0.0000	0.000	0.000	1121672.0	3796.4	-310.3148	1121672.0
10	19.1240	18.1901	0.0000	23394.2902	0.000	0.000	325449.2	11432.0	-309.6755	325449.2
11	19.1679	15.6188	0.0000	0.0000	0.000	0.000	11064177.1	3803.3	-351.4709	11064177.1
12	19.1709	15.4435	0.0000	23394.4215	0.000	0.000	1509660.2	11705.4	-350.8257	1509660.2
13	19.2147	12.8722	0.0000	0.0000	0.000	0.000	32637813.4	3811.4	-381.5959	32637813.4
14	19.2177	12.6969	0.0000	23394.5363	0.000	0.000	3346343.6	11963.7	-380.9463	3346343.6
15	19.2615	10.1256	0.0000	0.0000	0.000	0.000	61518268.7	3820.9	-400.7538	61518268.7
16	19.2645	9.9503	0.0000	23394.6352	0.000	0.000	5366235.6	12208.7	[illegible]	5366235.6
17	19.3084	7.3790	0.0000	0.0000	0.000	0.000	90251246.9	3831.7	-409.0043	90251246.9
18	19.3113	7.2037	0.0000	23394.7188	0.000	0.000	7035565.4	12441.8	[illegible]	7035565.4
19	19.3552	4.6324	0.0000	0.0000	0.000	0.000	111336114.3	3844.0	[illegible]	111336114.3
20	19.3582	4.4571	0.0000	23394.7874	0.000	0.000	7923630.1	12664.4	-405.7494	7923630.1
21	19.4020	1.8858	0.0000	0.0000	0.000	0.000	119391966.7	3857.8	-393.0022	119391966.7
22	19.4050	1.7105	0.0000	23394.8416	0.000	0.000	7809231.6	12877.6	-392.3500	7809231.6
23	19.4488	-0.8607	0.0000	0.0000	0.000	0.000	112431624.8	3873.1	-368.8507	112431624.8
24	19.4518	-1.0360	0.0000	23394.8817	0.000	0.000	6727706.5	13082.5	-368.2014	6727706.5
25	19.4956	-3.6073	0.0000	0.0000	0.000	0.000	92268461.6	3890.0	-333.9948	92268461.6
26	19.4986	-3.7826	0.0000	23394.9080	0.000	0.000	4960215.1	13279.9	-333.3498	4960215.1
27	19.5425	-6.3538	0.0000	0.0000	0.000	0.000	64080381.2	3908.5	-288.4782	64080381.2
28	19.5454	-6.5292	0.0000	23394.9209	0.000	0.000	2966908.4	13470.7	-287.8389	2966908.4
29	19.5893	-9.1004	0.0000	0.0000	0.000	0.000	35154694.1	3928.6	-232.3423	35154694.1
30	19.5923	-9.2757	0.0000	23394.9206	0.000	0.000	1265533.5	13655.5	-231.7100	1265533.5
31	19.6361	-11.8469	0.0000	0.0000	0.000	0.000	12837085.3	3950.4	-165.6266	12837085.3
32	19.6391	-12.0222	0.0000	23394.9075	0.000	0.000	256988.3	13835.2	-165.0025	256988.3
33	19.6829	-14.5935	0.0000	0.0000	0.000	0.000	1707330.0	[illegible]	-88.3684	1707330.0
34	19.6859	-14.7688	0.0000	23394.8817	0.000	0.000	-711.2	14010.2	-87.7539	711.2
35	19.7298	-17.3400	0.0000	0.0000	0.000	0.000	3895.5	3999.1	-0.6036	-3895.5

Figure 31.10. (a,b) Coil stress analysis

is bound to the bobbin surface with no risk of coil 'lift off' from the bobbin surface.

Figure 31.10 shows the result of superimposing cooldown and energization forces to the 1.5 T coil's initial winding force.

After cooldown to 4 K, the hoop stress in the bobbin increases to −11 403 psi with a −296 psi radial pressure. This is a result of the coil contracting more than the stainless steel bobbin. After energizing to 1.5 T, the positive B_z at the coil inner radius causes a radial outward Lorentz force F_r which reduces the bobbin's hoop stress to −4491 psi with resulting radial pressure reduction to −120 psi. This final stress in the bobbin cylinder is acceptable because the negative radial pressure ensures the coil module stays firmly in contact with the bobbin surface and does not 'lift off' of the bobbin surface. It should be noted that the winding tension could be increased if necessary to ensure a negative first layer radial pressure. As an increase in winding tension directly increases conductor stress a balance between radial pressure and conductor stress must be achieved. The maximum conductor stress is 14 010 psi (well below yield strength for the conductor at cryogenic temperature) and the maximum radial internal coil pressure is an acceptable −409 psi.

A summary of the coil stress analysis is shown for coil module #3 in our 1.5 T example in Figure 31.11.

	15T, M3 analysis
Bpk (kg) (ID->OD)	26.43->-17.34
Jm (A cm^{-2})	23396
Fwind (lbf)	20
Inside radial pressure after winding (psi)	−180
Inside radial pressure after winding and cooldown (psi)	−296
Inside radial pressure after wind/cool/ energization (psi)	−120
Max radial pressure in winding (psi)	−409
Bobbin hoop stress after winding (psi)	−6922
Bobbin hoop stress after wind/cool (psi)	−11403
Bobbin hoop stress after wind/cool/energization (psi)	−4491
Max conductor hoop stress after energization (psi)	14010

Figure 31.11. Coil stress analysis summary

31.8 MRI SUPERCONDUCTING MAGNET DESIGN

A modern MRI superconducting magnet comprises of the following main components: an external vacuum vessel with supporting frame, an internal helium vessel with coil and coil bobbin (former), a single thermal shield, persistent switch, low heat leak current leads, a two-stage GM cryocooler with associated cold head sleeve, and a LHe fill and vent stack with helium gas relief system. As will be discussed in detail in subsequent sections, the external vacuum vessel and thermal shields are necessary to minimize heat transfer to the internal helium vessel, the cryocooler and cold head sleeve extract heat from the thermal shield and reliquifies helium gas thus eliminating helium boil-off and the persistent switch and current leads allow for charging, discharging, and persistent operation of the magnet. Figure 31.12 shows a typical cross-section of a 1.5 T MRI superconducting magnet.

The vacuum vessel comprises of an outer cylinder, inner cylinder, and two end plates. Typical vacuum levels within the vacuum space are 10^{-10} atm or $\sim 10^{-7}$ Torr. The vacuum vessel is typically made from 304-grade stainless steel due to its low gas permeability, excellent weldability, and resistance to external gas leaks. The outer vacuum cylinder is sized to resist buckling due to a 15 psia external and 0 psia internal (vacuum) pressures. The inner warm bore cylinder is under the same pressure, but being internal pressure there is no buckling concern and thus the cylinder can often be thinner. End plates are also 304 stainless steel with typical thickness of about 12.7 mm or $^1/_2''$. The determining factor for vacuum vessel end plate thickness is not material stress but deformation or deflection under vacuum. Insufficient end plate thickness can lead to 'dishing' of the end plates making gradient coil

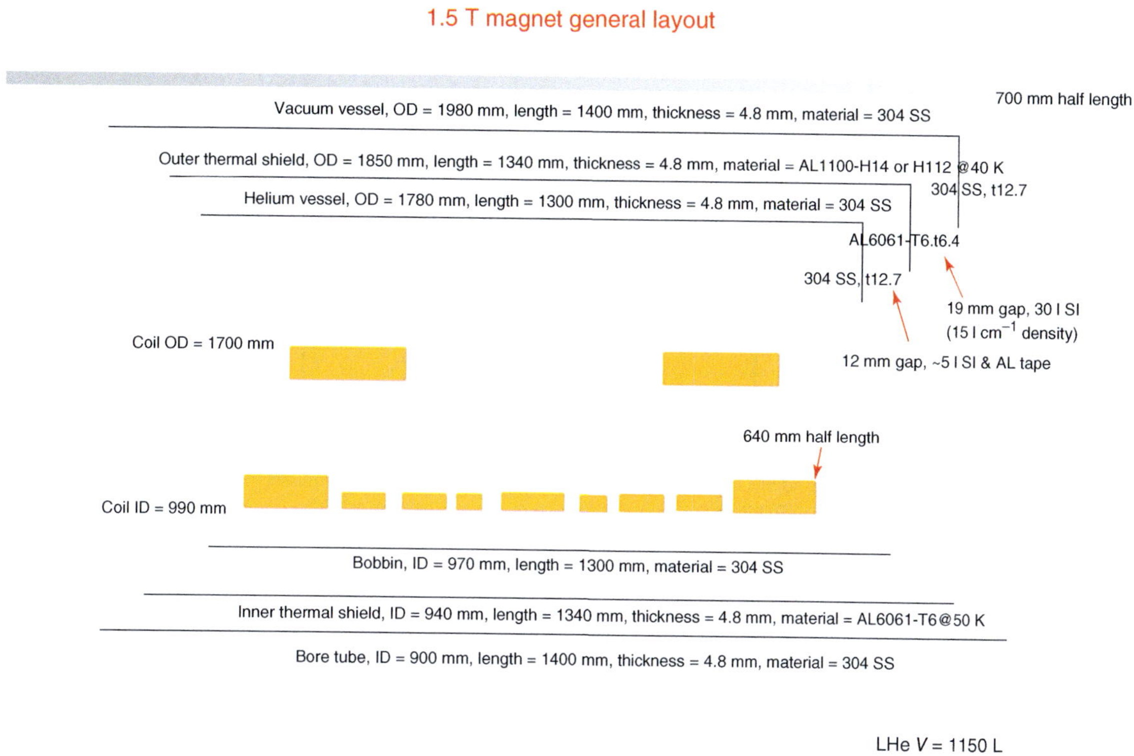

Figure 31.12. 1.5 T magnet layout

mounting unnecessarily difficult. Full penetration leak tight TIG welds are usually applied between cylinders and end plates.

The thermal shield also comprises an outer and inner cylinder with mating end plates. Typically, thermal shields are made of high purity, high conductivity (K), aluminum such as AL1050-0 or AL1100-0 to minimize the thermal temperature gradients across the thermal shield.

A key consideration in determining material type and thickness (besides temperature gradient) is the eddy current generated within the thermal shield's inner cylinder due to the changing field with respect to time (dB/dt) associated with the spatial encoding gradients. The inner shield time constant τ is given as (inductance/resistance):

$$\tau = \frac{L}{R}$$

where $R = (\rho l/A)$ and ρ = material resistivity at thermal shield's temperature at ~40 K, l = resistive length, A = resistive area.

Resistivity is inversely proportional to conductivity and thus high conductivity materials such as AL1100-0 have low resistivity. In addition, resistivity drops by as much as a factor of 10 between 300 and 40 K for many aluminum alloys. The result is a low resistance, high conductivity, inner thermal shield. Therefore, it is not uncommon for the characteristic time constant associated with the inner thermal shield to be in the 50–400 ms range. This long time constant and slow response, unfortunately, interferes with the desired pulsed gradient waveform as seen in Figure 31.13.

Traditionally, MRI system designers have solved the eddy current induced distorted waveform issue by careful choice of the thermal shield's inner cylinder thickness and material as well as applying a pre-emphasis to the gradient waveform resulting in a compensated eddy current with reduced system interference. Some manufacturers have also slit the inner thermal shield along the cylinder length thus causing an electrical 'break' circumferentially to reduce eddy current effects. Finally, one MRI supplier creatively solved this problem by actively shielding

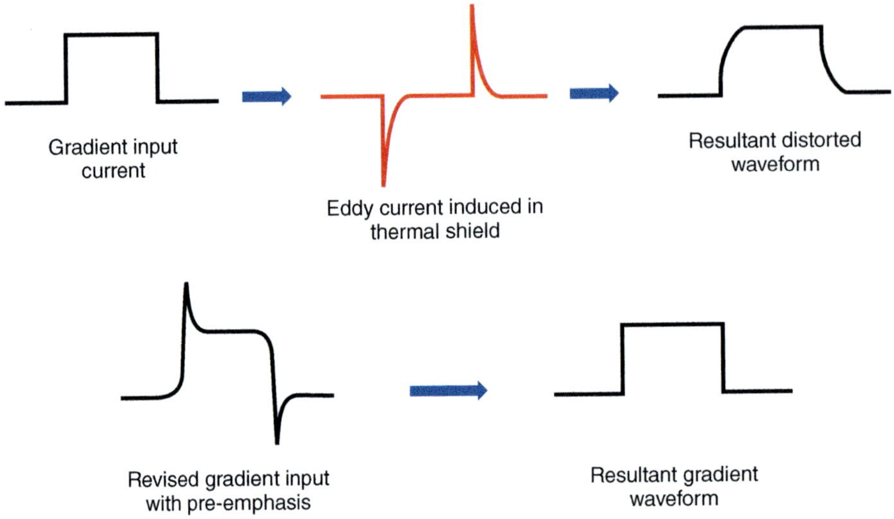

Figure 31.13. Gradient waveform and response

the gradient coil to reduce the dB/dt at the location of the inner thermal shield thereby reducing eddy current effects. It should be noted that the inner warm bore tube and helium vessel are typically made of high resistivity stainless steel with associated small time constant (a few milliseconds), and therefore the thermal shield's time constant dominates system eddy current behavior.

The thermal shield is an intermediate thermal barrier between the 300 K vacuum vessel and 4 K helium vessel. Heat transfer from the room temperature 300 K vacuum vessel to the cryogenic surfaces within the magnet occurs mainly via thermal conduction and thermal radiation. The magnet's thermal shield is often referred to as a radiation shield. Thermal radiation heat transfer is proportional to surface emissivity and ($T_H^4 - T_c^4$) where T_H is 300 K and T_c is ~40 K for the case of a single thermal shield. By utilizing a single thermal shield, the radiation heat transfer is divided into two segments with the thermal shield ($T_H^4 - T_c^4$) = ($300^4 - 40^4$) and the helium vessel ($T_H^4 - T_c^4$) = ($40^4 - 4^4$) or 0.03% of what would otherwise radiate from 300 to 4 K without the intermediate single thermal shield. This reduction in radiation heat to the helium system is critical to maintaining the cryogenic temperatures required for the superconducting magnet to operate and is the sole reason a radiation thermal shield is found in all superconducting MRI magnets.

Approximately 30 layers of aluminized Mylar, called superinsulation, or SI, are wrapped loosely around the thermal shield to provide a low emissivity surface, establish thermal gradient layers between the vacuum vessel and thermal shield as well as eliminate any potential 300–40 K direct 'shine through' radiation. In addition, heat transfer occurs via solid conduction through the thermal shield and helium vessel's supports, cryogenic venting, current leads, instrumentation and sensor leads, voltage taps, etc. Figure 31.14 shows the addition of superinsulation as well as the typical total heat loads to the thermal shields and helium vessel found in an MRI superconducting magnet.

Heat load to the thermal shield is of the order of 40–50 W, whereas the total heat load to the helium vessel is of the order of 0.5–1.0 W in a typical MRI superconducting magnet.

The helium vessel comprises of an outer cylinder, inner cylinder (or coil winding bobbin/former), and associated end plates. The helium vessel stores the 750–1500 l of LHe volume necessary to cool and maintain the superconducting coil operating at ~4.2 K. LHe changes state from liquid to gas when heated with volumetric expansion of approximately 750 times when 4.2 K LHe becomes 300 K helium gas. Thus, the helium vessel is a pressure vessel certified to international pressure vessel standards such as the American Society of Mechanical Engineer's ASME Section 8 Division 1 code and/or the European Pressure Equipment Directive PED code. Helium gas vent calculations are performed with helium gas rupture

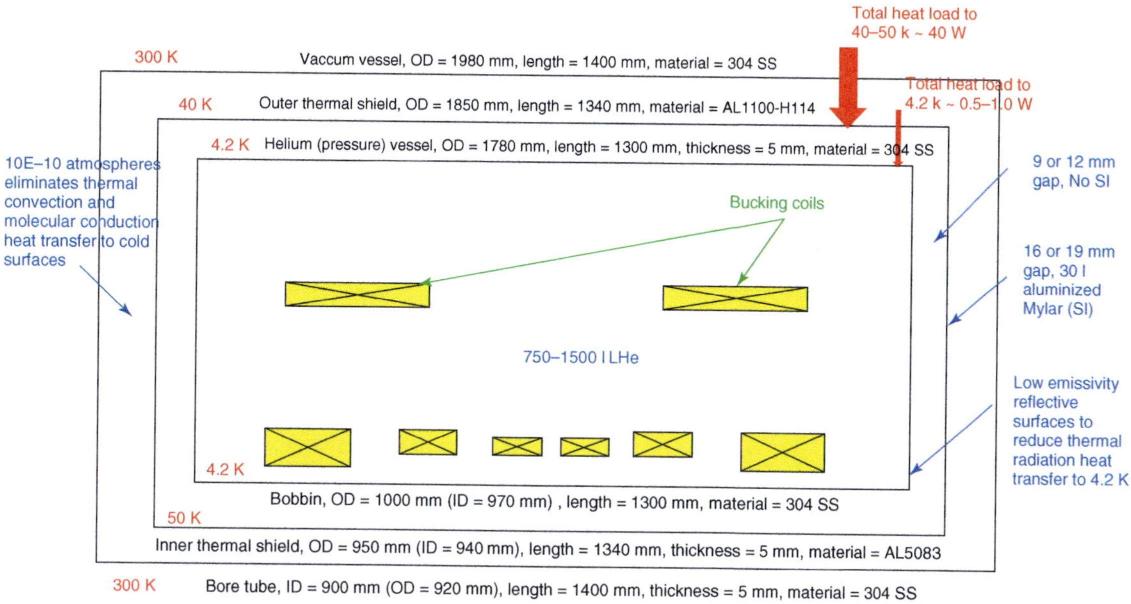

Figure 31.14. Superconducting magnet cross-section with heat loads

disks and safety relief valves installed to ensure over pressurization of the vessel does not occur. Low emissivity aluminum tape is often applied directly to the helium vessel with superinsulation used between thermal shield and helium vessel to minimize thermal radiation heat transfer.

The inner cylinder of the helium vessel is also part of the pressure vessel and is often simultaneously the winding bobbin (former) for the superconducting coil modules. Figure 31.15 shows a typical 3.0 T winding bobbin with outer helium vessel cylinder and end plates as modeled in a finite element analysis (FEA) stress analysis program. The geometry is modeled as axisymmetric with mirror symmetry about the horizontal axis. Note: the axisymmetric axis is shown vertical in Figure 31.15's model, whereas it can be appreciated this axis is horizontal in an actual MRI magnet.

Figure 31.16 shows the internal operating differential pressure of 18 psi (3 psig or 18 psia internal, 0 psia vacuum external pressure), the added axial Lorentz forces to all coil modules (per Figure 31.7) and the added radial pressure due to winding, cooldown, and energization (as exampled in Figures 31.9 and 31.10).

Figure 31.17 is the resulting FEA analysis of our fully loaded example showing radial displacement X, axial displacement Y, and displacement magnitude in inches. Deformations are examined and geometry revised as required to keep stress and strain within limits.

Figure 31.18 shows the three-dimensional Von Mises stress in the helium vessel and bobbin as well as within the coil modules. Helium vessel, bobbin, and coil stresses are all examined and verified to be mechanically acceptable.

Early superconducting MRI magnets ran 'open cycle' and vented the helium gas boil-off from the 0.5–1.0 W 4 K heat load directly to the atmosphere. Modern magnets use two-stage rare-earth GM cryocoolers with a cooling capacity of approximately 40–50 W at an upper cold head first stage operating temperature of ~40 K and 0.5–1.0 W at a lower second stage operating temperature of ~3.5–4.0 K. Often a permanently installed cold head 'sleeve' is employed in the magnet allowing the cold head to be removed from the magnet to be serviced or replaced at yearly intervals. A heat exchanger capable of re-liquefying helium gas to LHe is cooled by the second stage allowing the magnet to run 'closed cycle' with no helium gas venting to atmosphere. Figures 31.19 and 31.20 show an example of a cryocooler cold head and cold head sleeve.

Current leads allowing the magnet to be charged or discharged can take several forms. Early MRI superconducting magnets utilized vapor cooled resistive

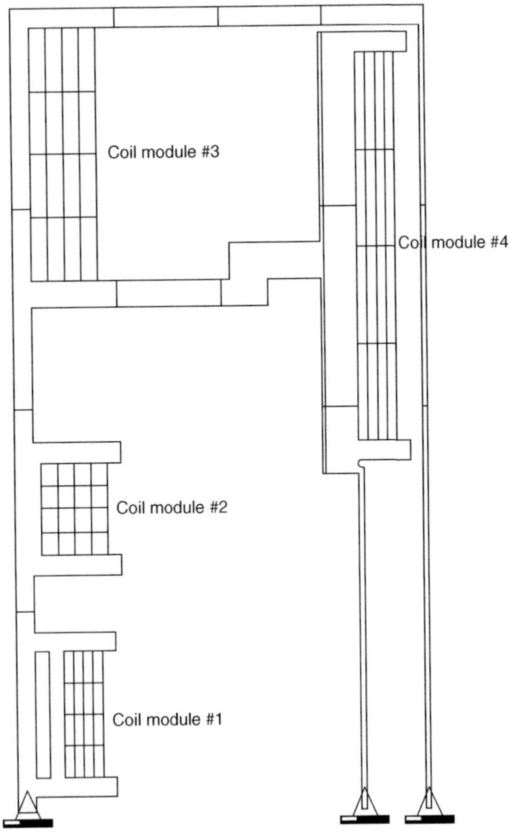

Figure 31.15. Axisymmetric FEA coil/bobbin model

leads with the enthalpy of boil-off helium gas cooling the leads when undergoing the natural I^2R heating associated with charging or discharging of the magnet. Removable or retractable current leads eliminated the leads in normal magnet persistent operation and were temporarily inserted only for charging or discharging of the magnet. Again these leads were vapor cooled to compensate for the I^2R heating when charging or discharging. Permanently installed low loss leads, such as those using high-temperature superconducting (HTS), have become more common as development and cost of these lead choices have become more attractive. These leads have essentially no I^2R heating to the 4 K helium vessel when charging or discharging. Figure 31.21 shows an example of a magnet current lead assembly.

Finally, located within the magnet's helium space is a persistent current switch or PCS. This is a small zero inductance superconducting coil that is connected electrically in series with the main magnet coils. Heaters located within the PCS can be 'turned on' thus heating the PCS from its superconducting state to its normal resistive state. When resistive, the PCS acts like an 'open switch' relative to the superconducting (zero resistance) main coils thus allowing the operator to gain control of the charge or discharge process. When the magnet is fully charged to the desired field (1.5 T or 3.0 T typically) the PCS is allowed to cool to its superconducting state thereby 'closing the switch' and creating an infinite loop current path from main coils to PCS. At that time, the current leads (if removable) can be retracted and the main power supply disconnected. An interesting design challenge of the persistent switch is the need for the PCS to be zero inductance and of relatively high resistance when warmed to its normal state. This is accomplished by bifilar winding of the PCS and use of high resistance stabilizer surrounding the NbTi wire within the PCS. The same voltage used to charge or discharge the main magnet coils is applied in parallel to the PCS causing V^2/R heating into the LHe. This additional heat load (along with that from the current leads) usually far exceeds the cooling capacity of the cold head's second stage causing open cycle LHe boil-off. Refilling with LHe is often required after a charge or discharge of the magnet.

31.9 MAGNET ELECTRICAL CIRCUIT AND POWER SUPPLY

Figure 31.22 illustrates the typical components associated with the MRI magnet's internal electrical circuit. The superconducting winding is comprised of coil modules which are connected in series with all modules then connected in parallel to the persistent switch (PCS). Resistive heaters are mounted internally to the PCS and cold (4 K) protection diodes (labeled D1) are also connected in parallel. The magnet's internal electrical circuit can and does operate detached from the external power supply circuit when in normal persistent operation.

When the magnet is in normal operation it is in 'persistent' mode where the magnet current flows in series through each coil module to the PCS and returns back through the coil modules thus forming a closed loop. MRI superconducting magnets typically are charged (energized) and left in normal persistent mode for 1–2 years at which time the magnet is discharged to permit routine servicing of the cryocoolers cold head

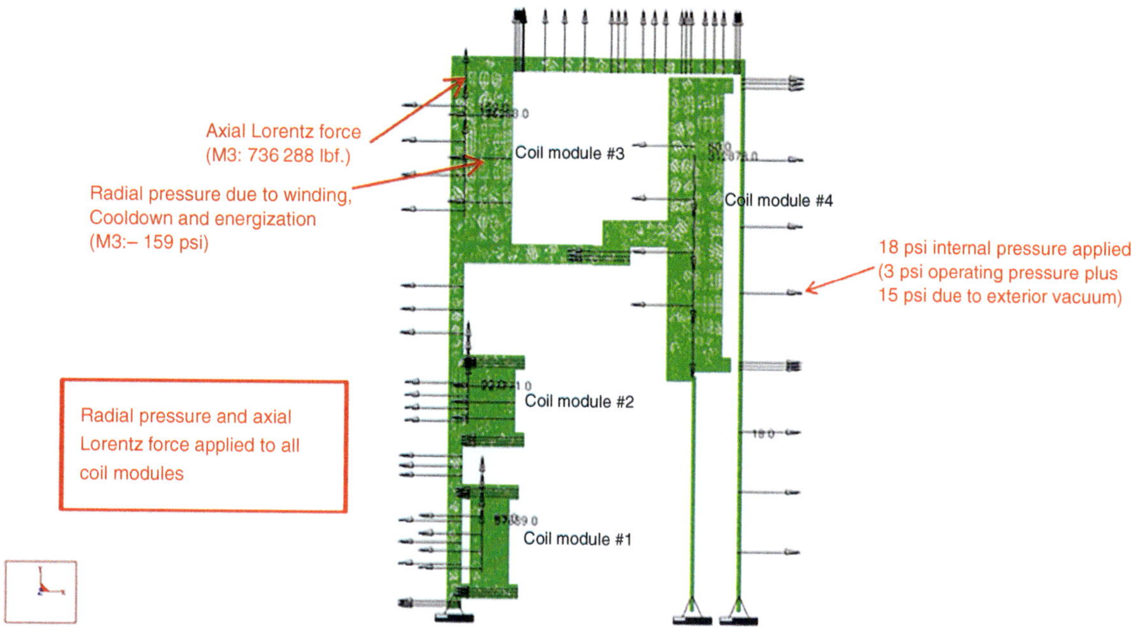

Figure 31.16. FEA coil/bobbin model with applied forces/pressures

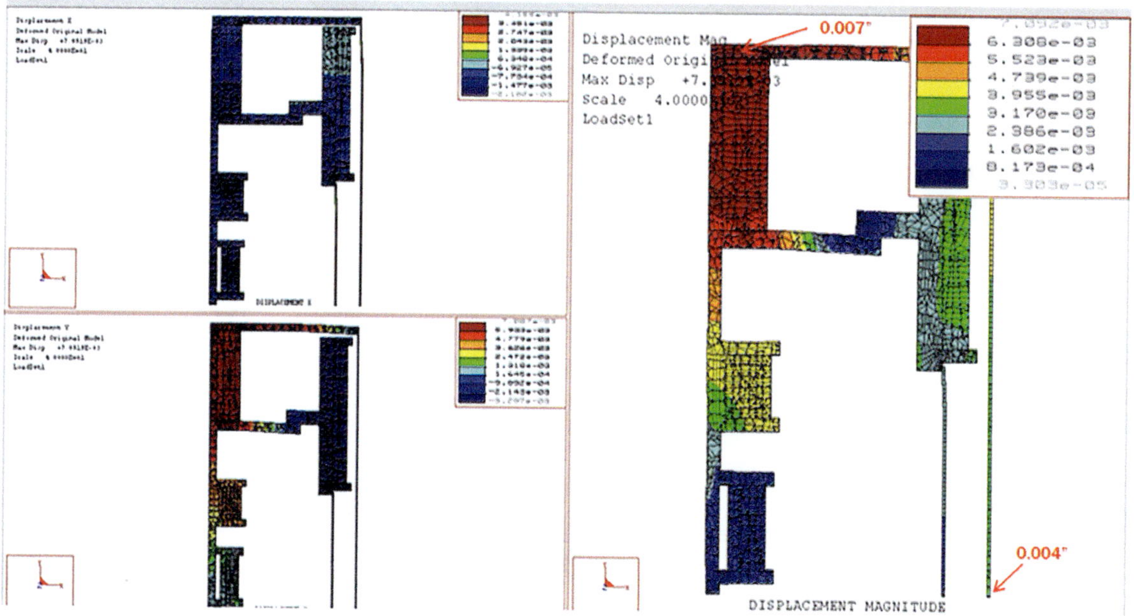

Figure 31.17. FEA coil/bobbin analysis

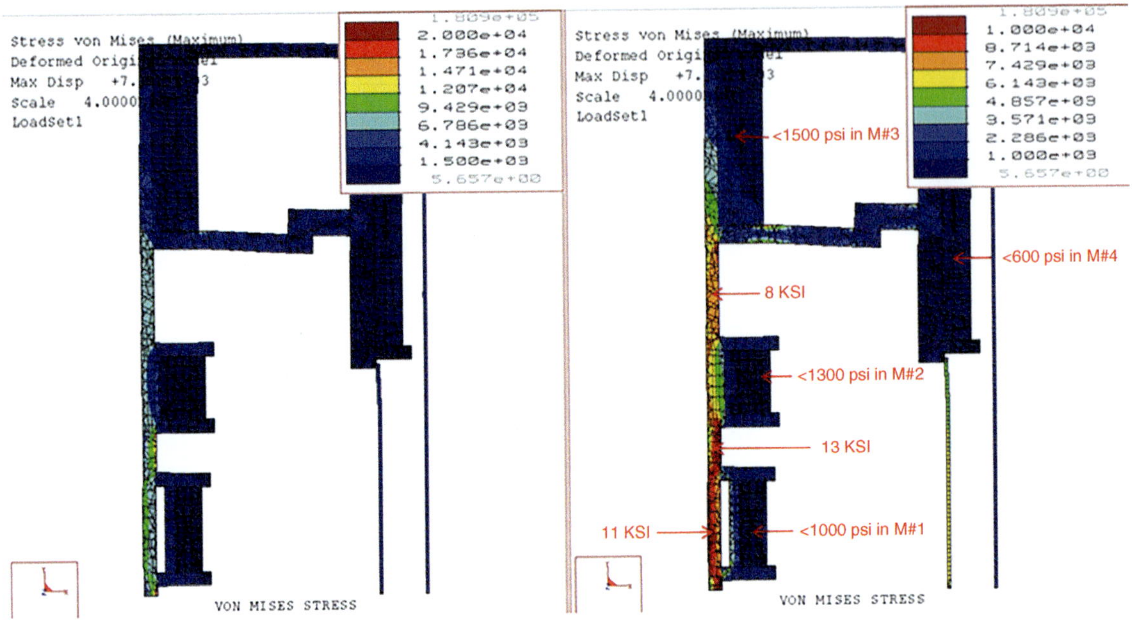

Figure 31.18. FEA coil/bobbin analysis

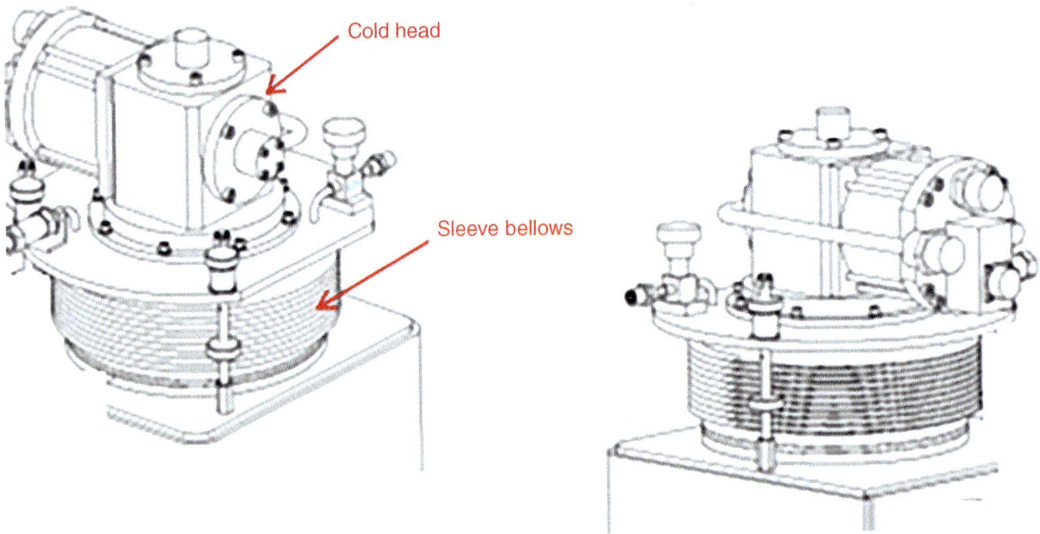

Figure 31.19. Cryocooler cold head and sleeve

and compressor. Figure 31.23 illustrates the current path of an energized magnet in persistent mode.

When the magnet is in persistent mode and detached from the external power supply, there must be an additional parallel pathway for the current in case the persistent switch becomes 'normal' or resistive. This also applies if the coil were to quench (also becomes resistive). Often the choice is made to install internal cold diodes that operate at 4 K. These diodes must be bench tested by repeated thermal cycling (300 K to

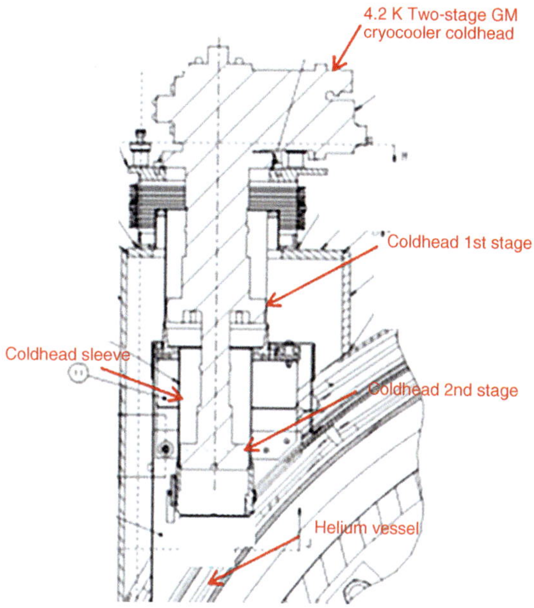

Figure 31.20. Cryocooler cold head and sleeve, side view

4 K to 300 K) to ensure safe operation at cryogenic temperature. As a group, the diode threshold voltage at 4 K must be well above the magnet charging voltage so these diodes are not activated during the charging process. In our example shown below the charging voltage is 6.6 V and the diode group threshold voltage is 12 V. Figure 31.24 shows the current path through the cold diode protection path.

An example of the fundamental components of an MRI superconducting magnet's power supply and charging/discharging circuit are shown in Figure 31.25. A DC power supply provides the charging voltage, usually between 5 and 25 VDC. A dump resistor or bank of dump diodes are used to dissipate the stored energy from the superconducting winding (coil modules) during magnet discharge. Alternatively, a four-quadrant power supply can be used so that the charging voltage polarity is reversed and the magnet discharged by essentially 'charging in reverse'.

The simplified charging process from zero field is as follows:

1. The magnet's LHe level and pressure is confirmed, thus allowing for safe charging.
2. Retractable current leads are installed (if permanent leads are not present).
3. Helium gas flow is allowed to vent to atmosphere and pass by the leads cooling them and providing the necessary enthalpy for removal of the current lead's subsequent I^2R heating.

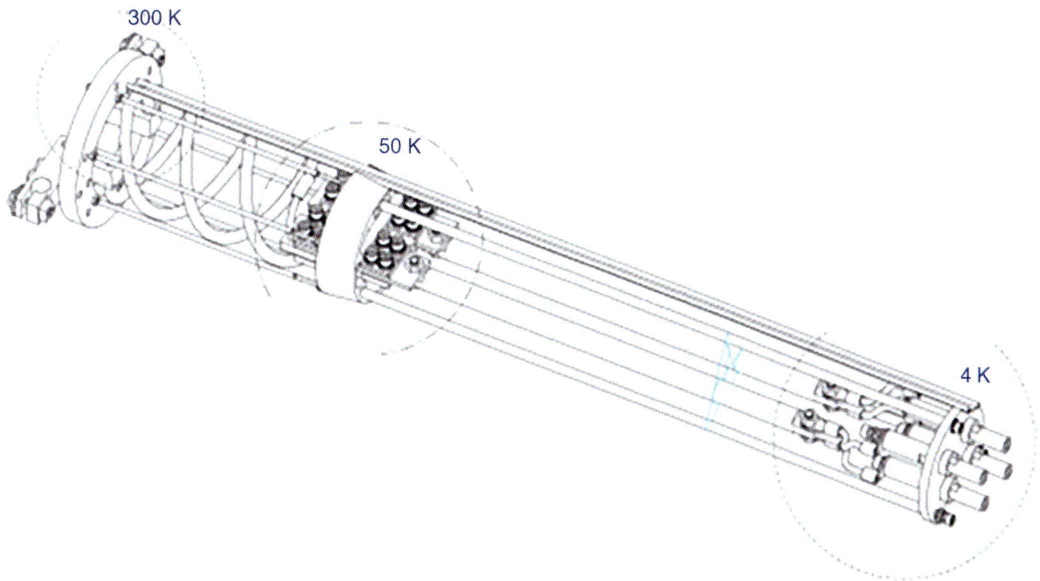

Figure 31.21. Magnet current lead assembly

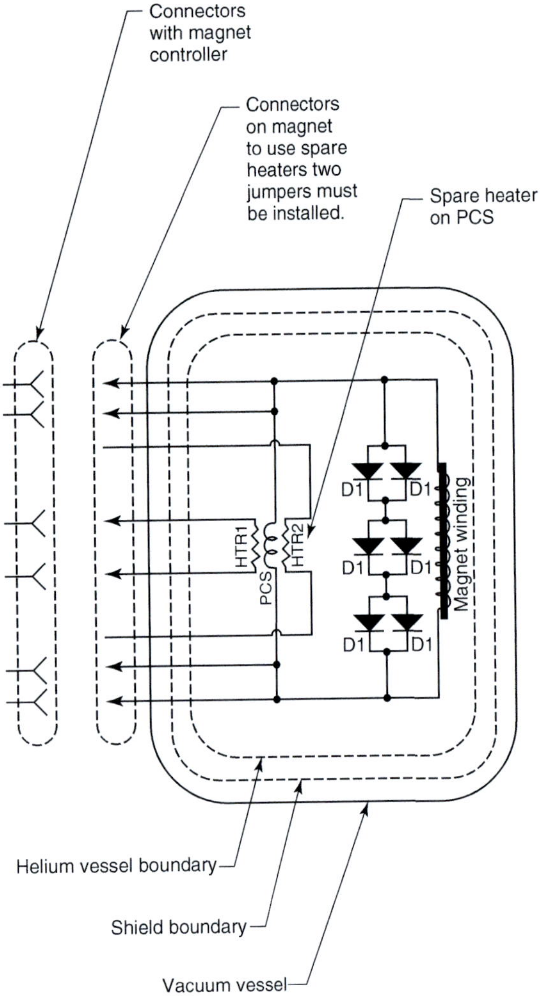

Figure 31.22. MRI magnet's internal electrical circuit

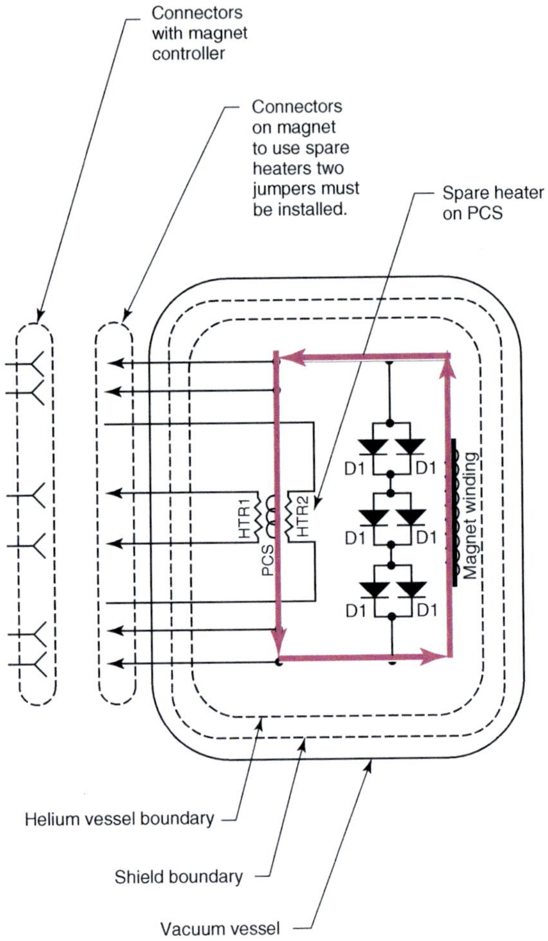

Figure 31.23. Energized magnet in persistent mode

4. The heater on the PCS is energized by separate external power supply, thus driving the PCS from superconducting to normal state.
5. A DC voltage (usually 5–10 VDC) is applied across the magnet terminals initiating the slow $V = LdI/dt$ inductive charging of the coil (Figure 31.26). The time, d*t*, required to charge the magnet is dictated by the coil module's total inductance, charging voltage, and magnet operational current and is typically 1–3 h.
6. The same voltage that is across the magnet terminals is also across the PCS thus providing additional PCS heating via V^2/R heating ensuring the PCS remains resistive in its normal state.
7. Once the desired magnet operational current (typically 400–600 A) is reached, the charging voltage is reduced to zero across the magnet terminals. The PCS heater voltage is then turned off and the PCS once again cools and becomes superconducting.
8. At this time, there is no net current in the PCS as the full operational magnet current flowing through the switch is nulled by the current from the power supply.
9. The current from the power supply is next reduced to zero allowing the magnet current to

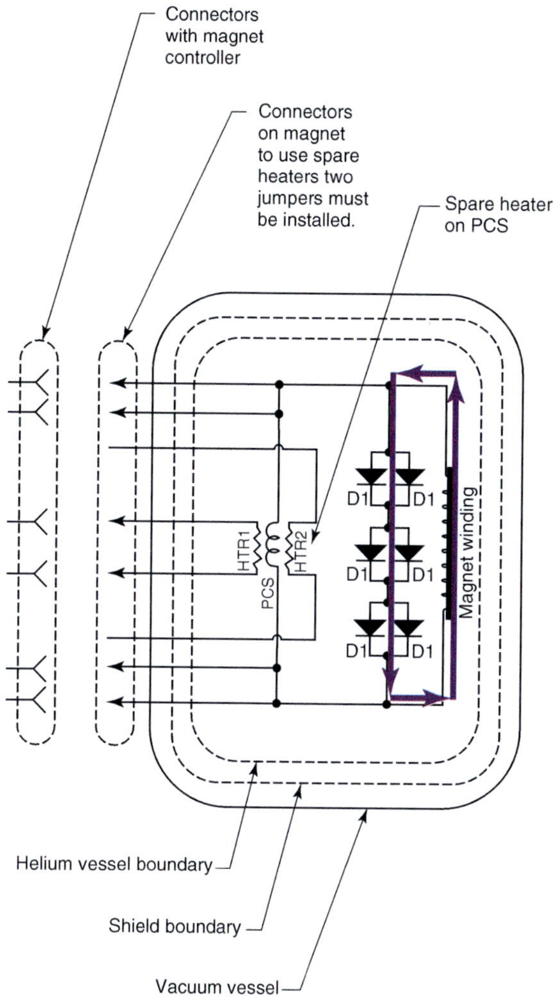

Figure 31.24. Current path through the cold diode protection path

become 'persistent' as shown in Figure 31.23. Full operational current now flows through the PCS.

10. After warming of the external current lead connections, the retractable current leads are removed.

The simplified discharging process is as follows:

1. The magnet's LHe level and pressure is confirmed thus allowing for safe discharging.
2. Retractable current leads are installed (if permanent leads are not present).
3. Helium gas flow is allowed to vent to atmosphere and pass by the leads, cooling them and providing the necessary enthalpy for removal of the current lead's subsequent I^2R heating.
4. The power supply's voltage is preset to 5–10 VDC and the current is raised to match the operational current within the magnet. As the PCS has zero inductance, this current can be increased from zero to operational current quickly, typically in a minute or two. This step nulls the current in the PCS to within a few amperes.
5. The heater on the PCS is energized by separate external power supply, thus driving the PCS from superconducting to normal state.
6. The power supply voltage is reduced to zero allowing discharge through the external dump resistor or diode bank. Alternatively, a four-quadrant power supply can be set with opposite voltage polarity allowing for quicker discharge (Figure 31.27).
7. The same voltage that is across the magnet terminals is also across the PCS, thus providing additional PCS heating via V^2/R heating ensuring the PCS remains resistive in its normal state.
8. Once the magnet operational current reaches zero, the PCS heater voltage is turned off and the PCS once again cools and becomes superconducting.
9. After warming of the external current lead connections, the retractable current leads are removed.

Finally, in addition to the main DC power supply, PCS power supply and discharge diode bank or dump resistor, there is a liquid helium level sensor meter, displays and/or controllers for the coil's internal voltage taps (used diagnostically by magnet vendor to determine location of quench if and when one occurs) and temperature sensors, a magnet helium vessel pressure controller and sensor display and emergency ramp-down power supply. These are usually contained collectively in what is termed the Magnet controller.

DISCLAIMER

The subject matter, content, and views presented do not represent the views of the Department of Health and Human Services (HHS), US Food and Drug Administration (FDA), and/or the United States.

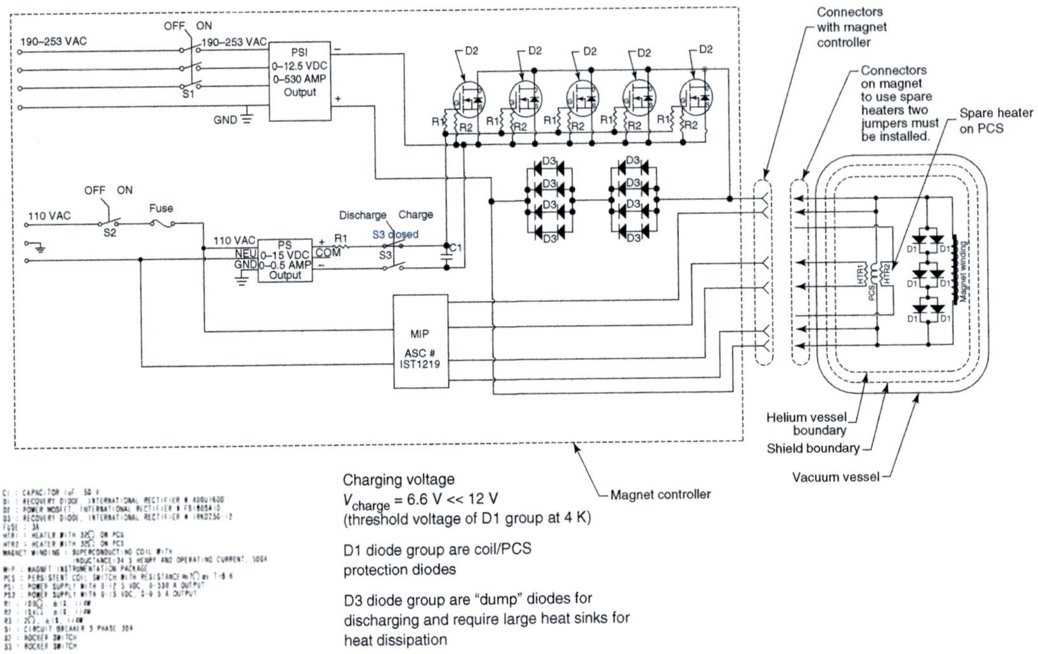

Figure 31.25. Magnet power supply and charging/discharging circuit

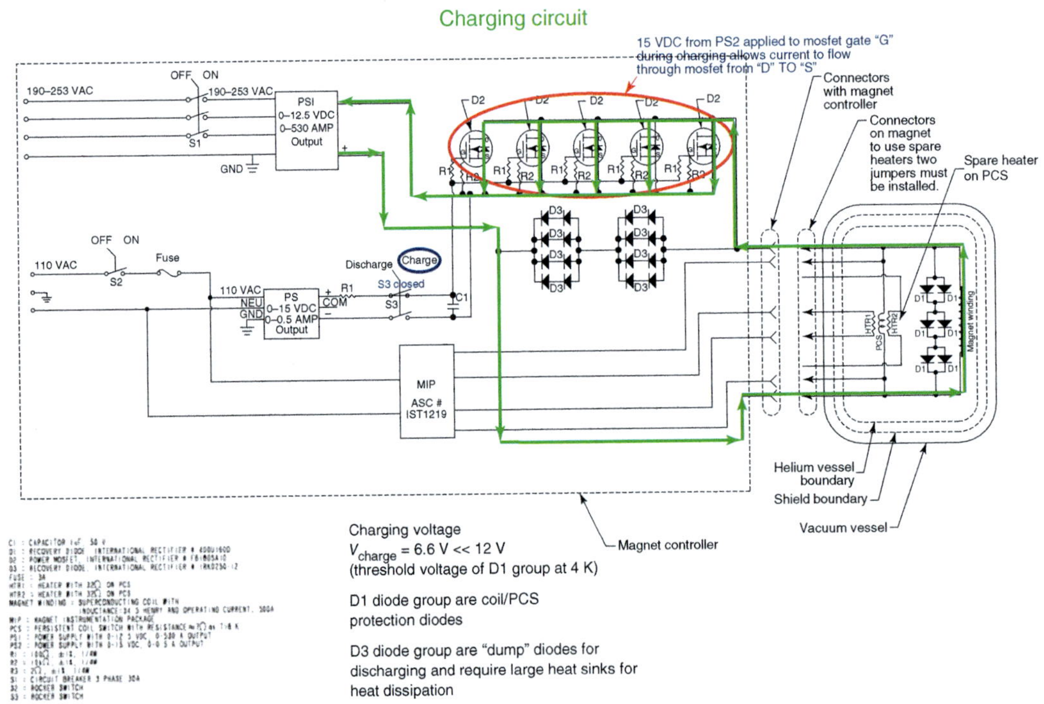

Figure 31.26. Charging circuit

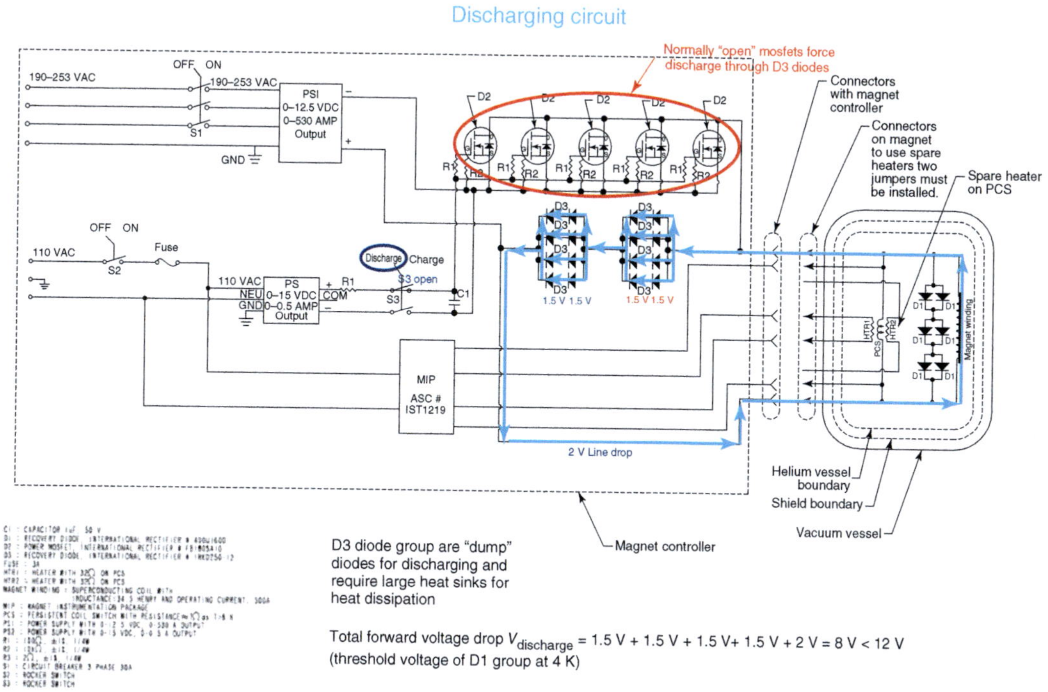

Figure 31.27. Discharging circuit

RELATED ARTICLES IN EMAGRES

Garroway, Allen N.: Origins of MRI—A Personal View

Hinshaw, Waldo: Notes on the History of MR Imaging from my Perspective

Lauterbur, Paul C.: One Path out of Many—How MRI Actually Began

Ramsey, Norman F.: Origins of Magnetic Resonance

Cryogenic Magnets for Whole-Body Magnetic Resonance Systems

High Temperature Superconductors

Magnetic Resonance Imaging: A Historical Overview

REFERENCES

1. M. H. Nayfeh and M. K. Brussel, Electricity and Magnetism, John Wiley & Sons, Inc: New York, 1985.
2. J. H. Kim, S. I. Park, T. D. Le, and H. M. Kim, *Prog. Superconduct. Cryogenics*, 2014, **16**, 47.

Chapter 32

Fabrication of Superconducting Magnets for MRI

Bruce Breneman

Breneman Consulting, Rancho Santa Fe, CA, USA

Safety and Biological Effects in MRI.
Edited by Devashish Shrivastava and J. Thomas Vaughan

ISBN: 978-1-118-82130-5
Also published in eMagRes (online edition)
DOI: 10.1002/9780470034590.emrstm1591

32.1 MAGNET CROSS SECTION

To review, a modern magnetic resonance imaging (MRI) superconducting magnet comprises of the following main components: an external vacuum vessel with frame, an internal helium vessel with coil and coil bobbin/former, a single thermal shield, persistent switch, low heat lead current leads, a two-stage GM Cryocooler with associated cold head sleeve, and a liquid helium (LHe) fill and vent stack with helium gas relief system. Figure 32.1 shows a pictorial representation of a 1.5 T MRI superconducting magnet cross section. Figure 32.2 shows a physical cross section of the same magnet.

32.2 HELIUM VESSEL WINDING BOBBIN

Magnet fabrication starts with the helium vessel inner cylinder, which in this 1.5 T example is also

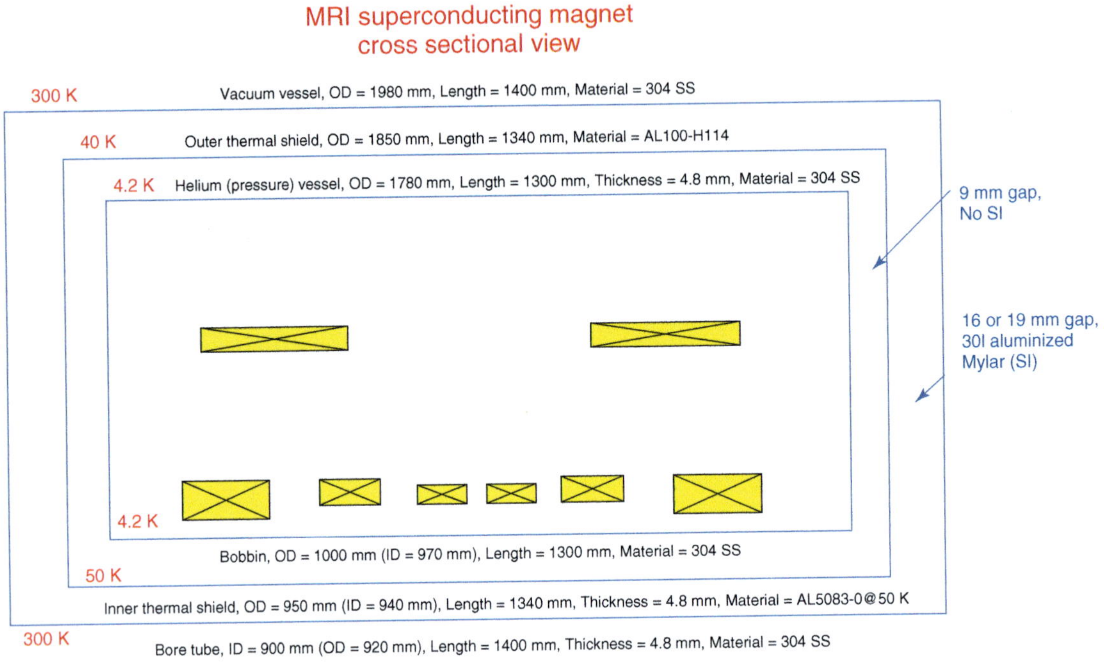

Figure 32.1. 1.5 T magnet pictorial cross section

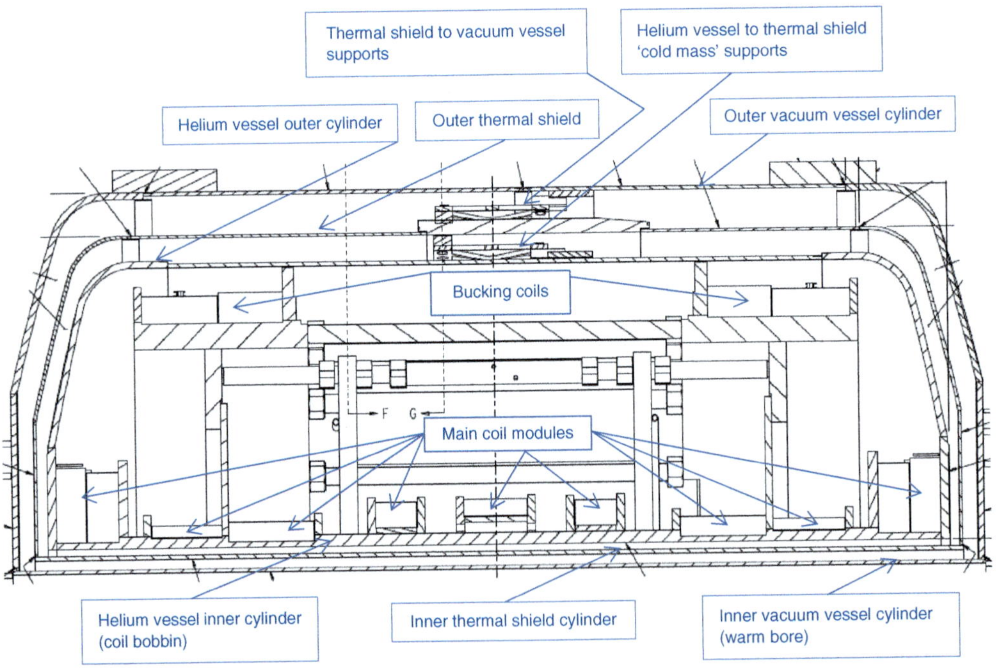

Figure 32.2. 1.5 T magnet cross section

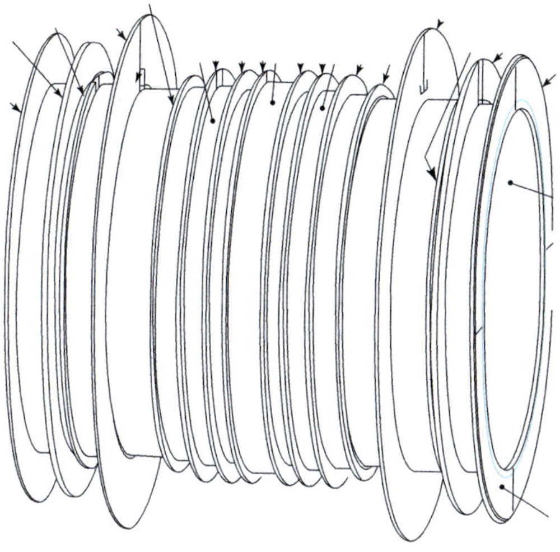

Figure 32.3. Bobbin assembly

the winding bobbin or coil former. The bobbin is machined from rolled and longitudinally welded 304 stainless steel and has tungsten inert gas (TIG) welded winding flanges to support the left and right sides of each coil module. As previously discussed, the axial Lorentz forces can approach a million pounds thus proper weld preparations are required for each flange. The bobbin far left and right flanges are eventually welded to the final helium vessel end plates after winding is complete. The surface of the bobbin is lathe machined to a diametrical and cylindricity tolerance of 0.5 mm. The axial location of the coil flanges, width, and perpendicularity are machined to a very tight tolerance of 0.1 mm to ensure accurate coil module placement. The bobbin longitudinal welds and end plate plates are radiographically or dye penetrant checked prior to winding as repair of a leaking bobbin weld is difficult to correct after winding is complete. Figures 32.3–32.6 show a typical bobbin assembly.

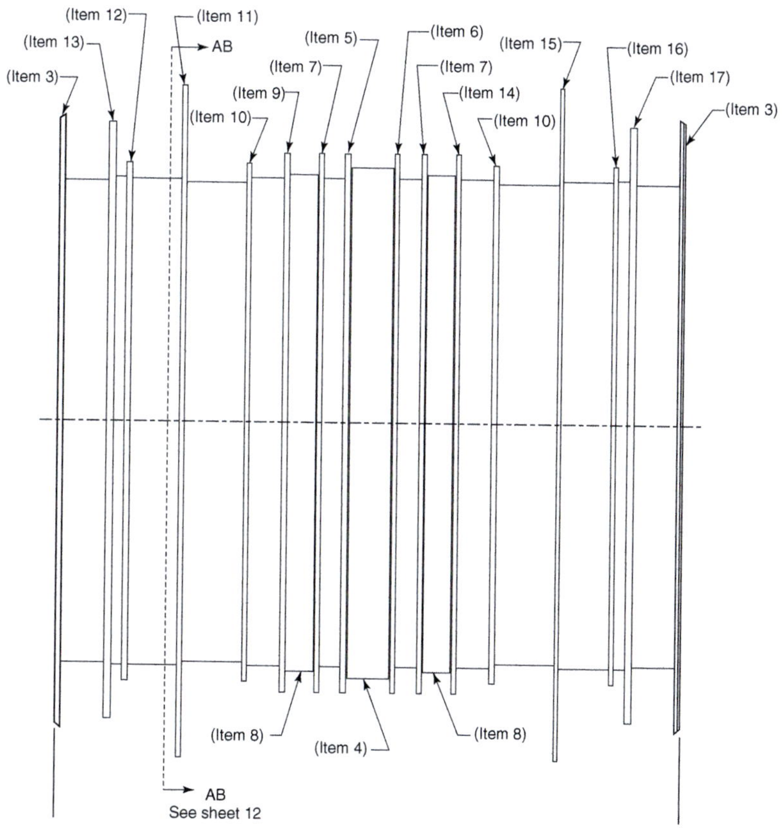

Figure 32.4. Bobbin assembly

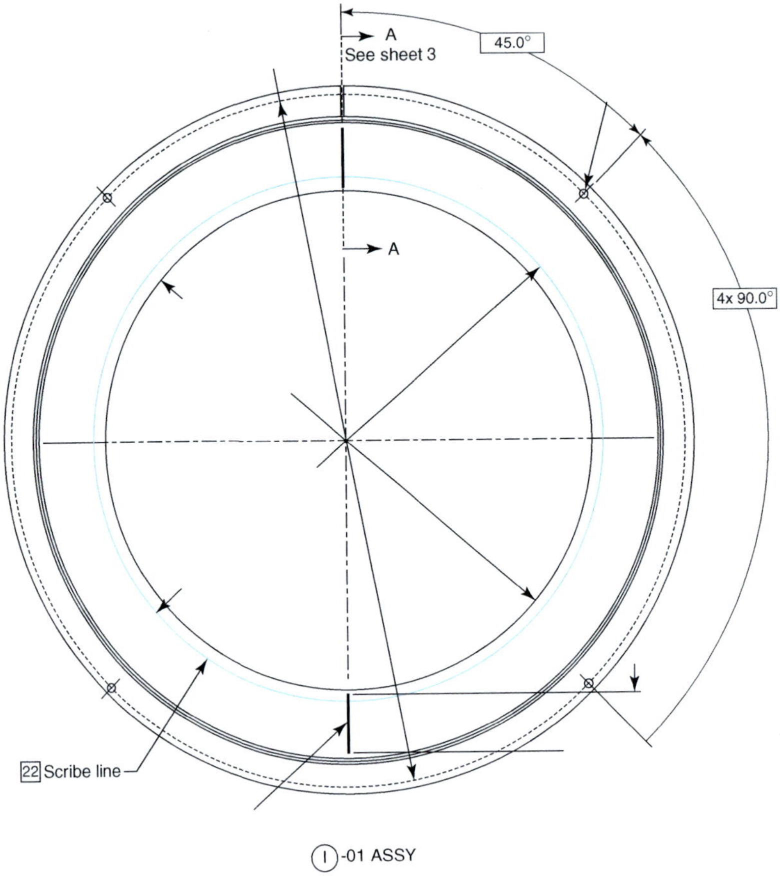

Figure 32.5. Bobbin assembly

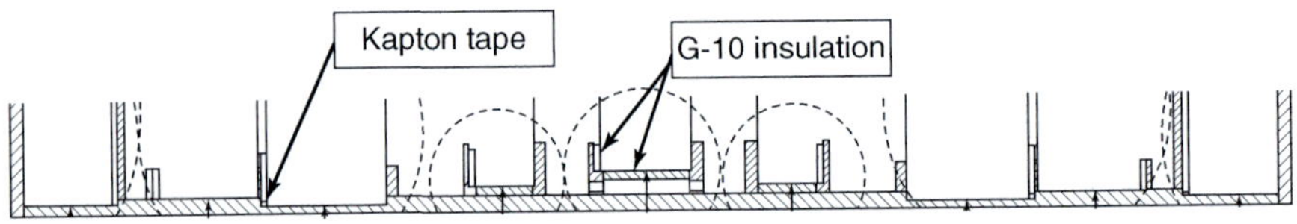

Figure 32.6. Bobbin insulation

Prior to winding, each bobbin surface/end plate edge is Kapton™ tape insulated and the winding surfaces and flanges are insulated with 0.3–0.5 mm thick G-10 fiberglass phenolic material (Figure 32.6).

32.3 COIL MODULE WINDING

The bobbin is mounted on the winding machine, the supply spool of superconducting wire mounted on the de-spooler and the start of the wire is fed through a G-10 wire transition on the coil module flange. A 10–75 lbf tension is applied to the wire (as determined in previously described coil stress analysis) and a base coat of two-part cryogenic grade, approximately 500 cps viscosity, epoxy is applied. As winding proceeds, epoxy is hand applied in what is referred to as a 'wet lay-up' process. It should be noted that some magnet manufacturers prefer to use Stycast epoxy in their wet lay-up winding while others wind dry and afterward

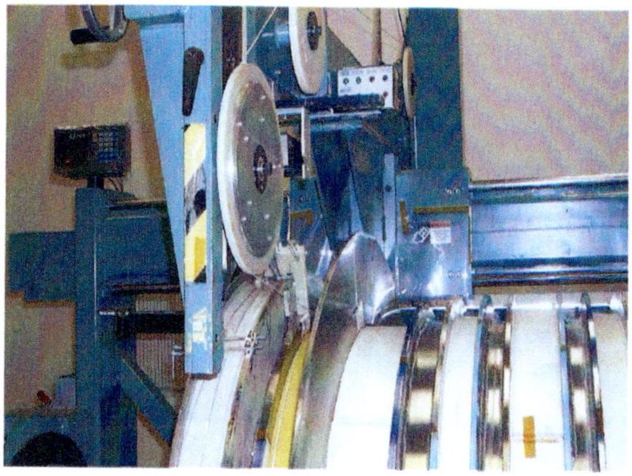

Figure 32.7. 1.5 T magnet coil winding

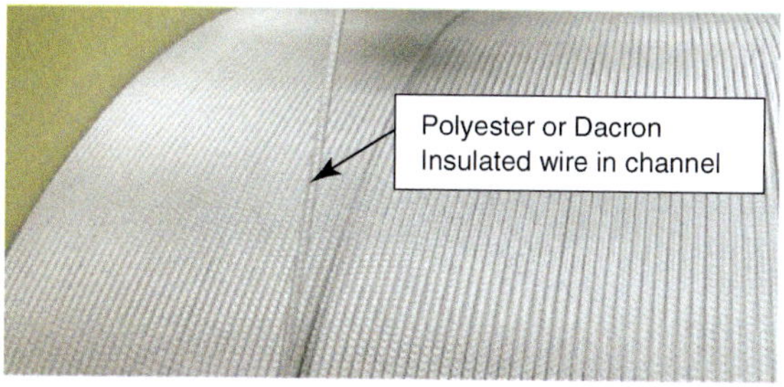

Figure 32.8. 1.5 T magnet coil winding

perform back pressure epoxy vacuum impregnation. Either of these methods can yield good results. To ensure the method's success, extensive test winding and destructive testing is performed prior to actual coil winding to prove proper epoxy penetration to all layers and turns of the winding.

As multiple winding layers are wound, the diametrical build is often measured using a pi tape with corrections made to ensure proper radial dimension. This can be done by adding or removing 0.05–0.1 mm perforated paper, S-glass, E-glass, or fiberglass which is often used during the winding process as additional interlayer insulation and/or to establish a good winding surface for subsequent winding layers.

Each coil module is wound in sequence, in this case using the wet lay-up method. Superconducting wire feed spools have finite length and thus logical end points must be predetermined. 'Lead in' and 'lead out' wires are left exposed at these locations and a low resistance wire joint made after winding is complete.

Figures 32.7–32.9 show actual coil winding of our 1.5 T example.

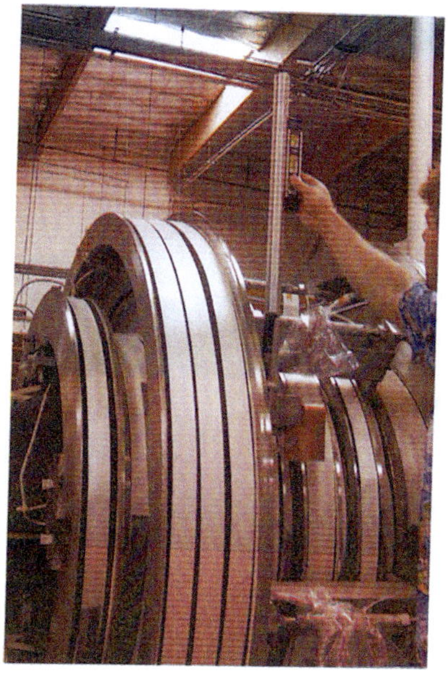

Figure 32.9. 1.5 T magnet coil winding

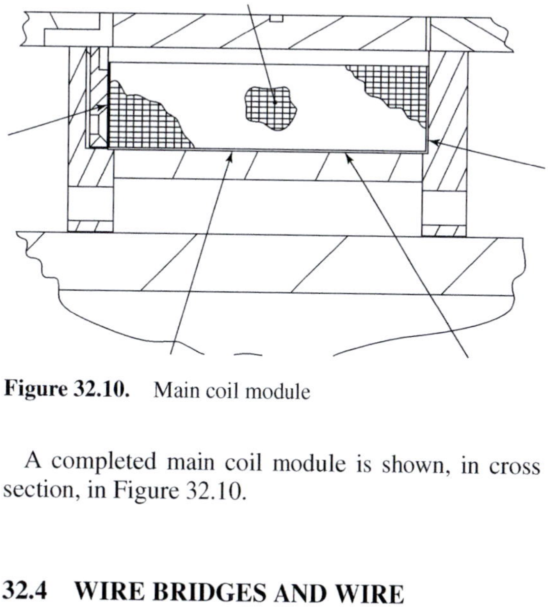

Figure 32.10. Main coil module

A completed main coil module is shown, in cross section, in Figure 32.10.

32.4 WIRE BRIDGES AND WIRE TRANSITIONS

The completed bucking coil module is shown in Figure 32.11. In this case, it can be observed that the start and end points of the coil module winding are on opposite ends. A G-10 'bridge' with wire inserted and epoxy fixed within a machined groove

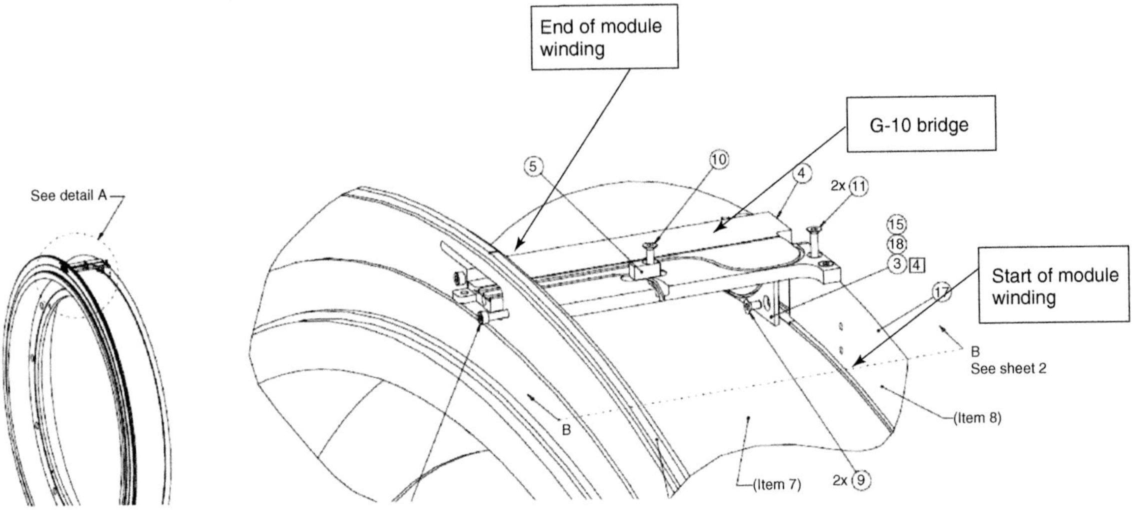

Figure 32.11. Bucking coil module

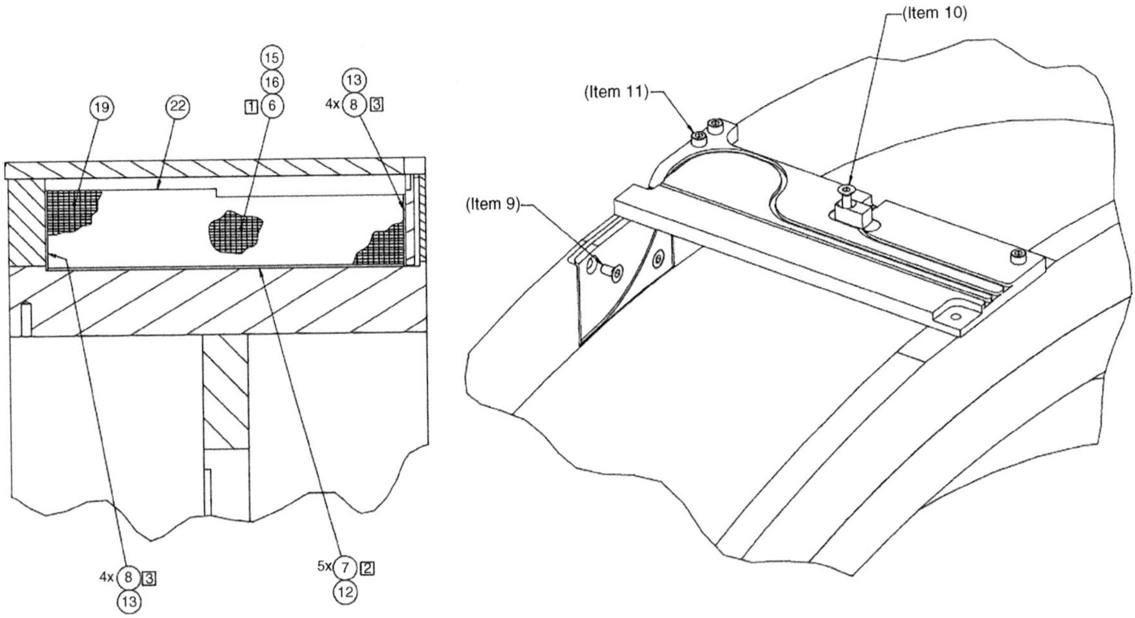

Figure 32.12. Opposing bucking coil module and wire transition

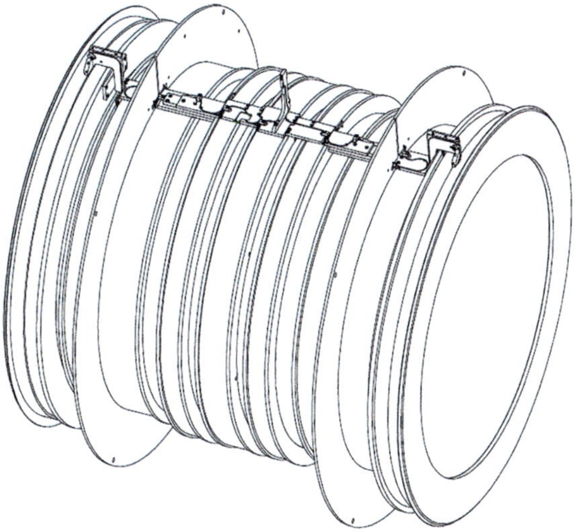

Figure 32.13. Completed coil modules with wire transitions

allows for a smooth, low strain, return to winding start location.

Figure 32.12 shows the opposing bucking module with G-10 bridge and wire transitions.

The coil winding with all modules wound and wire transitions performed is shown in Figures 32.13–32.15.

32.5 COIL INSTRUMENTATION

Instrumentation such as ruthenium oxide or Cernox temperature sensors are mounted at strategic locations such as the top of the bucking coil module as shown in Figure 32.16. Voltage taps are added to the lead

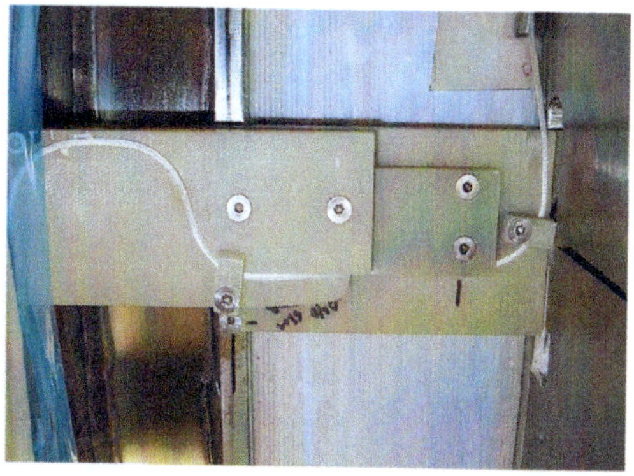

Figure 32.15. Completed coil module with wire transitions

in and lead out of all coil modules providing location information in the event of a coil quench. Finally, as seen in Figure 32.16, film resistors are surface mounted using epoxy allowing for Emergency Ramp Down capability as previously described as well as 'quench back' control. These quench back film resistors act as heaters and allow all modules to participate in a coil quench thus more equally distributing and depositing the coil's stored energy and minimizing temperature increase to any one coil module.

32.6 WIRE JOINTS

As previously mentioned, each superconducting wire feed spool has finite length which is less than the overall required length. Typically, 4–5 spools of wire are required to wind a 1.5 T coil. Logical end points for each spool are specified in the design phase with wire lengths specified by the magnet fabricator to the wire

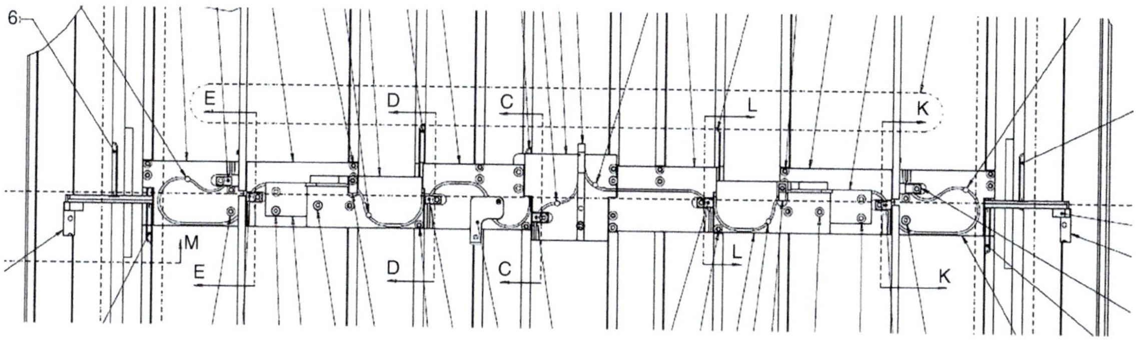

Figure 32.14. Completed coil modules with wire transitions

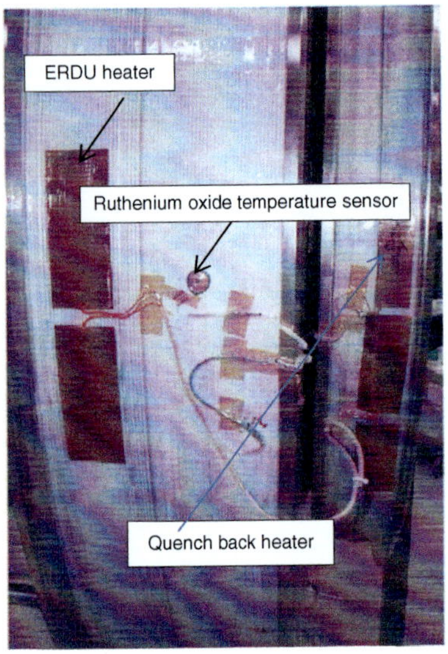

Figure 32.16. Coil instrumentation

manufacturer. 'Lead in' and 'lead out' wires are left exposed at these predetermined locations and a low resistance wire joint made after winding is complete. Each joint method is unique to each MRI magnet manufacturer. One technique is to etch and remove each of the mating wire's stabilizing copper over a 5 cm length, ultrasonically clean and braid the filaments of each end together, place the braided assembly in a copper substrate and the substrate pressed to form a solid junction. This mechanical joint is performed under high force, elevated temperature, and vacuum to ensure joint resistances of $<1E\text{-}09\ \Omega$. The joints are then mechanically and thermally supported by placing each in a copper joint cup with molten indium filling the cup's cavity thus securing the joint. Figure 32.17 shows the wire bridges and wire groove feeds to each copper joint cup.

32.7 PERSISTENT CURRENT SWITCH (PCS)

Located within the magnet's helium space is a persistent current switch or PCS. This is a small zero inductance superconducting coil that is connected electrically in series with the main magnet coils. Figure 32.18 depicts a PCS for our 1.5 T example.

The finished copper cups with joints and PCS are installed as shown in Figure 32.19.

32.8 PROTECTION DIODES

The PCS protection diode assembly can be seen in Figure 32.20.

Figure 32.21 is a photograph showing the diode assembly, the copper cups with joints and PCS, main lead assemblies and LHe level sensors.

32.9 POWER LEAD MULTI-CONTACT CONNECTORS

Mounted at the top of the coil is an assembly comprising of four male Multilam™ multi-contact power lead connectors as shown in Figures 32.22 and 32.23. One pair of connectors is for the positive voltage lead while the other pair is for the negative voltage lead. Matching female Multilam connectors are incorporated into the removable current lead assembly.

32.10 HELIUM VESSEL ASSEMBLY

Once the coil winding, wire bridge transitions and wire joints are completed and all instrumentation, PCS, protection diode assembly and Multilam multi-contact connectors are installed, the helium vessel assembly can be completed. As described previously, the helium vessel assembly comprises of the outer cylinder, inner cylinder (coil winding bobbin), and associated end plates.

The inner cylinder of the helium vessel is part of the pressure vessel and in this example simultaneously the winding bobbin/former for the superconducting coil modules. Support rods are installed and TIG welded (as seen in Figure 32.24) between the two bucking coils to support the very large axial Lorentz force previously discussed.

The outer helium vessel cylinder, helium vessel main neck tube and mounting brackets for the cold mass support system are next TIG welded together as shown in Figures 32.25–32.27. The entire helium vessel assembly next undergoes a leak check in which the interior

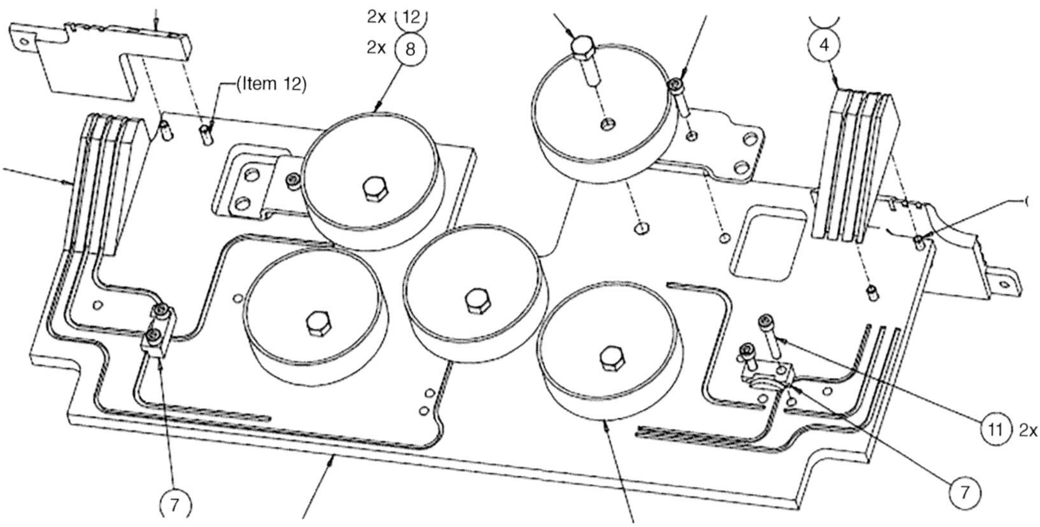

Figure 32.17. Wire bridges and joint cups

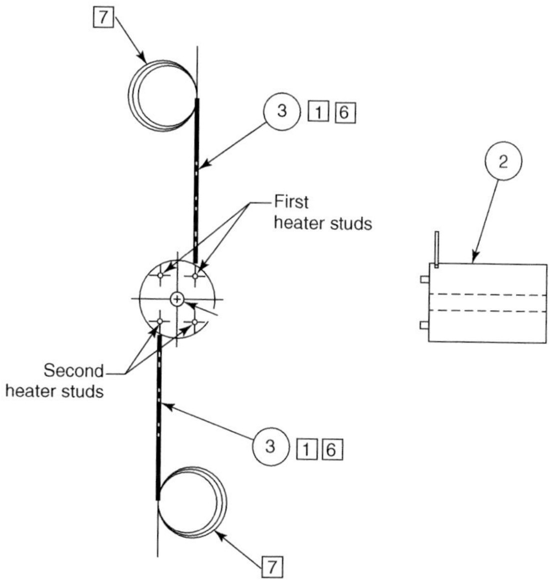

Figure 32.18. Persistent current switch (PCS)

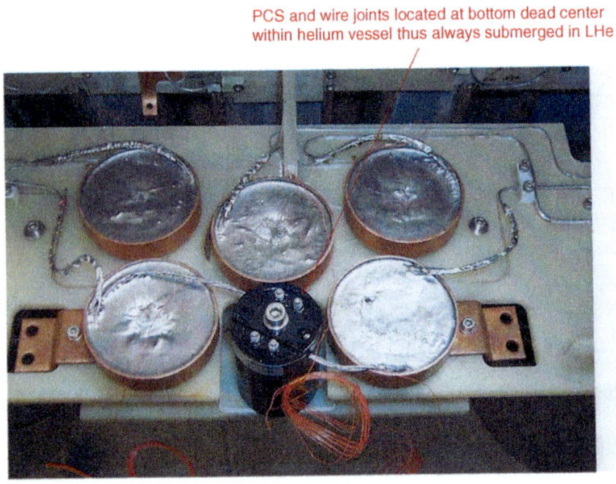

Figure 32.19. Completed joint cups and PCS

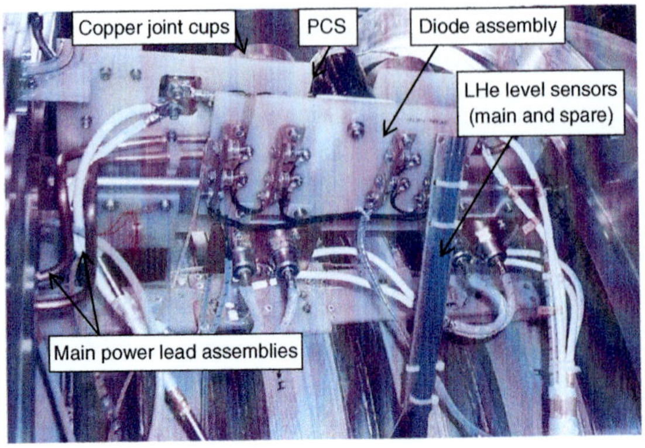

Figure 32.21. PCS protection diode assembly

of the helium vessel assembly is vacuum pumped and connected to a leak detector while the exterior of the helium vessel assembly is covered and sealed in a plastic bag which is flooded with helium gas. If any helium is detected inside, then each and every external helium vessel assembly weld is individually checked by local flooding with helium gas. The leak location is re-welded and once again leak checked.

Note, as discussed previously, now is not an acceptable time to find a leak in the inner helium vessel/winding bobbin/former cylinder longitudinal weld as this weld is in close proximity to the coil winding. Heat from repairing a leaking longitudinal inner cylinder weld could damage the wound coil modules. It is for this reason that these welds were previously checked.

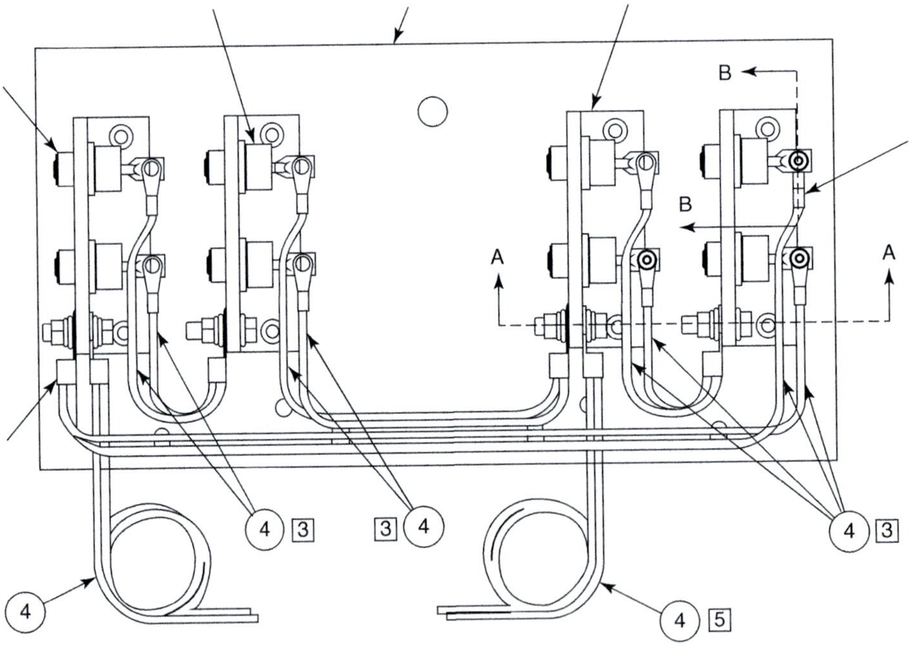

Figure 32.20. PCS protection diode assembly

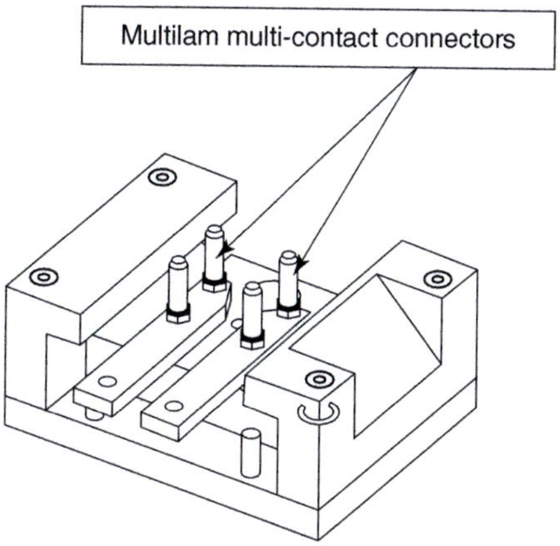

Figure 32.22. Multilam connectors

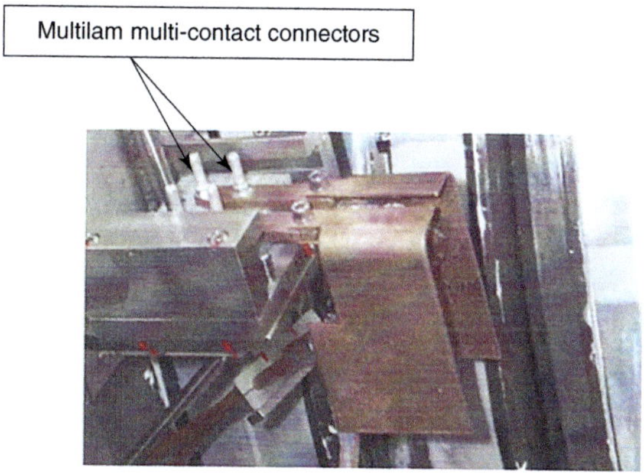

Figure 32.23. Multilam connectors

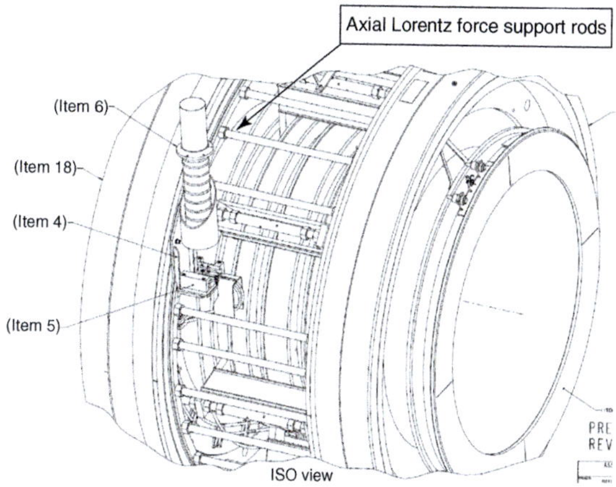

Figure 32.24. Axial Lorentz force supports

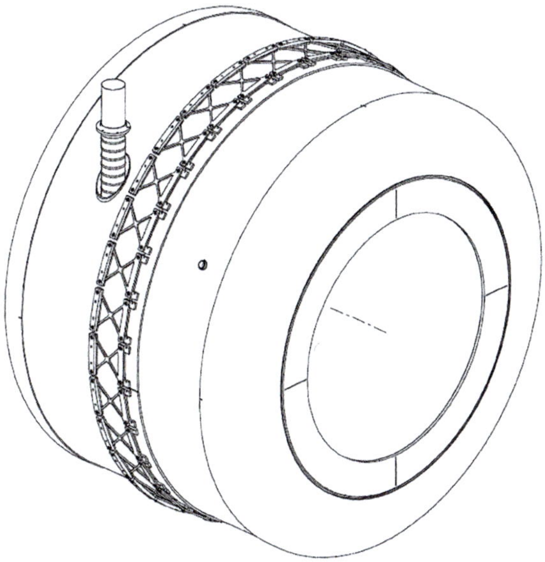

Figure 32.25. Cold mass supports

32.11 SUPPORT SYSTEM ASSEMBLY

Many types of 'cold mass' support systems can be deployed to support the helium vessel and shield. These supports react the normal static weight of the helium vessel and thermal shield and support the 1–3 G acceleration induced force that can occur during magnet transportation. The helium vessel can be directly or independently supported by the vacuum vessel. Alternately, the helium vessel can be supported by the thermal shield and the thermal shield supported to the vacuum vessel. Stiff, high modulus of elasticity materials such as S or E-glass reinforced plastic or carbon fiber are often used due to their high strength to thermal conductivity ratio. The cold mass support system in our 1.5 T case is a truss system shown in Figures 32.25–32.27. Approximately 40 G-10 trusses are installed between the helium vessel outer cylinder and outer thermal shield.

32.12 THERMAL RADIATION SHIELD ASSEMBLY

The magnet's thermal shield is often referred to as a radiation shield. Approximately 30 layers of

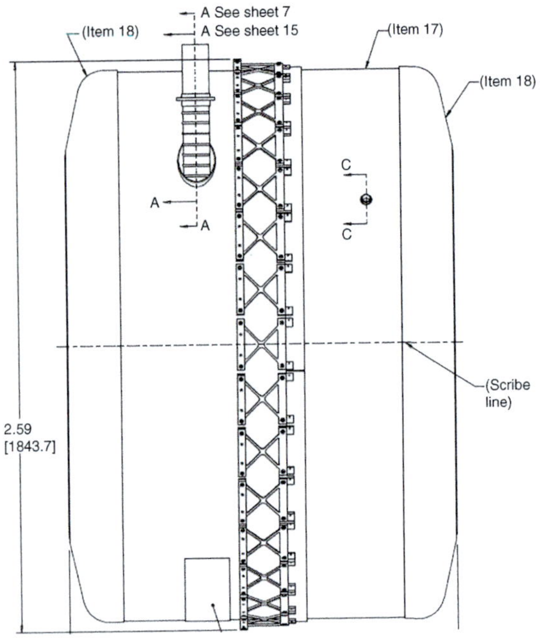

Figure 32.26. Cold mass supports

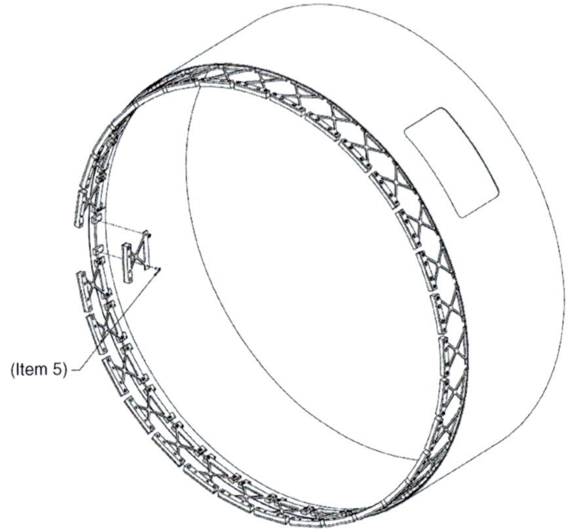

Figure 32.28. G-10 trusses

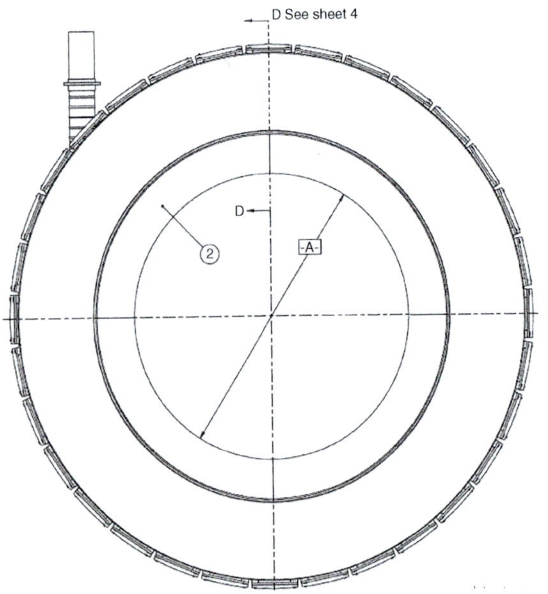

Figure 32.27. Cold mass supports

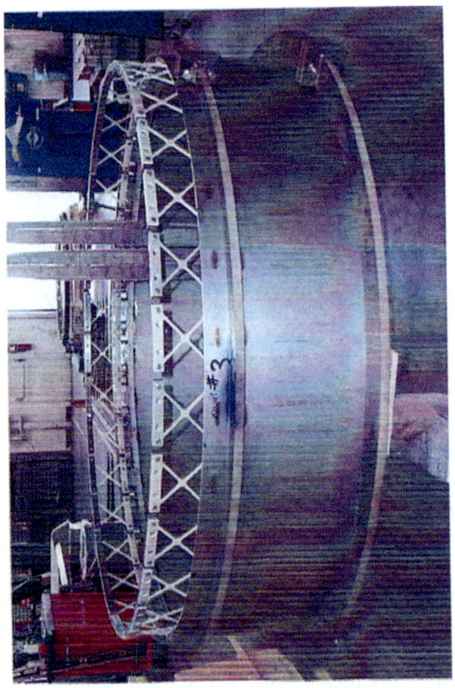

Figure 32.29. G-10 trusses

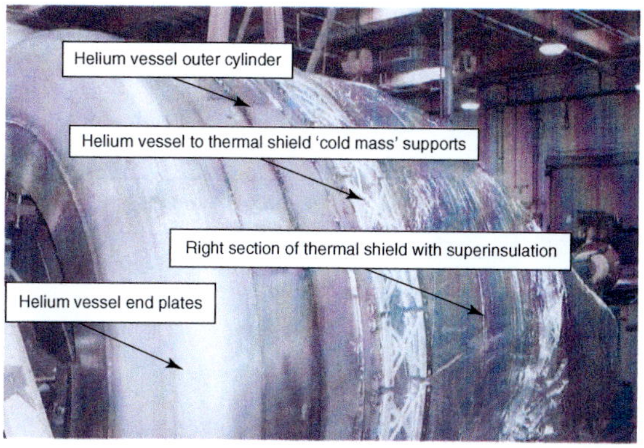

Figure 32.30. Completed helium vessel

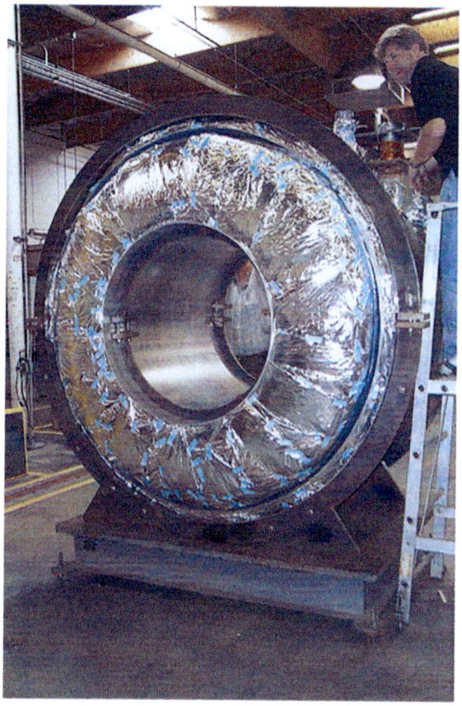

Figure 32.31. Helium vessel, thermal shield, and vacuum vessel assemblies

aluminized Mylar, called superinsulation or SI, are wrapped loosely surrounding the thermal shield to provide a low emissivity surface, establish thermal gradient layers between the vacuum vessel and

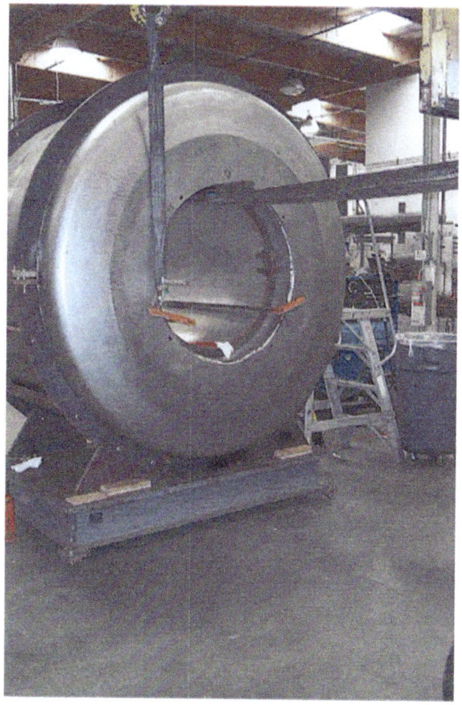

Figure 32.32. Completed vacuum vessel assembly

thermal shield as well as eliminate any potential 300 K to 40 K direct 'shine through' passage between warm and cold surfaces. Forty G-10 trusses are next installed between the outer thermal shield and outer vacuum vessel as seen in Figures 32.28 and 32.29.

32.13 COMPLETED OUTER THERMAL SHIELD AND HELIUM VESSEL ASSEMBLY

Figure 32.30 shows the completed helium vessel on the left end of the figure, the helium vessel outer cylinder to outer thermal shield truss system centrally located near magnet middle and the SI outer thermal shield on the right end. The left section of the thermal shield is TIG welded to a central stiffening ring in the following step.

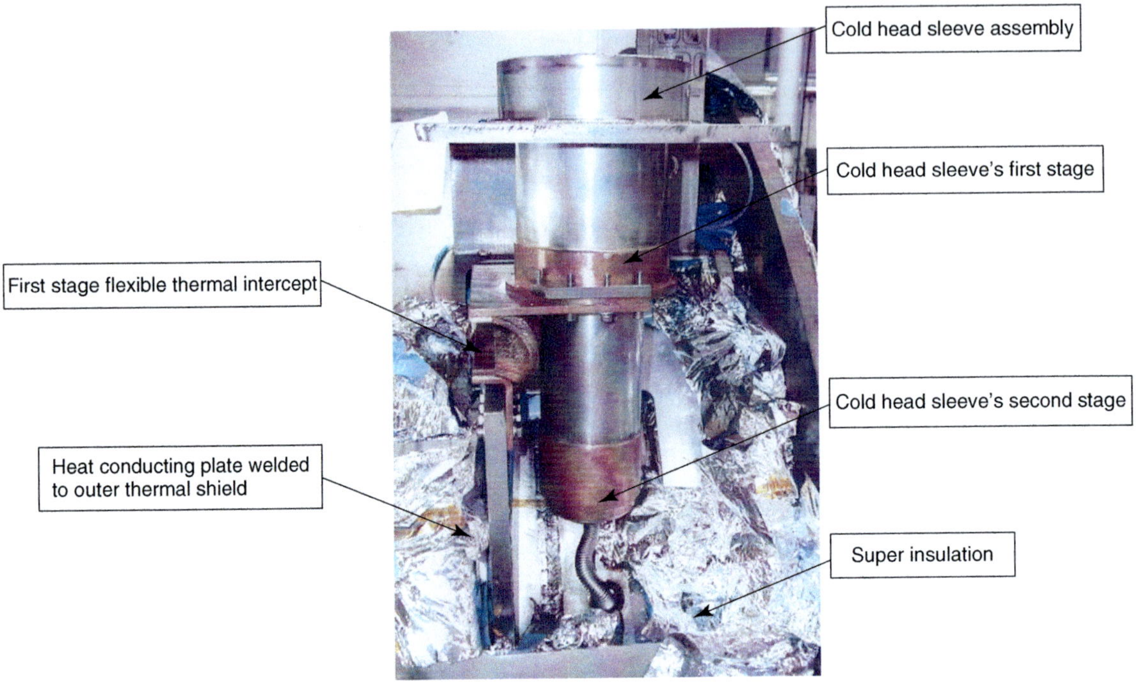

Figure 32.33. Cold head sleeve

32.14 INNER THERMAL SHIELD AND VACUUM BORE TUBE ASSEMBLY

Once the helium vessel, outer thermal shield, and outer vacuum vessel are assembled via their truss support systems, the inner thermal shield is brought into position. This inner thermal shield has temporary rounding rings at each end at the cylinder's inner diameter keeping the cylindricity to within 1.0 mm throughout and concentric near each end to approximately 0.5–1.0 mm. Again, 30 layers of SI are loosely wrapped around the outer diameter of the inner thermal shield. Each thermal shield end plate is positioned in place and TIG welds are made between each end plate and inner and outer thermal shield cylinders. Similarly, the vacuum vessel inner cylinder (referred to as the 'warm bore') is positioned and TIG welded to the vacuum vessel end plates. Rounding rings are employed in the warm bore tube inner diameter to keep it cylindrical throughout and concentric at each end. Figure 32.31 shows the helium vessel, thermal shield, and vacuum vessel assemblies prior to welding the vacuum vessel endplates. Note the carefully wrapped SI layers.

32.15 COMPLETED VACUUM VESSEL ASSEMBLY

The completed vacuum vessel assembly prior to TIG welding is shown in Figure 32.32.

32.16 COLD HEAD SLEEVE ASSEMBLY

Often a permanently installed 'cold head sleeve' is installed in the magnet allowing the Cryocooler cold head to be removed from the magnet when serviced at maintenance intervals. A heat exchanger capable of re-liquefying helium gas to LHe is associated with the second stage allowing the magnet to run 'closed cycle' with no helium gas venting to atmosphere. Figures 32.33 and 32.34 show a typical cold head sleeve. A flexible, high conductivity thermal intercept is shown connected between the sleeve's first stage

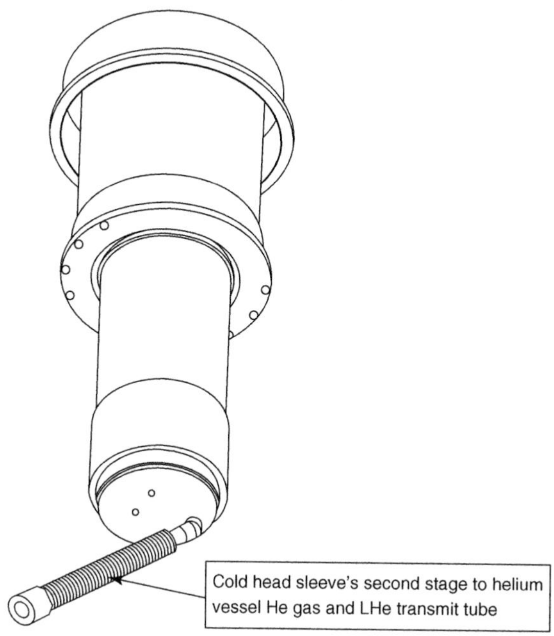

Figure 32.34. Cold head sleeve

and outer thermal shield. This thermal connection allows for approximately 40 W of cooling to the thermal shield assembly with an associated minimal temperature drop of only 1–3 K.

32.17 CRYOCOOLER COLD HEAD ASSEMBLY

A two-stage rare earth GM Cryocooler cold head, as shown in Figure 32.35, will eventually be mated with the cold head sleeve assembly above.

32.18 REMOVABLE CURRENT LEAD ASSEMBLY

Removable (retractable) current leads eliminate the need for permanently installed leads and are inserted only for charging or discharging of the magnet. These leads are shown in Figures 32.36–32.38 and are located within the 'lead/vent turret' as seen in Figure 32.39.

32.19 COLD HEAD SLEEVE THERMAL SHIELDING

Just as the main magnet has a thermal radiation shield, the lead and vent tube assembly, as well as the cold head sleeve assembly, must have thermal barriers

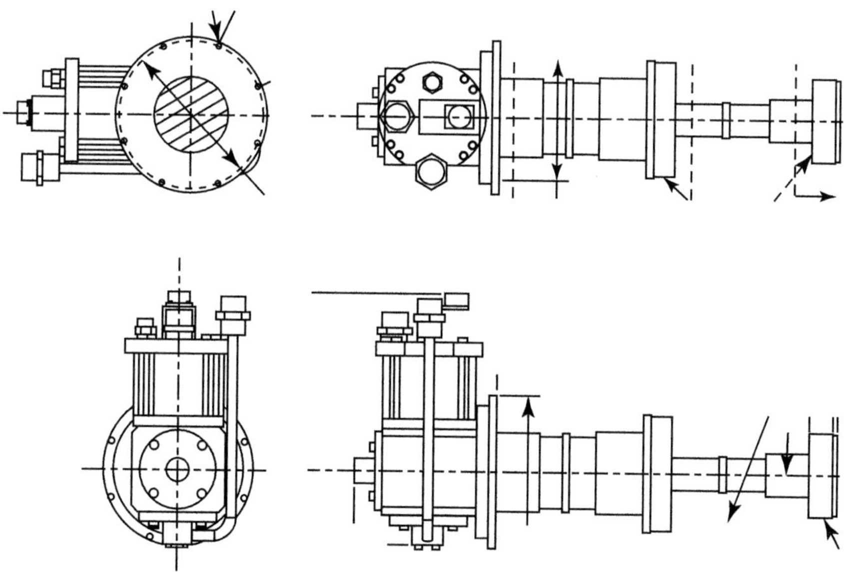

Figure 32.35. Two-stage rare earth GM Cryocooler cold head

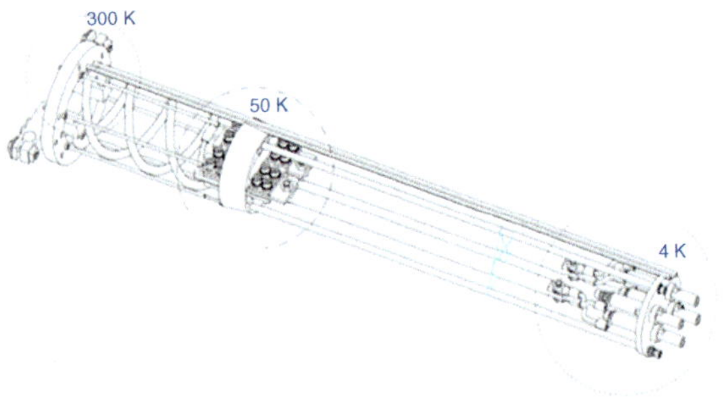

Figure 32.36. Removable (retractable) current leads

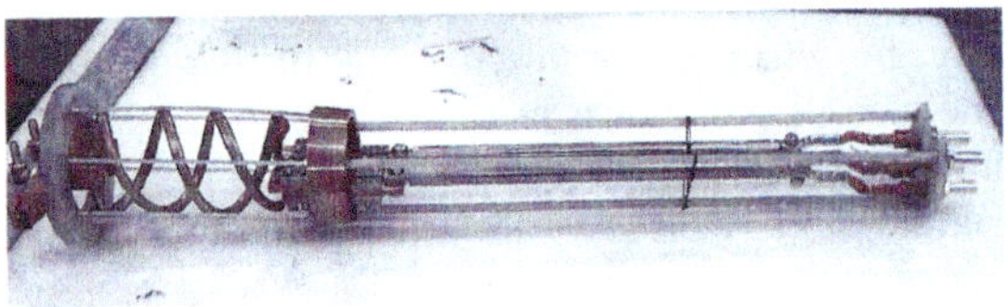

Figure 32.37. Removable (retractable) current leads

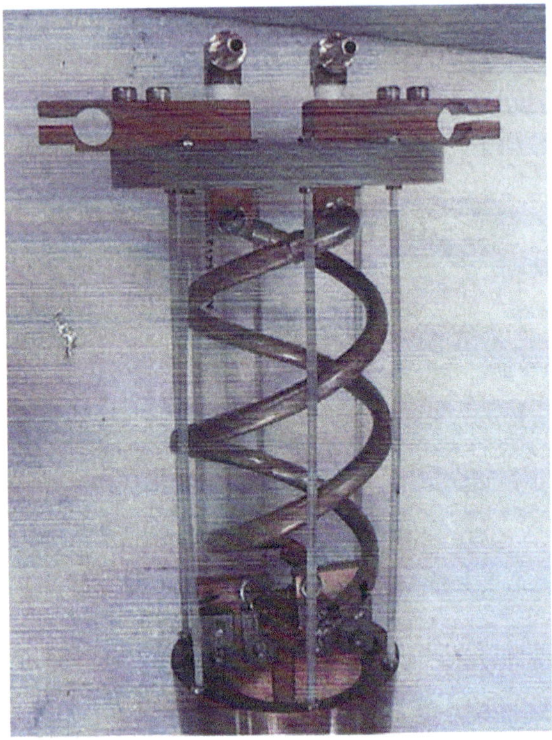

Figure 32.38. Removable (retractable) current leads

between room temperature and 4.2 K. Figure 32.40 shows the cold head sleeve assembly thermal shield. Once installed, as shown in Figure 32.41, the thermal shield must be wrapped with 15–30 layers of SI as shown in Figure 32.42.

The completed lead and cold head sleeve turrets are shown in Figure 32.43.

32.20 HELIUM GAS VENT SYSTEM

The helium gas vent system is very important for the safety of the magnet as well as personnel working near the magnet. If the LHe surrounding the magnet coil is heated due to a quench or vacuum space breach, it undergoes a change in state from liquid to a gas at 4.2 K. Subsequently, the helium gas is further heated from the excess stored energy in the magnet's coil. The helium gas warms and consequently expands by a factor of ~750 as the gas approaches room temperature. Insufficient flow diameter or flow impedance can cause large pressure differentials leading to unsafe pressure within the helium vessel. The main vent tube assembly previously shown in Figures 32.24–32.27 must be properly sized in diameter to permit the full helium gas flow rate.

Several parallel flow paths allow safe venting as the helium gas exits the magnet vent tube assembly. The first parallel flow path is for normal gas venting associated with LHe filling or charging/discharging of the magnet coil. A manual ball valve is used to open and close this path as both LHe filling and charging/discharging is a planned event. A second parallel flow path is via a large diameter safety relief check valve. This check valve may be

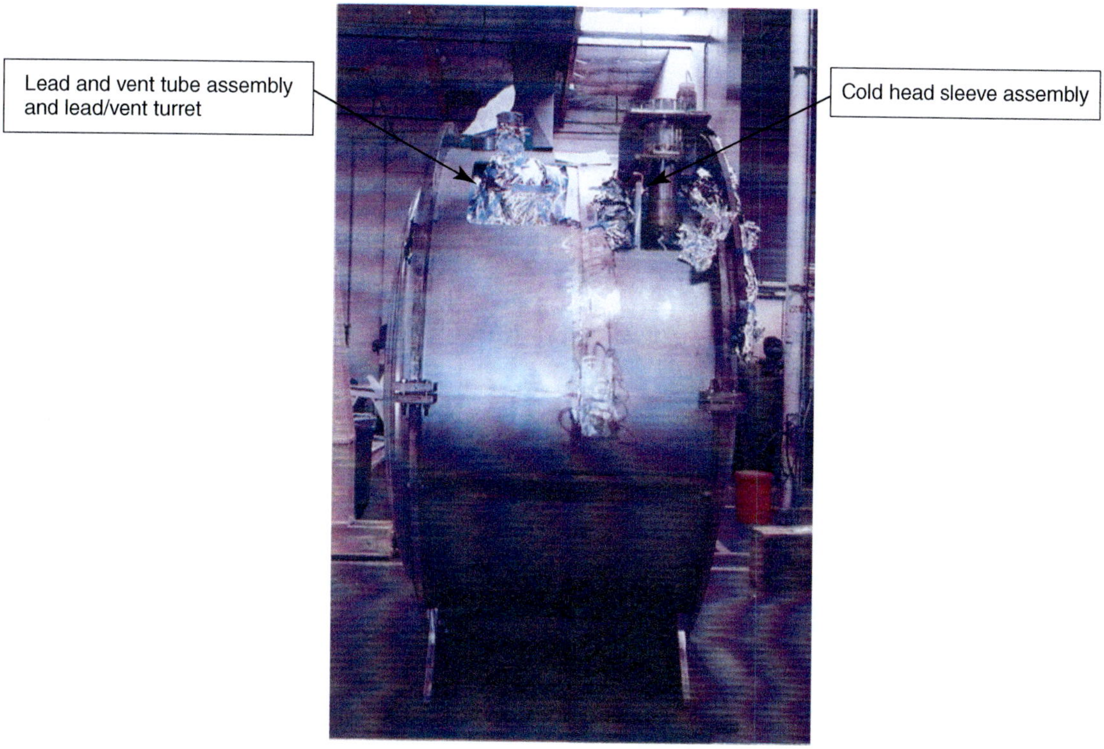

Figure 32.39. Lead/vent turret

set at 1–5 psig and opens and closes in the event of a magnet quench. Finally, a third parallel flow path is via a rupture disc set at 15–20 psig. In the event, the safety relief check valve does not fully open and is frozen closed or insufficient to allow proper venting of the helium gas, the thin-walled stainless steel disc mechanically ruptures allowing for full helium gas venting without large pressure build-up within the helium vessel assembly. After rupture, the disc must be manually removed and replaced.

The helium gas finally exits the magnet and is eventually vented to atmosphere via the site's helium vent pipe.

Figures 32.44–32.46 show the helium gas vent system for our 1.5 T example.

32.21 INSTRUMENTATION VACUUM CONNECTORS

Leads for instrumentation described in Figure 32.16 such as ruthenium oxide or Cernox temperature sensors, voltage taps, and film resistors as well as leads for the PCS heaters exit the vacuum vessel via vacuum use rated pin connectors. Figure 32.47 shows two such pin connectors after bolting to previously welded mounting brackets.

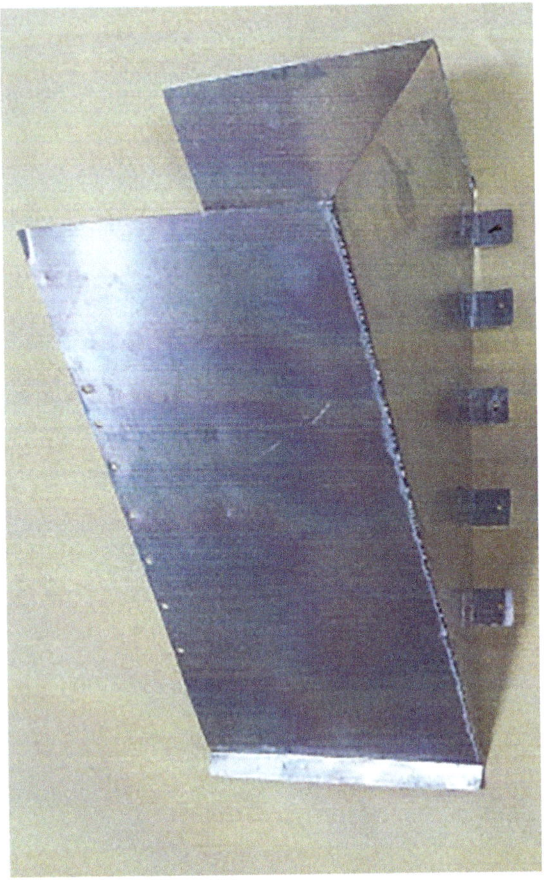

Figure 32.40. Sleeve shield

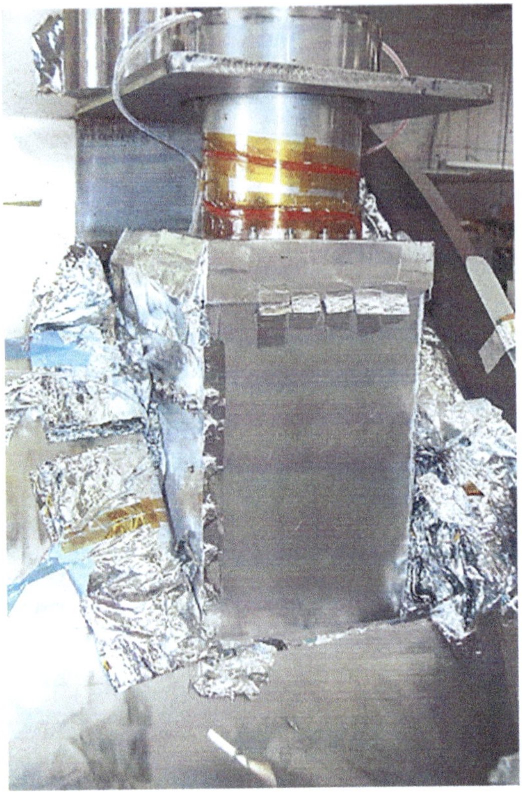

Figure 32.41. Sleeve shield

32.22 COMPLETED VENT SYSTEM

Figures 32.48 and 32.49 show the completed vent system with removable lead, Cryocooler cold head and LHe fill assembly installed.

32.23 VACUUM PUMPING AND LEAK DETECTION

Once assembly is complete the vacuum vessel is vacuum pumped to <10E−10 atm (~10E−07 Torr) and helium gas is pumped into the helium vessel. A mass spectrometer leak detector is connected to the vacuum vessel and once again the helium vessel assembly is leak checked. Once confirmation is obtained that no leakage rate is detected from the helium vessel, the entire vacuum vessel is bagged and helium gas is introduced into the bag thus saturating all external welds with helium gas. A leak check is performed again and once completed the cooldown is commenced. Initially, liquid nitrogen (LN_2) is transferred into the helium vessel to pre-cool the cold mass from 300 to 77 K. After a several days of 'soak time' the LN_2 is removed, the Cryocooler cold head is turned on and LHe is introduced into the helium vessel assembly. Initially, the LHe transfer is very slow so as to benefit from the cooling associated with the enthalpy of the cold helium gas. After several days, and approximately 3000–5000 l of LHe, the coil assembly reaches 4.2 K.

32.24 QUALITY ASSURANCE VERIFICATION

Finally, quality assurance and magnet parameter testing is performed verifying typical parameters as shown in Table 32.1.

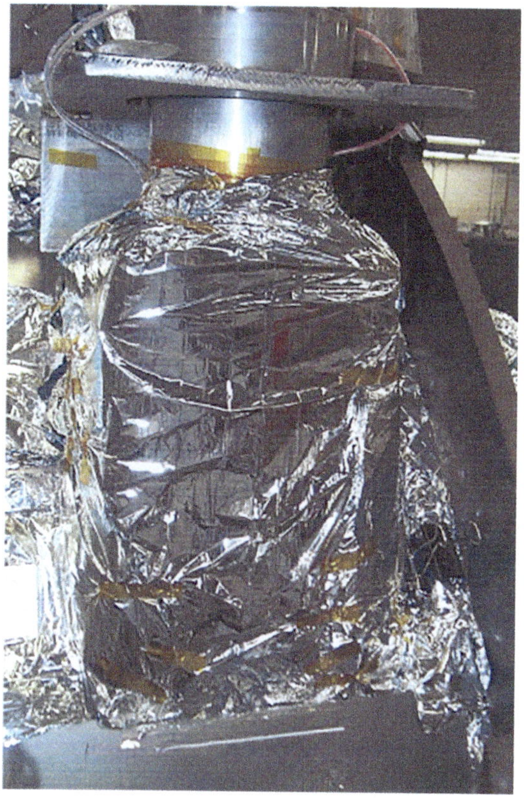

Figure 32.42. Sleeve shield w/SI

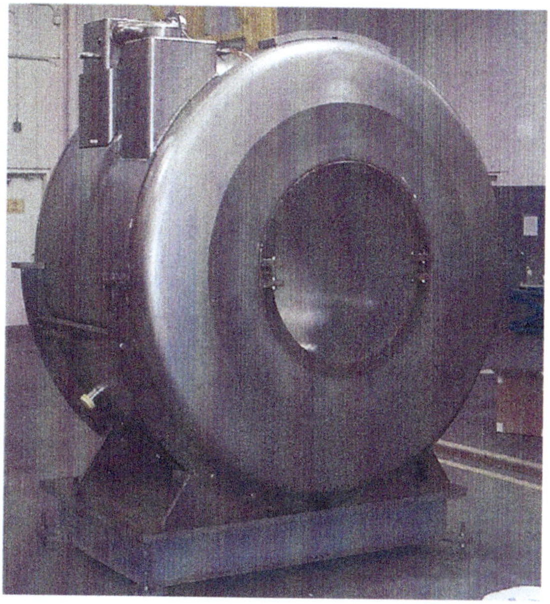

Figure 32.43. Completed lead and cold head sleeve turrets

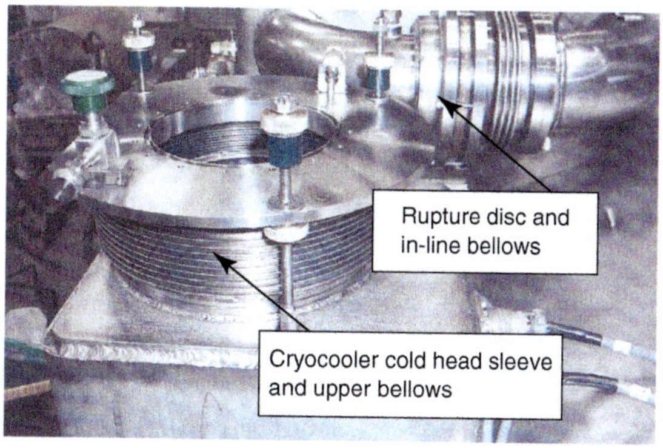

Figure 32.44. Helium gas vent system

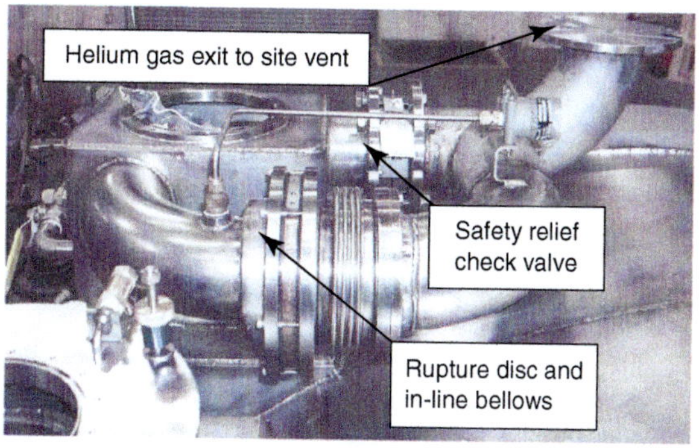

Figure 32.45. Helium gas vent system

DISCLAIMER

The subject matter, content, and views presented do not represent the views of the Department of Health and Human Services (HHS), US Food and Drug Administration (FDA), and/or the United States.

RELATED ARTICLES IN EMAGRES

Garroway, Allen N.: Origins of MRI—A Personal View

Hinshaw, Waldo: Notes on the History of MR Imaging from my Perspective

Lauterbur, Paul C.: One Path out of Many—How MRI Actually Began

Ramsey, Norman F.: Origins of Magnetic Resonance

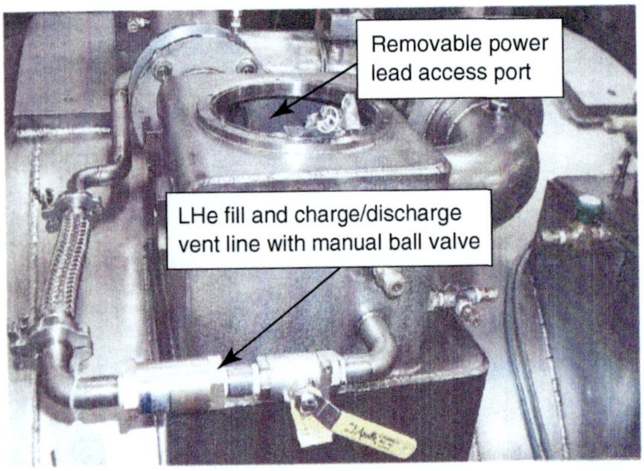

Figure 32.46. Helium gas vent system

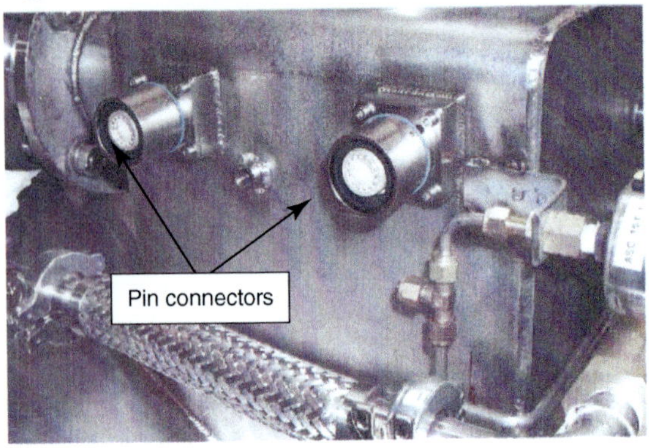

Figure 32.47. Pin connectors

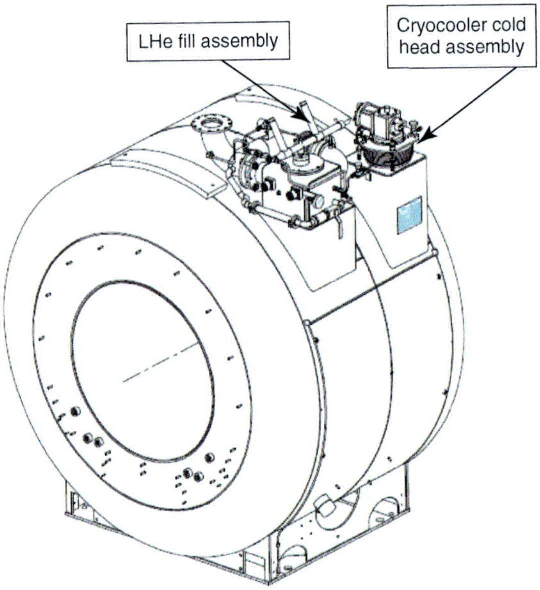

Figure 32.48. Completed vent system

Table 32.1. Typical 1.5 T MRI superconducting magnet specification

Dimensions	
Height	<2300 mm
Width	<1950 mm
Length	<1400 mm
Minimum required ceiling height	<2350 mm
Minimum service height	<2800 mm
Minimum doorway dimensions	2500 mm × 1500 mm
Warm bore diameter	900 mm
Magnet warm bore centerline height	1000 mm
Weight	<4000 kg
Magnetics	
Central field	1.5 T
Tested over field	1.53 T
Fringe fields, 5G, radial × axial	<2.5 m × <4.0 m
Operating current	500 A
Homogeneity, Vrms, 50 cm DSV, 40 cm DSV	<2.0 ppm, <1.0 ppm
Field decay rate	<0.1 ppm h^{-1}
Energization time	<60 min
Cryogenics	
2 Stage 4.2K GM Cryocooler with cold head sleeve	
Zero liquid helium boil-off	
Liquid helium hold time (100–30%)	>2 years
LHe volume	1000 l
LHe loss during charging or discharging	<20 l
Thermal shield operating temperature	~40 K

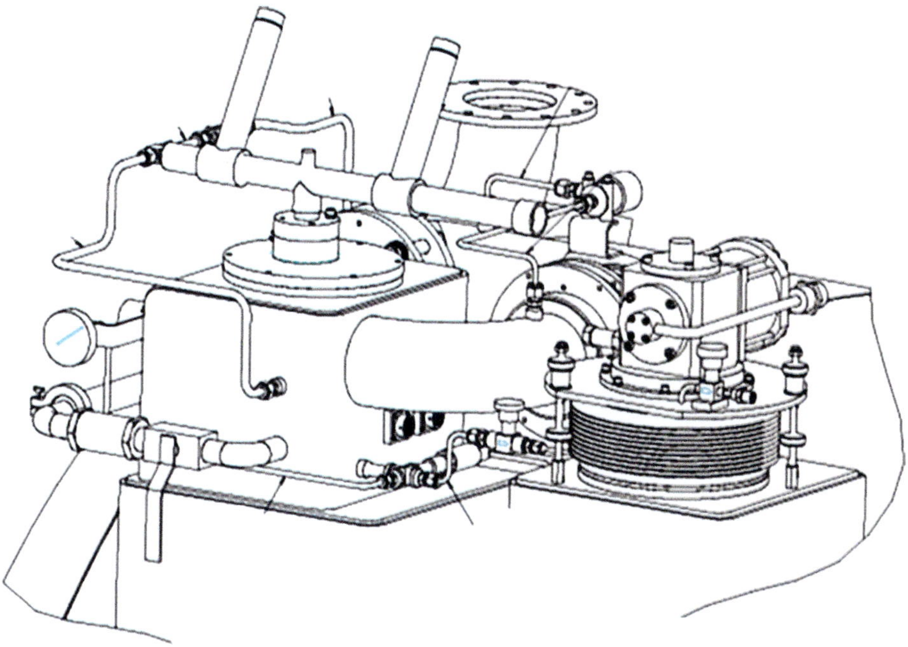

Figure 32.49. Completed vent system

Cryogenic Magnets for Whole-Body Magnetic Resonance Systems

High Temperature Superconductors

Magnetic Resonance Imaging: A Historical Overview

Quality Control and Quantification in Whole Body MRI and MRS

Safety Considerations in MRI

Chapter 33

Magnet Field Shimming and External Ferromagnetic Influences on the Homogeneity and Site Shielding of Superconducting MRI Magnets

Bruce Breneman

Breneman Consulting, Rancho Santa Fe, CA, USA

33.1 MRI SUPERCONDUCTING MAGNET FIELD SHIMMING

The goal of any MRI superconducting magnet is to provide a strong central magnetic field (typically 1.5 or 3.0 T) while simultaneously having a homogeneous magnetic field within a central volume corresponding to a 40 or 50 cm diameter. For our 1.5 T example, the requirement for homogeneity is <2.0 and <1.0 ppm VRMS (volume root mean square) over a 50 and 40 cm DSV (diameter spherical volume) respectively. Furthermore, it is desired to minimize low order magnetic field gradients across the entire DSV as well as higher-order gradients near the outer surface of the 40 or 50 cm diameter. These low- and high-order gradients will be defined and further discussed in the following sections.

There are several reasons why an 'as fabricated' magnet does not inherently have the exact homogeneity as specified and calculated by the coil designer. Manufacturing tolerances associated with the bobbin's diameter and cylindricity, coil module axial position tolerance, radial build tolerance of coil layers during winding and variation in conductor size can all lead to differences between fabricated and calculated results. Adding to these are environmental effects associated with ferromagnetic material located at the site location. These can be from carbon steel rebar or plates in the floor or ceiling, carbon or silicon steel wall shielding required by the site to control the position of the magnet's external 5G field, carbon steel I-beams in the floor, ceiling or walls, automobiles in nearby parking garages, elevators or nearby service equipment, etc.

During the final stages of magnet fabrication, the magnet undergoes testing and quality control/assurance verification. The magnet is initially field mapped and shimmed to best null all manufacturing induced field errors. When the magnet is on

Safety and Biological Effects in MRI.
Edited by Devashish Shrivastava and J. Thomas Vaughan

ISBN: 978-1-118-82130-5
Also published in eMagRes (online edition)
DOI: 10.1002/9780470034590.emrstm1594

RZ Coordiantes

Coordinate; Radius(cm) 25.00 OK

Plane	#1	#2	#3	#4	#5	#6	#7	#8	#9	#10	#11	#12
Z(cm)	24.54	22.60	19.25	14.68	9.20	3.13	-3.13	-9.20	-14.68	-19.25	-22.60	-24.54
R(cm)	4.78	10.68	15.95	20.23	23.25	24.80	24.80	23.25	20.23	15.95	10.68	4.78

Figure 33.1. 12 Plane plot coordinates

6775 mG

Magnetic Field Data

Field Value (Maximum 5 digits in 1 mG) OK

*\Plan	#1	#2	#3	#4	#5	#6	#7	#8	#9	#10	#11	#12
0	06775	06538	06563	07132	07158	06420	06026	06427	06291	05533	05070	04999
30	06737	06505	06575	07178	07198	06415	05948	06296	06148	05368	04919	04917
60	06716	06499	06594	07189	07165	06345	05873	06140	05935	05160	04765	04848
90	06716	06502	06583	07092	06840	05856	05411	05835	05801	05064	04699	04824
120	06733	06507	06537	07043	06989	06249	05893	06201	05987	05185	04786	04859
150	06779	06564	06592	07083	07036	06319	06061	06462	06299	05479	04997	04951
180	06837	06690	06773	07329	07294	06551	06272	06701	06587	05770	05210	05055
210	06900	06834	06987	07626	07794	07127	06726	06943	06640	05839	05323	05132
240	06937	06925	07065	07596	07548	06669	06161	06432	06304	05701	05329	05172
270	06936	06905	06977	07338	07112	06195	05725	06131	06084	05609	05299	05173
300	06890	06786	06823	07298	07334	06630	06242	06468	06265	05631	05258	05140
330	06829	06640	06648	07243	07449	06907	06551	06701	06366	05606	05177	05078
360	06775	06538	06563	07132	07158	06420	06026	06427	06291	05533	05070	04999
Delta	00221	00426	00528	00583	00954	01271	01315	01108	00839	00775	00630	00349

Figure 33.2. 12 Plane mapped 1.5 T field data

site, it is field mapped and re-shimmed to compensate for site ferromagnetic effects. This field mapping and shimming methodology used by the manufacturer and on-site is described below.

A magnetometer with multiple NMR probes is mounted to a mapping jig that, in turn, is mounted to the magnet's vacuum vessel end flanges. This NMR probe array is rotated every 15° or 30° within the central volume at which time the magnetic flux density is sampled. The probe array typically has 12 probes mounted at axial locations selected to maximize the mathematical usefulness of the mapped field data. Figure 33.1 shows typical 12 plane plot coordinates.

The 12 plane mapped 1.5 T field data are automatically imported into a field analysis and calculation/optimization algorithm as seen in Figure 33.2. Data imported are shown as the last 5 digits of the magnetic field, i.e., 15,0(06775) mG, for plane 1 at zero degrees.

These measured field values are sufficient to allow for the fields to be mathematically expressed. A mathematical equation is calculated which, in turn, describes the field at the locations defined above as well as everywhere within the DSV. In Cartesian coordinates, the magnetic flux density in the z-direction within the DSV is given by the Legendre expansion:

$$
\begin{aligned}
B_z = {} & A_1{}^0 + 2A_2{}^0 Z + 3A_2{}^1 X + 3B_2{}^1 Y \\
& + (3/2)A_3{}^0(2Z^2 - X^2 - Y^2) + 12A_3{}^1 ZX \\
& + 12B_3{}^1 ZY + 15A_3{}^2(X^2 - Y^2) + 30B_3{}^2 XY \\
& + 4A_4{}^0 Z(Z^2 - (Z/3)(X^2 + Y^2)) \\
& + 15A_4{}^1 X(4Z^2 - X^2 - Y^2) \\
& + 15B_4{}^1 Y(4Z^2 - X^2 - Y^2) + \cdots
\end{aligned}
$$

Figure 33.3 shows the first five orders of the Legendre expansion in Cartesian form (https://doi.org/10.1371/journal.pone.0181552.t001).

When the order is zero, the polynomials in the expansion are called *zonal harmonics*. These are the axial gradients of the field and are Z^1, Z^2, Z^3, Z^4, Z^5, Z^6, Z^7, Z^8, Z^9, Z^{10}, Z^{11} … It should be noted that only the even order zonal harmonics Z^2, Z^4, Z^6, Z^8, Z^{10} … exist in coil design due to mirror symmetry about the vertical axis. Undesirable odd order zonal harmonics Z^1, Z^3, Z^5, Z^7, Z^9 Z^{11} appear due to magnet manufacturing tolerance errors in coil winding and from site ferromagnetic effects.

The nonzero order polynomials are called *tesseral harmonics*. These are X, Y, ZX, $X^2 - Y^2$, etc. and are the off-axis/transverse components of the field. Tesseral harmonics do not exist in coil design but are present in the sited magnet due to magnet manufacturing tolerance errors and site ferromagnetic effects. These field 'errors' tend to produce 'low order' zonal and/or tesseral harmonics such as X, Y, and Z^1, Z^2. Typically, higher order zonal harmonics are nulled during the coil module design phase.

The zonal and tesseral Legendre coefficients are calculated by the calculation/optimization computer program and each coefficient is displayed in ppm as seen in Figure 33.4.

While it would be ideal for all locations within the DSV to be described only by $B_z^0 = A_1^0$ (with all other Legendre coefficients zero in magnitude), this is never the case for manufacturing and site reasons mentioned previously. Thus the computer-based program's algorithm must have one or more methods to 'shim the field'. Field shimming homogenizes fields within the DSV by minimizing the Legendre coefficients and thus minimizing field gradients. All methods shim the field by using small, precisely sized, pieces of ferromagnetic iron either attached to the surface of the vacuum vessel bore tube, attached to the surface of the gradient coil (mounted within the bore tube) or located within shim pockets internal to the gradient coil. These ferromagnetic shims act as 'magnetic dipole sinks' within

Degree (α)	Order (β)	Abbreviation	Coefficients	Spherical coordinates	Rectangular coordinates
0	0	Z^0	A_1^0	1	1
1	0	Z	$2A_2^0$	$r \cos \theta$	z
1	1	X	$3A_2^1$	$r \sin \theta \cos \phi$	x
1	1	Y	$3B_2^1$	$r \sin \theta \sin \phi$	y
2	0	Z^2	$3A_3^0$	$r^2 (3\cos^2 \theta - 1)/2$	$z^2 - (x^2 + y^2)/^2$
2	1	XZ	$12A_3^1$	$r^2 \cos \theta \sin \theta \cos \phi$	xz
2	1	YZ	$12B_3^1$	$r^2 \cos \theta \sin \theta \sin \phi$	yz
2	2	$X^2–Y^2$	$15A_3^2$	$r^2 \sin^2 \theta \cos2\phi$	$x^2 - y^2$
2	2	$2XY$	$15B_3^2$	$r^2 \sin^2 \theta \sin2\phi$	$2yz$
3	0	Z^3	$4A_4^0$	$r^3 \cos \theta (5\cos^2 \theta - 3)/2$	$z[z^2 - 3(x^2 + y^2)/2]$
3	1	XZ^2	$15A_4^1$	$r^3 \sin \theta \cos \phi (5\cos^2 \theta - 1)/2$	$x[4z^2 - (x^2 + y^2)]$
3	1	YZ^2	$15B_4^1$	$r^3 \sin \theta \sin \phi (5\cos^2 \theta - 1)/2$	$y[4z^2 - (x^2 + y^2)]$
3	2	$Z(X^2–Y^2)$	$90A_4^2$	$r^3 \cos \theta \sin^2\theta\cos2\phi$	$z(x^2 - y^2)$
3	2	XYZ	$90B_4^2$	$r^3 \cos \theta \sin^2\theta\sin2\phi$	$2xyz$
3	3	X^3	$105A_4^3$	$r^3 \sin^3\theta\cos3\phi$	$x^3 - 3xy^2$
3	3	Y^3	$105B_4^3$	$r^3 \sin^3\theta\sin3\phi$	$3x^2y - y^3$
4	0	Z^4	$5A_5^0/8$	$r^4(35\cos^4 \theta - 30\cos^2 \theta + 3)$	$8z^4 - 24z^2 (x^2 + y^2) +3(x^2 + y^2)^2$
4	1	XZ^3	$15A_5^1$	$r^3 \sin \theta \cos \phi \cos\theta(7\cos^2\theta - 3)$	$x[4z^3 - 3(x^2 + y^2)z]$
4	1	YZ^3	$15B_5^1$	$r^4 \sin \theta \sin \phi \cos\theta(7\cos^2\theta - 3)$	$y[4z^3 - 3(x^2 + y^2)z]$
4	2	$Z^2(X^2–Y^2)$	$105A_5^2/2$	$r^4 \sin^2 \theta \cos2\phi(7\cos^2\theta - 1)$	$[6z^2 - (x^2 + y^2)]\times(x^2 - y^2)$
4	2	XYZ^2	$105B_5^2/2$	$r^4 \sin^2\theta \sin2\phi(7\cos^2\theta - 1)$	$[6z^2 - (x^2 + y^2)]\times2xy$
4	3	ZX^3	$840A_5^3$	$r^4 \cos \theta \sin^3\theta \cos3\phi$	$z[x^3 - 3xy^2]$
4	3	ZY^3	$840B_5^3$	$r^4 \cos \theta\sin^3\theta\sin3\phi$	$z[y^3 - 3yx^2]$
4	4	$(X^2–Y^2)^2$	$945A_5^4$	$r^4 \sin^4\theta \cos4\phi$	$(x^2 - y^2)^2 - 4x^2y^2$
4	4	$XY(X^2–Y^2)$	$945B_5^4$	$r^4 \sin^4\theta \sin4\phi$	$4xy(x^2 - y^2)$
5	0	Z^5	$3A_6^0/4$	$r^5 \cos\theta(63\cos^4\theta - 70\cos^2\theta + 15)$	$8z^5 - 40z^3 (x^2 + y^2) +15z(x^2 + y^2)^2$

Figure 33.3. Legendre expansion

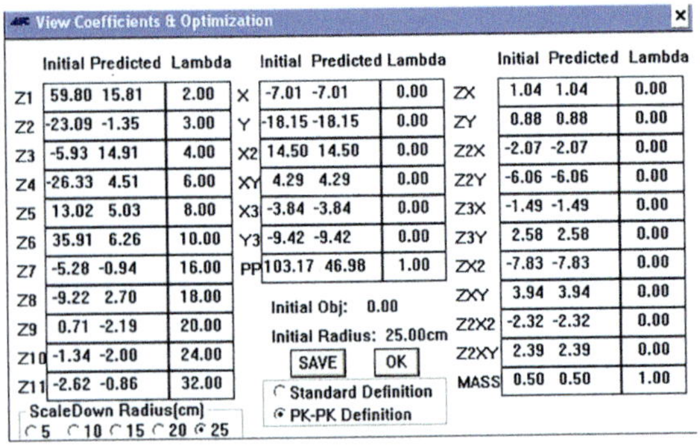

	Initial	Predicted	Lambda		Initial	Predicted	Lambda		Initial	Predicted	Lambda
Z1	59.80	15.81	2.00	X	-7.01	-7.01	0.00	ZX	1.04	1.04	0.00
Z2	-23.09	-1.35	3.00	Y	-18.15	-18.15	0.00	ZY	0.88	0.88	0.00
Z3	-5.93	14.91	4.00	X2	14.50	14.50	0.00	Z2X	-2.07	-2.07	0.00
Z4	-26.33	4.51	6.00	XY	4.29	4.29	0.00	Z2Y	-6.06	-6.06	0.00
Z5	13.02	5.03	8.00	X3	-3.84	-3.84	0.00	Z3X	-1.49	-1.49	0.00
Z6	35.91	6.26	10.00	Y3	-9.42	-9.42	0.00	Z3Y	2.58	2.58	0.00
Z7	-5.28	-0.94	16.00	PP	103.17	46.98	1.00	ZX2	-7.83	-7.83	0.00
Z8	-9.22	2.70	18.00					ZXY	3.94	3.94	0.00
Z9	0.71	-2.19	20.00					Z2X2	-2.32	-2.32	0.00
Z10	-1.34	-2.00	24.00					Z2XY	2.39	2.39	0.00
Z11	-2.62	-0.86	32.00					MASS	0.50	0.50	1.00

Figure 33.4. Legendre coefficients

the bore and thus locally reduce the field near each shim. Figure 33.5 shows the effect of placing a 1.0 cm cube ferromagnetic shim at an axial location 15 cm from the magnet center and at an angle of 180°.

The lower curve in red represents the calculated field effect of this dipole shim on the Z = 14.68 cm plane. As can be seen, the field is reduced due by the magnetic sink at 180° as expected. By contrast, fields are increased at 180° in planes mirrored about the magnet vertical axis. Each dipole sink effect is also evaluated mathematically as a net difference to the coefficients of the Legendre expansion. Therefore, multiple dipoles can be utilized thus either minimizing field differences within the DSV or minimizing the coefficients of the Legendre expansion.

If the mapped field data produce primarily zonal effects (Z^1, Z^3, Z^5, Z^7, Z^9, and Z^{11}) then a series of ferromagnetic dipole rings are useful. These rings can either be symmetric or nonsymmetric about magnet center (Z = 0). These calculated rings are practically divided into 12 individual dipoles at 30° spacing for placement on the bore, gradient coil ID or within the gradient coil. Figure 33.6 shows the auto zonal ring shim method.

If the mapped field data produces zonal and tesseral effects in somewhat equal amount then a number of individual ferromagnetic dipoles are useful. Auto dipole/harmonics simultaneously minimizes all zonal coefficients and tesseral coefficients which, in turn, also homogenizes the field within the DSV. Once again, this is done by applying ferrous dipole shims on the bore, gradient coil ID or within the gradient coil shim pockets.

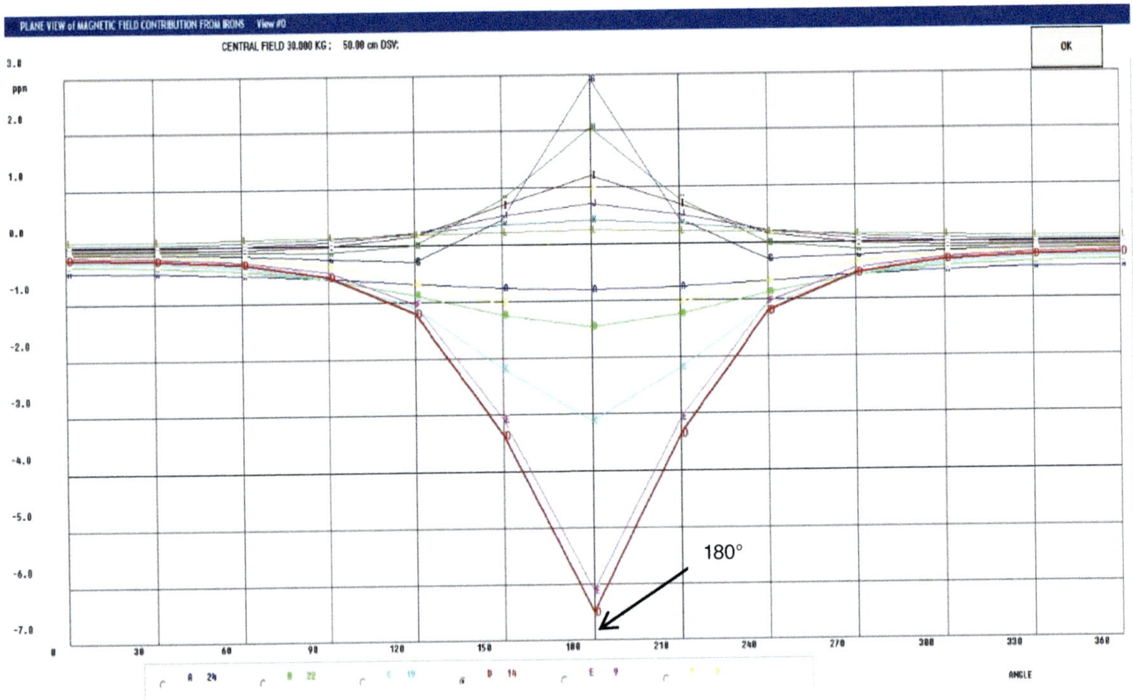

Figure 33.5. Magnetic dipole sink effect

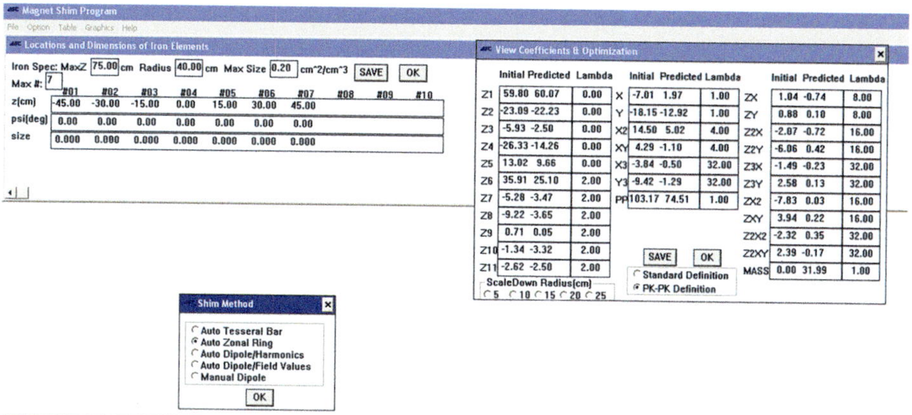

Figure 33.6. Auto zonal ring shim method

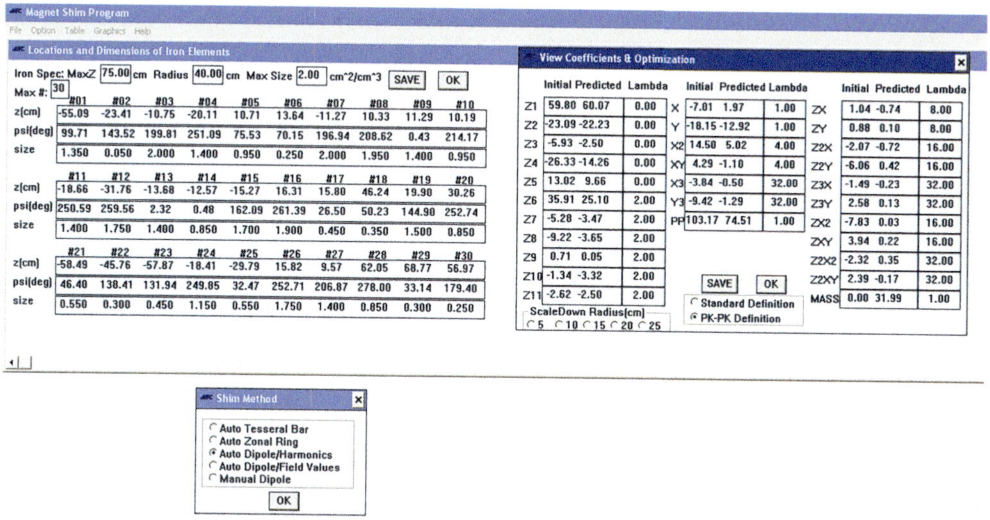

Figure 33.7. Auto dipole/harmonics method

Figure 33.7 displays this shim method.

Once the zonal and tesseral Legendre coefficients are reduced it is often helpful to further reduce the peak–peak field inhomogeneity within the DSV. Auto dipole/field values method is used in this situation. Individual ferromagnetic dipoles are calculated by auto dipole/field values in order to raise locations of low field or suppress locations of high field.

Figure 33.8 displays the auto dipole/field values shim method.

Finally, individual dipoles can be mathematically placed by the experienced magnet technician with each dipole's effect displayed as shown in the manual dipole method shown in Figures 33.9 and 33.10.

Plotting of the field data is often useful to visualize the peaks and valleys of the fields as shown in Figures 33.11 and 33.12. From this visualization, as well as the minimization of all zonal and tesseral coefficients, an experienced magnet technician can successfully shim any typical magnet installation by employing the full capabilities of the shimming algorithm.

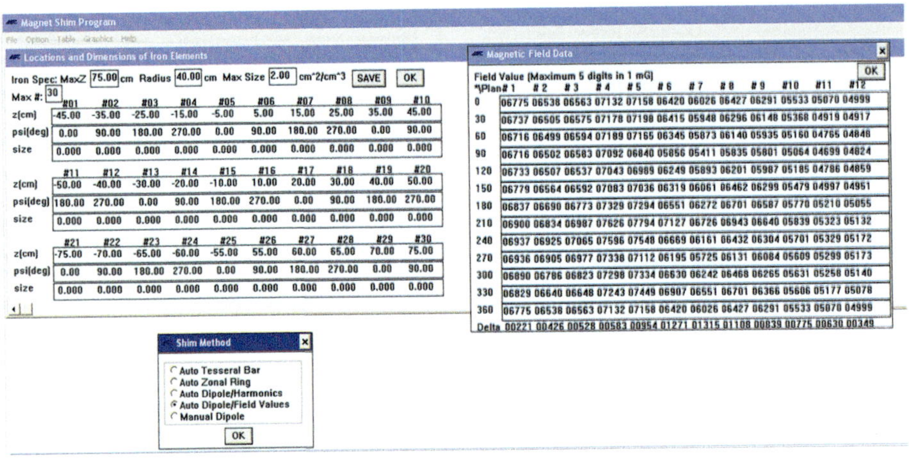

Figure 33.8. Auto dipole/field values method

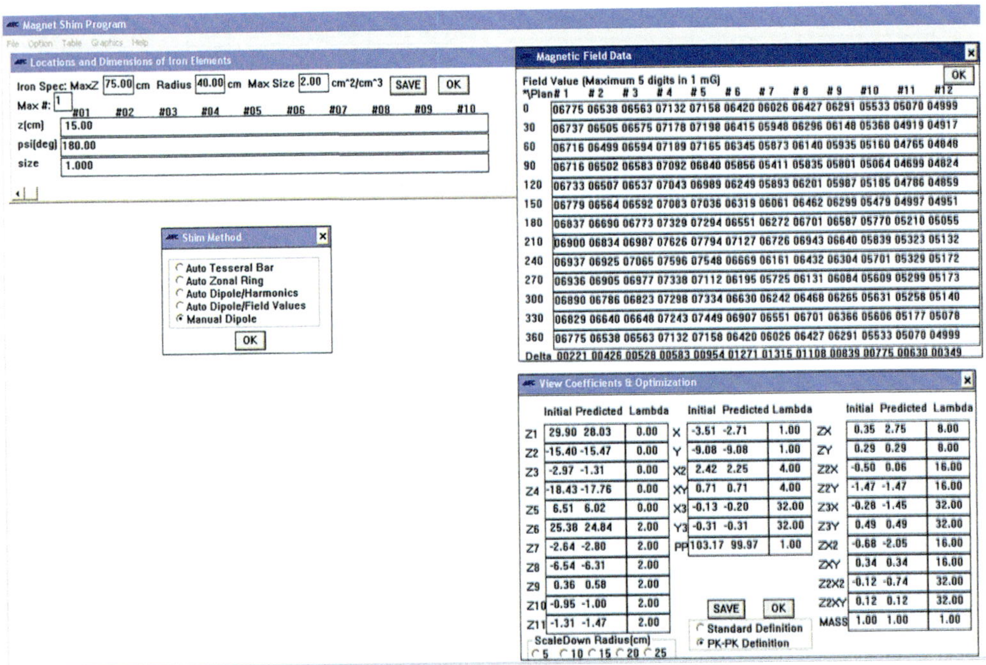

Figure 33.9. Manual dipole method

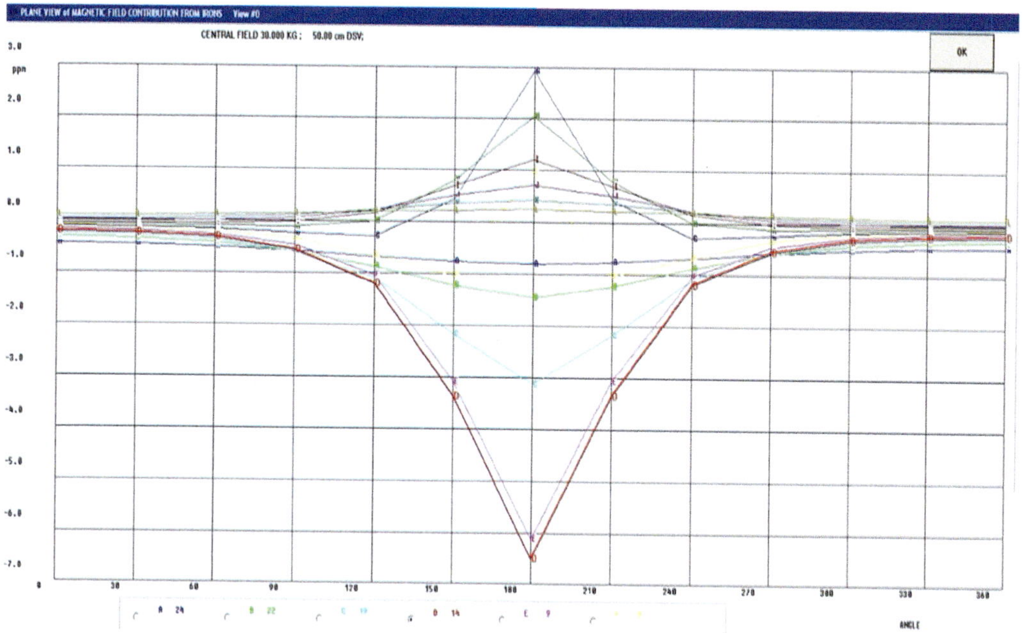

Figure 33.10. Manual dipole method

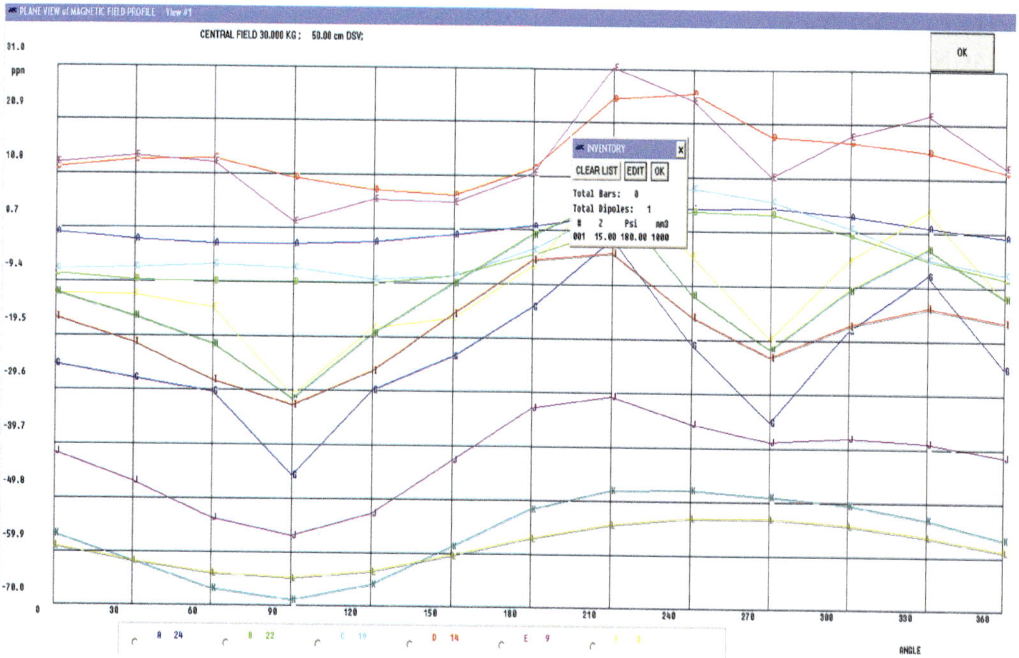

Figure 33.11. Field data planar view

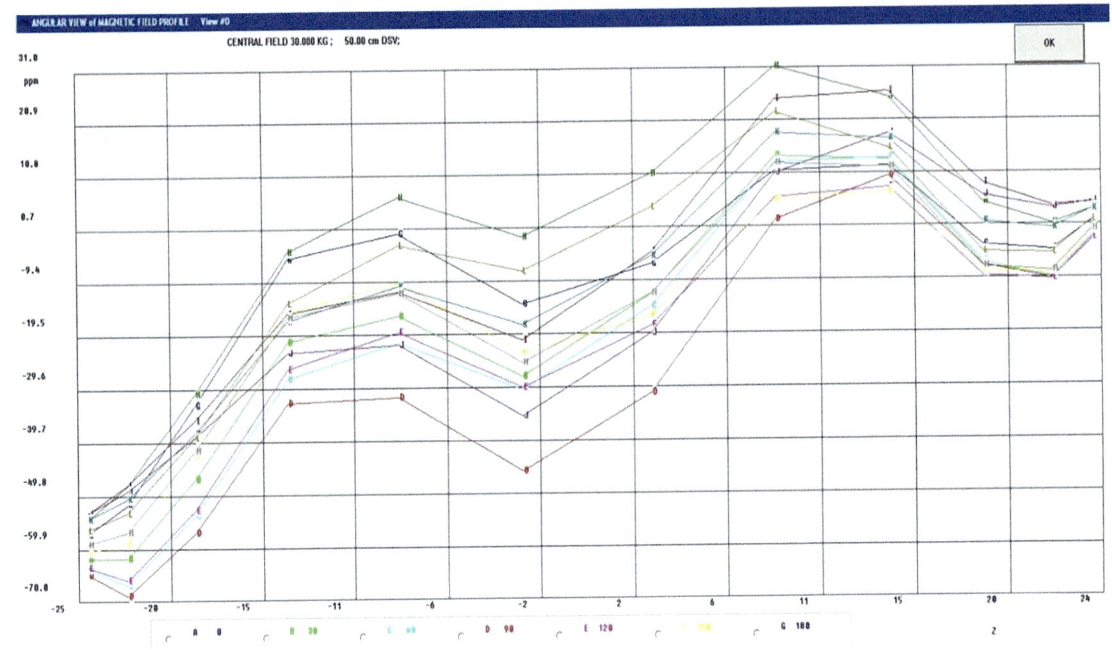

Figure 33.12. Field data angular view

33.2 EXTERNAL FERROMAGNETIC INFLUENCES ON MAGNET HOMOGENEITY

The MRI superconducting magnet site environment influences overall field homogeneity. These environmental effects are due to ferromagnetic material near the magnet and can be due to carbon steel rebar or plates in the floor or ceiling, carbon steel I-beams in the floor, ceiling or walls, automobiles in nearby parking garages or carbon steel side wall. In addition, floor and/or ceiling shielding may be required to control the 5G field position. These site issues typically create 'low order' gradients (Legendre coefficients) such as zonals Z, Z^2, or Z^3 and/or tesserals X, Y, ZX, ZY, $X^2 - Y^2$ and XY. The MRI magnet manufacturer has physical limits for the maximum site shim capacity which is often limited by space in the gradient coil pockets. The practical low order linear X, Y, and Z limits are <200 ppm/50 cm DSV, <80 ppm/50 cm DSV for Z^2, and <40 ppm/50 cm DSV for $X^2 - Y^2$ and XY.

Figure 33.13 shows the effect on magnet homogeneity from side and rear wall ferromagnetic shielding. It can be appreciated that similar steel in the form of I-beams, plates, automobiles, etc. would produce similar effects.

Figure 33.14 shows the effect on magnet homogeneity from ceiling and rear wall ferromagnetic shielding.

Figures 33.15 and 33.16 illustrate more complex site issues affecting magnet homogeneity. The site environment in Figure 33.15 has ferromagnetic I-beams, an asymmetrical left and rear carbon steel wall and a carbon steel floor with a central cut-out. Figure 33.16 has a large quantity of carbon steel 1″ diameter rebar embedded in the cement floor. For simplicity, this case was modeled as a grid of larger diameter rods having equivalent volume and mass. After determining that the Legendre coefficients were within the allowable shim limits, both sites were field mapped, fields analyzed and shims placed to minimize Legendre coefficients as well as minimize the peak-peak field difference within the DSV.

33.3 SHIELDING FUNDAMENTALS

It is a requirement of the MRI safety standard IEC 60601-2-33 that the MRI magnet external field not

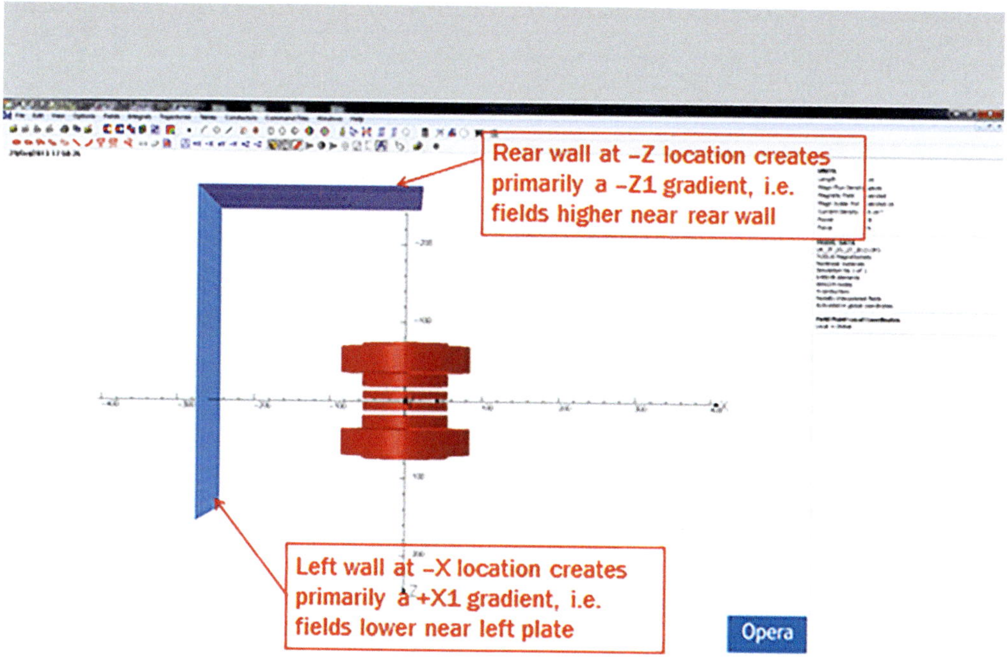

Figure 33.13. Side and rear wall shielding effect

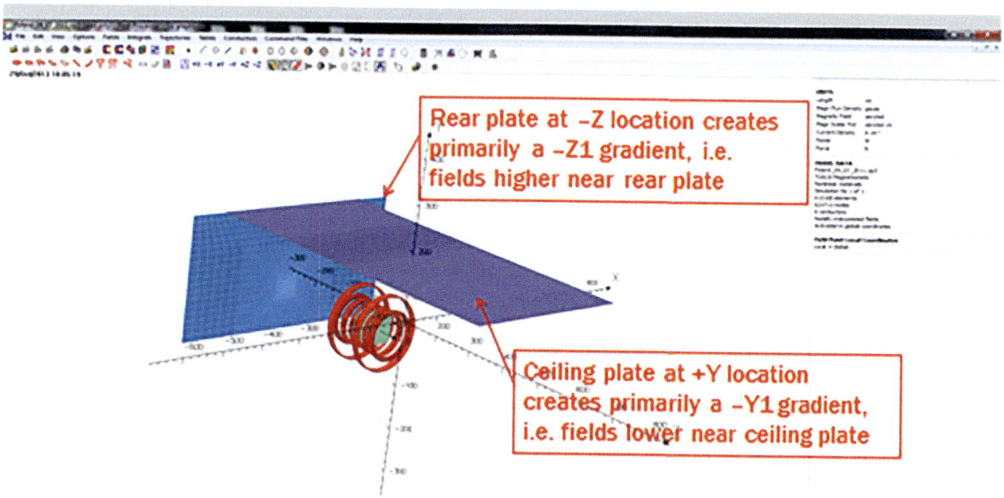

Figure 33.14. Ceiling and rear wall shielding effect

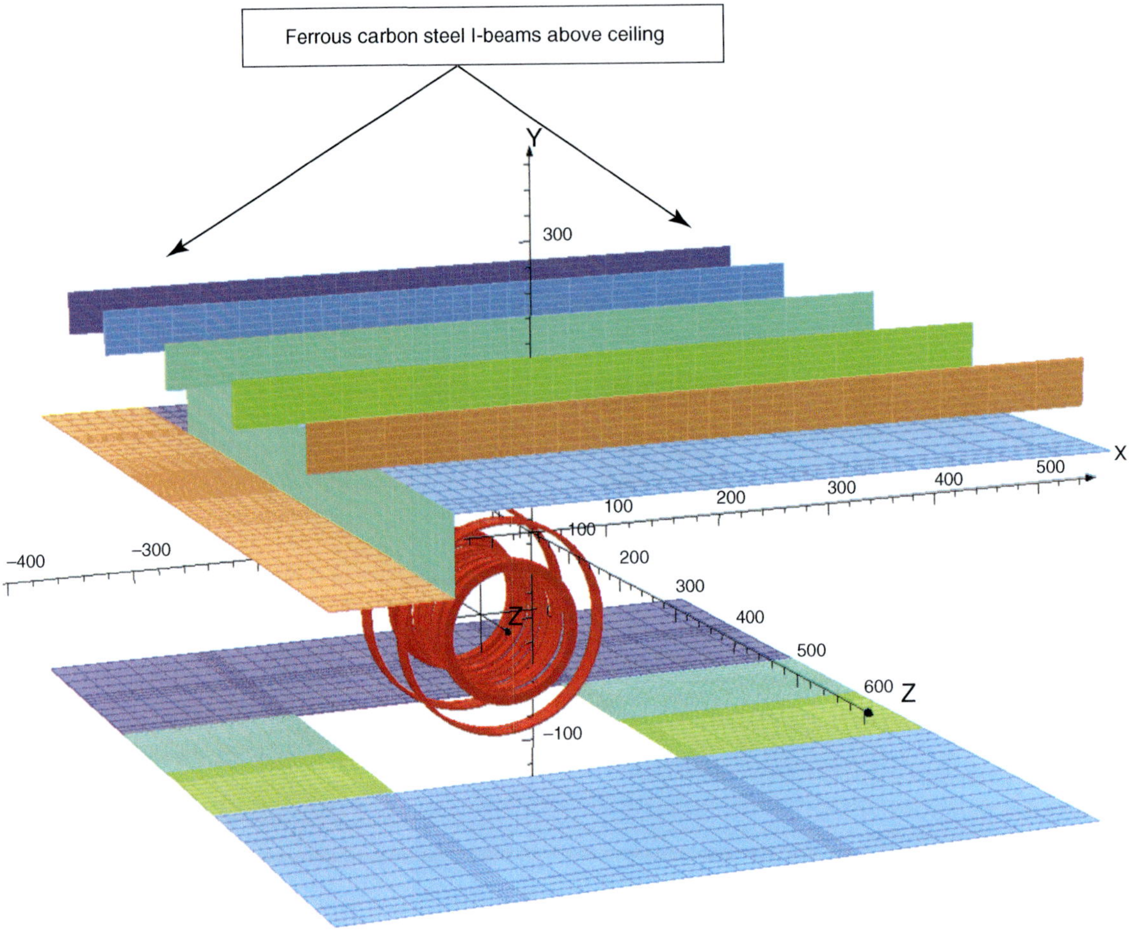

Figure 33.15. I-Beams in ceiling

exceed 5G in public areas because cardiac implantable electronic devices (CIED) have certain functions that are enabled in magnetic fields ≥10G (ISO 14117 Active implantable medical devices – electromagnetic compatibility – EMC test protocols for implantable cardiac pacemakers, implantable cardioverter defibrillators, and cardiac resynchronization devices). In addition, the 5G control is a beneficial buffer regarding attractive forces on ferrous tools, chairs, and oxygen tanks, etc. Some sites have even stricter self-imposed 1G limits when the magnet is in proximity to electron microscopes, CT scanners, or nearby MRI magnets.

Most modern MRI superconducting magnets have inherent 'active shielding' to reduce the 5G footprint size. In addition, room shielding using low carbon steel plates or silicon steel is often utilized to contain the 5G footprint.

In order to better understand room shielding, a bit of physics background is helpful. Below is a description of basic shielding theory.

$$\boldsymbol{B} = \mu^{*}\boldsymbol{H}$$

where

- μ = relative permeability

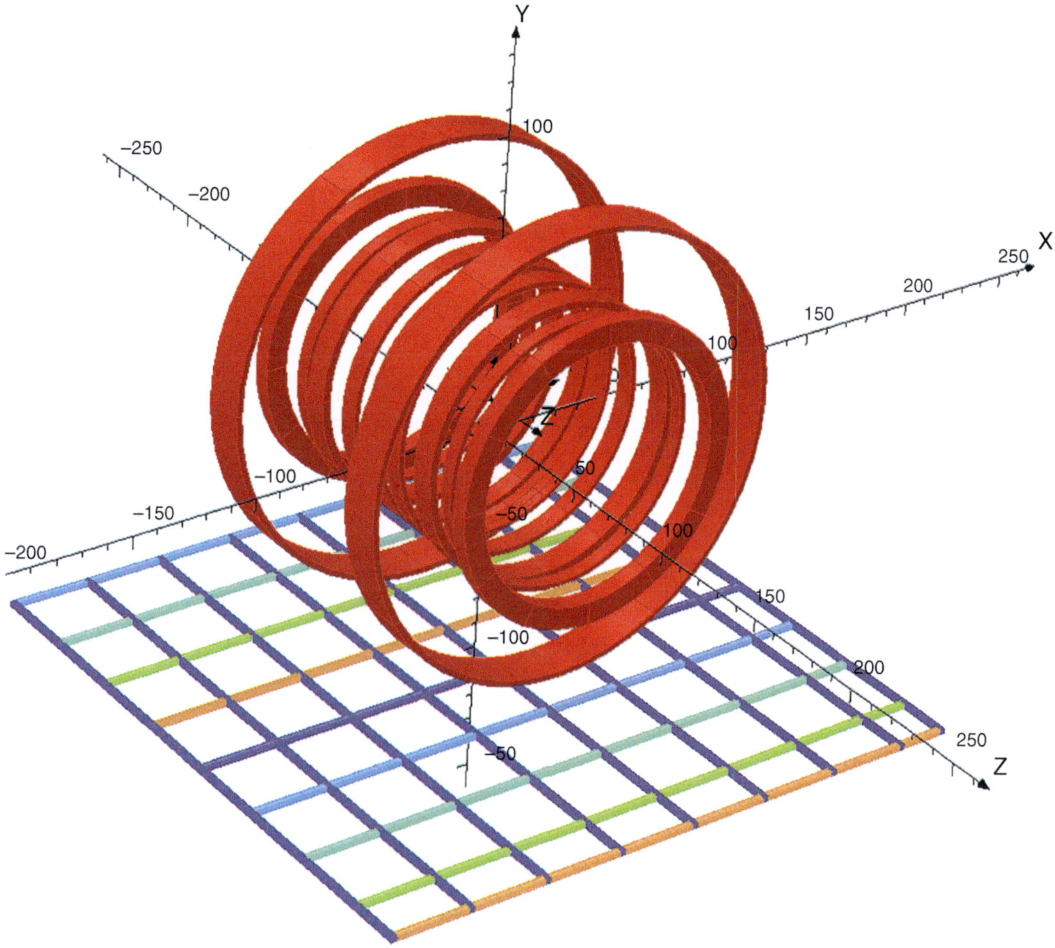

Figure 33.16. Rebar in floor

- $\mu = 1.0$ (cgs units) for vacuum, air, plastics (non-ferromagnetic materials) $1 < \mu < 100–200$ for higher permeable ferromagnetic materials;
- $\boldsymbol{B} = \boldsymbol{H}$ in air only (cgs units), $\boldsymbol{B} = \mu^*\boldsymbol{H}$ for all other materials;
- $\boldsymbol{H}$ = magnetic field strength or magnetic field intensity, in A m^{-1} (SI units) or Oersteds (cgs units). $\boldsymbol{H}$ has the same value independent of material it passes through. $\boldsymbol{H}$ drives $\boldsymbol{B}$ into ferrous materials. It is flux density, $\boldsymbol{B}$, generated within the shield wall that provides magnetic field shielding;
- $\boldsymbol{B}$ = total magnetic flux/area or magnetic flux density, in T (SI units) or G (cgs units):
  - 10 000 G = 1.0 T.
  - Earth's magnetic field is ~0.5 G.
  - $\boldsymbol{B}_{sat}$ is the maximum $\boldsymbol{B}$ attainable within a nonlinear material. Additional $\boldsymbol{H}$ will thus only add additional $\boldsymbol{B}$ as it would normally in air.
  - Magnetic flux density, $\boldsymbol{B}$, generated within the shield produces site magnetic shielding.
  - Relative permeability is the slope of the $\boldsymbol{B}$–$\boldsymbol{H}$ curve. Higher permeability materials generally

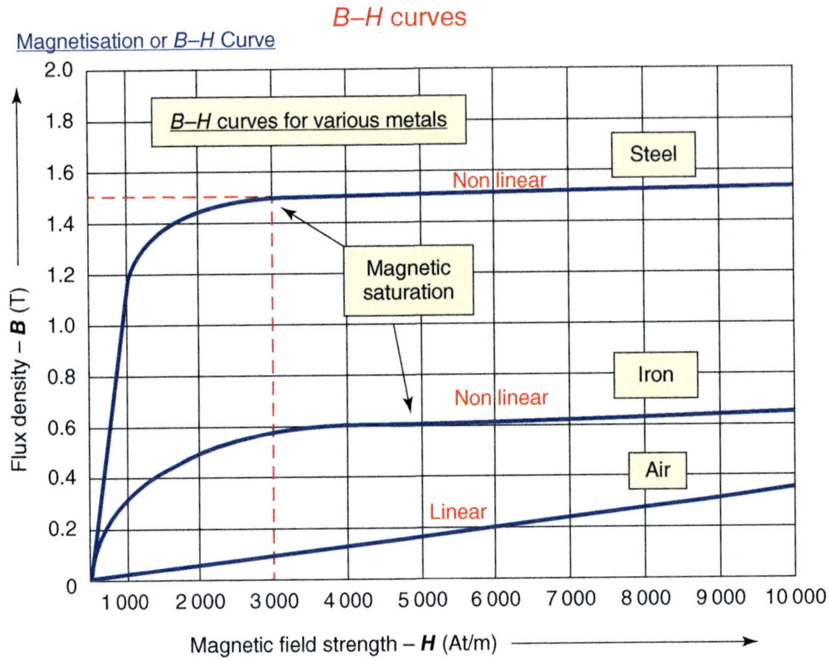

Figure 33.17. ***B–H*** curves

have lower B_{sat} but have the advantage of generating higher B values from lower H.

Carbon steel such as C1010 or A36 has a relative permeability 100–200 times that of air. This allows for a far greater amount of magnetic flux density, B, to be 'captured' within the material for any given magnetic field strength, H.

Figure 33.17 shows B–H curves for air, iron, and carbon steel (https://www.electronics-tutorials.ws/electromagnetism/magnetic-hysteresis.html). As magnetic field strength, H, increases in carbon the steel a significantly larger magnetic flux density, B, is generated. At magnetic saturation, the material can no longer 'hold' additional flux and at subsequent higher H values, the material is no more useful than air. It is this capturing of magnetic flux within carbon steel or silicon steel plates that provides useful magnetic field shielding.

As the shield wall gets closer to magnet isocenter, magnetic field intensity, H, is inherently higher which induces greater magnetic flux density, B, in the shielding thus thicker shielding is generally required. Lower permeability materials with higher B_{sat}, such as low carbon steels, can be used.

As the shield wall gets closer to magnet isocenter the effect on magnet homogeneity increases nonlinearly.

As the shield wall moves away from isocenter, magnetic field intensity, H, decreases so a better quality (higher permeability) material such as silicon steel is advantageous to drive higher magnetic flux density, B, in the shielding.

33.4 SITE SHIELDING EXAMPLES

In the simplest terms, a six-sided ferromagnetic or silicon steel box surrounding the magnet at the location of the site's interior walls can, and often, is used for site shielding. The type of material (carbon steel vs. silicon steel) and thickness of material (6–25 mm) is determined typically by simulating the actual magnet with proposed shielding in a 3D nonlinear finite element analysis (FEA) magnetostatic computer program. Material choice and thicknesses can then be optimized to control the 5G footprint as needed. Homogeneity

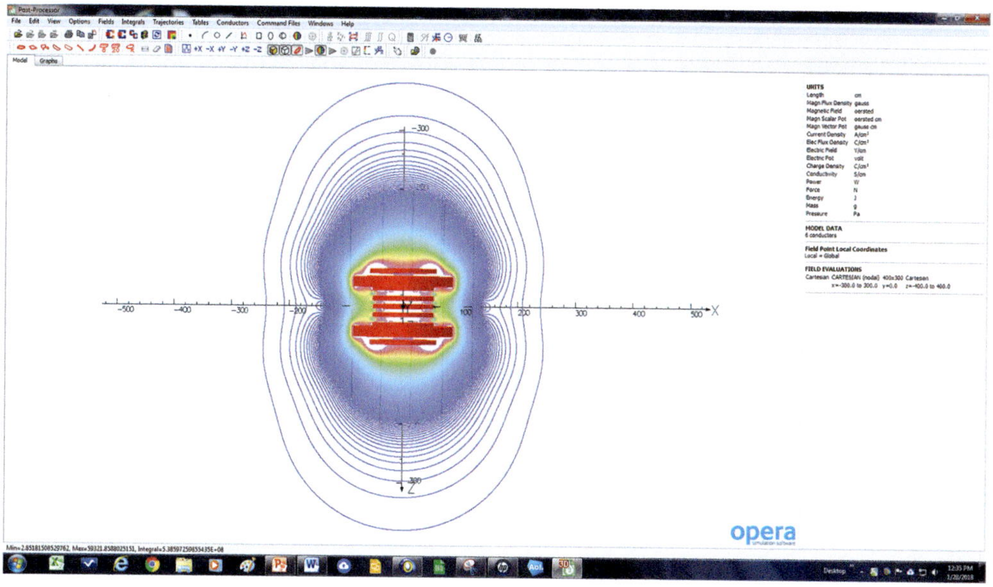

Figure 33.18. Flux lines – no shielding

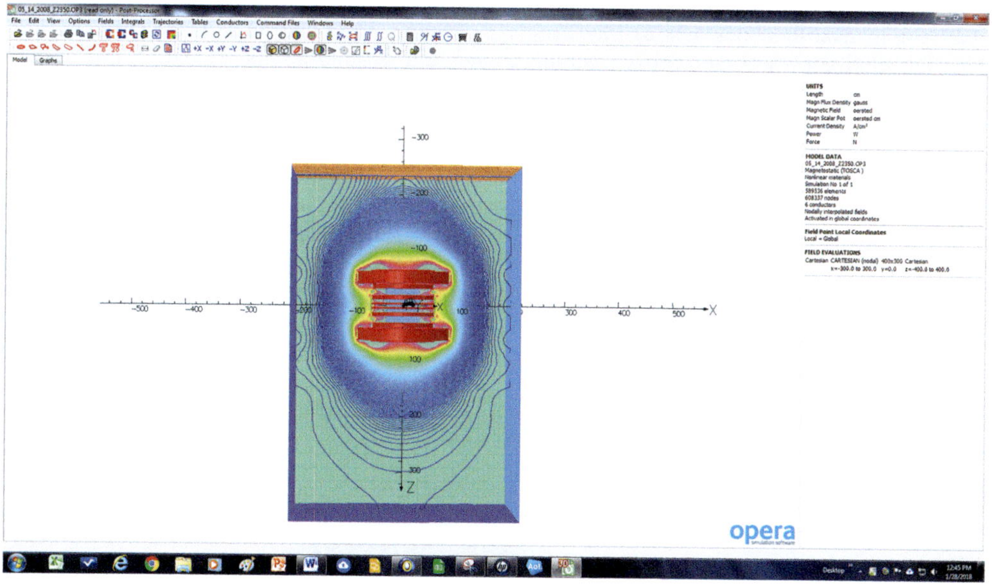

Figure 33.19. Flux lines – full six-sided shielding

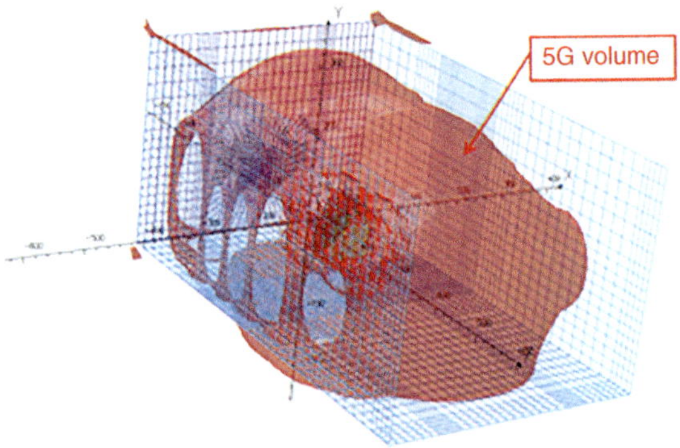

Figure 33.20. 5G flux lines

and Legendre coefficients are mathematically calculated within the DSV to ensure they are within shim capability as described previously.

Often the site does not require full six-sided shielding if for example, the site is sufficient large in one or more directions. Single story sites often do not require ceiling shielding and do not require floor shielding.

Figures 33.18 and 33.19 show the magnetic flux density, ***B***, flux lines ranging from 0 to 15 000 G for our 1.5 T example without shielding and with a six-sided ferromagnetic shield (*note*: ceiling plate is hidden in Figure 33.20 so as to make flux lines visible). Flux capturing in the high relative permeability carbon steel site shielding is evident.

Figure 33.20 shows the FEA analysis of a six-sided ferromagnetic room shield. The magnet is located within the shield walls nearest to the rear wall with magnet centerline approximately 1.0 m above floor elevation. For this case, the magnet's 5G flux lines are shown in red and can be seen to fully reside within the shield walls. Note some ballooning of the 5G was permitted below the magnet as can be observed.

Figure 33.21 shows the effect to the 5G flux line with rear and partial left wall shielding. Ballooning of 5G flux lines occur in front of the magnet. Warmer colors depict higher ***B*** fields; cooler colors depict lower ***B*** fields thus allowing the designer to optimize material thickness.

In the example shown in Figure 33.22, it was important to contain the 5G flux lines in the front and rear only. The Legendre coefficients for the actual magnet with shielding induced effect were calculated and displayed to the right.

The case shown in Figure 33.23 required full 5G containment at the floor below as this magnet was placed on the second floor with a medical office below. A unique floor design with end 'wings' was designed to meet the site's needs.

The case depicted on Figure 33.24 had the requirement that 5G be limited to the left, rear, and ceiling walls as well as head height on the floor below. Appropriate shielding was designed and installed. Note the central cut-out in the floor shielding directly under the magnet. This is required to keep the *Y* gradient within shim limits.

Figure 33.25 graphically shows the ***B*** field values at the surface of the shielding. Higher ***B*** fields can be observed as warmer colors which indicate regions potentially benefiting from thicker material while cooler colors indicate lower ***B*** fields where material thickness can be minimized.

In the case of Figure 33.26, only rear shielding was required.

Figures 33.27 and 33.28 represent a magnet placed nonorthogonally to the shield. While complexities arise in the FEA modeling of this case, the design of the shield and analysis is routine.

The case shown in Figure 33.29 required 5G field containment below the second-floor office space above the magnet. The magnet was sited on the ground floor with no other 5G requirements.

Figure 33.30 again shows the necessity for a central cut-out below the magnet in the closer carbon steel plate. A secondary lower silicon steel plate is used where ***H*** fields are naturally somewhat lower.

In Figure 33.31, a large door cut-out is modeled.

And finally, a three-sided shield configuration is seen in Figure 33.32.

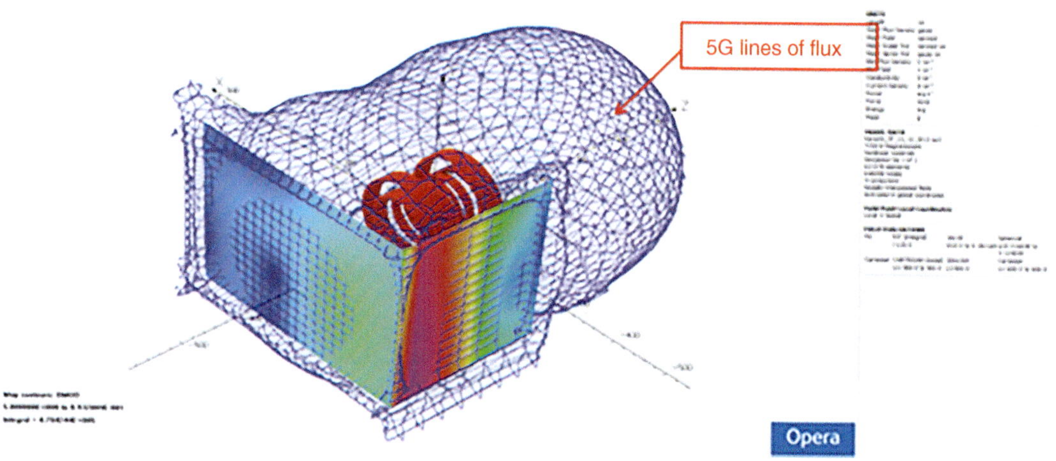

Figure 33.21. Shielding example

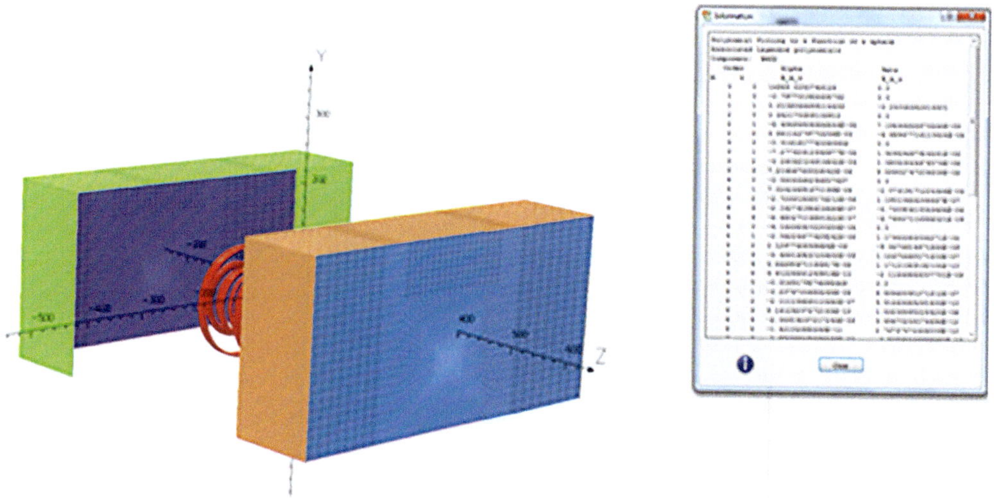

Figure 33.22. Shielding example

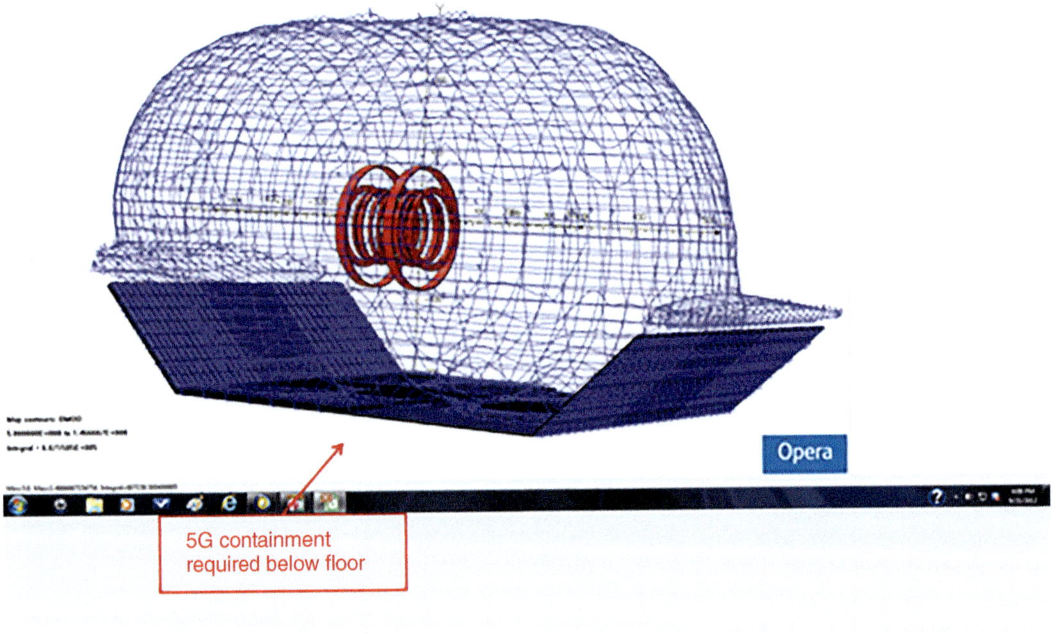

Figure 33.23. Shielding example

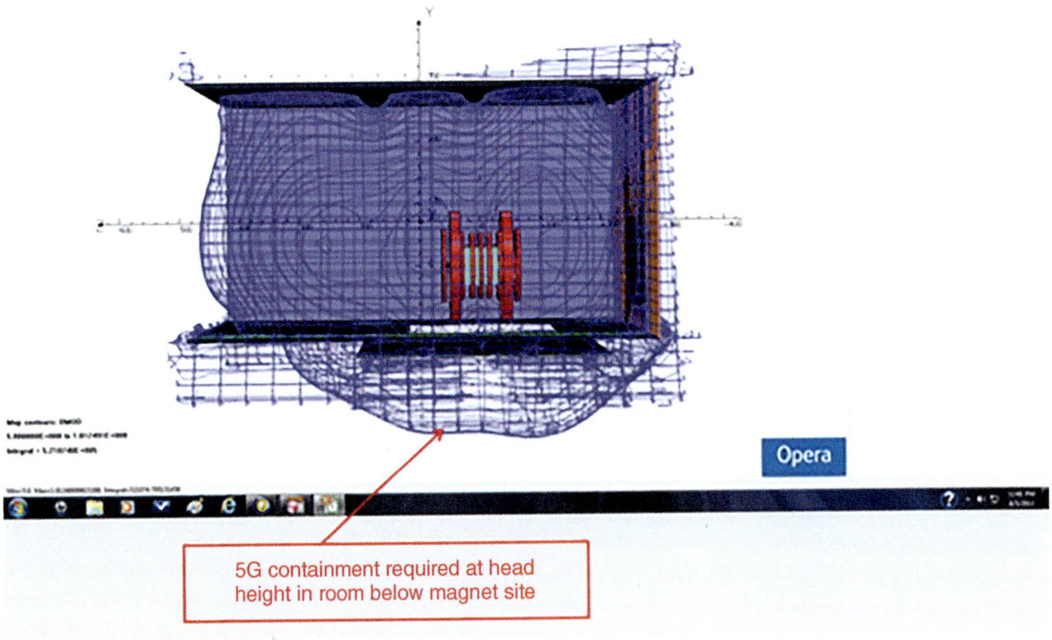

Figure 33.24. Shielding example

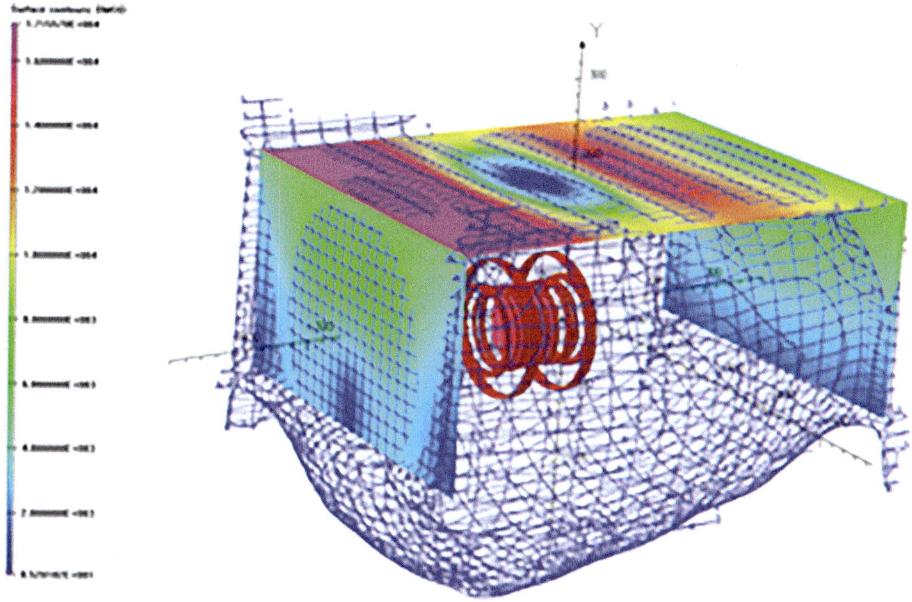

Figure 33.25. Shielding example

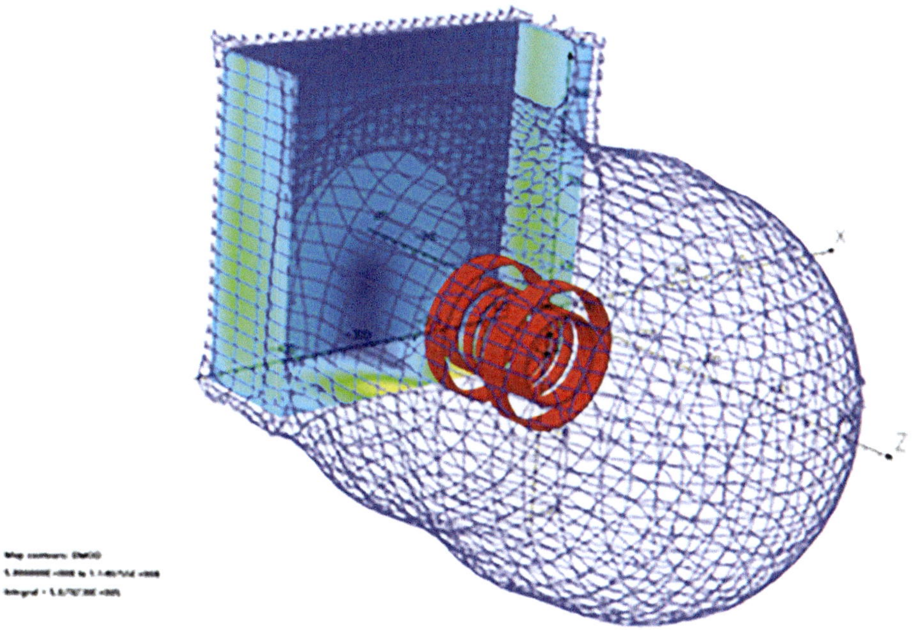

Figure 33.26. Shielding example

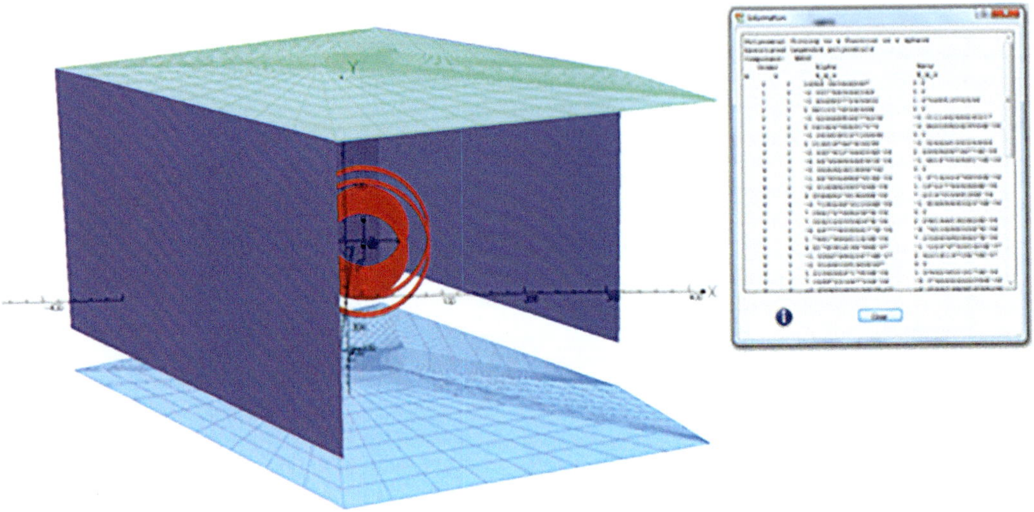

Figure 33.27. Shielding example

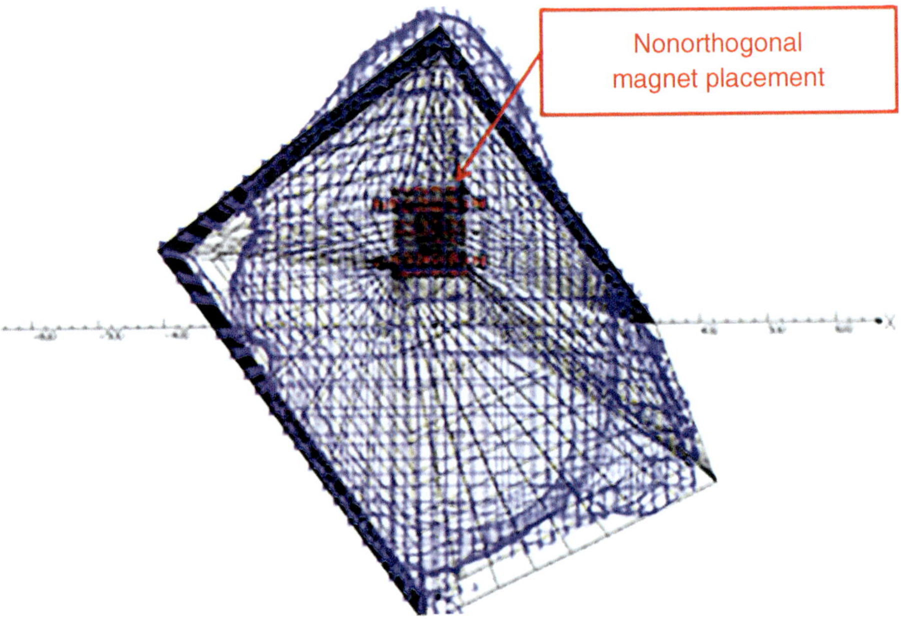

Figure 33.28. Shielding example, top view

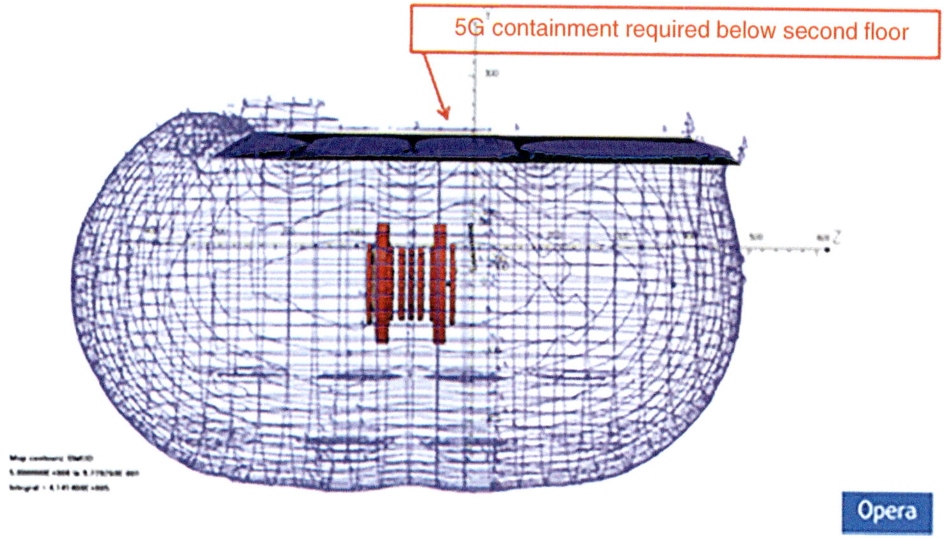

Figure 33.29. Shielding example

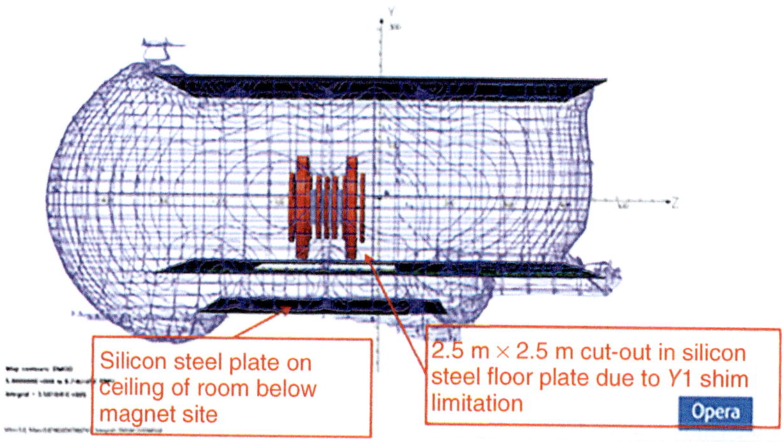

Figure 33.30. Shielding example

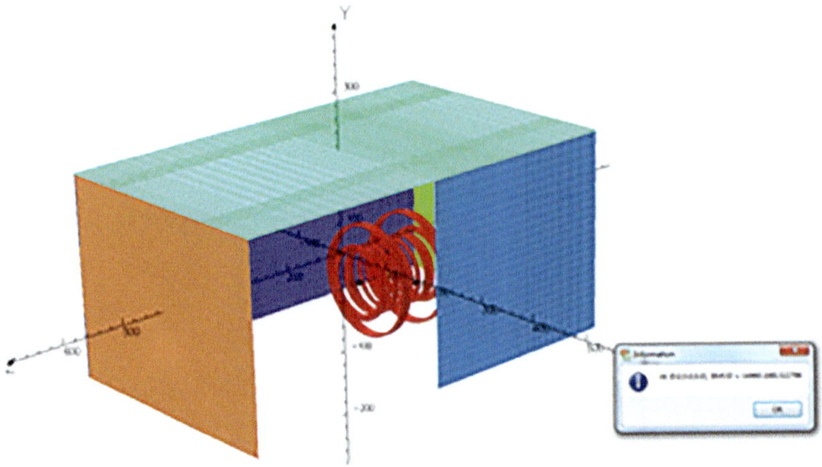

Figure 33.31. Shielding example

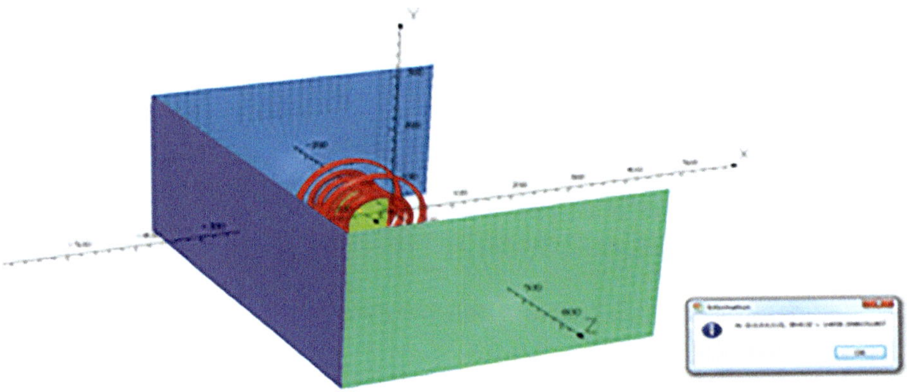

Figure 33.32. Shielding example

DISCLAIMER

The subject matter, content, and views presented do not represent the views of the Department of Health and Human Services (HHS), US Food and Drug Administration (FDA), and/or the United States.

RELATED ARTICLES IN EMAGRES

Shimming of Superconducting Magnets

Shimming for High-Resolution NMR Spectroscopy

Chapter 34
Gradient Coils

Maxim Zaitsev, Philipp Amrein, Feng Jia, and Sebastian Littin

University of Freiburg, Freiburg, Germany

34.1 INTRODUCTION

In magnetic resonance imaging (MRI), a substantial engineering effort is invested in creating a sufficiently homogeneous main magnetic field over the target imaging region. Laborious optimization steps are involved in magnet design and shimming to achieve stringent specifications for the field homogeneity of the unloaded magnet of few parts per million (ppm).[1] Introducing a sample, an animal, or a person into the magnet distorts the field, which is typically compensated for in part by the active shim system.[2]

To realize the spatial encoding, one needs a means of inducing spatially inhomogeneous distributions of Larmor frequency. The most straightforward spatial encoding, which is traditionally used in MRI, is based on inducing linear resonance frequency variations. These variations are effected by overlaying the main magnetic field with additional spacial encoding magnetic fields (SEMs) generated by specially designed electromagnets, the so-called gradient coils. Although it would be most natural to assess the gradient strength in units of $\mathrm{Hz\,m^{-1}}$,[3] traditionally, $\mathrm{mT\,m^{-1}}$ is used in clinical MRI, and G/cm (gauss per cm) is often used in small animal imaging and nuclear magnetic resonance (NMR) communities. Current whole-body human scanners are capable of reaching gradient strengths of $30-80\,\mathrm{mT\,m^{-1}}$, with up to $300\,\mathrm{mT\,m^{-1}}$ reported for experimental systems.[4] Animal and small-bore MRI systems often reach gradient strengths in the range or above several tesla per meter.

Noteworthy is the fact that for typical MRI settings, the magnitude of the magnetic fields created by the gradient coils is substantially lower than the main magnetic field. Considering a rather strong gradient field of $50\,\mathrm{mT\,m^{-1}}$ and the field of view (FOV) of 50 cm, and observing that the maximal field is produced at the periphery of the FOV, one arrives at the absolute field strength of about 12.5 mT, which is over two orders of magnitude lower than the typical clinical field of 1.5 T.

Fields created by the gradient coil are often referred to as *gradient fields* or *magnetic field gradients*, which is somewhat misleading. Strictly speaking, these magnetic fields are designed to create a linear variation of the Larmor frequency rather than the magnetic field itself. To avoid confusion, a term *gradient coil field* is used throughout this chapter to refer to the magnetic field created by a particular gradient coil. Note that the magnetic field is a vector quantity characterized by a

Safety and Biological Effects in MRI.
Edited by Devashish Shrivastava and J. Thomas Vaughan

ISBN: 978-1-118-82130-5
Also published in eMagRes (online edition)
DOI: 10.1002/9780470034590.emrstm1620

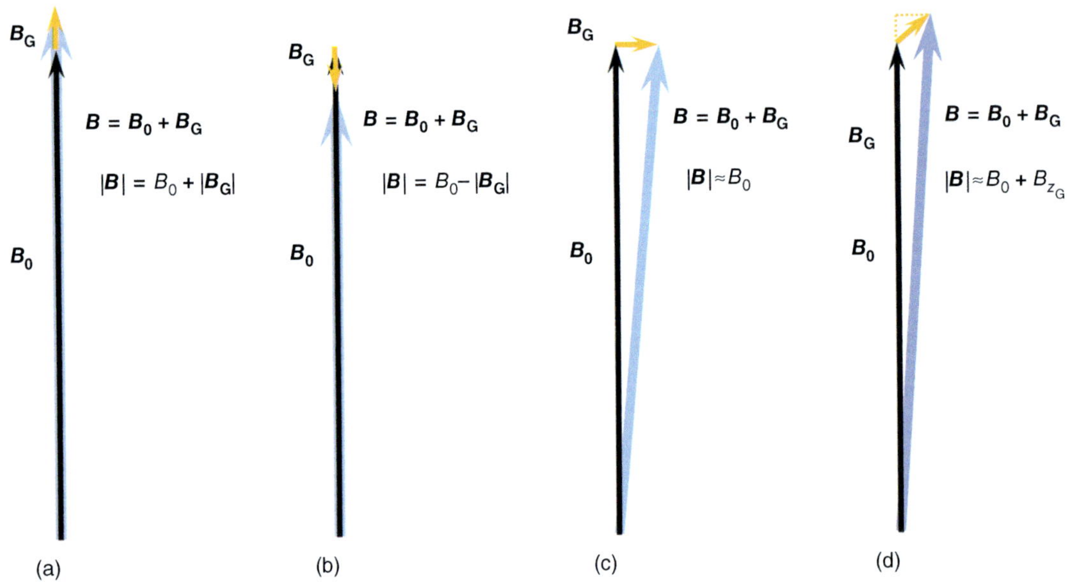

Figure 34.1. Cartoon demonstrating a vector addition of the strong main magnetic field $\boldsymbol{B}_0$ (black arrows) and a relatively weak gradient coil field (yellow arrows) under different conditions: (a) parallel, (b) antiparallel, (c) orthogonal, and (d) declined. The resulting vector is shown in light blue. In this demonstration, the ratio between the main field and the gradient coil field magnitudes is about 10. In typical MRI settings, this ratio is even higher, with the main field of the order of several tesla and the gradient coil field maximum of the order of several tens of millitesla

direction and strength at every point in space, whereas Larmor frequency is a scalar quantity, proportional to the magnitude of the local magnetic field. Upon the action of the gradient coils, the local magnetic field at every point in space becomes a vector sum of a strong and homogeneous main magnetic field $\boldsymbol{B}_0$, and spatially dependent magnetic fields induced by each gradient coil. Per convention, the main magnetic field $\boldsymbol{B}_0$ is oriented along the z-axis. Without loss of generality, consider the field of a single gradient coil, $\boldsymbol{B}_G$. As visualized in Figure 34.1 for a number of cases, bearing in mind that $|\boldsymbol{B}_0| \gg |\boldsymbol{B}_G|$, primarily the vector component of $\boldsymbol{B}_G$ that is collinear to $\boldsymbol{B}_0$ is able to change the magnitude of the resulting vector, whereas the vector components orthogonal to $\boldsymbol{B}_G$ have a much smaller, typically negligible, effect.

Due to the high homogeneity of the main magnetic field, the resonance frequency $\omega_0 = \gamma|\boldsymbol{B}_0|$ is typically assumed to have no spatial dependency. Under the action of the gradient coil field, the resonance frequency becomes

$$\omega(\mathbf{x}) = \gamma\,|\boldsymbol{B}_0 + \boldsymbol{B}_G(\mathbf{x})| \qquad (34.1)$$

where $\mathbf{x}$ is the three-dimensional vector corresponding to the spatial position, and γ is the gyromagnetic ratio. Considering $\boldsymbol{B}_0 = B_0\hat{\mathbf{z}}$, where $\hat{\mathbf{z}}$ is the unit vector along z-axis, and applying the second-order Taylor expansion, the Larmor frequency becomes[5]

$$\omega(\mathbf{x}) \approx \gamma B_0 + \gamma B_{z_G}(\mathbf{x}) + \frac{\gamma}{B_0} B^2_{xy_G}(\mathbf{x}) + \cdots \qquad (34.2)$$

where $B_{z_G} = \boldsymbol{B}_G \cdot \hat{\mathbf{z}}$ is the component of the gradient coil field parallel to the main magnetic field, and $B_{xy_G} = |\boldsymbol{B}_G \times \hat{\mathbf{z}}|$ is the magnitude of the transverse component. Under the typical for MRI condition $|\boldsymbol{B}_0| \gg |\boldsymbol{B}_G|$, the first-order term in equation (34.2) vastly dominates over the second-order one; therefore, during the design of the gradients, only the z-component of the gradient coil field, B_{z_G}, is considered. The second term in equation (34.2) is the so-called concomitant field,[5,6] which may contribute to artifacts in certain MRI pulse sequences but is commonly ignored in the majority of situations. The transverse components of the gradient coil field are often termed *Maxwell terms* or *concomitant components* and may become important in applications using very high gradient amplitudes, as diffusion or flow imaging, or at lower magnetic field strengths.[7,8] In the context of gradient coil design, the subscript 'G' is commonly dropped, and the corresponding 'useful' field component of the gradient coil field is denoted B_z. The linearization $\omega(\mathbf{x}) \approx \gamma B_0 + \gamma B_z(\mathbf{x})$ has a further important implication: fields of multiple gradient coils used simultaneously contribute linearly to the observed frequency variation. Therefore, it is possible to construct a so-called *gradient set* or *gradient system*, which individual channels produce linear Larmor frequency variations along the x, y, and z axes. It is further convenient to define the gradient vector as

$$\mathbf{G} = \frac{1}{\gamma}\nabla\omega(\mathbf{x}) \tag{34.3}$$

where individual components of the gradient vector G_i, with $i = \{x, y, z\}$, are related to the z-components of the corresponding gradient coils such that $B_{z_i}(\mathbf{x}) = G_i x_i$.

The gradient system of commercial MRI systems with a conventional geometry is a cylindrical structure with a relatively thick wall of about 5–10 cm, which occupies the space between the warm bore of the magnet (i.e., bore size defined by the outer wall of the magnet's cryostat) and the patient-accessible bore. It includes highly optimized copper winding patterns targeted at creating the desired gradient fields, while minimizing the switching time (reducing inductance) and the energy dissipation (keeping resistance of the windings low). Modern gradient systems are equipped with a water-cooling system to transport the generated heat away from the coil. Commercial MRI systems are driven by high-power gradient power amplifiers, capable of generating currents of about 500–1000 A and voltages of up to ~2.5 kV. High currents are required to achieve high gradient amplitudes, whereas high voltages are needed to enable fast switching (i.e., short rise times). Up-to-date, MRI scanners are typically equipped with whole-body gradients reaching 40–70 mT m^{-1} per channel with a switching time of about 200 μs. Another important characteristic of the gradient coil is the size of the homogeneous gradient region, which alternatively can be specified as a maximum gradient deviation over the target imaging volume.

It is instructive to examine the possible spatial field distributions of the magnetic field corresponding to the longitudinal (z-gradient) and transverse (x or y gradient) fields. It is very difficult to visualize filed vectors in three dimensions; therefore, we chose to consider the XZ-plane and only visualize the in-plane vector components. Based on the symmetry, the through-plane component of the magnetic field vector of the said coils is 0 in the entire plane. Figure 34.2 shows magnetic fields of a simple transverse and longitudinal gradient coil. Streamline plots give an intuitive picture of the spatial field distribution. Level lines of B_z are plotted as black dotted lines. The target homogeneous region is omitted for clarity purposes but can be easily identified as the central area where the level lines of B_z are particularly evenly spaced. The color map in Figure 34.2 represents the magnitude

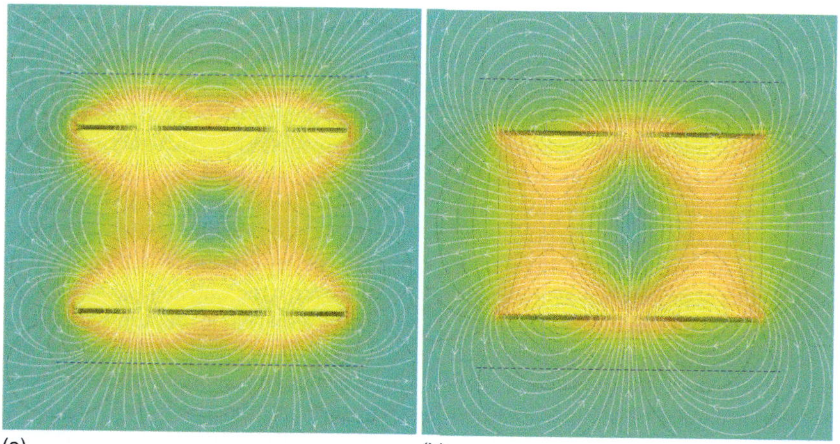

(a) (b)

Figure 34.2. Magnetic field of an unshielded transverse/x gradient coil (a) and an unshielded longitudinal/z gradient coil (b) in the XZ-plane. Color map indicates the magnitude of the magnetic field in an arbitrary scale common for both figures. White lines with arrows are the streamlines of the magnetic field vectors with too dense lines omitted for display purposes. Black dotted lines are level lines of the z-component of the magnetic field. Blue dashed lines indicate the approximate location of the cold surfaces in the cryostat

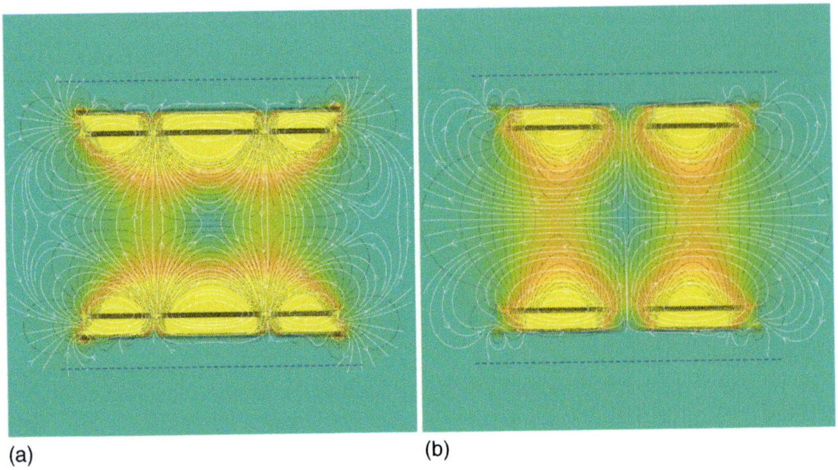

Figure 34.3. Magnetic field of an actively shielded transverse/*x* gradient coil (a) and a shielded longitudinal/*z* gradient coil (b). Color maps and all conventions concerning the line and plot styles correspond to those in Figure 34.2. As seen, active shielding 'squeezes' the majority of the stray fields of the gradient coil into the space between the primary and the secondary windings

of the magnetic field. As seen, the transverse coil produces a substantially higher magnitude of the magnetic field for the same gradient strength.

Note that the example coils in Figure 34.2 produce substantial magnetic fields at the location of the cold conductive structures inside the cryostat of the main magnet (indicated as a dashed line). When the current through the gradient coil is changed, long-lived eddy currents are induced in these structures, with life times on the order of seconds.[9–11] These eddy currents produce secondary fields in the target imaging region and distort both the temporal and spatial profiles of the encoding field. There was a solution proposed[12,13] to address this problem by predistorting the gradient-driving currents such that the superposition of the applied gradient fields and the eddy-current-induced fields would approximate the desired field variation in time. By applying a filter theory to this problem, this approach has evolved into the modern concept of preemphasis.[14,15] However, due to the fact that the eddy-current surface is located at a certain distance from the primary gradient coil windings, the spatial distribution of the field induced by eddy currents in the imaging volume generally differs substantially from linear gradients[16] and thus cannot be perfectly compensated for by preemphasis. Furthermore, eddy currents in the cold conductive structures dissipate their energy within the cryovessel, increasing the rate of helium boil-off.[17] Besides, the conductive surfaces carrying eddy currents experience Lenz forces both from the interaction with the main magnetic field and the switching gradient field, resulting in mechanical vibrations induced in the cryostat, which wear the magnet and increase the risk of a magnet quench.

A better way to avoid eddy currents is to use the active shielding principle.[18–20] The idea of active shielding consists in introducing additional windings exterior to the primary gradient coil windings. The current distribution in the shielding coil is designed to cancel the stray magnetic field of the primary coil outside the secondary coil. To ensure a perfect temporal synchronization of the primary and the secondary fields, the corresponding coils are switched in series. An example of the field distribution of the shielded coils can be seen in Figure 34.3. The secondary windings effectively confine the streamlines of the stray fields to the space between the primary and the secondary coils.

However, the advantageous properties of the shielded coil come at a price: the secondary coil also partially cancels the field of the primary coil in the imaging region, thereby reducing the coil efficiency. At the same time, due to the series connection of the primary and secondary windings, the inductance of the whole coil is increased. Similarly, due to the increased total length of the wire, the resistance and therefore the energy dissipated by the coil are increased. Nonetheless, all modern MRI systems use actively shielded gradients. Availability of whole-body actively shielded gradients in commercial

MRI scanners made it possible for the fast imaging sequences as echo-planar imaging (EPI)[21–23] or balanced steady state free precession (SSFP)[24,25] to enter clinical practice.

34.2 GRADIENT COIL DESIGN

The objective of the gradient design is to derive a technically realizable gradient coil winding pattern constrained to a predefined volume, capable of producing the desired partial variation of B_z within the target imaging region, subject to a number of additional technical constraints. These constraints typically include electrical load characteristics, such as resistance and inductance, maximum current, and breakdown voltages. The target field typically cannot be reached precisely in the entire imaging region, so a number of subregions with different tolerable deviations are often defined. Additional requirements, e.g., to reduce the likelihood of peripheral nerve stimulation (PNS), to control mechanical stress in the coil structure or the overall net forces and torques may also be specified.

If the winding pattern is known, the problem of calculating the magnetic field distribution can be solved relatively easily by integrating the Biot–Savart law along the conductor path. This forward problem can be solved directly numerically or semianalytically using a variety of methods, most commonly by either calculating the field components directly or via the magnetic vector potential. It is of interest to calculate B_z component of the gradient coil field in the target imaging volume, which is commonly termed a *region of uniformity* (ROU) of the gradient. Typically, this region is chosen to be a sphere of a certain diameter, which is referred to as diameter of a spherical volume (DSV). For shielded coils additional areas, typically cylindrical surfaces are defined, where the magnetic field contributions are reduced.

In contrast to the forward problem, the inverse magnetostatic problem, being the main objective of the gradient design, poses several challenges. First of all, there may not exist a precise solution, which exactly fulfills all desired conditions. This challenge is dealt with by accepting an approximate solution. Secondly, there may exist infinitely many solutions, which approximate the mathematical problem at hand equally well.

Gradient design problem belongs to a common class of the so-called ill-posed inverse problems. Mathematically, ill-posed problems present numerous challenges, e.g., by making it difficult to find the globally optimal solution or proofing that the solution found is close enough to the global optimum. However, the variability of the feasible solutions and the particular properties of the solution space present an excellent opportunity from the engineering perspective to optimize the resulting coils for further parameters and physical characteristics. This is achieved by introducing appropriate regularization factors and constraints to the initial inverse problem, intended to constrain the solution space and make it well behaving in some sense, e.g., convex. The latter allows for the efficient numerical solvers to be applied, to find appropriate solutions with an acceptable computation effort.[26]

The primary goal of the gradient design process is to construct a coil capable of creating a certain magnetic field distribution within the given volume. As mentioned above, the target magnetic field cannot be reached precisely in most cases, so a certain deviation needs to be accepted. The choice of the error function largely defines the properties of the designed coil as well as the possible trade-offs between its parameters. A popular error function, commonly used primarily due to its simplicity, is the field error at every point $\mathbf{x}$ within the target imaging region:

$$\Delta B_z(\mathbf{x}) = \frac{B_z(\mathbf{x}) - B_z^{\text{target}}(\mathbf{x})}{\max(|B_z^{\text{target}}(\mathbf{x})|)} \tag{34.4}$$

where $B_z(\mathbf{x})$ is the field achieved by the gradient coil, and $B_z^{\text{target}}(\mathbf{x})$ is the desired field profile, commonly defined for the given gradient vector $\mathbf{G}$ as $B_z^{\text{target}}(\mathbf{x}) = \mathbf{G} \cdot \mathbf{x}$. Gradient homogeneity is commonly specified as a maximum field error within a certain volume, e.g., 5% over the 20 cm DSV at the isocenter. The squared field error is commonly integrated over the target imaging volume to arrive to a single scalar, which can be used in the optimization algorithm. However, both maximum and the mean-squared field error are considered to be very weak homogeneity requirements, as both these conditions are strongly dominated by the highest field typically reached at the periphery of the imaging region and are not particularly sensitive to field deviations close to the isocenter. A substantially more precise control of the field behavior can be reached using the gradient error defined as

$$\Delta \mathbf{G}(\mathbf{x}) = \frac{\nabla B_z(\mathbf{x}) - \mathbf{G}}{|\mathbf{G}|} \tag{34.5}$$

Both magnetic field and the gradient produced by the coil are directly proportional to the applied electrical current. Therefore, equations (34.4) and (34.5) are typically evaluated at certain predefined current, e.g., unity current or the maximum nominal current. To avoid the dependency on the driving current, the gradient sensitivity, η, is defined as the ratio of the gradient magnitude produced at the iso-center to the applied current:

$$\eta = \frac{|\mathbf{G}|}{I} \tag{34.6}$$

The coil sensitivity is a very useful parameter when comparing gradient coils with the identical geometry. In a more general case it is, however, strongly dominated by the coil dimensions: smaller coils typically show much higher gradient sensitivity. Therefore, several more robust figures of merit were proposed. For the larger coils and fast imaging applications, the stored magnetic energy is often the most relevant parameter, which needs to be balanced against the coil sensitivity during the design process. For such situations, the inductive figure of merit is defined as[27]

$$\beta = \frac{\eta^2}{L} \tag{34.7}$$

where L is the inductance of the gradient coil. However, for smaller coils, such as local gradient coils or gradients in the high-resolution NMR spectrometers, the inductance is rarely the limiting parameter. It is rather the capacity of the cooling system to extract the thermal energy dissipated by the coil windings in the small volume of the coil. Similarly, for whole-body gradients targeted at diffusion imaging applications, which are driven by high currents sustained for hundreds of milliseconds, the resistance, R, of the coil needs to be balanced against the gradient sensitivity; therefore, the resistive figure of merit is used, defined as[28]

$$\gamma = \frac{\eta^2}{R} \tag{34.8}$$

Oftentimes, the abovementioned figures of merit are defined as a square root of equations (34.7) and (34.8), respectively.

Development of a gradient coil typically involves iterative optimization of the coil design parameters to approach the desired magnetic field pattern while fulfilling the specified constraints. This necessarily requires a parameterization of the coil design with a certain number of variables, which are then adapted by the optimization engine of choice. In the early works, discrete wire windings were parameterized and optimized.[29,30] The structure of the windings was primarily defined by the available manufacturing technology and some physical considerations, for instance the positions of the individual wire tracks or groups of wires. However, these coils could not reach particularly high-performance metrics, primarily due to either limitations of the predefined parameter space. More complex and flexible models face difficulties during the numerical optimization, oftentimes resulting in NP-hard (non-deterministic polynomial-time hardness) nonlinear optimization problems with complex topologies.[31,32] A commonly adopted alternative approach is to use a continuous current density optimization space. It is based on a simplification of the coil structure, where during the optimization the discrete windings are replaced with a continuous current density distribution confined to the corresponding spatial structure, e.g., two cylindrical surfaces corresponding to the primary and secondary (shielding) layers of the coil.[18,19,33] In the final design stage, the continuous current distribution is converted to discrete wire paths.

There are a variety of the methods in the literature, especially numerous in the past decade of the previous century, which model the current density in a variety of ways and link it to the field in the target imaging region.[34,35] They also differ in the way how the magnetic field within the target region is modeled. For a comprehensive historical review, the reader is referred to the corresponding review papers.[36,37] In the following section, we focus on the discretized stream function approach combined with the boundary element method, which emerged in the early 2000s. Both due to the high availability of the computing power and their conceptual simplicity, gradient design methods of this kind have mostly superseded the previous more mathematically involved techniques.

34.3 DISCRETIZED STREAM FUNCTION METHOD

It is advantageous to describe a surface current density by means of its scalar stream function. Stream function of the electrical current is closely related to the stream function in fluid dynamics introduced by Joseph Louis Lagrange for describing 2D flows of incompressible liquids. Stream function of the electrical current is a scalar function $\psi(\mathbf{r})$ defined on a smooth surface Γ such that

$$\mathbf{J}(\mathbf{r}) = \nabla \times [\psi(\mathbf{r})\mathbf{n}(\mathbf{r})], \text{ for } \mathbf{r} \in \Gamma \tag{34.9}$$

where $\mathbf{J}(\mathbf{r})$ is the local current density, tangential to Γ, and $\mathbf{n}(\mathbf{r})$ is the local normal vector of Γ. As the function

$\psi(\mathbf{r})$ is only defined on the surface, the differentiation in the rotation operator needs to be performed along the surface. The advantage of the above definition is that the current density $\mathbf{J}(\mathbf{r})$ automatically fulfills the charge preservation requirement, and the pure rotation field is guaranteed to be divergence free. A further advantage comes from the fact that $\psi(\mathbf{r})$ is a scalar function needing a single number at every point to describe the corresponding current density, so the number of degrees of freedom in the inverse problem is effectively reduced.

In its physical meaning, the stream function value at a certain point corresponds to the local circular current, flowing in an isolated infinitesimally small closed loop around that point. Noteworthy is that the stream function is defined up to an arbitrary additive constant, which is commonly conveniently selected such that the stream function at the external boundary of the current-carrying surface turns to 0. When the stream function is constant in a certain area, the neighboring opposing currents at the edges of the infinitesimally small cells cancel each other, so there is no net current flowing through that area. In the areas where the stream function shows a local gradient, there is a net current flowing orthogonal to that gradient. From the two abovementioned properties, it is clear that electrical currents may only flow along the level lines of the stream function. Furthermore, due to the fact that the local current density is proportional to the gradient of the stream function, the density of the level lines taken at equidistant values of the stream function closely corresponds to the magnitude of the local current density.

Due to the abovementioned relations between the stream function and the current density, the following procedure is commonly applied to convert the stream function to discrete windings.[38] In the first step, for the chosen number of turns the corresponding level lines are found. These are then taken as the center lines of the unconnected circular conductors carrying the same current. In the next step, the loops are cut open and interconnected in series. The feeding wire, which feeds the innermost loop, is then placed directly above or below the surface Γ, such that it overlaps the interconnection bridges. The close proximity of the feeding wire and the interconnection bridges effectively compensates for the far field created by the opposite currents flowing in these structures. In the majority of recent publications the described procedure appears to include at least some manual interaction, e.g., to account for certain technological constraints. Due to the very involved manual procedures required for this final design steps, oftentimes in publications the windings of the gradient coils are visualized as simple level lines of the stream function without interconnections.

Equation (34.9) links a continuous stream function to a continuous current density distribution. In real gradient design applications, the stream function needs to be discretized. For simple geometries, such as planar or cylindrical coils, a regular rectangular mesh can be employed.[38] However, the true power of the discretized stream function method is unfolded when it is used in combination with generic triangular meshes.[39–41] A dense triangular mesh can be derived for literally any arbitrary current-carrying surface associated with any practically feasible gradient coil using a variety of software algorithms and tools,[42,43] some of which are free and open source.[44] The values of the stream function on each of the nodes within the mesh are used as the design variables during the optimization process. The values of the stream function on the boundary nodes are forced to an arbitrary constant along each boundary. Assuming a constant current density within each patch, expressions were derived for both the current density and the stream function at any point within the surface Γ.[40] More importantly, analytic expressions were derived to precompute various system matrices. For the vector $\boldsymbol{\psi} = [\psi(\mathbf{r}_1), \psi(\mathbf{r}_2), \cdots, \psi(\mathbf{r}_n)]$ containing the values of the stream function samples at the locations of the mesh nodes for all the nodes in the mesh, it is then possible to express the z-component of the magnetic field at a series of test points as a vector as

$$\mathbf{b} = \mathbf{B}\boldsymbol{\psi} \qquad (34.10)$$

where matrix $\mathbf{B}$ contains weights which only depend on the geometry of the current-carrying surface and the test point locations within the target imaging region. Similar to that, vector components of the current density $\mathbf{j}_{\{x,y,z\}}$ for the axes $\boldsymbol{x}, \boldsymbol{y}$, and z, respectively, can be expressed in the matrix form as

$$\mathbf{j}_{\{x,y,z\}} = \mathbf{J}_{\{x,y,z\}}\boldsymbol{\psi} \qquad (34.11)$$

An analogous expression can be derived for the mechanical torque vector $\mathbf{m}$. The magnetic energy stored in the coil can be expressed as a quadratic form with respect to the stream function vector $\boldsymbol{\psi}$:

$$W = \boldsymbol{\psi}^{\mathrm{T}}\mathbf{L}\boldsymbol{\psi} \qquad (34.12)$$

where $\mathbf{L}$ is the precomputed inductance matrix, which only depends on the geometry of the mesh, and $\boldsymbol{\psi}^{\mathrm{T}}$ is

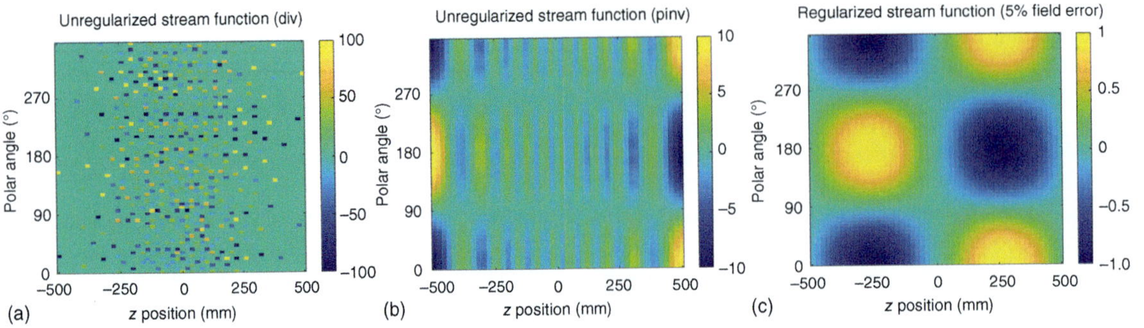

Figure 34.4. 2D plots of the surface stream functions for a hypothetical *x*-gradient coil designed by a direct inversion of equation (34.10) (a) using matrix division operation in Matlab; (b) using Moore–Penrose pseudoinverse implementation in Matlab; and (c) regularized for the dissipated power to achieve approximately 5% maximum field error. Note that in panel (a) the color range was enhanced by a factor of 100, in panel (b) by a factor of 10 with respect to panel (c)

the transposed vector containing the stream function values. Similarly, the power dissipated by the coil can be written as

$$P = \boldsymbol{\psi}^{\mathrm{T}}\mathbf{R}\boldsymbol{\psi} \tag{34.13}$$

where **R** is the resistance matrix associated with the coil structure. The gradient coil optimization problem can then be formulated as a minimization of the objective function Φ:

$$\Phi = \|\mathbf{b} - \mathbf{b}_{\text{target}}\|_2 + \lambda_P P + \lambda_W W + \lambda_m|\mathbf{m}| + \lambda_j\|\mathbf{j}\|_{\mathrm{p}} \tag{34.14}$$

The minimization of the functional Φ diminishes the difference between the achieved and the target field, while at the same time minimizing the dissipated power P, the stored magnetic energy W, and the net torque acting on the coil $|\mathbf{m}|$. The additional term in the equation above, $\|\mathbf{j}\|_{\mathrm{p}}$, is the p-norm of the electric current density, which is a smooth approximation of the maximum current density, which is introduced to control the minimum wire spacing.[28] The relative weights of all these regularization factors are controlled by the corresponding Lagrange multipliers. Typically, the Lagrange multipliers are iteratively adjusted to arrive to a desired field error while fulfilling other coil specifications, such as inductance, resistance, dissipated power, or maximum torque. Oftentimes, these requirements can be formulated as constraints instead of regularization terms to avoid a tedious search of the appropriate weighting factors. In this case, however, constrained optimization engines need to be used, which are generally slower than the unconstrained ones and require a careful initialization since many engines, such as the penalty method, transform the original constrained problem into a sequence of unconstrained problems and solve these unconstrained problems sequentially.[45]

The importance of the regularization during the gradient coil design is underlined by the following example. As mentioned above, the problem of finding a current distribution capable of generating a certain magnetic field in a constrained region of space is mathematically ill-posed. To demonstrate the point, a hypothetical transverse gradient coil was designed without any regularization, which corresponds to setting all Lagrange multipliers in equation (34.14) to 0. Alternatively, it can be seen as a direct inversion of equation (34.10). As seen in Figure 34.4(a), the direct inversion of equation (34.10) produces a nonsense result dominated by the numerical errors. Using Moore–Penrose pseudoinverse as implemented in Matlab (MathWorks Inc., Natick, MA, USA) by the pinv() function (see Figure 34.4b) produces a physically correct but totally unreasonable coil, requiring extremely high current densities (high stream function values with steep gradients) as well as the oscillating patterns, leading to a lower efficiency and a higher inductance. Adding a power-regularizing term produces a stream function map with a familiar appearance (Figure 34.4c). The same stream function with the level lines added to visualize the winding layout is shown in Figure 34.5 mapped to the three-dimensional cylindrical surface corresponding to the current-carrying surface used in the design.

As mentioned above, for the practical fast imaging applications it is necessary to control eddy current performance of the coil during the gradient coil design. This is typically achieved by introducing additional terms to equation (34.14), which model the magnetic

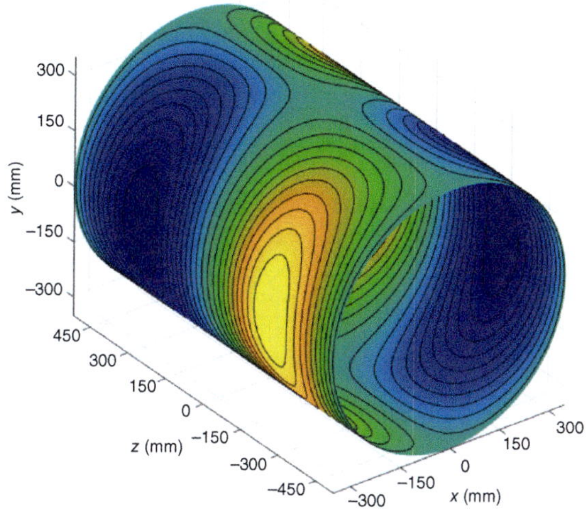

Figure 34.5. 3D representation of the stream function along with the wire tracks for the regularized design in Figure 34.4(c)

field effects of the eddy currents induced in the cold magnet structures.[28,38] Another reason for controlling the magnetic fields of the gradient coil escaping into the cryostat is to reduce interactions of the gradient fields with the magnet, e.g., to suppress accelerated helium boil-off. Strictly speaking, only the field components normal to the cold conductive surface contribute to the eddy currents and Lorenz forces, but typically if any component of the incident field is suppressed, others disappear as well, as the stray field components are connected by the Maxwell/Laplace equations. Therefore, suppressing a single component is computationally advantageous as it results in a linear equation added to the objective function. Exemplary shielded coil wire tracks can be seen in Figure 34.6.

34.4 MECHANICAL VIBRATIONS AND ACOUSTIC NOISE

Any conductor carrying an electric current and exposed to an external magnetic field nonparallel to the conductor direction experiences a Lorenz force. This force acts in a direction orthogonal to both the direction of the magnetic field and the current flowing through the conductor, with the magnitude proportional to both parameters. For a curved conductor, an elementary force contribution acting at the conductor segment $\mathbf{dl}$ carrying current I is expressed as

$$\mathrm{d}\mathbf{F} = I\,\boldsymbol{B}(\mathbf{r}) \times \mathrm{d}\mathbf{l} \qquad (34.15)$$

The net force acting at the entire conductor is acquired as a path integral of equation (34.15) along the conductor length. As typical gradient coil windings can be considered as approximately closed conductors, in a perfectly homogeneous magnetic field $\boldsymbol{B}(\mathbf{r}) = \boldsymbol{B}_0$, the net force acting at the entire gradient coil approaches zero. For symmetrical coils, such as used in classical whole-body gradient systems, the net torque acting at the whole coil is also zero. As mentioned above, in coils with asymmetric windings, such as gradient inserts, the net torque can be considered and effectively minimized during the gradient design process according to equation (34.14). However, in modern actively shielded magnets, the magnetic field at the location of the whole-body gradient coil cannot be considered perfectly homogeneous, and the actual field distribution of the main magnet needs to be taken into account in equation (34.15).

Because the effects of Lorentz forces scale with main magnetic field strength, they have to be managed properly for safe in vivo operation. The forces acting at each half-turn of the conductor within the coil correspond to the weight action of several metric tons. Therefore, advanced engineering models and construction techniques have been presented for a proper management of forces and torques. This becomes especially important at ultrahigh field strengths of 7 T and above. Vibrational simulations may include, but are not limited to, vibrations in the magnet-gradient assembly, mechanical resonances, and vibration of connector cables.[17] For the typical gradient coil dimensions, low-frequency regime is defined for the gradient switching frequencies below 100 Hz. In this range only the net forces and torques need to be considered, which can be well managed during the gradient design process. For higher frequencies, the internal mechanical oscillations of the gradient coil cylinder become important. The gradient coil structure, being a thick-walled cylinder, exposes under these conditions a variety of its natural resonances or eigenmodes, such as bending (the so-called banana mode), breathing (radial compression), ovaling, or torsion deformations. These mechanical resonance modes typically correspond to distinct frequencies. These resonances need to be managed at the design stage by applying advanced multiphysics modeling and modifying the mechanical structure of the coil accordingly. Furthermore, final vibrations and acoustic noise levels can

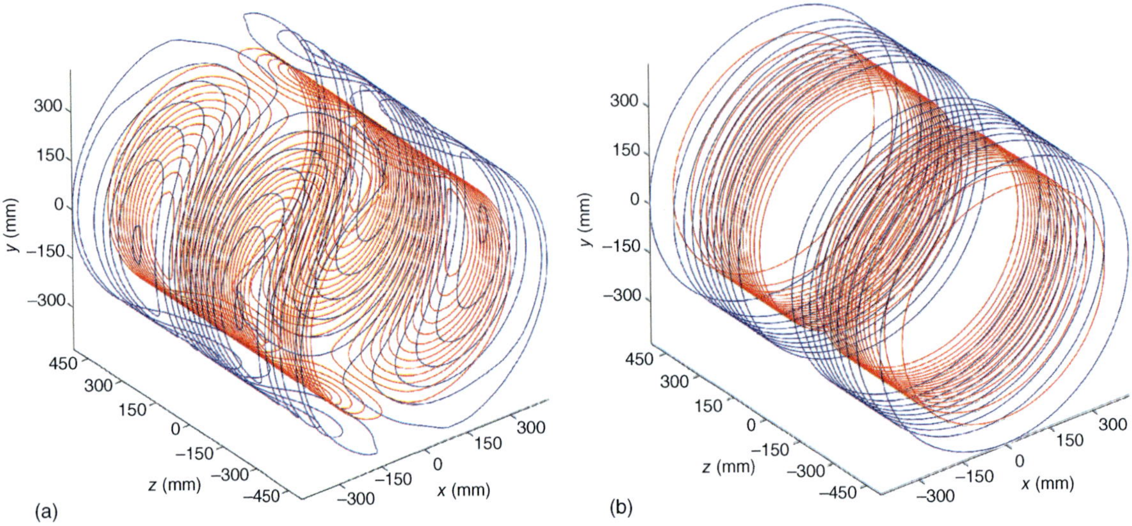

Figure 34.6. 3D representations of the wire tracks exemplary shielded coil designs: (a) transverse (x) gradient coil; (b) longitudinal (z) gradient coil. Primary layer windings are shown in red, whereas shielding windings are shown in blue

be further managed from the pulse sequence side by avoiding or reducing the corresponding frequency contributions in the applied gradient waveforms. On one hand, this is necessary to ensure a mechanical stability of the gradient system, e.g., to avoid delamination and disintegration of the gradient coil assembly. On the other hand, it helps to manage the acoustic noise to keep the sound pressure level (SPL) acceptable for the safe in vivo operation. Safety aspects associated with the high SPL in MR imaging are treated in much detail elsewhere (see Chapter 7).

34.5 PERIPHERAL NERVE STIMULATION

Time-varying magnetic fields, such as generated by the gradient coils, may potentially induce electric fields in living tissues, strong enough to cause neuronal discharges. The most relevant in the context of MRI effect observed in human subjects is the peripheral nerve stimulation (PNS).[46–48] The majority of the current clinical MRI systems are capable of exceeding sensible PNS thresholds, at least based on their maximum gradient and slew rate specifications. Therefore, all MRI systems implement PNS safety monitoring mechanisms, which in fact notably limit the achievable imaging speed. Detailed mechanisms of interactions between the gradient coil fields and the nerve tissue are discussed at length in the literature.[48–50] Here, we only briefly mention PNS considerations in the context of gradient coil design.

When considering PNS it is important to take into account not only the B_z component of the gradient coil field used for spatial encoding. According to the Maxwell equations, the transverse components B_x and B_y also contribute to the induced electric fields. As seen in Figures 34.2 and 34.3, for both unshielded and shielded gradient coils, respectively, the magnitude of the magnetic field reaches its highest values outside of the target imaging region and close to the magnet bore. It is therefore intuitively clear that smaller coils with a reduced region of gradient uniformity, as well as coils with lower linearity specifications, are likely to induce less PNS.[51,52] This was confirmed in the recent high-performance breast[53] and head-only designs.[54,55] It was further hypothesized that using nonlinear encoding fields, as in PatLoc,[56] O-Space,[57] or FRONSAC,[58] approaches may offset PNS constraints. Experimental validation of this assumption faces, however, difficulties due to the absence of gradient hardware with a sufficiently high performance. Another potential way of managing PNS is to tailor the field to the imaging region using additional gradient channels.[59,60] At its extreme, this approach was realized in the matrix gradient coil,[61] capable of creating a variety of spatial encoding magnetic fields as a superposition of the fields of its 84 elements.

34.6 MANUFACTURING CONSIDERATIONS

A practical implementation of high-performance gradient coils for human MRI presents a number of substantial engineering challenges. The gradient windings are supposed to carry currents on the order of 1000 A, which necessarily requires handling conductor tracks of with cross sections on the order of 1 cm^2 to safely endure high direct currents as required for diffusion weighting. The requirement of fast switching of the currents, however, limits the maximum wire width due to the skin effect and internal eddy currents. To partially avoid those, multiple filaments or slotted conductors need to be used. Furthermore, due to the substantial inductance of typical whole-body gradient coils (on the order of 1000 nH), fast changes of the currents require an application of high transient voltages, on the order of 2 kV and above. This sets stringent requirements on the electrical insulation within each of the coil channels (e.g., between the windings and the bridged return paths, as well as between the gradient channels). For typical duty cycles, whole-body gradient coils can dissipate up to 50 kW of thermal power, which need to be safely removed from the magnet bore by an appropriately scaled water-cooling system. Last but not least, a typical whole-body gradient coil, when fully assembled, weighs between 500 and 1000 kg, requiring industrial-grade lifting equipment for mechanical handling. Typically the coils are fully assembled and in the final step impregnated into epoxy resin under vacuum to glue the coil parts together for mechanical stiffness and fill all empty spaces to avoid building up of static surface charges.

A typical gradient coil is realized as a thick-walled cylindrical structure where individual conductive layers are placed on cylinders of varying radii to form the final sandwich-like structure (see Figure 34.7). Each layer is typically premanufactured and then sequentially assembled to form the final coil structure. An important factor is the mechanical precision of the assembly process, which only allows for extremely low tolerances, especially for the relative alignment between the primary and the shielding layers.

There are several established (but still competing) technologies for manufacturing individual coil windings. Z-coil is typically wound directly from a discrete wire. For the transverse gradient channels there are two competing approaches: winding from discrete wires and cutting from a solid conductor. Discrete wires are typically glued on thin glass-reinforced plastic (GRP) carrier plates using computer-controlled winding machines. Solid conductor technology typically relies on cutting groves in copper plates by water jetting, laser cutting, or etching. Thereafter, the plane structures are rolled to the required diameter using corresponding machinery. As this final step may introduce deformations into the winding structure, some manufacturers prefer to cut coil elements from curved copper sheets or pipes. Partly-assembled coils can be seen in Figure 34.8. Water-cooling layers are typically applied between the current-carrying surfaces. An interesting but technologically challenging option is to use hollow conductor, with the water flow applied directly inside of the windings. Due to the direct thermal contact between the wires and

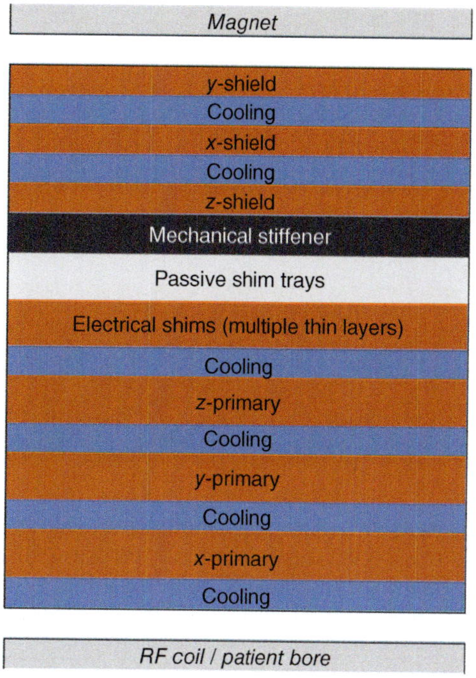

Figure 34.7. Multilayered sandwich structure of a typical gradient coil. The particular sequence of primary and secondary gradient coil windings is subject to a number of engineering decisions and varies between different coils and manufacturers. Some of the cooling layers may be avoided or integrated with the electrical windings using the hollow conductor technology. Fiber glass fabric is applied between the depicted layers to provide both additional mechanical reinforcement and electrical insulation. The whole gradient coil assembly is impregnated with epoxy resin under vacuum to fill all residual empty spaces

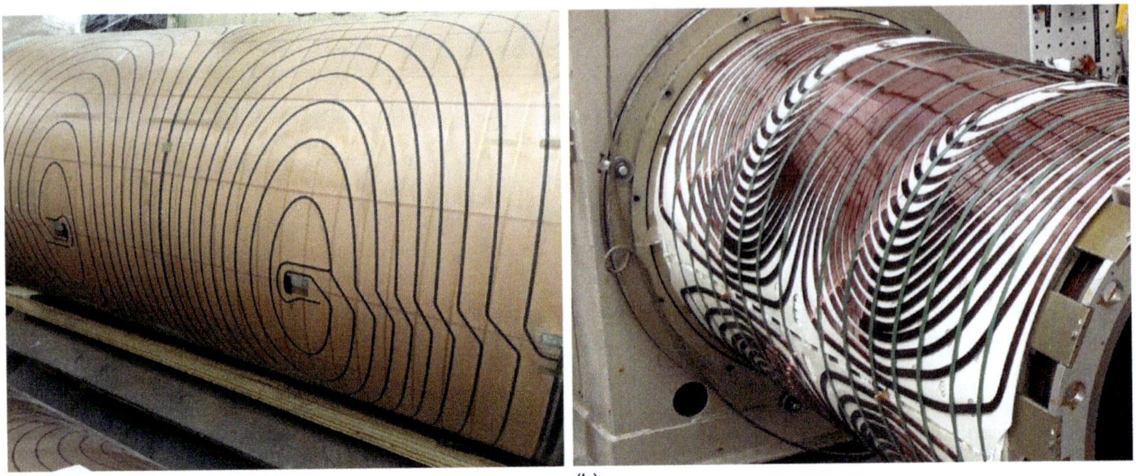

(a) (b)

Figure 34.8. Transverse gradient coils built using different manufacturing technologies: (a) with coil elements etched from copper plates or (b) with coils wound from a discrete conductor, readily glued to a carrier plate. (a) Photograph of a GE whole-body XRMb gradient coil providing 50 mT m^{-1} at 200 T m^{-1} s^{-1} and is used in 60 cm patient bore systems. (Courtesy of GE Healthcare.) (b) Gradient coil of the 3 T wide-bore Skyra system providing 45 mT m^{-1} at 200 T m^{-1} s^{-1} within the 70 cm patient bore (Courtesy of Siemens Healthineers)

the coolant, this provides a very efficient cooling option. However, as the typical wire length of the gradient coil can reach up to several hundred meters, the single electrical winding needs to be split into several parallel water-cooling circles. Due to the substantial voltage differences between the water entry/exit points, highly deionized water is required as coolant to prevent electrocorrosion inside the conductors.

Due to the abovementioned challenges the majority of the gradient coils are realized by the industry. Traditional gradient research at the universities was limited to methodologic aspects and realization of proof-of-concept models. However, several recent high-performance coils were presented with substantial contributions from research institutions.[54,55,62]

ACKNOWLEDGMENTS

The authors gracefully acknowledge Drs. Thomas Foo of GE Global Research and Andrew Dewdney of Siemens Healthineers for their help with acquiring photographs of industrial gradient coils in production.

REFERENCES

1. B. Breneman, in 'eMagRes', American Cancer Society, John Wiley and Sons: New York, 2019, p 137. DOI: 10.1002/9781119441649.emrstm1590.
2. J. P. Stockmann and L. L. Wald, *NeuroImage*, 2018, **168**, 71. DOI: 10.1016/j.neuroimage.2017.06.013.
3. K. J. Layton, S. Kroboth, F. Jia, S. Littin, H. Yu, J. Leupold, J. F. Nielsen, T. Stöcker, and M. Zaitsev, *Magn. Reson. Med.*, 2017, **77**, 1544. DOI: 10.1002/mrm.26235.
4. K. Setsompop, R. Kimmlingen, E. Eberlein, T. Witzel, J. Cohen-Adad, M. N. JA, B. Keil, M. D. Tisdall, P. Hoecht, P. Dietz, S. F. Cauley, V. Tountcheva, V. Matschl, V. H. Lenz, K. Heberlein, A. Potthast, H. Thein, J. Van Horn, A. Toga, F. Schmitt, D. Lehne, B. R. Rosen, V. Wedeen, and L. L. Wald, *NeuroImage*, 2013, **80**, 220. DOI: 10.1016/j.neuroimage.2013.05.078.
5. M. A. Bernstein, X. J. Zhou, J. A. Polzin, K. F. King, A. Ganin, N. J. Pelc, and G. H. Glover, *Magn. Reson. Med.*, 1998, **39**, 300. DOI: 10.1002/mrm.1910390218.
6. K. F. King, A. Ganin, X. J. Zhou, and M. A. Bernstein, *Magn. Reson. Med.*, 1999, **41**, 103. DOI: 10.1002/(sici)1522-2594(199901)41:1<103::aid-mrm15>3.0.co;2-m.

7. C. Meier, M. Zwanger, T. Feiweier, and D. Porter, *Magn. Reson. Med.*, 2008, **60**, 128. DOI: 10.1002/mrm.21615.
8. W. R. Myers, M. Mössle, and J. Clarke, *J. Magn. Reson.*, 2005, **177**, 274. DOI: 10.1016/j.jmr.2005.08.003.
9. E. A. Badea and O. Craiu, *IEEE Trans. Magn.*, 1997, **33**, 1330. DOI: 10.1109/20.582501.
10. G. Ries, *IEEE Trans. Magn.*, 1988, **24**, 516. DOI: 10.1109/20.43970.
11. A. Trakic, H. Wang, F. Liu, H. S. Lopez, and S. Crozier, *IEEE Trans. Appl. Supercond.*, 2006, **16**, 1924. DOI: 10.1109/TASC.2006.874000.
12. J. J. van Vaals and A. H. Bergman, *J. Magn. Reson.*, 1990, **90**, 52. DOI: 10.1016/0022-2364(90)90365-g.
13. M. A. Martens, L. S. Petropoulos, R. W. Brown, J. H. Andrews, M. A. Morich, and J. L. Patrick, *Rev. Sci. Instrum.*, 1991, **62**, 2639. DOI: 10.1063/1.1142245.
14. M. A. Morich, D. A. Lampman, W. R. Dannels, and F. D. Goldie, *IEEE Trans. Med. Imaging*, 1988, **7**, 247. DOI: 10.1109/42.7789.
15. P. D. Majors, J. L. Blackley, S. A. Altobelli, A. Caprihan, and E. Fukushima, *J. Magn. Reson.*, 1990, **87**, 548. DOI: 10.1016/0022-2364(90)90311-V.
16. S. J. Vannesjo, M. Haeberlin, L. Kasper, M. Pavan, B. J. Wilm, C. Barmet, and K. P. Pruessmann, *Magn. Reson. Med.*, 2013, **69**, 583. DOI: 10.1002/mrm.24263.
17. S. A. Winkler, F. Schmitt, H. Landes, J. de Bever, T. Wade, A. Alejski, and B. K. Rutt, *NeuroImage*, 2018, **168**, 59. DOI: 10.1016/j.neuroimage.2016.11.033.
18. P. Mansfield and B. Chapman, *J. Phys. E*, 1986, **19**, 540. DOI: 10.1088/0022-3735/19/7/008.
19. R. Bowtell and P. Mansfield, *Magn. Reson. Med.*, 1991, **17**, 15–; discussion 19–21. DOI: 10.1002/mrm.1910170105.
20. P. Roemer, W. Edelstein, and J. Hickey. Self-shielded gradient coils. Book of abstracts, In *5th Annual Meeting of the Society of Magnetic Resonance in Medicine*, 1986.
21. P. Mansfield, *J. Phys. C - Solid State Phys.*, 1977, **10**, L55.
22. R. Ordidge, *MAGMA*, 1999, **9**, 117. DOI: 10.1007/BF02594607.
23. M. S. Cohen and F. Schmitt, *NeuroImage*, 2012, **62**, 652. DOI: 10.1016/wj.neuroimage.2012.01.038.
24. O. Bieri and K. Scheffler, *J. Magn. Reson. Imaging*, 2013, **38**, 2. DOI: 10.1002/jmri.24163.
25. B. A. Hargreaves, *J. Magn. Reson. Imaging*, 2012, **36**, 1300. DOI: 10.1002/jmri.23742.
26. M. S. Poole and N. J. Shah, *J. Magn. Reson.*, 2014, **244**, 36. DOI: 10.1016/j.jmr.2014.04.015.
27. B. A. Chronik and B. K. Rutt, *Magn. Reson. Med.*, 1998, **39**, 270. DOI: 10.1002/mrm.1910390214.
28. M. S. Poole, P. T. While, H. S. Lopez, and S. Crozier, *Magn. Reson. Med.*, 2012, **68**, 639. DOI: 10.1002/mrm.23248.
29. K. C. Chu and B. K. Rutt, *Magn. Reson. Med.*, 1994, **31**, 652. DOI: 10.1002/mrm.1910310611.
30. E. C. Wong, A. Jesmanowicz, and J. S. Hyde, *Magn. Reson. Med.*, 1991, **21**, 39. DOI: 10.1002/mrm.1910210107.
31. S. Crozier, L. K. Forbes, and D. M. Doddrell, *J. Magn. Reson. Ser. A*, 1994, **107**, 126. DOI: 10.1006/jmra.1994.1058.
32. S. Shvartsman and M. C. Steckner, *Concepts Magn. Reson. Part B: Magn. Reson. Eng.*, 2007, **31B**, 95. DOI: 10.1002/cmr.b.20084.
33. B. L. W. Chapman, *MAGMA*, 1999, **9**, 146. DOI: 10.1007/BF02594613.
34. R. Turner, *J. Phys. D. Appl. Phys.*, 1986, **19**, L147. DOI: 10.1088/0022-3727/19/8/001.
35. R. Turner, *J. Phys. E: Sci. Instrum.*, 1988, **21**, 948. DOI: 10.1088/0022-3735/21/10/008.
36. R. Turner, *Magn. Reson. Imaging*, 1993, **11**, 903. DOI: 10.1016/0730-725X(93)90209-V.
37. S. S. Hidalgo-Tobon, *Concepts Magn. Reson. A*, 2010, **36A**, 223. DOI: 10.1002/cmr.a.20163.
38. G. N. Peeren, *J. Comput. Phys.*, 2003, **191**, 305. DOI: 10.1016/S0021-9991(03)00320-6.
39. S. Pissanetzky, *Meas. Sci. Technol.*, 1992, **3**, 667. DOI: 10.1088/0957-0233/3/7/007.
40. R. A. Lemdiasov and R. Ludwig, *Concepts Magn. Reson. Part B: Magn. Reson. Eng.*, 2005, **26B**, 67. DOI: 10.1002/cmr.b.20040.
41. M. Poole and R. Bowtell, *Concepts Magn. Reson. Part B: Magn. Reson. Eng.*, 2007, **31B**, 162. DOI: 10.1002/cmr.b.20091.
42. S.-W. Cheng, T. K. Dey, and J. Shewchuk, Delaunay Mesh Generation, CRC Press: Boca Raton, 2013.
43. D. Lo, Finite Element Mesh Generation, CRC Press, Taylor & Francis Group: Boca Raton, 2015.
44. Blender. http://blender.org (accessed 20 August 2019).

45. J. Nocedal and S. J. Wright, in 'Numerical Optimization', Springer Series in Operations Research and Financial Engineering, eds T. V. Mikosch, S. I. Resnick, and S. M. Robinson, Springer: New York, NY, 2006, p 497. DOI: 10.1007/978-0-387-40065-5_17.

46. T. F. Budinger, *IEEE Trans. Nucl. Sci.*, 1979, **26**, 2821. DOI: 10.1109/TNS.1979.4330543.

47. M. S. Cohen, R. M. Weisskoff, R. R. Rzedzian, and H. L. Kantor, *Magn. Reson. Med.*, 1990, **14**, 409. DOI: 10.1002/mrm.1910140226.

48. J. F. Schenck, in 'eMagRes', American Cancer Society, John Wiley and Sons: New York, 2015. DOI: 10.1002/9781119441649.emrstm1324.

49. J. Nyenhuis and D. Gross, in 'eMagRes', American Cancer Society, John Wiley and Sons: New York, 2019, p 29. DOI: 10.1002/9781119441649.emrstm1575.

50. M. Davids, B. Guérin, L. R. Schad, and L. L. Wald, in 'eMagRes', American Cancer Society, John Wiley and Sons: New York, 2019, p 87. DOI: 10.1002/9781119441649.emrstm1586.

51. E. C. Wong, in 'eMagRes', American Cancer Society, John Wiley and Sons: New York, 2007. DOI: 10.1002/9781119441649.emrstm0599.

52. M. Zhu, L. Xia, and F. Liu, *Crit. Rev. Biomed. Eng.*, 2014, **42**, 493.

53. H. S. Lopez, M. Poole, and S. Crozier, *J. Magn. Reson.*, 2009, **199**, 48. DOI: 10.1016/j.jmr.2009.03.011.

54. M. Weiger, J. Overweg, M. B. Rösler, R. Froidevaux, F. Hennel, B. J. Wilm, A. Penn, U. Sturzenegger, W. Schuth, M. Mathlener, M. Borgo, P. Börnert, C. Leussler, R. Luechinger, B. E. Dietrich, J. Reber, D. O. Brunner, T. Schmid, L. Vionnet, and K. P. Pruessmann, *Magn. Reson. Med.*, 2018, **79**, 3256. DOI: 10.1002/mrm.26954.

55. E. T. Tan, Y. Hua, E. W. Fiveland, M. E. Vermilyea, J. E. Piel, K. J. Park, V. B. Ho, and F. TKF, *Magn. Reson. Med.*, 2019, **83**, 352. DOI: 10.1002/mrm.27909.

56. J. Hennig, A. M. Welz, G. Schultz, J. Korvink, Z. Liu, O. Speck, and M. Zaitsev, *MAGMA*, 2008, **21**, 5.

57. J. P. Stockmann, P. A. Ciris, G. Galiana, L. Tam, and R. T. Constable, *Magn. Reson. Med.*, 2010, **64**, 447. DOI: 10.1002/mrm.22425.

58. N. L. Dispenza, S. Littin, M. Zaitsev, R. T. Constable, and G. Galiana, *Sci. Rep.*, 2019, **9**, 1912. DOI: 10.1038/s41598-018-36802-5.

59. E. Smith, F. Freschi, M. Repetto, and S. Crozier, *Magn. Reson. Med.*, 2017, **78**, 784. DOI: 10.1002/mrm.26404.

60. S. M. Moon, K. C. Goodrich, J. R. Hadley, S. E. Kim, G. L. Zeng, G. R. Morrell, M. A. MA, B. A. Chronik, and D. L. Parker, *Magn. Reson. Med.*, 2011, **65**, 863. DOI: 10.1002/mrm.22639.

61. S. Littin, F. Jia, K. J. Layton, S. Kroboth, H. Yu, J. Hennig, and M. Zaitsev, *Magn. Reson. Med.*, 2018, **79**, 1181. DOI: 10.1002/mrm.26700.

62. S.-K. Lee, J.-B. Mathieu, D. Graziani, J. Piel, E. Budesheim, E. Fiveland, C. J. Hardy, E. T. Tan, B. Amm, T. K. Foo, M. A. Bernstein, J. Huston 3rd, Y. Shu, and J. F. Schenck, *Magn. Reson. Med.*, 2016, **76**, 1939. DOI: 10.1002/mrm.26044.

Chapter 35
RF Coil Construction for MRI

J. Thomas Vaughan[1] and Russell Lagore[2]

[1]*Columbia University in the City of New York, New York, NY, USA*
[2]*University of Minnesota, Minneapolis, MN, USA*

35.1 INTRODUCTION

A radio-frequency (RF) detection coil for magnetic resonance spectroscopy (MRS) is a transducer device that inductively couples RF energy to excite and then receive a free induction decay (FID) nuclear magnetic resonance (NMR) signal from a desired sample typically adjacent to or within the volume of this RF coil.[1] This coil is placed about a sample, or a sample is placed within the coil, both within the homogeneous center of a superconducting magnet as shown in Figure 35.1.

The RF detection circuit or probe is most often an RF coil, which is an electrical circuit sometimes called a tank circuit, designed to store energy in an electromagnetic (EM) field, mostly within a wavelength of its confines. This energy storage oscillates at an RF between electrical field storage in the capacitance of the circuit and magnetic field storage in the inductance of the circuit. It is this RF magnetic induction field of the coil that couples to the nuclear magnetic spins of the measured sample, most efficiently at the Larmor frequency of the atomic nuclei under study. Therefore, the inductive reactance and capacitive reactance of a coil are chosen to tune the frequency of the coil to match the Larmor frequency of a desired nuclear species. Ohmic and conductance losses to the circuit and sample conductors and dielectrics result in noise and heat, degrading the signal-to-noise ratio (SNR) of the measurement and increasing the heating of the circuit and sample.

Physically, the RF coil or probe head is mounted atop a nonmagnetic, ideally nonconducting structural column inserted into the center of a magnet as shown in Figure 35.1(a), or on a moving table that introduces the sample and coil to the magnet in a horizontal bore system as shown in Figure 35.1(b). The coil, often a cylindrical cage-type circuit structure or a surface coil, is surrounded by a Faraday shield as shown in Figure 35.2. This shield can be part of the probe head, or it can be integrated into the bore of the magnet. The Faraday cage is designed through the use of appropriate materials, circuit, and/or geometry to efficiently conduct RF current in order to effectively shield the RF coil from the gradient, shim, and magnet coils within the magnet bore, but to attenuate lower frequency switched gradient currents that might generate $\boldsymbol{B}_0$ field perturbing eddy currents in the sample under study.

This chapter is dedicated specifically to RF detection coils for MRS. While there can be as many RF coil designs as there are applications for them, 23 of the

Safety and Biological Effects in MRI.
Edited by Devashish Shrivastava and J. Thomas Vaughan
 ISBN: 978-1-118-82130-5
Also published in eMagRes (online edition)
DOI: 10.1002/9780470034590.emrstm1572

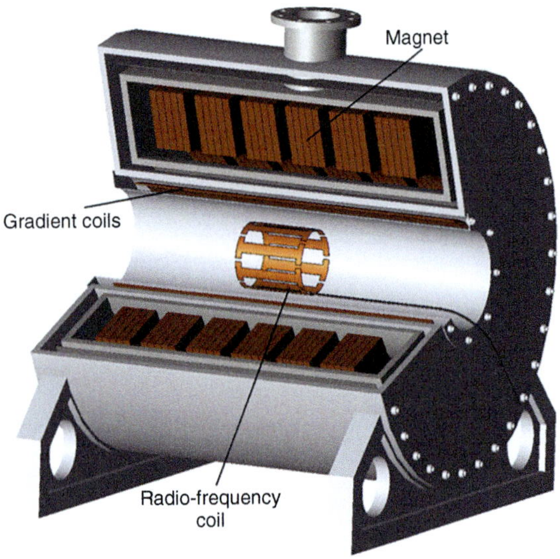

Figure 35.1. MRI magnets. Horizontal bore magnets are used for MRI. While scaled to different sizes, the coils used in each are of similar designs covered in this chapter

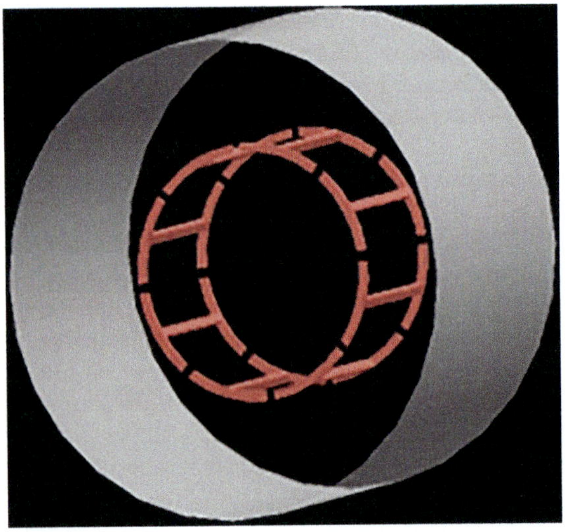

Figure 35.2. MRI coil within a cylindrical Faraday shield

more common design variations most often used are presented. Background, description, circuit drawings, field plots, application notes, and references accompany each design. The intent is to provide the reader with enough information to select appropriate coils for their applications and to direct the coil user to additional references for building and/or obtaining and applying said coils. For convenience of classification, RF detection coils for MRS might be divided into two design categories that originate with the two Nobel fathers of NMR, Felix Bloch's wire coils[2,3] and Ed Purcell's transmission line coils.[4]

35.1.1 Wire Coils

'Wire' is a lay term for coils made of lumped elements, or discrete capacitors in resonance with discrete wire or foil inductors. The simplest of these coils is typified by single- or multiple-looped wire-wound solenoids, and they are easy to build and use, and often the most effective designs, especially in applications for which the coil circuit is shorter than one tenth of the Larmor wavelength where ohmic and radiative losses are negligible and coil currents are uniform and well behaved. These wire designs include Felix Bloch's first crossed pairs,[3] single-loop solenoid 'surface coils',[5] Helmholtz pairs[6] and loop arrays.[7] 'Cage' coils are another lumped element design typically consisting of a ladder network of rungs wrapped around an ellipsoidal volume form, with the rails or rungs joined to form 'end rings'.[8,9] As with other lumped element or wire coils, birdcages are most effective when they are electrically small compared to the wavelength at which they operate. These coils are especially useful for uniform measurements from larger sample volumes within the bore of cylindrical, superconducting electromagnets. Cage designs include the Alderman–Grant resonator, birdcages, millipede coils, and Litz designs.[8,10–13] These ubiquitous coils are readily available commercially and are relatively easy to build.

35.1.2 Transmission Line Coils

Transmission line [transverse electromagnetic (TEM)] coils are the distributed circuit analogs of lumped element coils. Their inductance and capacitance, as well as their conductance and resistance, are uniformly distributed over the coil circuit. Transmission lines consisting of two or more parallel conductors within close proximity are often the best way to achieve this distributed circuit. Examples of transmission lines are cavities, waveguides, slotted tubes, coaxial, microstrips, and striplines.[14–19] Robert Pound and Ed Purcell's first coil was a re-entrant 'klystron' cavity.[4]

Coils built by transmission line principles are less inductive and less radiative and thereby more efficient for applications where the coil circuit exceeds one tenth of the Larmor wavelength. This condition often exists at higher field strengths and for larger sample volumes.

35.1.3 Antennas

Whereas coils are near-field tank circuits or energy storage transducers, antennas are designed for radiating to the far field, beyond a wave length. This condition is rarely realized within high-resolution or small-bore horizontal MRS magnets today. However, because MRS detection is performed in human bore-sized magnets up to 10.5 T where far-field measurements can be made, antennas are included in this chapter. The simple dipole antenna and dipole arrays are examples.[20]

35.2 WIRE COILS

35.2.1 Surface Coils

35.2.1.1 Single-loop Solenoids

The simplest coil circuit can be depicted as the *RLC* single-loop solenoid shown in Figure 35.3. '*R*' is the electrical resistance, in ohms of the wire, '*L*' is the inductance of the wire loop, in henrys and '*C*' is the capacitance schematized as two capacitive plates, in farads. The inductance in this simple coil is typically determined by the sample volume to which this coil is applied. Larger samples require longer more inductive wire circuits. This design may surround a sample or be placed adjacent to the surface of a sample; hence it is commonly called 'surface coil'. For the most efficient energy transfer and band-pass filter function, the coil is tuned to resonate at the Larmor frequency of the nuclear species of interest by adjusting a variable capacitor '*C*' in the coil circuit $f = 1/(2\pi\sqrt{LC})$. This coil can be used in transmission mode, receive mode, or with a transmit–receive (TR) switch as a transceiver. Two central spatial planes to which the RF magnetic ($\boldsymbol{B}_1$) field of this coil inductively couples are shown in Figure 35.4. The red color indicates higher intensity and the yellow and green lower intensity in these linear-scale contour plots. An RF current loop like this is also known as an RF magnetic dipole because of the RF field it generates. These single-loop surface coils couple to approximately one coil radius hemisphere from the plane of the coil as applied to a sample surface.

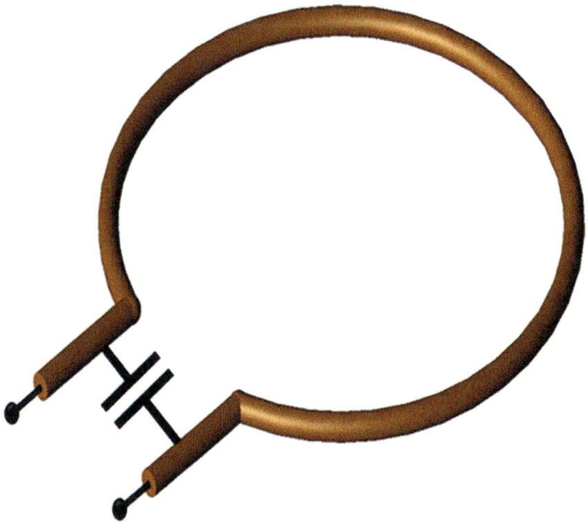

Figure 35.3. Single-loop wire solenoid, 'surface coil'

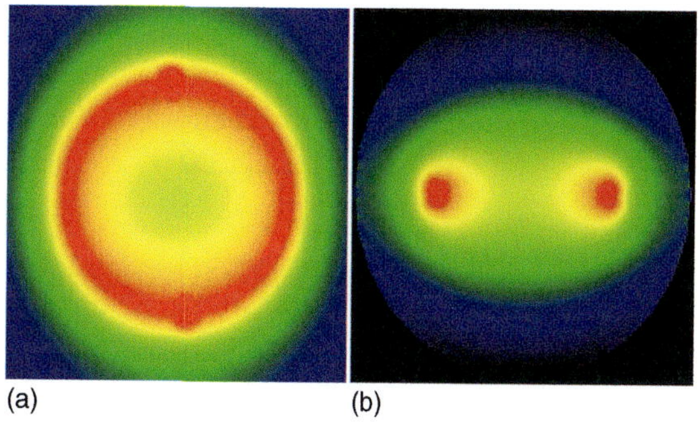

Figure 35.4. $\boldsymbol{B}_1$ field, transaxial (a), and axial (b), center planes for single-loop solenoid

Construction of these single-loop coils is quite simple, requiring only a few centimeters of ±18 gage transformer wire formed into a sample-sized loop and a nonmagnetic variable capacitor in the 2–25 pF range soldered into the parallel position shown in Figure 35.3. This capacitor is the tuning capacitor and is used to tune the inductive loop resonance to the Larmor frequency. Figure 35.5 shows the typical double-balanced, impedance-matching circuit used to match the 50 Ω coaxial cable to the unknown, variable impedance of an RF coil with a sample load. Shown is the coil tuning capacitor, C_t, and two

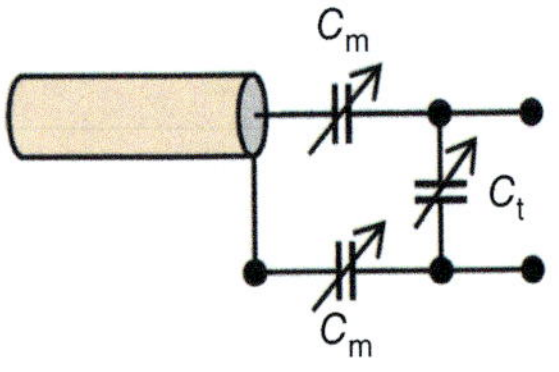

Figure 35.5. Coil-cable, double-balanced matching circuit

variable impedance-matching capacitors, C_m, of an approximately equal range, soldered in series with the terminals of the coil. One of these capacitors is soldered to the shield of a coaxial cable and the other is soldered to the center conductor of this cable as shown. Either directly or via the coaxial cable, the coil terminals are connected to a transmitter and/or receiver often through a TR switch.[21] To scale up the resonant frequency and/or size of this coil, capacitive splits can be added to the coil as shown in Figure 35.6. This coil is constructed of foil as well. The $\boldsymbol{B}_1$ fields of this split coil in Figure 35.7 are expectedly similar to those shown in Figure 35.4. This approach of adding lumped capacitance across multiple splits in the coil loop costs efficiency due to increased $\boldsymbol{E}$ field losses to the capacitors and to the sample space and the sample.

A sampling of surface coils built for different applications follows. These surface coils may be constructed of wire or foil and may be shaped in 3D geometry and size to best fit and couple to a region of interest (ROI) as in Figure 35.8. Cryogenically cooled and superconducting versions of a single-loop

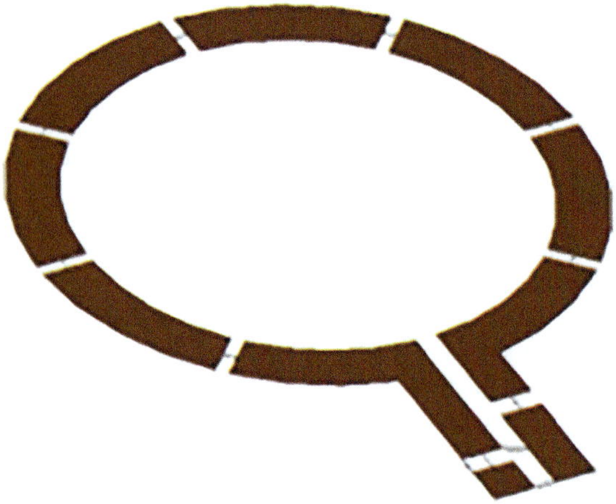

Figure 35.6. Single-loop, capacitively split, foil solenoid surface coil. Capacitors are not shown

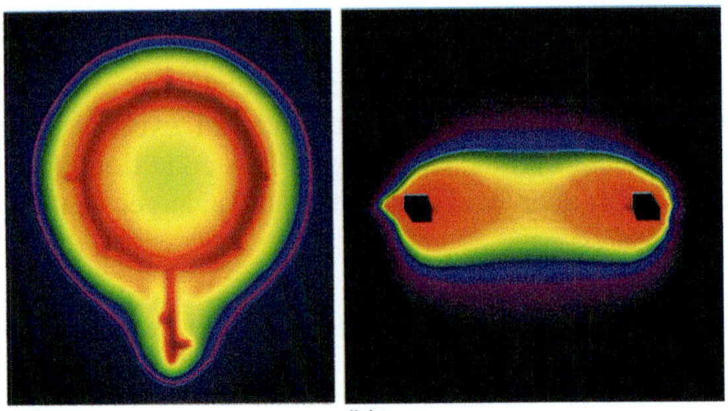

Figure 35.7. $\boldsymbol{B}_1$ field, transaxial (a), and axial (b), center planes for single-loop, split solenoid

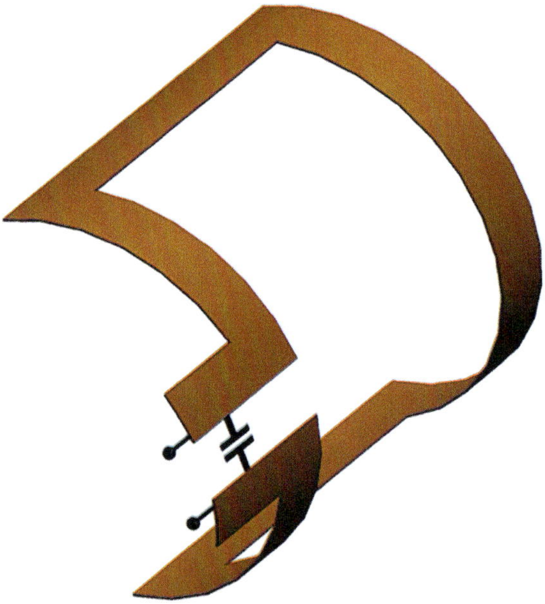

Figure 35.8. Rectangular, sample conforming, foil solenoid surface coil

coil for significantly enhanced SNR can be bought commercially.[22–24] One constraint to keep in mind is that these coils will be oriented such that the axis of the coil will generally be perpendicular to the axis of the magnet bore for the maximum transmit and/or receive efficiency. These loops can also be double-tuned for observing two nuclei serially, or simultaneously, in an experiment, depending on the way the coil is interfaced to the MRS system and the pulse protocols used.[25]

35.2.1.2 Multiple-loop Arrays

Multiple-loop elements may be configured in an array about a sample space to accomplish a number of objectives as will be described in some of the designs that follow. Concentric loops as shown in Figure 35.9 can be used for localizing an ROI by field profiling or for multinuclear MRS by tuning each loop to a different nuclear species–specific Larmor frequency.[26] For the multinuclear design, the larger of the two loops is typically used for proton scout imaging and shimming, while the smaller one is used to acquire the signal from a second nuclear species. Both coils are used in transceiver mode, and each is connected to its tuned TR switch, filter, and preamplifier/power amplifier.

Multiple loops can also be configured into phased arrays as shown in Figure 35.10.[7] Phased arrays, used as surface or volume coils, extend the performance of an electrically small and efficient loop to an arbitrarily large field of view (FOV). Phased arrays are most often used as application-specific, ROI local receivers together with a larger, uniform transmit coil such as a body coil in the clinical magnetic resonance imaging/magnetic resonance spectroscopy (MRI/MRS) systems. Each loop is connected to its own receiver channel often beginning as a gallium arsenide field-effect transistor (GaAsFET) decoupling preamplifier embedded in the each loop. Each loop must be actively detuned during RF transmit pulse periods by an integrated PIN diode circuit as shown in Figure 35.11. Figure 35.10 shows a single diode in each loop to represent this detuning circuit and capacitive splitting. The loops must in the array also be isolated from their neighbors to decouple correlated sample noise and to increase parallel imaging performance depending on multiple channels of independent signals from discrete sample spaces. This isolation or decoupling between receiver loops is accomplished by canceling the mutual inductance between neighboring loops. This can be done with capacitance or inductance executed by critically overlapping adjacent loops as shown in Figure 35.10. The larger transmit volume coil must also be detuned during the receive period. This detuning is achieved by active PIN diode circuits in the transmit coil. These transmit coil detuning circuits can have the PIN diode in the shunt to ground position as shown in Figure 35.11, or in the series position shown in Figure 35.12.

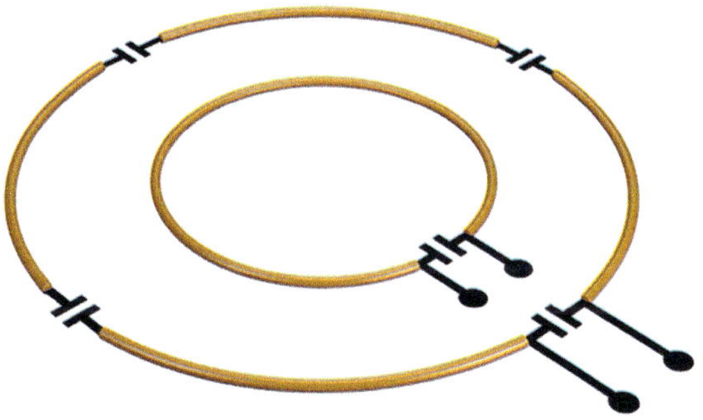

Figure 35.9. Concentric loops surface coil

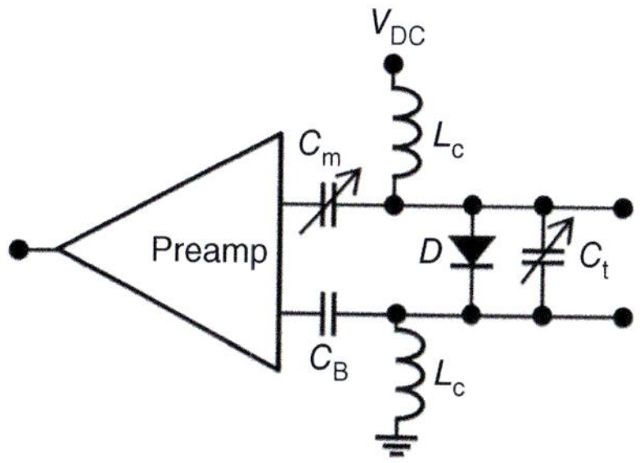

Figure 35.11. Parallel PIN diode and preamplifier detuning circuit for receive array loops

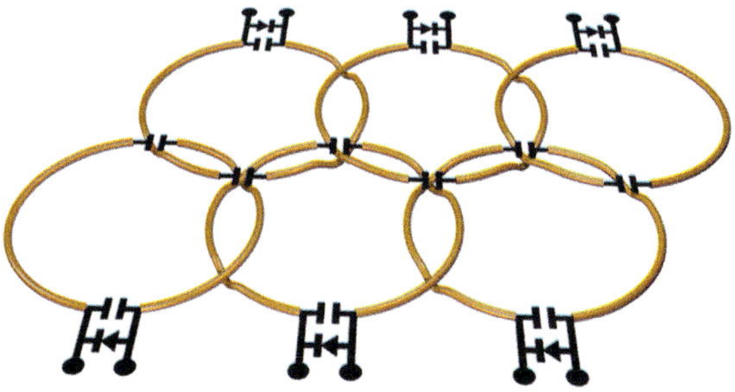

Figure 35.10. Phased array surface coil. (From Ref. 7)

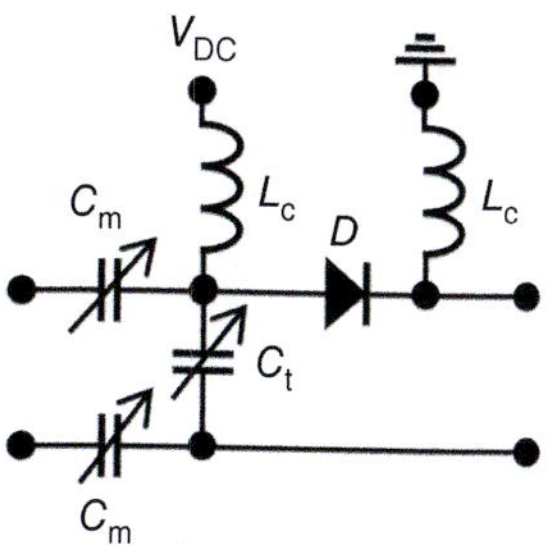

Figure 35.12. Series PIN diode detuning circuit for transmit array elements

35.2.2 Volume Coils

35.2.2.1 Solenoids

As with surface coils, wire-wound solenoids can be used as volume coils too. Figure 35.13 shows a multiturn solenoid whose purpose is to extend and intensify the linear $\boldsymbol{B}_1$ field of the coil along the axis of the RF coil. Such a coil with multiple turns around a volume has significantly higher coil inductance than other designs, and thereby requires a proportionately lower tuning capacitance. Due to its high inductance, this design is most effectively used as a simple transceiver coil for small laboratory animals, excised tissue samples, or test-tube or capillary samples of lower gamma nuclei where a lower Larmor frequency coil is required. In addition to being a good performer for small samples and lower frequencies, this is a simple and easy coil to build and use in the laboratory.

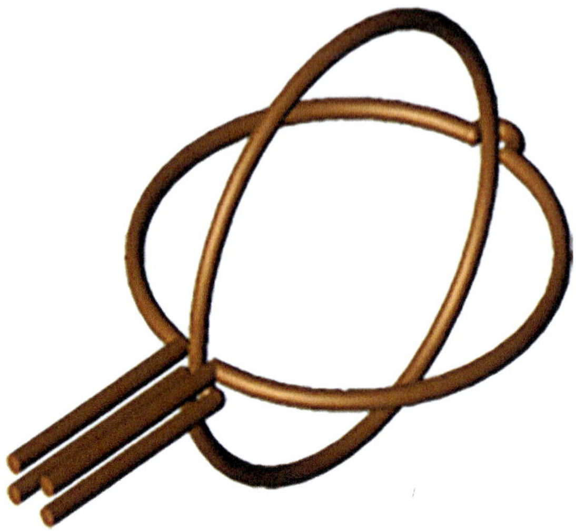

Figure 35.14. Crossed-wire loops. (From Ref. 3)

35.2.2.2 Crossed Pairs

Felix Bloch's crossed-coil design is shown in Figure 35.14.[3] This design is composed of a pair of independent loops and can be used in two ways. Bloch connected one loop to his transmitter and the other loop to his receiver. When the loop planes are crossed or perpendicular as shown, the transmit field of one loop is geometrically isolated from the received field of the other loop. Another use of this loop pair is to generate a quadrature or circularly polarized transmit and/or receive field. In such a coil, the transmit field will be more uniform over a larger FOV in the sample, and the SNR of the NMR signal detected from the sample will be improved by as much as a $\sqrt{2}$ factor. Finally, a third way to use this coil is as a double-tuned or multinuclear coil. In this case, one of the two loops could be tuned to the Larmor frequency of a first nuclear species and the second loop could be tuned to a second Larmor frequency of a second nuclear species. The crossed pair could then be used to detect two different MRS signals from two different species. These coils could be used as transmit only coils, receive only coils, or transmit and receive coils. Again, the axes of this coil pair would be oriented about a sample, perpendicular to the axis of the MRS magnet. Despite the many potential uses and modes of operation for this coil, access to its central sample space is somewhat inaccessible in a fixed probe structure.

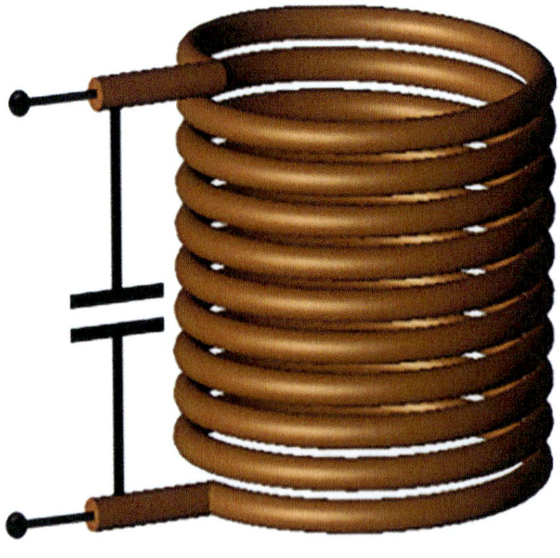

Figure 35.13. Multiloop wire solenoid

However, a particularly useful variation of this crossed-coil design is shown in Figure 35.15. The crossed pair can be opened and spread to fit a curved, anatomic surface or partial volume, while still achieving quadrature field over at least a portion of the sample space. While this crossed pair can be useful as a quadrature transceiver for imaging, this design has proven particularly useful when combined with a second transceiver loop tuned to a low gamma Larmor frequency and nested at the intersection of the larger crossed pair. This multinuclear design is proven to

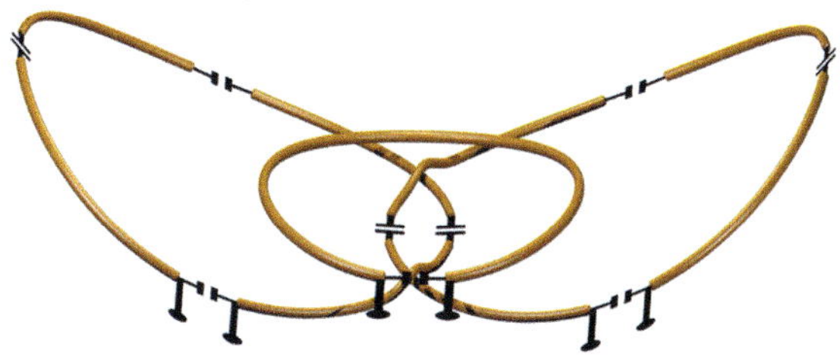

Figure 35.15. Quadrature surface coil with nested loop for receiver or X-nucleus

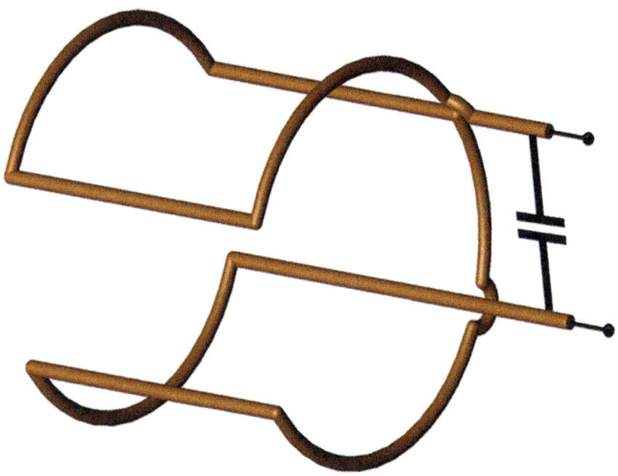

Figure 35.16. Series-wound saddle pair

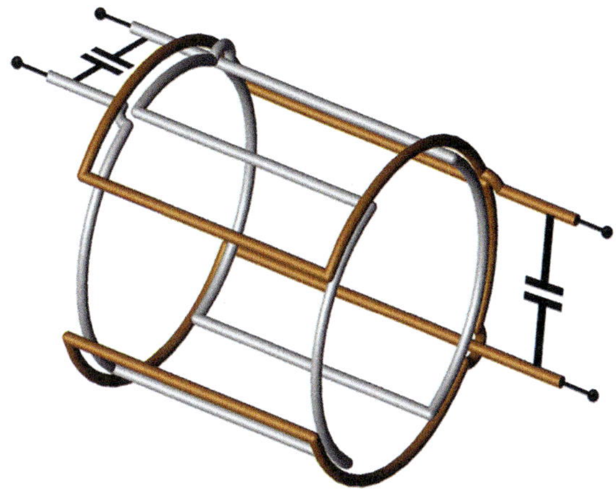

Figure 35.17. Crossed-wire saddle pairs

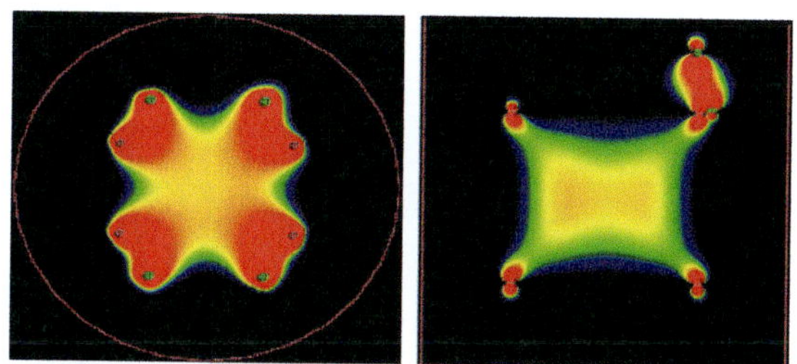

(a) (b)

Figure 35.18. $\boldsymbol{B}_1$ field, transaxial (a) and axial (b) center planes for circularly polarized crossed-wire saddle pairs

give efficient, local MRI performance and highly sensitive X-nucleus MRS.[27,28]

35.2.2.3 Saddle Pairs

The series-wound saddle pair shown in Figure 35.16 can be viewed as a two-loop solenoid, but wound to efficiently and conveniently accommodate a sample in a linear $\boldsymbol{B}_1$ field perpendicular to the magnet's $\boldsymbol{B}_0$ field as desired.[6,29–31] More desirable for most applications, however, is the combination of two of these saddle pairs in a crossed-pair configuration as shown in Figure 35.17. The crossed saddle pair can be used in all of the ways possible with the crossed pair of Figure 35.14, but is a more space-efficient design. This coil generates a large, circularly polarized field perpendicular to the magnet bore while allowing easy access to the full sample volume of the coil. To minimize coupling and maximize isolation between the two saddle pairs for best SNR performance, and to cover the largest volume FOV, the two saddle pairs will be overlapped as shown such that the mutual inductance between the loops is critically cancelled. The amount of overlap is dependent on coil design and sample loading parameters and is typically empirically determined by adjusting the size and position of overlapping coils until a maximum isolation point (S12 > 12 dB) is achieved between the two. As with the crossed pair, each saddle pair can be used as a transmit and a separate receive coil, respectively, or can be tuned to the Larmor frequencies of two separate nuclei for multinuclear signal acquisition. Many modern MRS detector coils use variations of the crossed saddle pair design. The fields in the transaxial and axial central planes for the coil are shown in Figure 35.18.

Saddle pairs can be constructed from foil as well, as shown in Figure 35.19. Foil may be used for ease-of-fabrication reasons. For example, foil coil elements can be milled or etched with ease, accuracy, and precision from circuit board material. This board material can add to the stability of the coil circuit as well. To avoid parasitic capacitance between the

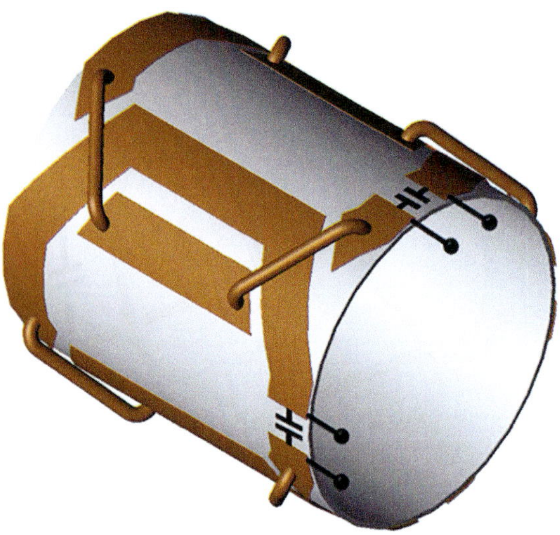

Figure 35.19. Crossed-foil saddle pairs

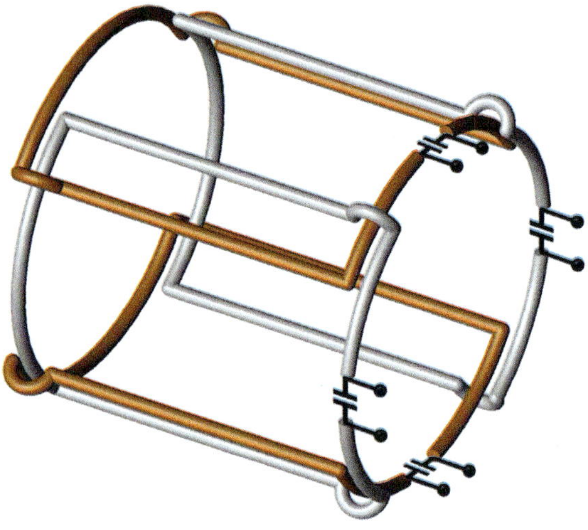

Figure 35.21. Four-loop wire array

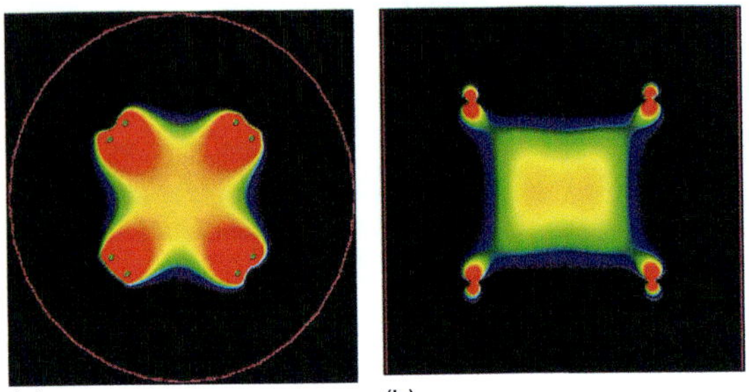

(a) (b)

Figure 35.20. B_1 field, transaxial and axial center planes for circularly polarized crossed-foil pairs

overlapping loops, wire jumpers can be used as shown in Figure 35.19. While the electrical quality Q, a measure of the efficiency of an RF circuit, will be a bit lower with foil loops vs wire loops, the field coverage of a wire-wound coil compared to a foil-etched coil of the same dimensions are very similar as can be seen by comparing Figures 35.18 and 35.20.

35.2.2.4 Phased Arrays

The next step in the evolution of the saddle pair designs are the multiloop or phased array designs where every loop has its own independent terminals for connecting to a preamplifier, a power amplifier, or a TR switch.[7,32–34] Examples of wire and foil, four-loop coils are shown in Figures 35.21 and 35.22. These

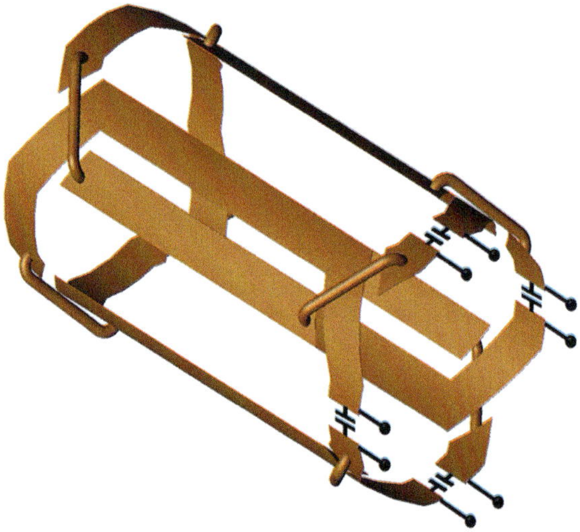

Figure 35.22. Four-loop foil array

arrays are typically composed of two or more wire or foil loops critically overlapping to minimize coupling from nearest neighbors as in the surface array of Figure 35.10. This decoupling can be achieved with capacitive cancelation of mutual inductance as well. The loops should be decoupled or isolated from each other as determined by the S12 network analyzer measurement, by 12 dB or more for best coil operation. Arrays can be used as receive-only coils, transmit-only coils, or transceiver coils and can be formed to any volume or surface. Arrays are most often used as application-specific receivers in clinical applications where a whole-body cage-type coil is used as a homogeneous transmitter. This combination of coils is used to achieve a uniform excite field and high SNR signal detection from a local ROI. As with surface arrays, volume receivers must also be decoupled from the transmit coils. This decoupling is achieved in the same way as the surface array of Figure 35.10, by detuning the receive arrays during transmit by switched PIN diodes in detuning circuits embedded in the receive array loops, and by detuning the transmit coil during the signal detection period by similar PIN diode detuning of the transmit coil (see Figures 35.11 and 35.12). Decoupling preamplifiers at the loop element terminals C_t further increase the receive array isolation from the transmit coil. Transceiver arrays, however, make use of a PIN diode TR switch only, switching the coil terminals alternately in time between the power amplifier during transmit mode and the receiver during receiver mode.

For MRS specific use, arrays may be tuned to the Larmor frequency of any nuclei by tuning each loop by the same method described for a single-loop coil of Figure 35.3. The $\boldsymbol{B}_1$ fields of the four-loop arrays in Figures 35.21 and 35.22 will be very similar to those shown in Figures 35.18 and 35.20, respectively. Arrays can be tuned to more than one nucleus as well, by double-tuning each loop or by tuning alternating loops to alternating frequencies.

Arrays bring a number of advantages. They facilitate enhanced signal and speed of data acquisition through parallel imaging and multiband techniques. They can be used for optimizing SNR or homogeneity and minimizing specific absorption rate (SAR) over an ROI by field profiling, $\boldsymbol{B}_1$ shimming, and beam steering techniques. These techniques are especially useful with high-field applications to correct for EM interference patterns and $\boldsymbol{B}_0$ inhomogeneities that can be problematic with shortening Larmor wavelengths and increasing susceptibility artifacts, respectively. Arrays also offer a means to cover larger regions of interest more efficiently using arrays of electrically smaller, less radiating coil elements. For all of these reasons, arrays are a popular choice for MRS coils today. However, there are many older MR systems in use with only a single transmit and/or receive port per nucleus. These will not accommodate multichannel array coils.

35.2.2.5 Cage Coils

Cage coils are wire- or foil-wound, lumped element coil circuits based on ladder rather than loop or solenoid circuits.[8,10–13,35–38] This coil circuit type achieves a uniform $\boldsymbol{B}_1$ field within its typically cylindrical volume by a 360° azimuthal distribution of linear currents surrounding this volume. The return path for these linear current elements is on end rings, current paths connecting the ends of the linear elements or ‘rungs’. While the theoretical limit of infinite length would achieve perfect field uniformity within the volume of this coil, a ‘square’ coil for which the length equals the diameter is sufficient for most MRI and MRS, FOVs.

Birdcages

An early example of the cage coil is the Alderman–Grant design shown in Figure 35.23.[8] Its current paths approximate those of a linear, six-rung, high-pass birdcage, with two missing zero current rungs and split capacitive end rings. Named for their filter circuit analogs, cage coils can be tuned with lumped tuning capacitance distributed in the rungs (low pass), with capacitance distributed in the rings (high pass), or with lumped capacitance distributed in the rungs and rings (band pass). Because the high-pass design displaces the capacitors and therefore parasitic $\boldsymbol{E}$ fields from the center of the sample space to the ends of the coil, the high-pass design as pictured in Figure 35.24 is the most favored of the birdcage coils.[10,11,38] The high-pass coil achieves higher frequencies as well, an important feature for

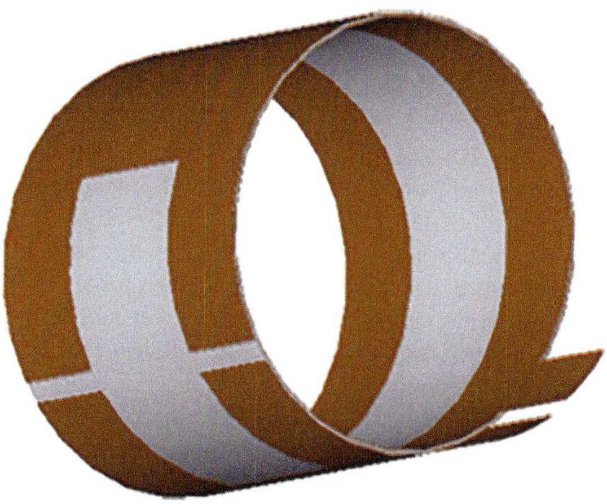

Figure 35.23. Alderman–Grant coil. (From Ref. 8)

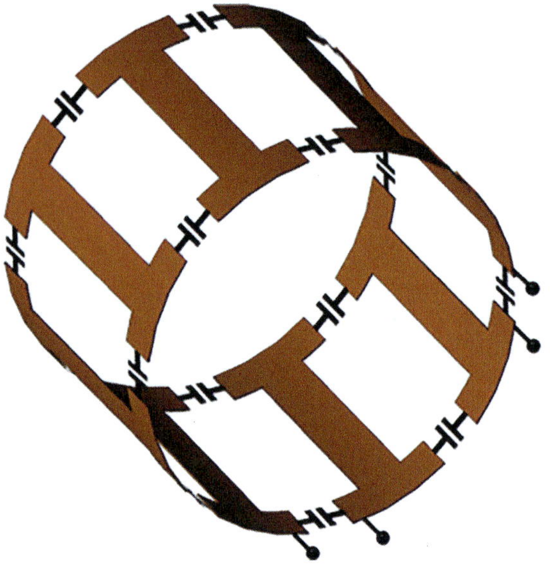

Figure 35.24. High-pass birdcage

the large whole-body coils often employing this design. This symmetric coil structure can be driven and/or received as a circularly polarized coil for best SNR and FOV coverage. For quadrature operation, transmit and/or receive cables are attached 90° apart at the terminal positions shown, using the matching circuit of Figure 35.5. A quadrature hybrid is a useful circuit for splitting a single power amplifier channel into two 90° phased transmit feeds. The same hybrid can recombine the $\boldsymbol{B}_1+$, 90° phased receive channels to feed a single receiver channel in the most simple transmit and receive interface for these coils.

While ubiquitous transceiver head coils are still in use, the most common modern application for the birdcage is for uniform transmit coils to accompany phased array receiver coils. Because clinical transmit coils are very large, these big monolithic resonators require a significant number of capacitive breaks in the rings and rungs rendering a band-pass coil. These physically and electrically large coils operating on the edge of self-resonance are very radiative and therefore inefficient, requiring large, 32 kW pulsed power amplifiers to drive them. SAR from these lossy radiators presents significant limitations to RF protocols. Accordingly, the utility of birdcage transmitters becomes limited for most larger preclinical and human applications at 3 T and above, the field in which most MRS applications begin. Birdcages almost always operate inside a Faraday shield as shown in Figure 35.2. The center-plane

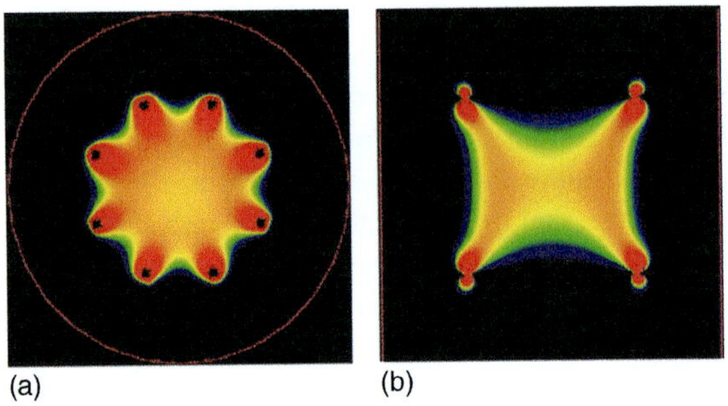

Figure 35.25. $\boldsymbol{B}_1$ field, transaxial (a) and axial (b) center planes for circularly polarized birdcage

birdcage $\boldsymbol{B}_1$ fields calculated in Figure 35.25 show the characteristic FOV for this uniform transmitter. End ring currents destroy MR signals and cause a sharp, concave $\boldsymbol{B}_1$ field cut-off at the ends of the coil. This can be an advantage, preventing signal wrap from beyond the coil's volume.

Birdcage coils too can be double-tuned to more than one Larmor frequency for multinuclear MRS. The most common design approach for double-tuning a birdcage is to add a second set of end rings, effectively creating two coils of different electrical lengths in one circuit.[35]

Millipede Coils

Before Varian left the MRS field, their millipede coil was a favorite.[13,37] It is still produced privately by

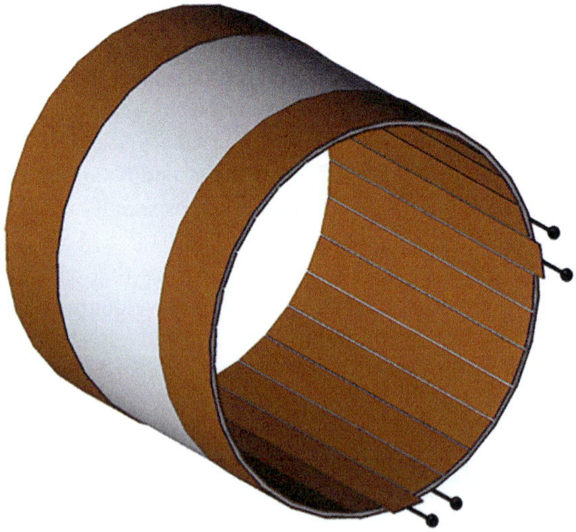

Figure 35.26. Millipede coil

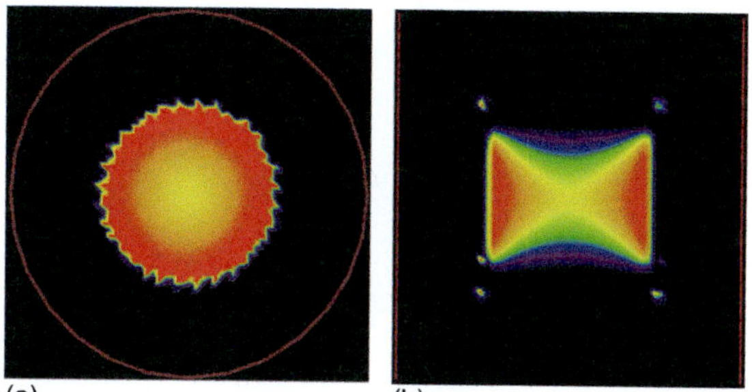

(a) (b)

Figure 35.27. $\boldsymbol{B}_1$ field, transaxial (a) and axial (b) for circularly polarized millipede coil

its inventor, Ernest Wong at Extend MR, LLC. The millipede coil is basically a foil made in birdcage design that maximizes the number of rungs. Its tuning capacitance is in the low-pass position, but displaced to each end of the coil rather than in the middle. The capacitance is distributed in the foil rung–ring overlap at the ends of each rung. The benefit of this design is its high uniformity over most of the volume of the coil. The millipede coil and its field contours are shown in Figures 35.26 and 35.27. It is operated mostly as a circularly polarized, transceiver coil. As with a birdcage, its transmit and receive terminals are 90° apart.

35.2.2.6 *Litz Coils*

Litz coils are a wire- or foil-wound, lumped element cage coil variant that are produced and sold to many users by Doty Scientific, Inc., Columbia SC.[12,36] 'Litz' meaning braided or woven refers to the woven appearance of these coils. This design uses capacitive overlaps by its foil rungs and rings to achieve a

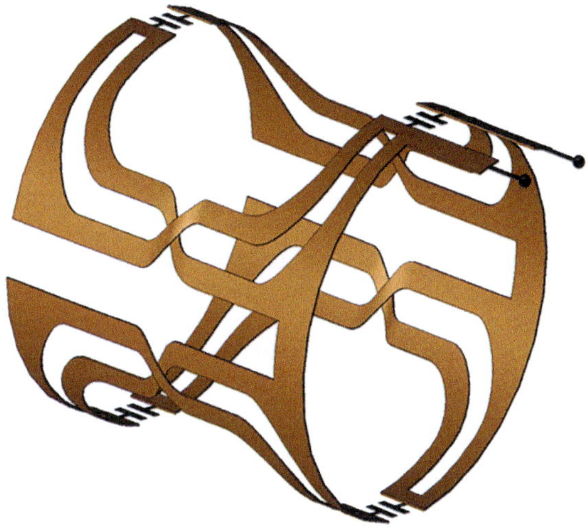

Figure 35.28. Litz coil, linear

tuned cage-like mode of operation. While few MRS experimentalists build these intricate coils, they well made by their manufacturer and are widely used in the mostly vertical bore and preclinical horizontal bore markets. For simplicity of viewing, a linear Litz coil is shown in Figure 35.28 with the $\boldsymbol{B}_1$ fields produced in Figure 35.29. Circularly polarized and double-tuned Litz coils are more common and show good performance.[36] A linear cage-like field contour is apparent.

35.3 TRANSMISSION LINE COILS

The first MRS coil built, by Robert Pound for Ed Purcell, was a transmission line coil. It was

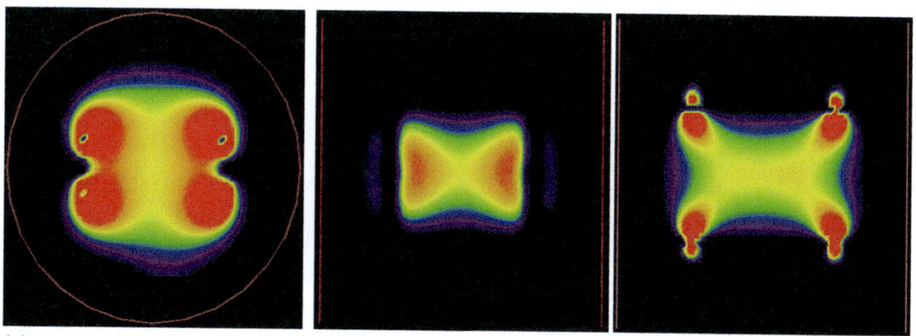

(a) (b) (c)

Figure 35.29. Transaxial (a), *xz* (b), and *yz* (c) axial, center planes for linearly polarized Litz coil. (From Ref. 36) specifically a reentrant cavity of a klystron design used for microwave radar research.[4] Any circuit that propagates a TEM wave defines a transmission line, hence the name 'TEM' given to this class of coil circuits. TEM coils include coaxial, stripline and microstrip transmission lines, as well as resonant cavities and waveguides.[17–19,39–43] The primary objective of employing these designs is to achieve higher efficiency and more uniform current and field distribution, especially at higher field strengths and Larmor frequencies. Lumped element circuits as used in the wire-wound coils are inherently low-frequency devices. They are built with discrete inductors and capacitors. Their design equations are based on Thevenin's and Kirchoff's circuit equations. And their fields are approximated by Biot Savart. When circuit wavelengths exceed a tenth of a wavelength, however, they begin to radiate energy increasingly like an antenna. To conserve this energy, we must abandon lumped element design in favor of transmission line designs and Maxwell's time-dependent EM field calculations. As with ultra-high-frequency (UHF) circuits in telecommunications industry, UHF coils benefit from transmission line (TEM) design. In this design, there are no lumped elements other than trimmer caps and chokes. The bulk inductance, capacitance, conductance, and small resistances are parameters in the transmission line equations and are integrally distributed throughout the TEM circuit. Energy is conserved. The coil is more efficient as evidenced by significantly higher Q values. This increased efficiency at higher operating frequencies is especially appreciated at higher magnetic fields where MRS becomes more useful.

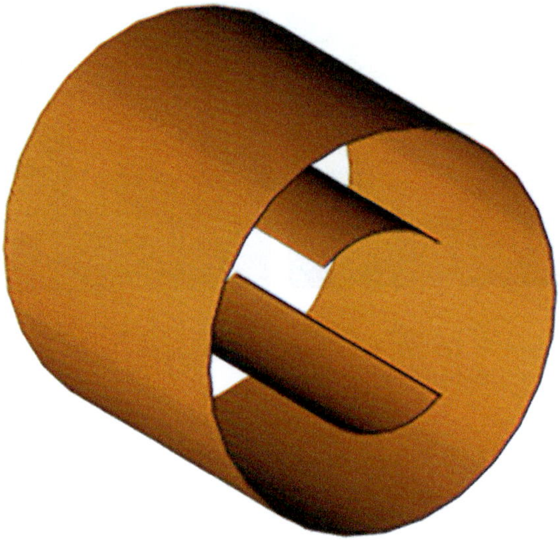

Figure 35.30. Slotted tube. (From Refs. 14, 15)

35.3.1 Slotted Tube Resonators

An early example of a transmission line coil for MRS is the Schneider and Dullenkopf, slotted tube resonator pictured in Figure 35.30.[14,15] The transmission line nature of this coil is easy to see as an outer conductor serving also as the shield and a coaxial, hollow center conductor containing the sample space. The transmission line parameters are distributed over the length of this structure, between the shield and the center conductor plates. While this design was used in both early vertical small bore and horizontal clinical bore magnets, it has evolved into a more useful and widely used 'TEM' design as pictured in Figures 35.31 and 35.32.[17,18,39]

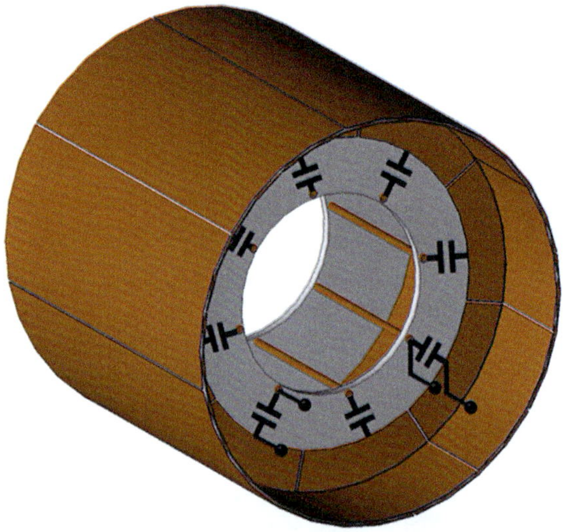

Figure 35.31. TEM coil, inductively coupled, coaxial line variant. (From Refs. 17, 18, 39)

35.3.2 TEM Coils: Coaxial Lines, Striplines, and Microstrips

Modern TEM coils are capacitively shortened and tuned, half-wave transmission line resonators very similar to the slotted tube resonator in concept but with a number of practical features that lend themselves to modern utility.[19,39–43] Among these features,

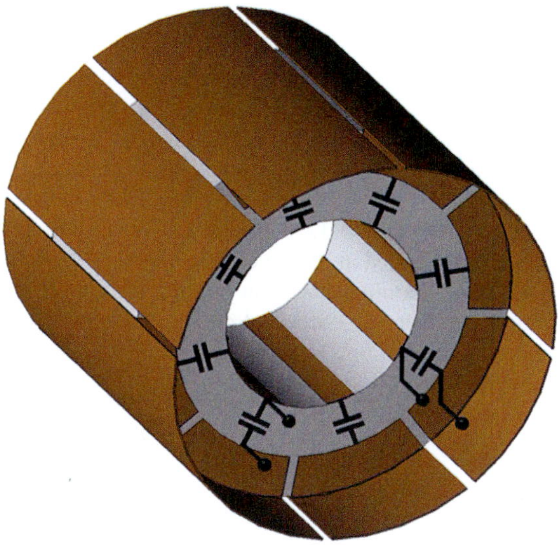

Figure 35.32. TEM coil, actively coupled, stripline variant. (From Refs. 17, 8, 39)

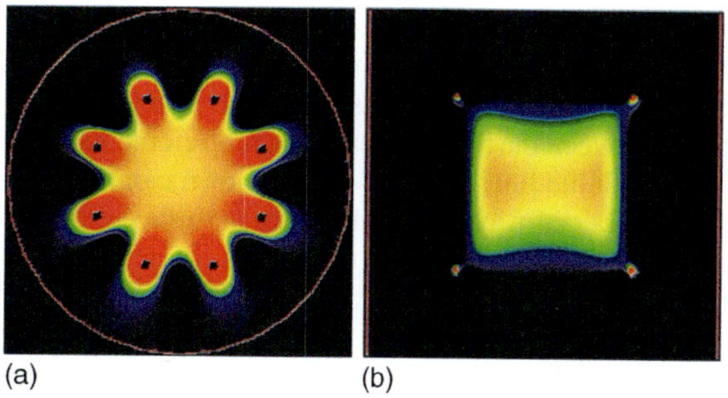

Figure 35.33. $\boldsymbol{B}_1$ field, transaxial (a) and axial (b) center planes for circularly polarized TEM coils

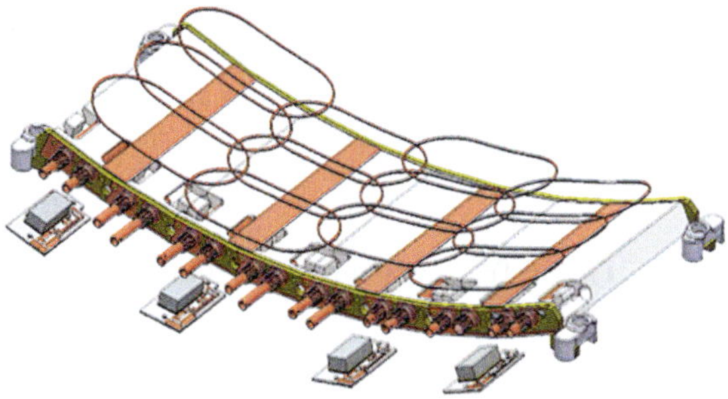

Figure 35.34. TEM surface array with nested loop phased array. (From Ref. 39)

the center conductor 'rungs' of these coils generate a highly uniform field like the rungs of a birdcage. Unlike the end-ring-connected birdcage coils, however, the rung conductors of the TEM coil are not connected at all. Their current return path is on the shield of the coil, in transmission line fashion. This feature, in turn, produces several benefits. Each rung in the TEM is an electrically short and efficient, independent resonator, the TEM coil being an array of these discrete resonant units. The useful frequency of this coil is therefore dependent on the inductance of a single rung only and not on the circuit size of the whole coil as for the end-ring-coupled birdcage. TEM coils have been shown to produce efficient body coils to 8 T and above.[39,44] Because each element operates independently of the next, each element can be driven with a different transmit signal with five degrees of freedom, namely, phase, magnitude, frequency, space, and time. This allows for $\boldsymbol{B}_1$ shimming, beam steering, and parallel imaging and multiband operation benefits. And because there are no end ring field cancelations, the FOV for a TEM is longer and more uniform than that of a birdcage of equal length. Compare the TEM field contours of Figure 35.33 to the birdcage contours of Figure 35.25. As with the birdcage, these coils can be used as receivers, transmitters, or transceivers. For the reasons above, TEM volume coils are coming into popular use as multichannel transmitters in modern MRI and MRS systems. While cylindrical volume coils are pictured, because TEM coils are essentially an array of independent transmission line elements, they can assume any spatial form. A common example is the TEM surface array (Figure 35.34) used for efficient, ultra-high-field body MRI and MRS.[39]

The TEM coil can be double-tuned as well by tuning alternating rungs to alternating Larmor frequencies of the desired nuclei. As with most double-tuned coils, the proton frequency is typically chosen for scout imaging, landmarking, shimming, and, sometimes, decoupling. A second 'x' nucleus is tuned for spectroscopic acquisition. This coil works quite well because the coil couples to the same sample volumes for scout imaging, $\boldsymbol{B}_0$ shimming at the proton frequency, and the x-nuclear MRS. The coil is also nearly as sensitive operating at two frequencies as its single-tuned counterpart.

Figure 35.34 shows a commonly used TEM configuration of linear transmit elements paired with a loop array receiver. Linear transmit elements in a surface array such as this, or in a volume coil, are relied upon for generating a more uniform $\boldsymbol{B}_1$ excite field, while the close-fitting phased array next to the sample is a more sensitive signal detector. Additionally, in an application like this where linear transmission line elements are used, there exists a geometric field decoupling between the line elements and loop elements centered with the lines. The assembly shown can be used in a number of ways. It can be used as surface coil for covering larger and deeper regions of interest. When paired with another similar assembly on the opposing side of a body, for example, the pair is very effective for efficient body imaging, conserving a factor of 6× or more RF transmit power compared to a full-bore body coil of a similar design. The TEM elements of the coil can be tuned to the proton frequency and used as a transceiver for imaging and shimming, while the phased array can be tuned to a second frequency for MRS applications. The TEM elements in this type of array are usually driven directly, which also allows for multichannel transmit applications and $\boldsymbol{B}_1$ shimming.

35.3.3 Other Transmission Line Coils

TEM coils can take other forms as well, mimicking almost any lumped element coil in form and function, albeit employing more efficient, transmission line circuit analogs. For example, the double-tuned surface coil pictured in Figure 35.35 is constructed from a section of a semirigid coax cable, though the same coil would be executed with stripline or microstrip just the same. In this coil, the continuous center conductor is tuned by circuit length and trimmer caps to a lower frequency, and the split shield is tuned with trimmer capacitors to a higher frequency. Most of the reactance of the coil is integrally distributed in transmission line fashion, making for a nicely balanced and efficient multinuclear surface coil.[1]

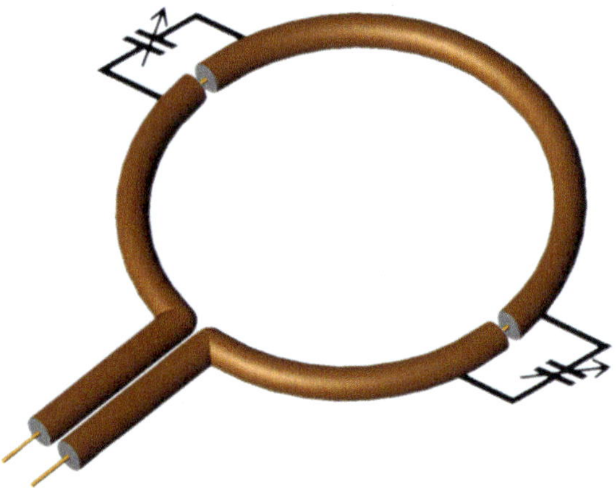

Figure 35.35. Transmission line, double-tuned surface coil

Another interesting transmission line design works especially well for high-resolution MRS.[19] This design can be formed to any volume or surface. As seen in Figures 35.36 and 35.37, a $\boldsymbol{B}_1$ field of maximum intensity is generated at the tip of a resonant, half-wave coaxial line. Sample space can be drilled into the dielectric between the outer and center conductor of a semirigid coaxial line section. This dielectric can be

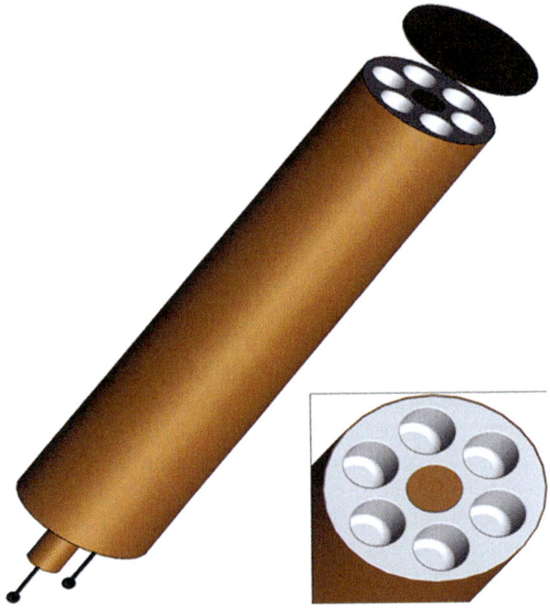

Figure 35.36. Open and short stubline coils

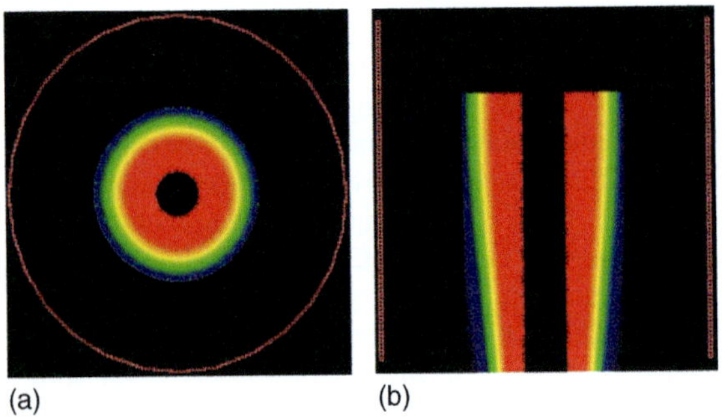

Figure 35.37. $\boldsymbol{B}_1$ field, transaxial (a) and axial (b) for stubline coils

selected to match the sample for minimum impedance gradient and maximum efficiency. This 'stubline' coil would be ideally suited for high-resolution, vertical bore magnets. This same approach, however, can be extended to horizontal bore, preclinical and clinical applications by using dielectric wave guides with access holes or apertures cut through the waveguide sidewalls at current nodes to couple to anatomy at those points with maximum efficiency. These structures can be double-tuned by choice of dielectric inside and outside of the cavity.[19] The inside of the cavity 'sees' one wavelength and the outside of the cavity sees another, typically either air or tissue determined.[45]

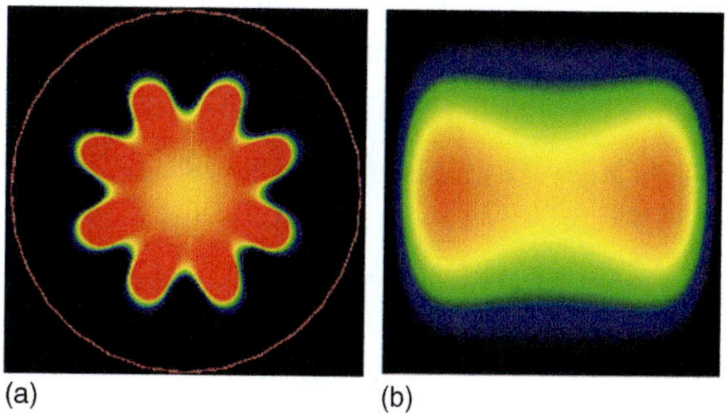

Figure 35.39. B_1 field, transaxial (a) and axial (b) center planes for dipole array

35.4 ANTENNAS

Finally, we conclude this chapter with a third coil circuit class, the antenna.[20] While the wire and transmission line coils are designed to store an RF magnetic field within or adjacent to their circuit, an antenna is designed to radiate its energy efficiently to the far field. The condition for antenna use applies when a sample ROI is in the far field, more than a full wavelength from the antenna. This condition occurs for MRI and MRS at the highest field strengths and largest physiological samples. This class of detectors has proven successful for reaching deep body ROIs at field strengths from 7 T (300 MHz) to 10.5 T (450 MHz), for example. Antennas composed of arrays of center-fed dipoles as pictured in Figure 35.38 have been built and tested to perform favorable in comparison to TEM coil arrays under these highest field conditions for human MRS. Compare the field contours of the dipole in Figure 35.39 to the TEM contours in Figure 35.33. Because these arrays have no end rings, like the TEM coils, the axial field extends further and more uniformly than a birdcage of equal physical length. The birdcage would not work at these highest frequencies and largest dimensions. Similar to TEM coils and other array structures, these dipole antennas can be double-tuned by tuning alternating elements in the array to alternating frequencies.

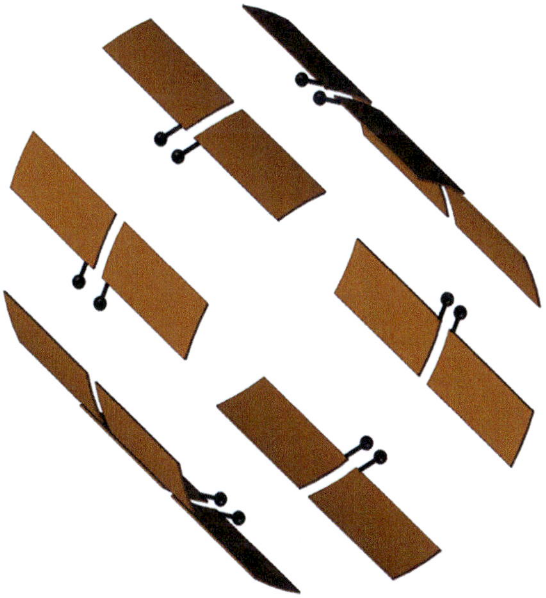

Figure 35.38. Dipole array

RELATED ARTICLES IN EMAGRES

Birdcage Resonators: Highly Homogeneous Radiofrequency Coils for Magnetic Resonance

Coils for Insertion into the Human Body

Design and Use of Internal Receiver Coils for Magnetic Resonance Imaging

Multifrequency Coils for Whole Body Studies

Radiofrequency Systems and Coils for MRI and MRS

Refrigerated and Superconducting Receiver Coils in Whole Body Magnetic Resonance

Spatial Encoding Using Multiple rf Coils: SMASH Imaging and Parallel MRI

Surface Coil NMR: Detection with Inhomogeneous Radiofrequency Field Antennas

Surface and Other Local Coils for In Vivo Studies

Whole Body Machines: NMR Phased Array Coil Systems

TEM Transceiver Head Array Coils for Ultra High Magnetic Fields

TEM Arrays, Design and Implementation

Quadrature Surface Coils

Double-Tuned Surface Coils

Quadrature Transverse Electromagnetic (TEM) Surface Coils

Radiofrequency Fields and SAR for Transverse Electromagnetic (TEM) Surface Coils

Double-Tuned Birdcage Coils: Construction and Tuning

Radiofrequency Fields and SAR for Bird Cage Coils

TEM Body Coils

Transverse Electromagnetic (TEM) Surface Coils for Extremities

Receiver Loop Arrays

Coil Array Design for Parallel Imaging: Theory and Applications

Millipede Coils

Microcoils

Catheter Coils

Radiofrequency Heating Models and Measurements

Characterization of Multichannel Coil Arrays on the Benchtop

A Standard Procedure for Analyzing Radio Frequency MRI Coils

Litz Coils for High Resolution and Animal Probes, Especially for Double Resonance

RF Field Modeling for Double-Tuned Volume Coils

An Historical Introduction to Surface Coils: The Early Days

Transceiver Loop Arrays

Radiofrequency Coils for NMR: A Peripatetic History of Their Twists and Turns

Nested Surface Coils for Multinuclear NMR

Birdcage Volume Coil Design

Bioeffects and Safety of Radiofrequency Electromagnetic Fields

Radiofrequency Fields: Interactions, Biological Effects, and Safety Issues

RF Device Safety and Compatibility

Safety Considerations in MRI

REFERENCES

1. J. T. Vaughan, in 'Ultra High Field Magnetic Resonance Imaging', ed P. Robitaille, Springer Academic/Plenum Publishers: New York, NY, 2006, Chapter 6.
2. F. Bloch, *Phys. Rev.*, 1946, **70**, 460.
3. F. Bloch, W. W. Hansen, and M. Packard, *Phys. Rev.*, 1946, **70**, 474.
4. E. M. Purcell, H. C. Torrey, and R. V. Pound, *Phys. Rev.*, 1946, **69**, 37.
5. J. J. Ackerman, T. H. Grove, G. G. Wong, D. G. Gadian, and G. K. Radda, *Nature*, 1980, **283**, 167.
6. D. I. Hoult, C. N. Chen, and V. J. Sank, *Magn. Reson. Med.*, 1984, **1**, 339.
7. P. B. Roemer, W. A. Edelstein, C. E. Hayes, S. P. Souza, and O. M. Mueller, *Magn. Reson. Med.*, 1990, **16**, 192.
8. D. W. Alderman and D. M. Grant, *J. Magn. Reson.*, 1979, **36**, 447.
9. C. E. Hayes, *Magn. Reson. Imaging*, 1993, **11**, 81.
10. C. E. Hayes, *NMR Biomed.*, 2009, **22**, 908.
11. C. E. Hayes, W. A. Edelstein, J. F. Schenck, O. M. Mueller, and M. Eash, *J. Magn. Reson.*, 1985, **63**, 622.
12. F. D. Doty, G. Entzminger Jr., and C. D. Hauck, *J. Magn. Reson.*, 1999, **140**, 17.
13. W. H. Wong, (San Jose, CA), Inventor Varian, Inc. (Palo Alto, CA), assignee, Millipede coils, U.S. Pat. 6,285,189, 2001.
14. H. J. Schneider and P. Dullenkopf, *Rev. Sci. Instrum.*, 1977, **48**, 68.

15. H. J. Schneider and P. Dullenkopf, *Rev. Sci. Instrum.*, 1977, **48**, 832.
16. P. H. Röschmann, (DE), Inventor U.S. Philips Corp. (New York, NY), assignee, Surface coil for high-frequency magnetic fields for magnetic resonance examinations, U.S. Pat. 4,775,837, 1988.
17. J. T. Vaughn Jr., (Birmingham, AL), Inventor UAB Research Foundation (Birmingham, AL), assignee, Radio frequency volume coils for imaging and spectroscopy, U.S. Pat. 5,557,247, 1996.
18. J. T. Vaughan, H. P. Hetherington, J. O. Otu, J. W. Pan, and G. M. Pohost, *Magn. Reson. Med.*, 1994, **32**, 206.
19. J. T. Vaughan, Inventor Massachusetts General Hospital, assignee, RF Coil for Imaging System, US patent no. US7268554B2, USA, 2003.
20. A. J. E. Raaijmakers and C. A. T. van den Berg, in 'RF Coils for MRI', eds J. T. Vaughan and J. Griffiths, John Wiley & Sons, Ltd.: Chichester, 2012, Chapter 17.
21. D. M. Petersen, in 'RF Coils for MRI', eds J. T. Vaughan and J. Griffiths, John Wiley & Sons, Ltd.: Chichester, 2012.
22. S. Junge, in 'RF Coils for MRI', eds J. T. Vaughan and J. Griffiths, John Wiley & Sons, Ltd.: Chichester, 2012, Chapter 20.
23. H. Kovacs, D. Moskau, and M. Spraul, *Prog. Nucl. Magn. Reson. Spectrosc.*, 2005, **46**, 131.
24. P. Styles, N. F. Soffe, and C. A. Scott, *J. Magn. Reson.*, 1989, **84**, 376.
25. B. L. Beck, in 'RF Coils for MRI', eds J. T. Vaughan and J. Griffiths, John Wiley & Sons, Ltd.: Chichester, 2012, Chapter 4.
26. M. Bendall, *Magn. Reson. Med.*, 1988, **8**, 380.
27. A. W. Magill and R. Grueter, in 'RF Coils for MRI', eds J. T. Vaughan and J. Griffiths, John Wiley & Sons, Ltd.: Chichester, 2012, Chapter 5.
28. C. M. Collin and A. G. Webb, in 'RF Coils for MRI', eds J. T. Vaughan and J. Griffiths, John Wiley & Sons, Ltd.: Chichester, 2012, Chapter 3.
29. C. N. Chen, D. I. Hoult, and V. J. Sank, *J. Magn. Reson.*, 1983, **54**, 324.
30. D. I. Hoult, C. N. Chen, and V. J. Sank, *Magn. Reson. Med.*, 1984, **1**, 171.
31. V. J. Sank, C. N. Chen, and D. I. Hoult, *J. Magn. Reson.*, 1986, **69**, 236.
32. D. K. Sodickson, M. A. Ohliger, R. Lattanzi, and G. C. Wiggins, in 'RF Coils for MRI', eds J. T. Vaughan and J. Griffiths, John Wiley & Sons, Ltd.: Chichester, 2012, Chapter 8.
33. M. A. Griswold, in 'RF Coils for MRI', eds J. T. Vaughan and J. Griffiths, John Wiley & Sons, Ltd.: Chichester, 2012, Chapter 10.
34. R. Duensing, in 'RF Coils for MRI', eds J. T. Vaughan and J. Griffiths, John Wiley & Sons, Ltd.: Chichester, 2012, Chapter 9.
35. J. Murphy-Boesch, in 'RF Coils for MRI', eds J. T. Vaughan and J. Griffiths, John Wiley & Sons, Ltd.: Chichester, 2012.
36. F. D. Doty and G. Entzminger, in 'RF Coils for MRI', eds J. T. Vaughan and J. Griffiths, John Wiley & Sons, Ltd.: Chichester, 2012, Chapter 21.
37. E. W. H. Wong, in 'RF Coils for MRI', eds J. T. Vaughan and J. Griffiths, John Wiley & Sons, Ltd.: Chichester, 2012, Chapter 22.
38. N. De Zanche, in 'RF Coils for MRI', eds J. T. Vaughan and J. Griffiths, John Wiley & Sons, Ltd.: Chichester, 2012, Chapter 11.
39. J. T. Vaughan, in 'RF Coils for MRI', eds J. T. Vaughan and J. Griffiths, John Wiley & Sons, Ltd.: Chichester, 2012, Chapter 13.
40. G. Adriany, in 'RF Coils for MRI', eds J. T. Vaughan and J. Griffiths, John Wiley & Sons, Ltd.: Chichester, 2012, Chapter 15.
41. G. Adriany, P. F. Van de Moortele, F. Wiesinger, S. Moeller, J. P. Strupp, P. Andersen, C. Snyder, X. Zhang, W. Chen, K. P. Pruessmann, P. Boesiger, T. Vaughan, and K. Ugurbil, *Magn. Reson. Med.*, 2005, **53**, 434.
42. N. I. Avdievich, in 'RF Coils for MRI', eds J. T. Vaughan and J. Griffiths, John Wiley & Sons, Ltd.: Chichester, 2012, Chapter 6.
43. N. I. Avdievich, in 'Transverse Electromagnetic (TEM) Surface Coils for Extremities, RF Coils for MRI', eds J. T. Vaughan and J. Griffiths, John Wiley & Sons, Ltd.: Chichester, 2012, Chapter 16.
44. J. T. Vaughan, G. Adriany, C. Snyder, L. Bolinger, H. Liu, J. Tian, and K. Ugurbil, *Magn. Reson. Med.*, 2004, **52**, 851.
45. J. T. Vaughan, Inventor University of Alabama at Birmingham, assignee, Cavity resonator for NMR system, US patent no. US5744957A, 1998.

Index

Abbreviations and Acronyms

2D	two-dimensional
AAA	abdominal aortic aneurysm
AAMI	Association for the Advancement of Medical Instrumentation
ABC	absorbing boundary condition
ABR	auditory brain stem response
ACR	American College of Radiology
ADC	Analog-to-Digital Converter
ADC	apparent diffusion coefficient
ADI	alternating direction implicit
AEP	auditory evoked potential
AIMD	active implantable medical device
ANC	active noise canceling
ANR	active noise reducing
ANSI	American National Standards Institute
APD	apparent proton density
ASC	applied superconetics
ASRS	Aviation Safety Reporting System
ASTM	American Society for Testing Materials
BBB	blood brain barrier
BEM-SF	Boundary Element Method Stream-Function
BHTE	Bioheat transfer equation
CEE	convective energy equation
CFL	Courant–Friedrich–Lewy
CFR	Code of Federal Regulations
CIED	cardiac implantable electronic devices
CMRR	Center for Magnetic Resonance Research
CNS	central nervous system
CP	circularly polarized
CP	commercially pure
CSF	cerebrospinal fluid
CSS	computational solid stress
CT	computed tomography
DAEN	Database of Adverse Event Notifications
DBS	deep brain stimulator
DNA	deoxyribonucleic acid
DRG	dorsal root ganglia
DSV	diameter of a spherical volume
ECG	electrocardiogram
ELM	extreme learning machine
EM	electromagnetic
EMF	electromagnetic fields
EMI	electromagnetic interferences
EPA	Environmental Protection Agency
EPG	extended phase graph
EPI	echo-planar imaging
ERB	Ethical Review Board
ETL	echo train length
EU	European Union
FAA	Federal Aviation Administration
FDA	Food and Drug Administration
FDTD	finite-difference time-domain
FEA	finite element analysis
FEM	finite element method
FFR	field-free region
FFT	fast Fourier transform
FHD	ferrohydrodynamics
FID	free induction decay
FIT	finite-integration technique
FLASH	fast low angle shot
FOV	field of view
FPO	fixed parameter option
FSE	fast spin echo
FSI	fluid structure interaction
GaAsFET	gallium arsenide field-effect transistor
GBCAs	gadolinium-based contrast agents
GBHTM	generic bioheat transfer model
GPU	general processing unit
GRE	gradient-recalled echo
GRP	glass-reinforced plastic
GVS	Galvanic vestibular stimulation
HD	heating duration
HIFU	high-intensity focused ultrasound
HIPAA	Health Insurance Portability and Accountability Act
HML	high-middle-low rating
HPA	Health Protection Agency
HSE	health and safety executive
HTS	high-critical temperature superconductors
IACUC	Institutional Animal Care and Usage Committee
ICD	implantable cardioverter defibrillator
ICNIRP	International Commission on Non-Ionizing Radiation Protection
IDE	investigational device exemption
IEC	Independent Ethics Committee
IEC	International Electrotechnical Commission
IFU	instructions for use
Ig	immunoglobulin
IGC	Intermagnetics General Corporation
IONPs	iron oxide nanoparticles
IPG	implantable pulse generator
IQ	image quality
IR	infrared
IR	inversion recovery
IRB	Institutional Review Board
ISMRM	International Society for Magnetic Resonance in Medicine
ISMRMRD	ISMRM Raw Data
JIRA	Japan Medical Imaging and Radiological Systems Industries Association
JSMRM	Japanese Society for Magnetic Resonance in Medicine
L-SAR	local specific absorption rate

LHe liquid helium
LMW low molecular weight
LP linear programming
MAUDE Manufacturer and User Facility Device Experience
MCAN maximum clinical acoustic noise
MDT magnetic drug targeting
ME medical electrical
MEMS microelectromechanical
MFH magnetic fluid hyperthermia
MFIV magnetic-field-induced vertigo
MGAN maximum gradient acoustic noise
MHD magnetohydrodynamics
MHRA Medicines and Healthcare products Regulatory Agency
MITA Medical Imaging and Technology Alliance
MoM method of moment
MoTLiM Modified transmission line method
MPI magnetic particle imaging
MR magnetic resonance
MRG McIntyre–Richardson–Grill
MRI magnetic resonance imaging
MRS magnetic resonance spectroscopy
MRT magnetic resonance thermometry
MRTI magnetic-resonance temperature imaging
MRU magnet run-down unit
MSHA Mine Safety and Health Administration
MT magnetization transfer
MTBF mean free time between failure
NbTi niobium titanium
NEMA/MITA National Electrical Manufacturers Association/Medical Imaging and Technology Alliance
NIH National Institutes of Health
NIOSH National Institute for Occupational Safety and Health
NIST National Institute of Standards and Technology
NITE noninvasive temperature estimation
NMRs nuclear magnetic resonance
NP nanoparticles
NRLS National Reporting and Learning System
NRR noise reduction rating
NS north-south
NSF nephrogenic systemic fibrosis
NTBI non-transferrin bound iron
NWIP new work item proposal
OAE otoacoustic emission
OEM original equipment manufacturer
OMT Oxford Magnet Technologies
OSHA Occupational Safety and Health Administration
Pa Pascal
PBA perfect boundary approximation
PCS persistent current switch
PD proton density
PE phase error
PEC perfect electric conductor
PET positron emission tomography
PI principal investigator
PIMD passive implanted medical device
PMA premarket approval
PML perfectly matched layer
PNS peripheral nerve stimulation
PPE personal protective equipment
ppm parts per million
PRE-TAPS pre-saturation targeting the potassium system
PRF proton resonance frequency
PRFS proton resonance frequency shift
psd positive semidefinite
PVC polyvinyl chloride
QSM quantitative susceptibility mapping
REB Research Ethics Board
RES reticuloendothelial system
RF radio frequency
RIL Radiologic Imaging Laboratory
ROI region of interest
ROS reactive oxygen species
ROU region of uniformity
RT ramp time
RWG Rao–Wilton–Gleason
SAR specific absorption rate
SCS spinal cord stimulator
SDO Standards Developing Organization
SE spin echo
SEM spacial encoding magnetic field
SFG spatial field gradients
SI International System of Units
SLC sound level conversion
SLP specific loss power
SMRT Society for Magnetic Resonance Radiographers and Technologists
SN south-north
SNR signal-to-noise ratio
SOR successive overrelaxation
SPGR spoiled gradient-recalled echo
SPL sound or acoustic pressure level
SR saturation recovery
SSCD superior semicircular canal dehiscence
SSFP steady-state free precession sequences
SVT supraventricular tachycardia
SWIFT sweep imaging with Fourier transformation
TAG Technical Advisory Group
TAMI Toshiba America MRI
TD thermal damage
TD thermal dose
TE echo time
TE transverse electric
TEM transverse electromagnetic
TIG tungsten inert gas
TIVA total intravenous anesthesia
TM transverse magnetic

TMS	transcranial magnetic stimulation
TOMROP	T_1 by multiple readout pulses
TR	repetition time
TR	technical report
TR	transmit–receive
TRUFI	true fast imaging
TS	technical specification
TSE	turbo spin echo
TSI	temperature sensor implant
TWA	time-weighted average
UHF	ultra-high-frequency
US FDA	US Food and Drug Administration
UTE	ultrashort time echo
VHM	visible human male
VNA	vector network analyzer
VOP	virtual observation point
VRMS	volume root mean square
WHO	World Health Organization
WIC	wire in channel

Printed and bound by CPI Group (UK) Ltd, Croydon, CR0 4YY
17/09/2026
14964269-0007